THE JOHNS HOPKINS WHITE PAPERS

2003

Hypertension and Stroke

Lung Disorders

Memory

Nutrition and Weight Control

Prostate Disorders

Vision

VOLUME 2

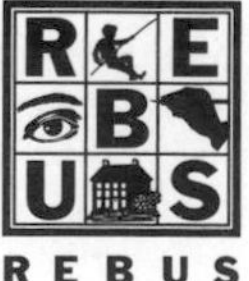

Prepared by the Editors of
The Johns Hopkins White Papers
Published by Rebus, Inc., New York

JOHNS HOPKINS MEDICINE
BALTIMORE, MARYLAND

THE JOHNS HOPKINS MEDICAL LETTER
HEALTH AFTER 50

THE JOHNS HOPKINS WHITE PAPERS *are published in association with* THE JOHNS HOPKINS MEDICAL LETTER: HEALTH AFTER 50. *This monthly eight-page newsletter provides practical, timely information for anyone concerned with taking control of his or her own health care. The newsletter is written in clear, nontechnical, easy-to-understand language and comes from the century-old tradition of Johns Hopkins excellence. For information on how to subscribe to this newsletter, please write to Health After 50, P.O. Box 420179, Palm Coast, FL 32142.*

Get subscription information online—along with the latest perspectives from our experts—at our Web site:

www.hopkinsafter50.com

Published in the United States in 2003 by Medletter Associates, an imprint of Rebus, Inc.,
632 Broadway, 11th Floor, New York, NY 10012

ISBN: 0-929661-72-9 Johns Hopkins White Papers, Volume Two

Printed in the United States

Note
This book is not intended as an alternative to personal medical advice. The reader should consult a physician in all matters relating to health and particularly in respect of any symptoms which may require diagnosis or medical attention. While the advice and information are believed to be accurate and true at the time of going to press, neither the authors nor the publisher can accept any legal responsibility or liability for any errors or omissions which may have occurred.

HYPERTENSION AND STROKE

Lawrence Appel, M.D.,

Rafael H. Llinas, M.D.,

and

Simeon Margolis, M.D., Ph.D.

2003

HYPERTENSION AND STROKE

Hypertension (high blood pressure) is one of the most common disorders in the United States. Because it often produces few symptoms before causing a major complication, such as a stroke, detection and treatment of hypertension are especially important. The past year has brought advances in hypertension and stroke research, including new techniques to identify people at high risk for stroke and new medications to help people lower their blood pressure. This White Paper discusses ways to prevent and manage hypertension, as well as how strokes can be prevented and treated.

■ ■ ■

Highlights:

- Can **eating oatmeal** reduce your blood pressure? (page 11)
- The controversy over **removing mercury from blood pressure gauges**. (page 14)
- **Ambulatory blood pressure monitoring**: The best way to get an accurate picture of your blood pressure. (page 17)
- What to do if standard treatment **doesn't control your high blood pressure**. (page 32)
- **Calcium channel blockers** as an alternative to diuretics and beta-blockers. (page 35)
- **Getting more folate** in your diet appears to reduce the risk of stroke. (page 44)
- New dangers from the **herbal supplement ephedrine (ma huang)**. (page 47)
- **Carotid endarterectomy,** the surgical procedure that can help prevent a stroke. (page 61)
- How **magnetic resonance imaging** may be able to identify people at increased risk for stroke. (page 63)
- Take this **questionnaire** to see whether **caring for a stroke patient** is affecting your health. (page 67)
- Treatments for **pain and muscle spasms** after a stroke. (page 72)

■ ■ ■

www.HopkinsAfter50.com
Visit us for the latest news on hypertension, stroke, and other information that will complement your Johns Hopkins White Paper.

THE AUTHORS

Lawrence Appel, M.D., received his M.D. from the New York University School of Medicine and performed his residency at Baltimore City Hospital. He is an associate professor at the Johns Hopkins University School of Medicine, with adjunct appointments in the departments of epidemiology and international health (human nutrition division) of the Johns Hopkins School of Hygiene and Public Health. He is also a practicing internist.

The focus of Dr. Appel's career is clinical research on the prevention of hypertension and cardiovascular and renal diseases, through both nonpharmacological and pharmacological approaches. During the course of his career, he has served on several national policy-making bodies, including the National Heart, Lung, and Blood Institute (NHLBI) Primary Prevention of Hypertension Working Group, the Nutrition Committee of the American Heart Association, and the Institute of Medicine Committee on Evaluation Coverage of Nutrition Services for the Medicare Population.

▪ ▪ ▪

Rafael H. Llinas, M.D., received his B.A. from Washington University in St. Louis and his M.D. from New York University. He completed his residency in neurology at the Harvard Longwood Program based at the Brigham and Women's Hospital. He also completed a two-year fellowship in cerebrovascular medicine at the Beth Israel Hospital in Boston. Currently he is an assistant professor of neurology and the director of stroke neurology at Johns Hopkins-Bayview Medical Center. He is a member of the Johns Hopkins acute stroke team, headed by Robert J. Wityk, M.D.

Dr. Llinas is a member of the American Heart Association stroke division and the Maryland stroke task force. His research interests involve neurosonology, diffusion/perfusion imaging, the use of neuroprotective agents, and secondary stroke prevention. He has published articles in such journals as *Stroke, Neurology,* and *Progress in Cardiovascular Diseases.*

▪ ▪ ▪

Simeon Margolis, M.D., Ph.D., received his B.A., M.D., and Ph.D. from the Johns Hopkins University School of Medicine and performed his internship and residency at Johns Hopkins Hospital. He is currently a professor of medicine and biological chemistry at the Johns Hopkins University School of Medicine and medical editor of *The Johns Hopkins Medical Letter, Health After 50.* He has served on various committees for the Department of Health, Education, and Welfare, including the National Diabetes Advisory Board and the Arteriosclerosis Specialized Centers of Research Review Committees. In addition, he has acted as a member of the Endocrinology and Metabolism Panel of the U.S. Food and Drug Administration.

A former weekly columnist for the *Baltimore Sun,* Dr. Margolis lectures regularly to medical students, physicians, and the general public on a wide variety of topics, such as the prevention of coronary heart disease, controlling cholesterol levels, the treatment of diabetes, and alternative medicine.

CONTENTS

HYPERTENSION AND STROKE

High blood pressure (hypertension) is one of the most prevalent disorders in the United States and the most important risk factor for stroke. Stroke is the third leading cause of death in the United States and the leading cause of disability. Because of the close relationship between hypertension and stroke, both topics are addressed here in a single White Paper.

Hypertension

Hypertension is sometimes referred to as the silent killer because it produces few, if any, symptoms but causes or contributes to the deaths of 210,000 Americans a year. The condition affects 50 million Americans and is a primary cause of stroke, heart disease, heart failure, kidney disease, and blindness. Fortunately, in most cases, the condition is easily detected and usually controllable with diet, exercise, and medication.

WHAT IS BLOOD PRESSURE?

Blood does not flow through the circulatory system in a steady stream; instead, it is pushed through the blood vessels with every heartbeat. Each time the heart contracts—a period known as *systole*—blood pressure rises as more blood is forced through the arteries. Each systole is followed by a moment of relaxation, or *diastole,* when blood pressure drops as the heart refills with blood and rests before its next contraction. Thus, pressure in the arteries rises and falls with each heartbeat. For this reason, blood pressure readings include two values: Systolic pressure, the higher number, corresponds with the peak pressure in the arteries during the heart's contraction; diastolic pressure, the lower number, reflects the lowest pressure in the arteries as the heart relaxes.

Blood pressure fluctuates throughout the day under the direct influence of three parts of the body: the heart, the arteries, and the kidneys. Variations in the strength of each heartbeat can lower or raise blood pressure—a more powerful contraction produces greater pressure. During exercise, for example, increased blood flow is needed to provide extra oxygen and nutrients to the muscles, so the heart beats faster and more forcefully to raise blood pressure and keep up with the demand. On the other hand, blood pressure drops as the heart slows during sleep. In addition, small arteries are encircled by smooth muscle cells that permit arteries to expand (dilate) to decrease blood pressure or narrow (constrict) to increase it. Stress or anger can raise blood pressure by triggering the release of hormones that constrict blood vessels. Finally, the volume of blood depends largely on how much water it contains; the kidneys can reduce blood pressure by eliminating excess salt and water.

These processes are controlled through an elaborate network of nerves and hormones. Special nerve endings called baroreceptors, residing in the walls of arteries, monitor blood pressure. When pressure increases, the artery wall stretches and the baroreceptors signal the central nervous system to lower the pressure. Blood pressure is similarly monitored at sites in the kidneys where blood is filtered (the glomeruli).

Several hormones help to regulate blood pressure. Three of these hormones act in concert: renin, angiotensin, and aldosterone. Renin, an enzyme produced by cells in the kidney, acts on a protein (angiotensinogen) secreted by the liver to form angiotensin I. As blood passes through the lungs, angiotensin I is transformed into angiotensin II, which raises blood pressure by causing arteries to constrict. (Renin and angiotensinogen are also manufactured in artery walls and other organs, where they constrict blood vessels to control blood pressure locally.) Angiotensin II also stimulates the release of aldosterone from the adrenal glands located above each kidney.

Aldosterone increases blood pressure by signaling the kidneys to retain sodium, which increases the volume of blood and thereby increases the amount of blood pumped by the heart. (Because the amount of water in the body depends on its content of sodium, the kidneys control the amount of water in the blood—and therefore blood pressure—by increasing or decreasing excretion of sodium into the urine.) A rise in blood pressure signals the kidneys to stop secreting renin. Dietary potassium inhibits the release of renin but stimulates the production of aldosterone.

Other hormones also affect blood pressure. Epinephrine (adrenaline) and norepinephrine increase blood pressure, for example, in times of stress, while calcitriol (formed from dietary vitamin D) and parathyroid hormone play less important roles in the regulation of blood pressure. Calcitriol constricts small arteries; parathyroid hormone dilates them. Though triggered mainly by low blood calcium levels, parathyroid hormone release also responds to sodium and potassium levels.

The Complications of Hypertension

Blood pressure is the amount of tension that blood exerts on the walls of arteries as it is pumped through the circulatory system. Prolonged elevations in blood pressure, a condition called hypertension, can damage various organs by injuring the walls of blood vessels. The complications of hypertension typically occur in the following five areas:

Arteries. The walls of arteries, which carry blood from the heart to the rest of the body, are normally strong and elastic. Hypertension accelerates the progression of atherosclerosis, a narrowing and stiffening of the arteries as a result of accumulations of plaques (composed mainly of cholesterol, fibrous tissue, and calcium) within the artery walls. Excess pressure on a weak spot in an artery can cause an outward bulge (an aneurysm) of its wall. Rupture of an aneurysm in the aorta (the main artery in the body) is almost always fatal unless recognized and treated promptly. A narrowed artery from atherosclerosis can limit blood flow through the arteries to the brain, heart, and other organs.

Brain. Formation of a blood clot in an artery already narrowed by atherosclerotic plaque can completely block the flow of blood through the artery and cause an ischemic stroke. Rupture of a weakened blood vessel in the brain causes a hemorrhagic stroke; brain tissue is damaged directly when blood leaks into the brain and indirectly when the break in the artery prevents blood from reaching areas beyond the rupture.

Heart. Atherosclerotic narrowing in the coronary arteries can limit the supply of oxygen-rich blood to the heart and lead to a type of chest pain called angina. Complete blockage of a coronary artery can cause a heart attack.

In hypertension, the heart works harder to pump against the higher pressures in the arteries. This excess workload thickens and increases the size of the heart's left ventricle (left ventricular hypertrophy), which elevates the risk of heart attacks, heart failure (an inability of the heart to pump enough blood to meet the body's needs), and sudden death.

Kidneys. Hypertension damages the small blood vessels in the kidneys, which remove waste products and water from the blood. Injury to these blood vessels interferes with kidney function so that waste products and fluid accumulate in the body (uremia). If kidney damage is severe enough (renal failure), dialysis treatment or a kidney transplant may become necessary. Kidney disease, in turn, worsens hypertension.

Eyes. The small arteries in the eye are susceptible to injury by hypertension. Blockage or leakage of blood from these arteries can lead to vision problems.

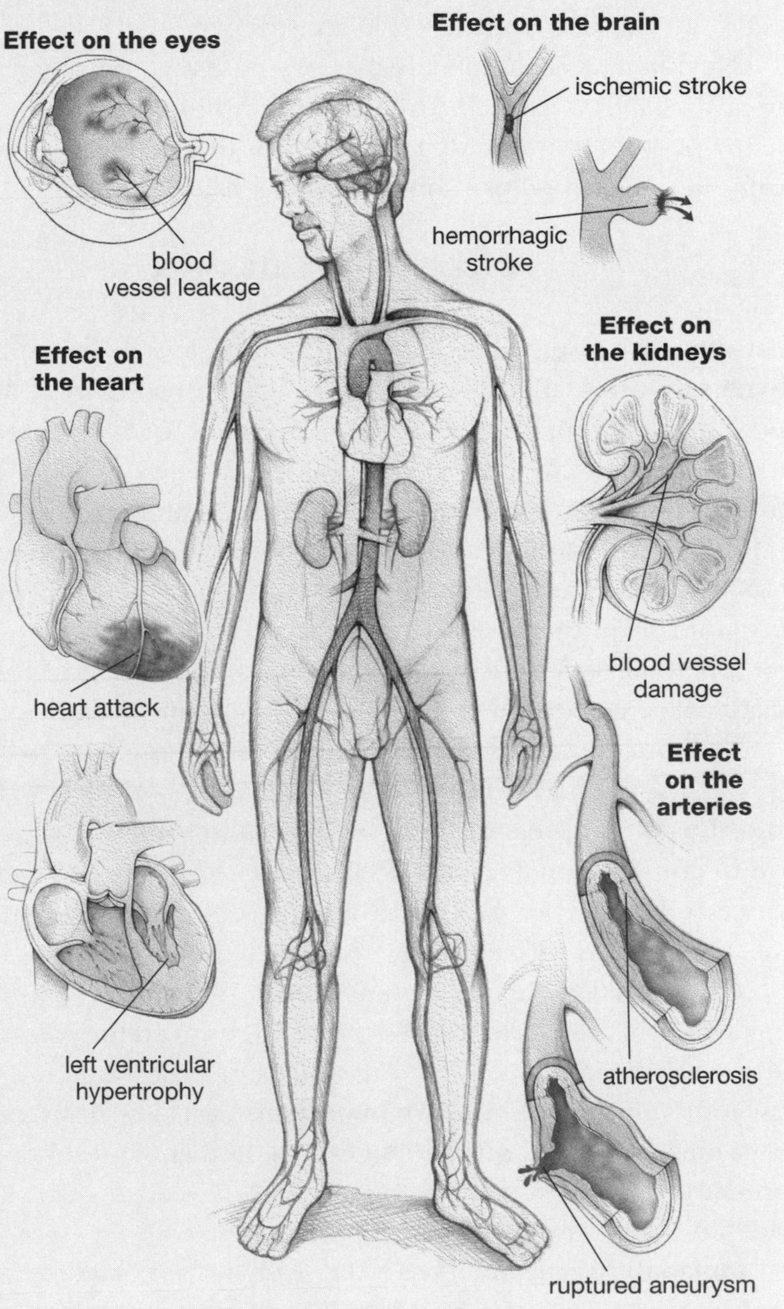

Atrial natriuretic factor, nitric oxide, and endothelin are additional substances involved in blood pressure regulation. Atrial natriuretic factor, produced by the atrium of the heart, causes the kidneys to excrete more sodium (and thus water) and inhibits aldosterone and renin production. Nitric oxide, secreted by cells lining blood vessel walls, relaxes smooth muscle cells and causes the arteries to dilate. Endothelin is a hormone released by endothelial cells that causes blood vessels to constrict.

Normally, this complex regulatory system allows blood pressure to rise or fall as needed while staying within a desirable range. In many people, however, abnormalities in this system lead to chronically elevated blood pressure, or hypertension.

CAUSES OF HYPERTENSION

No specific cause can be identified in 90% to 95% of patients with hypertension—called essential, or primary, hypertension. While hypertension is common in virtually all economically developed countries, it is uncommon in several isolated societies. When individuals from those societies migrate to developed countries, they often develop hypertension. These findings suggest that environmental factors, such as eating habits and level of physical activity, play an important role in the development of hypertension.

Essential hypertension results from one or more of the following factors, possibly in combination with unknown causes.

Sodium. Higher sodium levels raise blood pressure in two ways. By causing the body to retain water, sodium increases blood volume and thus blood pressure. Sodium also causes vascular smooth muscle to constrict small blood vessels, which produces a greater resistance to blood flow. Still controversial, however, is the underlying mechanism by which sodium constricts blood vessels.

Other dietary factors. In addition to sodium, several other dietary factors affect blood pressure. A high intake of potassium can lower blood pressure, while the effects of other minerals, such as calcium and magnesium, are uncertain. Diets low in fruits, vegetables, and dairy products and high in fat and cholesterol raise blood pressure. Obesity is associated with high blood pressure. Excessive alcohol intake also raises blood pressure.

Metabolic syndrome. Over the past decade, medical scientists and physicians have directed more attention to a common constellation of abnormalities—obesity, hypertension, high triglyceride levels (hypertriglyceridemia) and low HDL (high density lipoprotein) cholesterol levels, and premature coronary heart disease (CHD). The name given to this cluster of health problems is metabolic syndrome (previously called insulin resistance syndrome or syndrome X).

Triglycerides are blood lipids associated with an increased risk of CHD, while HDL cholesterol protects against CHD. Obesity, especially a significant accumulation of fat in the abdomen, launches the abnormalities of this syndrome by producing tissue resistance to the actions of insulin, which regulates blood levels of glucose (sugar). To overcome this resistance, the pancreas increases its production of insulin, and blood levels of insulin rise. High blood insulin levels promote hypertriglyceridemia by increasing the release of triglyceride-carrying lipoproteins from the liver. Blood glucose levels tend to rise despite the higher levels of blood insulin; diabetes (which is characterized by abnormally high blood glucose levels) results when insulin production by the pancreas can no longer keep up with the insulin resistance. Hypertension is not a direct result of the increased insulin levels, but insulin does heighten the activity of the sympathetic nervous system and cause sodium retention by the kidneys—both of which raise blood pressure.

Taken together, the abnormalities associated with metabolic syndrome increase the incidence of angina and heart attack. According to long-term studies, the higher the fasting blood insulin levels and the larger the amount of abdominal fat, the greater the likelihood of death from CHD. Although these risks exist even when blood glucose levels are only slightly elevated, they are magnified in people with diabetes.

Genetics. Studies of twins and other members of the same family have shown that essential hypertension has a genetic component. Researchers have identified a number of genetic mutations that result in inherited forms of hypertension. These mutations, however, account for only a small minority of all cases of hypertension. Future research may find additional mutations that are associated with more common forms of hypertension.

Exercise. Numerous studies show that increased physical activity can lower blood pressure. The type of exercise that is most effective is aerobic exercise, which involves repeated movement of large muscle groups. Moderate-intensity aerobic exercise (such as brisk walking) on most days of the week is recommended.

Secondary Hypertension

A number of disorders, as well as drugs, can cause secondary hypertension, which affects less than 5% of people with hypertension. It

NEW RESEARCH

Most Middle-Aged Individuals Eventually Develop Hypertension

About 90% of middle-aged people will eventually be diagnosed with hypertension, a new report illustrates.

Researchers studied data from 1,298 people in the Framingham Heart Study who were 55 to 65 years old and did not have hypertension when the study began in 1976. Participants underwent a medical evaluation, including blood pressure measurement, every two years until 1998.

Hypertension developed in 90% of people during the study; the rate was similar for men and women. Also, 60% eventually took antihypertensive medication. The risk of hypertension was about 60% higher for men studied between 1976 and 1998 than for those studied from 1952 to 1975. For women, the risk of hypertension remained constant over time. The percentages of people treated with antihypertensive drugs increased two- to threefold from the earlier to the later time period.

The rise in hypertension in men may be related to an increase in weight that occurred in men, but not in women, in the study across the two time periods. "The finding that 9 out of 10 middle-aged and older adults are likely to develop elevated blood pressure over their remaining lifetime reemphasizes that hypertension poses a major public health burden," the authors conclude.

JOURNAL OF THE AMERICAN MEDICAL ASSOCIATION
Volume 287, page 1003
February 27, 2002

is particularly important to identify secondary causes of hypertension because the high blood pressure might be cured or better controlled by eliminating the underlying problem.

Kidney disorders. Kidney disease that leads to chronic kidney (renal) failure almost always produces hypertension due to excessive retention of salt and water in the body. In addition, narrowing of the arteries supplying blood to one or both kidneys, and the resulting reduction in blood flow to the kidneys, causes a form of high blood pressure termed renovascular hypertension. In this disorder, the affected kidney senses an inadequate blood supply and secretes excessive amounts of renin, which acts on angiotensinogen to initiate the formation of angiotensin II. In many patients, renovascular hypertension can be cured or controlled by surgical repair of the narrowed arteries.

Adrenal tumors. Three types of adrenal tumors can cause hypertension: primary aldosteronism, Cushing syndrome, and pheochromocytoma. Primary aldosteronism is caused by a tumor or overgrowth of cells (hyperplasia) in the cortex of the adrenal gland, which can lead to hypertension due to an overproduction of aldosterone unrelated to angiotensin II stimulation. Cushing syndrome involves a tumor of the adrenal cortex that secretes excessive amounts of cortisone and related hormones, which raise blood pressure and cause a number of other problems. Treatment for high levels of aldosterone and Cushing syndrome is complicated and does not always control blood pressure. Pheochromocytoma, a tumor arising in the central, or medullary, portion of the adrenal gland, secretes large amounts of epinephrine or norepinephrine, which can cause hypertension. Removal of the tumor may cure the hypertension.

Other hormonal causes. Overproduction or inadequate production of thyroid hormone (hyperthyroidism or hypothyroidism, respectively), excessive growth hormone release by a pituitary tumor, or increased blood calcium levels associated with a parathyroid gland tumor can all cause hypertension.

Coarctation of the aorta. Narrowing of a portion of the aorta in the chest is associated with hypertension in the upper part of the body and low blood pressure in the abdomen and legs. This disorder, which can be corrected by surgery, is the most common secondary cause of hypertension in young individuals.

Drugs. The following drugs can raise blood pressure: corticosteroids, cyclosporine (Sandimmune, Neoral), epoetin (Epogen, Procrit), monoamine oxidase (MAO) inhibitors, tricyclic antidepres-

Evaluating Blood Pressure Levels

The blood pressure classifications listed below, developed by the Joint National Committee on Prevention, Detection, Evaluation, and Treatment of High Blood Pressure, apply to adult men and women who are not currently taking antihypertensive medications and are not acutely ill.

Category*	Systolic (mm Hg)	Diastolic (mm Hg)	Recommended Follow-up
Optimal	≤120	≤80	Recheck in two years
Normal	<130	<85	Recheck in two years
High-normal	130-139	85-89	Recheck in one year†
Hypertension			
Stage 1 (Mild)	140-159	90-99	Confirm within two months†
Stage 2 (Moderate)	160-179	100-109	Undergo complete medical evaluation and/or begin treatment within one month
Stage 3 (Severe)	≥180	≥110	Undergo complete medical evaluation and/or begin treatment immediately or within one week, depending on the severity of hypertension
Isolated systolic hypertension	≥140	<90	Confirm within two months†

* When determining which category a person falls into, use the more elevated number in the blood pressure reading. For example, someone with a reading of 140 mm Hg systolic and 100 mm Hg diastolic would fall into the Stage 2 (moderate) category.

† Applies only to initial blood pressure readings. Multiple readings at these levels may require more aggressive management.

sants, trimipramine (Surmontil), venlafaxine (Effexor), cocaine, and amphetamines. Cold remedies, nasal decongestants, and appetite suppressants that contain phenylpropanolamine (PPA) were banned by the U.S. Food and Drug Administration (FDA) because of their side effects. People should also be aware that some dietary supplements and weight loss products contain ephedra (ma huang), which can raise blood pressure and increase the risk of heart attack and stroke (see the sidebar on page 47).

In addition, nonsteroidal anti-inflammatory drugs (NSAIDs) have been linked to an increased need to start treatment of hypertension. These drugs, which include ibuprofen (Advil, Motrin), naproxen (Aleve), and indomethacin (Indocin), are commonly used for the treatment of arthritis and other conditions. One analysis of data pooled from published reports found that NSAIDs caused about a 5-mm Hg rise in both systolic and diastolic blood pressures in patients with high blood pressure. In another study, those taking

NSAIDs were 66% more likely to begin treatment with antihypertensive drugs than those not taking NSAIDs.

In light of these findings, patients with hypertension should use NSAIDs on a regular basis only when there are no potentially safer alternatives, such as acetaminophen (Tylenol), which can relieve pain for some arthritis patients. When NSAIDs are necessary, the lowest possible dose should be taken for as short a time as possible. In addition, NSAIDs may blunt the effect of certain antihypertensive medications (calcium channel blockers, ACE inhibitors, or diuretics) more than others, such as beta-blockers. A recent study, however, found that a newer NSAID called celecoxib (Celebrex) did not interfere with the effectiveness of the ACE inhibitor lisinopril (Prinivil, Zestril; see the sidebar on page 29).

SYMPTOMS AND SIGNS OF HYPERTENSION

Hypertension may produce no early symptoms and can go undetected for many years. Although some people complain of headaches, most often hypertension is discovered during a routine physical examination or, less commonly, when a patient experiences one of its complications: transient ischemic attack (TIA), stroke, visual abnormalities, angina, heart attack, heart failure, claudication (intermittent pain in the leg muscles associated with physical exertion), or symptoms of kidney disease.

Another situation in which a person may experience symptoms from hypertension is a hypertensive crisis. In a hypertensive crisis, blood pressure reaches very high levels (diastolic pressure above 120 mm Hg). This condition occurs in about 1% of people with hypertension—usually around age 40—and may be precipitated by abrupt cessation of antihypertensive medication. The two types of hypertensive crises are hypertensive emergency (also called malignant hypertension) and hypertensive urgency.

A hypertensive emergency is accompanied by one or more symptoms that indicate damage is occurring in the body's organs. These symptoms include chest pain, shortness of breath, seizures, back pain, headache with confusion and blurred vision, nausea, vomiting, and unresponsiveness. If people suspect they are experiencing a hypertensive emergency, they should not eat or drink anything. They should lie down until they can be driven to the hospital or until an ambulance arrives.

The more common form of hypertensive crisis—a hypertensive urgency—is not accompanied by symptoms indicative of organ damage. Instead, headache and nosebleed are the two most common symptoms of hypertensive urgency. Although this condition requires medical attention relatively soon, treatment is not needed immediately as is the case with a hypertensive emergency. Within a few hours of no treatment, a hypertensive urgency could become an emergency. However, immediate organ damage is unlikely if diastolic pressure remains below 130 mm Hg.

CLASSIFYING BLOOD PRESSURE

Published in November 1997, the Sixth Report of the Joint National Committee (JNC) on Prevention, Detection, Evaluation, and Treatment of High Blood Pressure was sponsored by the National Heart, Lung, and Blood Institute. The JNC report provides guidelines on diagnosing and treating hypertension (see the chart on page 7).

Systolic vs. Diastolic Pressure

Historically, doctors had focused on diastolic blood pressure for the diagnosis and treatment of hypertension. But according to a new advisory from the National High Blood Pressure Education Program, which is coordinated by the National Institutes of Health, systolic blood pressure may be a more important determinant of blood pressure-related complications than diastolic blood pressure.

In contrast to diastolic blood pressure, which tends to rise until about age 55 and then begins to fall, systolic blood pressure continues to rise with age. Previously, such elevations were thought to be a normal part of aging, caused by a gradual loss of elasticity in the arterial walls. Now, however, a substantial body of evidence has shown that high systolic blood pressure with a diastolic blood pressure under 90 mm Hg carries a high risk of heart attack and stroke. For example, in the long-term Framingham Heart Study, systolic blood pressure alone accurately identified the stage of hypertension in 91% of the participants, while diastolic blood pressure alone identified the correct stage in only 22%. In those over age 60, the results were even more striking: systolic blood pressure correctly staged hypertension in 99% of subjects.

In light of such findings, the National Heart, Lung, and Blood Institute recommends systolic blood pressure as the standard measure for the detection, evaluation, and treatment of hypertension, especially for middle-aged and older adults. In addition, blood pressure should be kept below 140/90 mm Hg, regardless of age. In

NEW RESEARCH

Coffee Not a Significant Factor in The Development of Hypertension

While drinking coffee can cause short-term increases in blood pressure, regular coffee drinkers do not have an elevated risk of hypertension, according to a new study.

Researchers from Johns Hopkins measured the blood pressure of 1,017 male medical school students (average age 26) and followed them for about 33 years. The participants provided information about their blood pressure and coffee intake during the follow-up period.

After adjusting for numerous factors that could affect blood pressure, such as a family history of hypertension, cigarette smoking, and alcohol intake, drinking one cup of coffee per day was found to raise blood pressure only slightly (by 0.19/0.27 mm Hg). And after adjusting for confounding factors, men who drank coffee in medical school were no more likely to be diagnosed with hypertension by age 60 than men who did not drink coffee.

Although coffee drinking did not increase the rate of hypertension in this study, the authors note that previous research has shown that people with established hypertension can lower their blood pressure by stopping coffee consumption.

ARCHIVES OF INTERNAL MEDICINE
Volume 162, page 657
March 25, 2002

people with diabetes, blood pressure should be maintained below 130/80 mm Hg; in people with heart or kidney failure, blood pressure should be kept as low as possible.

Isolated Systolic Hypertension

A high systolic blood pressure is very common in older adults. In fact, 65% of people over age 60 with hypertension have a condition called isolated systolic hypertension. Isolated systolic hypertension, defined as a systolic blood pressure of 140 mm Hg or higher and a diastolic blood pressure under 90 mm Hg, is associated with an increased risk of stroke, CHD, and kidney disease. In fact, some studies have shown that systolic blood pressure is a better predictor of complications and death than diastolic blood pressure.

Pulse Pressure

Another possible predictor of cardiovascular complications that is related to isolated systolic hypertension is pulse pressure, defined as the difference between systolic blood pressure and diastolic blood pressure. Pulse pressure reflects the stiffness of arteries, which may be just as important as blocked arteries in determining the risk of a heart attack.

In a study published in 2000, researchers pooled the results from three major hypertension studies involving a total of 7,929 patients. They found that the higher the pulse pressure, the greater the risk of cardiovascular complications and death from any cause.

White Coat Hypertension

Some people exhibit "white coat hypertension," consistently high blood pressure readings that are present only when patients are examined by a physician or are in a medical environment. Blood pressure measurements are normal when taken at home by the patients themselves, family members, or friends. As many as 20% of people with mild hypertension may have white coat hypertension.

Whether to treat white coat hypertension with antihypertensive drugs is a controversial issue. In general, people with white coat hypertension and no other risk factors for cardiovascular disease (disease of the arteries supplying the heart or other organs) may not require aggressive treatment but should be especially careful to avoid other risk factors and, like all adults, to adopt healthy lifestyle habits. However, any person with white coat hypertension who has organ damage from hypertension (for example, kidney or heart damage) requires treatment.

Some patients experience the opposite problem: Their average daytime blood pressure is high, but it is normal when measured in a medical setting. Such patients are unlikely to be treated for high blood pressure and therefore may miss out on the benefits of treatment. People with borderline in-office measurements are at greater risk for inaccurate diagnoses.

COMPLICATIONS OF HYPERTENSION

Excessive force of blood moving through arteries can damage both large and small arteries, leading to disease in the tissues or organs supplied by these damaged blood vessels.

Stroke and coronary heart disease. Hypertension accelerates the development of atherosclerosis, the narrowing of large arteries by deposits called plaques. Plaques are composed of cholesterol, smooth muscle cells, fibrous proteins, and calcium. Atherosclerosis can develop in large blood vessels, such as the aorta, and in arteries supplying blood to the brain, heart, kidneys, and legs.

Atherosclerotic plaques can cause the following: TIAs ("ministrokes" that subside within a few minutes to an hour) due to diminished blood flow (ischemia) to parts of the brain; angina resulting from partially obstructed coronary arteries; and pain in leg muscles when walking due to poor blood supply to the legs.

Blood clots, which tend to occur at sites of atherosclerotic narrowing of arteries, can totally block a blood vessel supplying the heart muscle and cause a heart attack. When this same process occurs in an artery to the brain, it may cause an ischemic stroke. (For a detailed discussion of stroke, see the section starting on page 37.) Even if reduced blood flow to the brain does not result in a stroke, it may have a more subtle impact on mental function. In one study, every 10-point rise in systolic pressure was associated with a 9% greater risk of impaired cognitive function (for example, attention, concentration, or short- and long-term memory). However, a more recent report found no association between blood pressure and cognitive changes.

Just why people with hypertension develop accelerated atherosclerosis is unclear. The stress of high blood pressure on arteries may injure the endothelial cells lining the arterial wall. This injury causes changes in endothelial cells that set off a chain of adverse reactions. In addition, the production of free radicals (unstable oxygen molecules) within the artery wall promotes oxidation of the fatty acids of low density lipoproteins (LDLs). Oxidized LDL further

NEW RESEARCH

Oats Help Lower Blood Pressure

Researchers know that adding oats to the diet can help reduce elevated blood cholesterol levels. Now two reports suggest that oats may also help lower blood pressure and reduce the need for blood pressure medication.

In the first study, researchers asked 88 adults (age 33 to 67) receiving treatment for hypertension to eat a daily serving of a breakfast cereal containing whole-grain oats or refined-grain wheat. After four weeks, 73% of the oats group was able to stop or cut in half the dose of their medication compared with 42% of the wheat group. After four weeks, blood pressure decreased by 6/3 mm Hg in the oats group but by only 2/1 mm Hg in the wheat group. However, blood pressure began to rise when cereal consumption was discontinued after 12 weeks.

In the second study, investigators randomized 18 patients (age 27 to 59) who had untreated hypertension to an oat-cereal group or a low-fiber cereal group. After six weeks, the oats group experienced an 8/6 mm Hg reduction in blood pressure, while those in the low-fiber group had almost no blood pressure reduction.

Because oats appear to lower blood pressure in addition to their proven ability to lower elevated cholesterol levels, the authors of the first study suggest that oats may help reduce the overall risk of cardiovascular disease.

THE JOURNAL OF FAMILY PRACTICE
Volume 51, pages 353 and 369
April 2002

damages endothelial cells, attracts white blood cells into the arterial wall, promotes the overgrowth of smooth muscle cells, and leads to the deposition of the cholesterol portion of LDL in the artery—thus forming an atherosclerotic plaque.

Hypertension is also an important risk factor for atrial fibrillation (a type of irregular heartbeat that originates in the atria, the upper chambers of the heart). For example, in one study, hypertension increased the risk of developing atrial fibrillation by 50% in men and by 40% in women.

Left ventricular hypertrophy. In people with hypertension, the heart must work harder to pump against the increased resistance of blood vessels. Like any muscle required to do more work, the muscular wall of the left ventricle, which supplies blood to all parts of the body except the lungs, grows thicker. This condition, called left ventricular hypertrophy, affects 30% of those with hypertension. The enlarged left ventricle requires a greater blood supply, which may not be met by coronary arteries already narrowed by atherosclerosis. Thus, patients with left ventricular hypertrophy are more likely to have angina, heart attacks, and heart failure.

In addition, left ventricular hypertrophy may cause abnormalities in the heart's electrical system. Women may need to pay special attention to left ventricular hypertrophy. In a study of black men and women, women with left ventricular hypertrophy but without significant CHD had a four times greater risk of dying of any cause than women without left ventricular hypertrophy. The risk of heart-related deaths was seven times greater among women with left ventricular hypertrophy than in those without the condition. Lifestyle modifications or medication to control hypertension can improve left ventricular hypertrophy but do not appear to reduce all the risks associated with the condition.

Aneurysm. By weakening arterial walls, high blood pressure can promote the development of an aneurysm (a sac-like bulging) in an artery of the brain or in the abdominal aorta. Rupture of an aneurysm can lead to catastrophic bleeding into the area of the brain surrounding the aneurysm (called a hemorrhagic stroke) or into the abdomen. Hypertension also predisposes people to a highly dangerous complication called a dissecting aneurysm, in which a tear in the aorta allows blood to enter the wall of the aorta itself.

Kidney damage. Hypertension can damage the kidneys in two ways: by fostering atherosclerotic narrowing of the main arteries supplying the kidneys (the renal arteries) and by damaging the small arteries within the kidneys. Either of these effects can lead to progressive loss of kidney function and, eventually, kidney failure with retention of waste products in the body (uremia). Such kidney damage illustrates the vicious circle of hypertension: High blood pressure can lead to kidney disease and atherosclerosis; kidney disease and atherosclerosis further elevate blood pressure; and higher blood pressure causes further kidney damage.

Even mild hypertension greatly increases the risk of kidney damage. In a 16-year study, men with Stage 1 hypertension had three times the risk of kidney failure compared with those whose blood pressures were 120/80 mm Hg or lower. Men with pressures of 210/120 mm Hg or higher had a 22 times greater risk of kidney failure than men with normal blood pressure.

Retinopathy. Persistent elevation of blood pressure can also damage the tiny arteries that supply blood to the retina—the light-sensitive layer of nerve tissue that lines the back of the eye. In the early stages of this disorder, known as hypertensive retinopathy, the retinal arteries thicken and narrow. Eventually, these vessels may develop blockages or begin to leak blood (hemorrhage) and fluid (exudate) into the surrounding tissue; in very severe cases, the optic nerve (the nerve that carries visual impulses to the brain) may swell and cause profound loss of sight. (These same changes also occur in the blood vessels of the brain.)

Hypertensive retinopathy typically evolves gradually, and many years may pass before people notice any visual symptoms. In general, the extent of retinopathy correlates closely with the severity and duration of hypertension. For this reason, eye examinations can provide clues to the duration of high blood pressure and the success of treatment. Treating high blood pressure usually prevents further damage to the retina. In patients with a hypertensive emergency, prompt antihypertensive treatment may reverse damage to the retina and restore lost vision.

PREVENTION OF HYPERTENSION

Prevention of *any* rise in blood pressure is important because organ damage can begin when pressures exceed 110 mm Hg systolic and 70 mm Hg diastolic—long before hypertension is present. Prevention of hypertension also eliminates the possible side effects and substantial costs of antihypertensive medications. Moreover, even when medications significantly lower blood pressure, studies have shown that treated hypertensive patients maintain a much higher

NEW RESEARCH

Treatment of Sleep Apnea Lowers Blood Pressure

People with sleep apnea—a disorder in which breathing stops periodically throughout the night—tend to have hypertension and therefore an elevated risk of cardiovascular disease. Now a study shows that effective treatment for sleep apnea can lower elevated blood pressure.

Researchers randomly assigned 118 men with sleep apnea either to a control group or to therapeutic treatment with nasal continuous positive airway pressure (CPAP) at night. CPAP involves wearing a mask hooked up to a machine that pumps air through the nose to keep the airways open. Patients in the control group used the same CPAP equipment, but the air pressure was insufficient to keep the airways open. Blood pressure was monitored throughout the study.

After one month of nightly CPAP treatment, blood pressure decreased by 2.3/2.4 mm Hg in the therapeutic CPAP group and increased 1.0/0.8 mm Hg in the control group. The improvements in blood pressure with CPAP occurred regardless of the patients' blood pressure at the beginning of the study; those with the most severe sleep apnea had the greatest reduction in blood pressure.

The lowered blood pressure observed with CPAP might reduce the risk of heart attack and stroke by about 15% and 20%, respectively, the authors write.

THE LANCET
Volume 359, page 204
January 19, 2002

The Controversy Over Mercury Blood Pressure Gauges

Blood pressure is measured using a sphygmomanometer, an instrument consisting of an inflatable cuff, an inflating bulb, and a gauge that has traditionally contained mercury. The cuff is placed around the patient's upper arm and inflated with the bulb. Then the level of mercury in the gauge rises according to how much pressure is required for the cuff to compress the brachial artery (the major blood vessel in the arm). Because mercury gauges are extremely reliable and require little maintenance, they have long been considered the gold standard for measuring blood pressure. However, many doctors have switched (or are in the process of switching) to other methods of measuring blood pressure, which may not be as reliable.

Moving Away From Mercury

In 1998, the Environmental Protection Agency (EPA) began urging hospitals and doctors' offices to reduce their use of mercury because of concerns about contaminating the environment. Mercury, which is also used in other medical devices such as thermometers, is a toxic metal that can damage the brain, nervous system, and kidneys. People can be exposed to mercury by inhaling it, touching it, or ingesting it (usually by eating fish from mercury-contaminated waters).

Mercury sphygmomanometers contain the least toxic form of mercury, and they are not responsible for the majority of mercury pollution. In addition, mercury sphygmomanometers and thermometers are highly unlikely to leak or spill. Regardless, the American Hospital Association and the EPA have agreed to remove as much mercury as possible from hospitals by 2005.

Uncertainty About Newer Devices

Mercury sphygmomanometers are being replaced with either aneroid or electronic devices. Aneroid (meaning "without liquid") devices use a set of pins and springs instead of mercury to measure how much pressure is required to compress the brachial artery. Electronic sphygmomanometers use mathematical formulas to calculate blood pressure from measurements such as pulse pressure, which reflects the stiffness of the arteries.

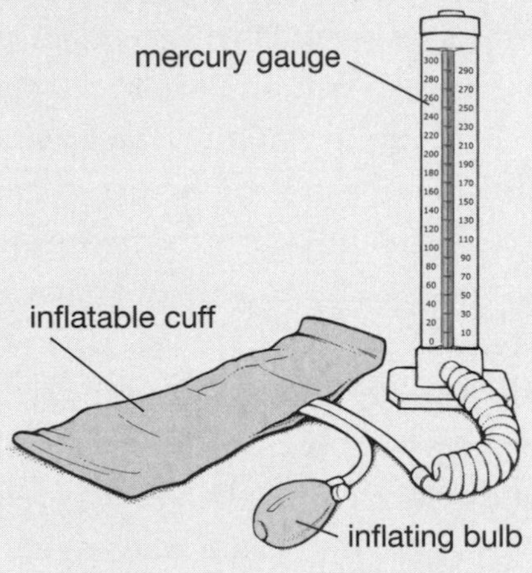

Mercury blood pressure monitor

Compared to mercury sphygmomanometers, aneroid and electronic devices can be easier to use and can reduce human error in taking measurements. However, the following concerns are making some experts uneasy about these newer devices:

- No good studies have compared the accuracy and reliability of aneroid or electronic sphygmomanometers with those of mercury devices.
- Aneroid and electronic sphygmomanometers have more working parts than mercury devices, so they are more likely to break and give inaccurate readings after extended use.
- Aneroid and electronic devices need to be calibrated (often by the manufacturer) every six months, something few hospitals and doctors' offices do.
- Little information is available on how electronic sphygmomanometers

risk of hypertensive complications than their normotensive counterparts with similar blood pressures. Therefore, prevention is the best way to reduce the risk of hypertensive complications.

The keys to preventing hypertension are weight loss, regular exercise, a diet rich in fruits and vegetables and low in sodium, and moderate alcohol consumption. Such relatively simple steps can have a considerable impact. Even a moderate weight loss, for example, decreased the development of hypertension by 50% in one study of individuals with high-normal blood pressure. The benefits of prevention are likely to be more substantial when several lifestyle changes are maintained for a prolonged period. According to a recent study, such lifestyle modifications are both feasible and effective.

work because manufacturers are allowed to keep their designs secret from competitors.

• A few doctors have reported that newer devices gave inaccurate readings that caused overtreatment or undertreatment of hypertension, resulting in illness or death.

The Experts' Opinions

As a result, the American Heart Association's Council for High Blood Pressure Research has issued a statement advising doctors and hospitals not to replace mercury sphygmomanometers until the newer devices are proven to be just as reliable.

Mercury sphygmomanometers are the most reliable tools available for measuring blood pressure, says Dr. Daniel Jones, a blood pressure expert at the University of Mississippi and the lead author of the American Heart Association statement. "We aren't prepared for the total replacement of mercury in blood pressure gauges, and there's no appropriate policy for maintaining the newer gauges."

Dr. Jones is hopeful that studies soon will examine how well aneroid and electronic sphygmomanometers compare with mercury devices so that hospitals and doctors can make more informed decisions about which type to use. So far, there is some evidence that well-maintained aneroid devices can be accurate. As part of the Mayo Clinic's annual inspection of its medical devices in 1999, 248 (17%) of its 1,500 aneroid sphygmomanometers were checked against a device known to be of high accuracy. Only one of the aneroid devices needed to be replaced or repaired. The remaining 247 gave accurate readings.

Both Dr. Jones and Dr. Lawrence Appel, coauthor of this White Paper, think that most hospitals and doctors will follow the EPA's recommendation, so that mercury devices will no longer be the standard for taking blood pressure measurements in the future. In addition, both feel that if evidence shows that aneroid and electronic devices are accurate, and if proper calibration procedures are put in place, these devices could be effective substitutes for mercury devices.

The Bottom Line

Dr. Jones cautions people with hypertension not to let this debate discourage them from getting regular blood pressure readings at their doctor's office. He says that if you are concerned about the accuracy of your blood pressure measurement, ask what kind of device your doctor is using and when it was last calibrated.

Patients also should keep in mind that while the device is important, so is the technique of taking the blood pressure. Resting while seated for five minutes before the reading, using the appropriate size cuff, taking the reading on the right arm, and taking at least two readings are all necessary to get an accurate blood pressure reading.

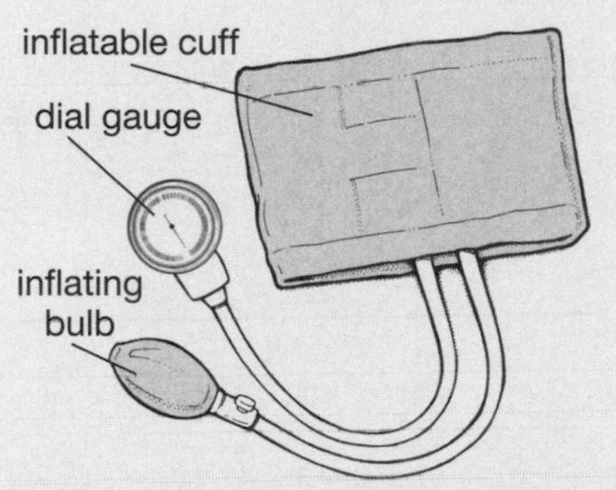

Aneroid blood pressure monitor

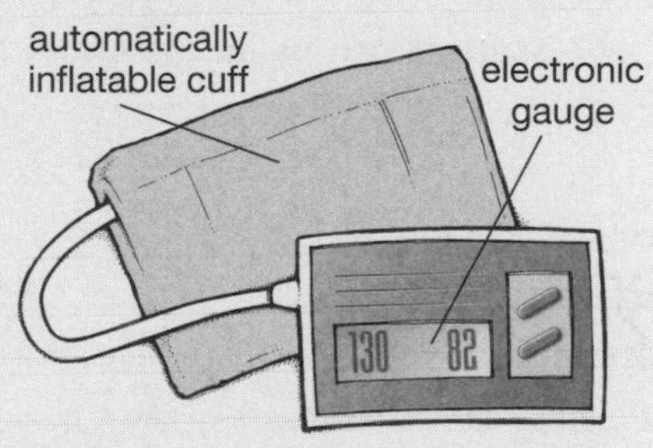

Electronic blood pressure monitor

DIAGNOSIS OF HYPERTENSION

Hypertension is discovered most often during a routine visit to the doctor. The instrument used to evaluate blood pressure in a doctor's office, known as a sphygmomanometer, typically consists of an inflating bulb, an inflatable cuff, and a mercury column gauge. Blood pressure is measured by wrapping the cuff around the upper arm and determining how much pressure is needed to compress the brachial artery—the major artery in the arm. The amount of pressure is equivalent to the height of the mercury in the gauge. Thus, blood pressures are expressed in millimeters of mercury, or mm Hg. In many instances, mercury sphygmomanometers are being replaced by aneroid or electronic devices. (For more information about mercury vs. aneroid or electronic blood pressure devices, see the feature on pages 14–15.)

Unless initial blood pressure readings are very high (systolic pressure of 210 mm Hg or higher, or diastolic of 120 mm Hg or higher), diagnosis of the presence and the severity of hypertension requires accurate measurements of elevated blood pressure on at least three occasions over a period of a week or more. To obtain representative values, patients should not smoke or ingest caffeine in the 30 minutes prior to blood pressure measurement. Patients should also be seated and at rest for at least five minutes before the measurement. The results of two or more readings, taken at least one minute apart, should be averaged.

Home Monitoring of Blood Pressure

Home monitoring of blood pressure can be useful in determining the presence of white coat hypertension (see page 10) and can help people with established hypertension keep track of the effects of lifestyle changes and medication. Two types of devices are available for home measurements: mechanical aneroid monitors and electronic monitors with a digital readout. Both types of monitors should be checked annually against a standard mercury sphygmomanometer to ensure continuing accuracy.

Traditionally, the best way to measure blood pressure at home has been with a manually operated aneroid sphygmomanometer that consists of a cuff, bulb, and gauge to register blood pressure levels. A stethoscope is also required (most monitors come with one). Advantages of aneroid monitors are their accuracy, consistency, and low price. To use the device, however, you must be able to squeeze the bulb rapidly to inflate the cuff, hear the thumping sounds of blood flow with the stethoscope, read the gauge that records the pressure, and loosen a valve to let out the air slowly. Thus, individuals with hearing or vision impairment or limited hand movement—from arthritis, for example—may not be able to use an aneroid monitor.

Many electronic home monitors have not been adequately tested, but fortunately, these monitors are improving. Some types have a cuff that inflates automatically, and even those with manually inflated cuffs will deflate automatically. You need only record the numbers that appear on a digital screen. Electronic monitors are more expensive than aneroid monitors; those with automatic cuff inflation are the most expensive. In general, prices of monitors range from $30 to $130.

Ambulatory Blood Pressure Monitoring

Blood pressure readings taken in the doctor's office are important for the diagnosis and treatment of high blood pressure. However, isolated readings may not accurately or completely reflect a patient's blood pressure, which fluctuates with time of day, physical activity, diet, medications, and stress. A technique called ambulatory blood pressure monitoring (ABPM) can document these fluctuations in blood pressure and provide additional information about a patient's true blood pressure over time.

How ABPM Works

ABPM measures blood pressure frequently throughout the day and night, typically every 15 to 30 minutes during the day and every 30 to 60 minutes during the night. The monitoring period is usually 24 or 48 hours. An inflatable cuff, worn around the arm, is connected to a blood pressure monitor about the size of a Walkman. The monitor is placed in a pouch and can be worn at the waist in a holster. At predetermined times, the cuff inflates automatically and takes blood pressure readings that are stored in the monitor and interpreted by your doctor. The monitor is lightweight and quiet, and most people are able to sleep and carry out their normal activities while wearing it. Rarely, people may experience minor bruising, swelling, or rash from the cuff.

In addition to wearing the monitor, patients may be asked to keep a diary of what time they woke up and went to sleep, when and what they ate, any strong emotions they experienced, medications they took, and exercise they performed. This information may help explain fluctuations in blood pressure.

ABPM measures blood pressure in one of two ways, and sometimes with a combination of both. The auscultatory method "hears" the flow of blood through the brachial artery (the main blood vessel in the arm) using microphones under the cuff; the oscillometric method "feels" the movement of the blood after closing off the brachial artery. No data are available to show which method is more effective. Most of the currently available devices are oscillometric. Each method has limitations: auscultatory monitors may be affected by background noise (such as cars or large machinery) and oscillometric monitors may give inaccurate readings due to vibrations or muscle tremors under the cuff.

Who Needs ABPM?

ABPM usually is not needed to diagnose hypertension in people who clearly have high blood pressure as determined by office or home blood pressure measurements. But ABPM may be helpful for people with:

White coat hypertension. About 20% of people have white coat hypertension—an elevated blood pressure only in the doctor's office. Because ABPM records blood pressure during daily activities, when the patient is not under stress associated with visiting the doctor, it can help identify white coat hypertension. It remains unclear whether people wlth this condition should be treated with medication. Some physicians do not treat individuals with white coat hypertension unless they have other risk factors for heart disease or have had a stroke or heart attack. Other physicians use medication to treat all patients with white coat hypertension.

Drug-resistant hypertension. Some people continue to have high blood pressure, according to measurements in the doctor's office, despite taking multiple medications to control the condition. However, office blood pressure readings may not be able to determine the true effect of the medications. ABPM can show the effect of medications on blood pressure and the duration of the effect.

Hypotension caused by blood pressure medication. Medication for high blood pressure can sometimes cause the pressure to drop too low. ABPM can determine how low the pressure falls after the patient takes the drug, and the doctor can adjust the dosage to prevent overmedication.

Episodic hypertension. ABPM can detect a rise in blood pressure that occurs sporadically in some people, often due to anxiety or another medical problem.

Borderline hypertension. Some people have high-normal blood pressure readings (systolic of 130 to 139 mm Hg or diastolic of 85 to 89 mm Hg) in the doctor's office but have evidence of hypertension-related damage to the heart, kidneys, or eyes. ABPM can show whether events such as physical activity or stress are causing blood pressure to rise to higher levels than those seen in the doctor's office.

Paying for ABPM

ABPM equipment can be purchased by consumers, but it is best used under a doctor's supervision. Medicare has recently begun paying for ABPM for patients who have suspected white coat hypertension. However, Medicare does not reimburse for ABPM in patients with the other conditions mentioned above, because the evidence of its benefit is inconclusive. Most private insurance companies do not cover ABPM at this time.

Ambulatory Blood Pressure Monitoring

Ambulatory blood pressure monitors automatically measure and record blood pressures throughout a 24- or 48-hour period. Such measurements may be useful for certain hypertensive patients, such as those with white coat hypertension, who have high blood pressure in a doctor's office but normal blood pressure outside of the office. Ambulatory monitoring is not necessary when office blood pressure readings are well beyond the threshold for treatment (multiple office readings above 140 mm Hg systolic or 90 mm Hg diastolic) or for those whose hypertension is confirmed by home monitoring. In terms of treatment, however, many experts feel strongly that office blood pressures, not ambulatory readings, should be the guide. For more information about ambulatory blood pressure monitoring, see the feature on page 17.

Medical Evaluation of Blood Pressure

Proper diagnosis of hypertension requires a thorough medical history, a physical examination, and laboratory tests. Blood pressure levels determined by a doctor to be lower than 130 mm Hg systolic and 85 mm Hg diastolic should be rechecked within two years. Pressures between 130 and 139 mm Hg systolic or 85 and 89 mm Hg diastolic should be rechecked within one year.

When blood pressures are consistently 140/90 mm Hg or above, the next step is to determine whether the hypertension is primary or secondary. Although secondary hypertension is uncommon, the possibility of secondary causes of high blood pressure should always be considered, since these forms of hypertension are potentially correctable and their identification may spare the patient a lifetime of antihypertensive medication.

Precise diagnosis of a secondary cause usually requires special laboratory tests and procedures. Because these tests are expensive and inconvenient, they are not performed in every patient. Instead, they are done only when a thorough medical history and physical examination—or the results of routine laboratory tests—raise a strong suspicion for a secondary cause of hypertension. The chance that an underlying disorder is responsible for hypertension is particularly likely under the following circumstances: failure to control blood pressure despite lifestyle changes and a combination of three antihypertensive medications; an unexplained increase in blood pressure in an individual whose blood pressure was previously well controlled; a hypertensive emergency (see page 8); new onset of hypertension, especially with blood pressures greater than

180/110 mm Hg; a spontaneously low blood potassium level; or headache, perspiration, and palpitations suggesting a pheochromocytoma (a tumor of the adrenal gland).

The other aims of a careful medical history, physical examination, and routine tests are to determine whether hypertension has caused tissue or organ damage, to detect lifestyle habits that may be contributing to hypertension, and to identify the presence of additional risk factors for cardiovascular disease.

TREATMENT OF HYPERTENSION

The treatment of primary hypertension is aimed directly at lowering blood pressure. If a cause of secondary hypertension is found, ideal management involves treating the underlying disorder. If such treatment is not possible or fails to control blood pressure, the treatment is the same as for primary hypertension.

In general, therapy for primary hypertension follows a stepwise approach. Unless an individual's blood pressure is extremely high (Stage 3), doctors usually start treatment with lifestyle modifications, such as weight loss, regular exercise, and improved diet. If blood pressure does not respond after six months to one year, a single medication is added to the lifestyle measures. (It is important to continue lifestyle changes throughout treatment.) If the first drug is inadequate, the doctor will increase its dosage, substitute another drug, or add a second drug. If necessary, a third drug can be added later.

In addition, the JNC report includes a system to help doctors make treatment decisions by classifying patients according to their overall cardiovascular risk. For instance, hypertensive individuals with diabetes or a prior heart attack or stroke should begin drug therapy at the same time as lifestyle modification. Also, the threshold for starting therapy is more stringent in these individuals—specifically, a systolic pressure of 135 mm Hg or higher and/or a diastolic blood pressure of 85 mm Hg or higher.

Treating high blood pressure in older adults requires lowering the blood pressure neither too far nor too rapidly. An abrupt drop in blood pressure on standing (orthostatic hypotension) is more common in elderly people when elevated systolic pressure is reduced too much or too fast. Orthostatic hypertension can cause dizziness and may lead to falls that could result in broken bones. Organ damage may also occur when blood pressure is reduced too quickly in older people. To prevent these complications, blood pressure should be reduced cautiously in elderly patients. For example, medications may

NEW RESEARCH

Hypertension Is Often Undertreated

Many patients with hypertension receive inadequate treatment for their condition, a new study shows.

Researchers examined the treatment of 270 people (age 25 to 96) who had hypertension for at least six months. After each patient's visit to the doctor, the investigators surveyed the physicians to determine what treatment they recommended and why.

More than 90% of the subjects had a systolic blood pressure exceeding 140 mm Hg, the cutoff point for initiation of antihypertensive treatment, according to current recommendations. Nonetheless, doctors recommended new drug therapy or increased the dosage of current medication in only 38% of the cases. On average, doctors reported that they typically recommend antihypertensive treatment when a patient's systolic blood pressure is above 149 mm Hg or the diastolic blood pressure is above 90 mm Hg. Yet evidence indicates that a systolic blood pressure of 140 mm Hg or more is a more important predictor of cardiovascular events than the diastolic blood pressure.

One of the main reasons doctors gave for not initiating or adjusting antihypertensive treatment was that they were often "willing to accept an elevated systolic [blood pressure] in their patients," the authors write.

ARCHIVES OF INTERNAL MEDICINE
Volume 162, page 413
February 25, 2002

be started at half the usual dosage, and increases in dosage made more slowly.

Someone experiencing a hypertensive emergency (see page 8) must seek immediate medical attention to have his or her blood pressure lowered. This reduction is done in a controlled manner, however, and initially to levels such as 110 mm Hg diastolic, to lessen the possibility of precipitating a stroke.

Lifestyle Modifications

Lifestyle modifications proven to lower blood pressure include weight loss, reduced dietary sodium, increased physical activity, and moderation in alcohol intake. An ample dietary intake of potassium also can lower blood pressure.

Adopting these lifestyle changes not only may prevent hypertension but also may eliminate or reduce the amount of medication needed to treat established hypertension. Whenever possible, an attempt should be made to control blood pressure by altering lifestyle before starting medication. If this is not possible, institution of lifestyle changes should coincide with starting medication.

Results from the DASH (Dietary Approaches to Stop Hypertension) trial provide a dietary approach to reducing blood pressure that might be as effective as a single antihypertensive drug. The DASH trial lasted eight weeks and illustrated the benefits of a healthy diet. During the study, 459 individuals with blood pressures averaging 131/85 mm Hg followed one of three diets: a control diet low in fruits and vegetables, with a fat intake typical of an American diet (37%); a diet with a similar fat intake to the control diet but with plenty of fruits and vegetables (8 to 10 servings a day); or the DASH diet, which is low in both saturated and total fat and rich in fruits, vegetables, and low-fat dairy foods.

The DASH diet was both quick and effective in lowering blood pressure. Within two weeks, average blood pressure dropped by 6/3 mm Hg on the DASH diet and by 3/1 mm Hg on the fruits and vegetables diet, in comparison to the typical American diet. These reductions were sustained over the eight-week period: By the end of the study, the DASH diet had reduced blood pressure by an average of 5.5/3 mm Hg compared with the control diet.

While the DASH diet is highly effective for prevention of hypertension, some of the most impressive results were in people who already had hypertension. These individuals, with blood pressures of 140/90 mm Hg or greater, lowered their levels by 11/5.5 mm Hg, which is as low as (or lower than) the results produced by a single

NEW RESEARCH

Weight Loss, Sodium Reduction Appear To Have Lasting Benefit

Losing weight and reducing sodium intake can help older people get off antihypertensive medication and stay off it in the long term, according to a new study.

The study looked at obese and nonobese people with high blood pressure that was controlled using one antihypertensive drug. A total of 141 obese people were randomized to weight loss, sodium restriction, combined weight loss and sodium restriction, or usual care. Three months later, antihypertensive medication was discontinued if blood pressure was controlled and reinstated if blood pressure exceeded 149/89 mm Hg. The interventions lasted about 2½ years.

An average of four years after the intervention ended, medication was no longer required by 23% of people in the combined weight loss and sodium reduction group, 17% of those in the weight loss group, and 15% of those in the sodium reduction group. By contrast, only 7% of those in the usual care group remained off medication. The groups did not differ in rates of cardiovascular events.

The finding that weight loss and sodium reduction programs provide persistent benefits may make such programs especially worthwhile, the authors note.

AMERICAN JOURNAL OF HYPERTENSION
Volume 15, page 732
August 2002

State-by-State Hypertension Rates

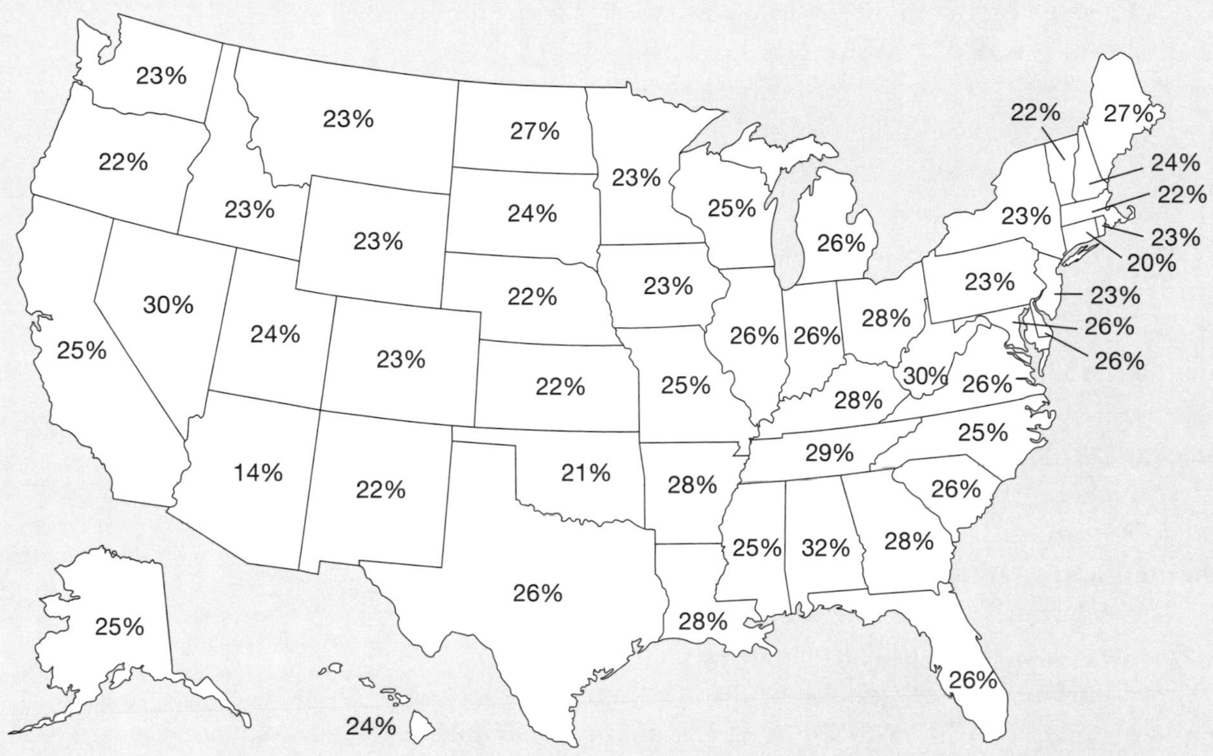

Source: *Morbidity and Mortality Weekly*, May 31, 2002, p. 456.

Beginning in 1972, the National Heart, Lung, and Blood Institute began to recommend that everyone age 20 and over have their blood pressure checked at least every two years. Subsequently, the percentage of adults with hypertension dropped from nearly 40% in the early 1970s to about 24% in the early 1990s. However, new statistics from the Centers for Disease Control and Prevention (CDC) indicate that the prevalence of hypertension is once again on the rise.

CDC researchers conducted telephone surveys of thousands of adults (age 20 and older) in each U.S. state and the District of Columbia every other year from 1991 to 1999. After tabulating the most recent statistics, the investigators did find some encouraging news: Nearly 95% of adults had their blood pressure checked within the last two years, a percentage that remained consistent throughout the 1990s. However, they also uncovered a significant increase in the number of people who said that they had ever been told they had hypertension—from 23% in 1991 to 25% in 1999.

The percentages differed somewhat by state. People living in Arizona were the least likely to have ever been told they had hypertension (14%), while Alabama residents were the most likely (32%) to have hypertension. Significant increases in hypertension since 1991 were found in 17 states (many in the South), while decreases were seen in only three states (Arizona, Connecticut, and Oklahoma). Demographic groups reporting the highest rate of hypertension included those age 65 and older (49%), blacks (36%), and people who did not graduate from high school (30%).

The CDC researchers attribute the increase in the prevalence of hypertension to two possible causes. First, increases in hypertension rates may be the result of rises in the number of people who are overweight or obese. In the United States, obesity rates in the adult population increased from 23% in the years 1988 to 1994 to 31% in 1999 and 2000. Second, the study's authors note that health care professionals may be getting better at detecting hypertension and communicating this diagnosis to their patients.

antihypertensive medication. In a separate analysis of the data, those with mild isolated systolic hypertension (between 140 and 159 mm Hg systolic) achieved a reduction in systolic pressure of 11 mm Hg.

Results from the DASH-Sodium trial published in *The New England Journal of Medicine* in 2001 indicate that combining the DASH diet with a reduced sodium intake can lower blood pressure more than either measure alone. In the study, investigators randomly assigned 412 people to eat either a typical American diet or the DASH diet. Participants followed their assigned diet at one of three sodium levels (3,300 mg, 2,400 mg, or 1,500 mg per day). People with hypertension who consumed the DASH diet with a low sodium level had a systolic blood pressure that was almost 12 mm Hg lower than that of people who ate the typical American diet with a high sodium level.

Lifestyle changes can be especially effective in older individuals. Weight loss, sodium reduction, and exercise lowered blood pressure in men and women age 60 to 85 by an average of 8.7 mm Hg systolic and 6.8 mm Hg diastolic during a recent six-month study. (Subjects started with diastolic levels between 85 and 100 mm Hg and were otherwise in good general health.) In another study, 43% of people over age 60 who reduced their sodium intake achieved a blood pressure of less than 150/90 mm Hg. Other beneficial lifestyle modifications for the elderly include reduced alcohol consumption (no more than two drinks per day), smoking cessation, elimination of caffeine, and increased potassium intake. (For tips on quitting smoking, see the feature on pages 52–53).

Medication

In people with Stage 1 hypertension (140 to 159 mm Hg systolic or 90 to 99 mm Hg diastolic) who have no evidence of organ or tissue damage and no other risk factors for CHD, lifestyle modifications are the initial approach. If blood pressure remains elevated after 6 to 12 months of lifestyle modifications, a single medication is typically started. In those with evidence of organ damage or with other cardiovascular risk factors besides hypertension, medication is initiated within six months or sooner. In the absence of organ damage or other risk factors, some doctors choose careful follow-up, rather than drug treatment, in patients with systolic pressures of up to 160 mm Hg and diastolic pressures between 90 and 94 mm Hg.

Medication should be started simultaneously with lifestyle modifications in those with Stage 2 or Stage 3 hypertension. When hypertension is especially severe, it may be necessary to start treatment with two drugs. Lower dosages of antihypertensive medications are usually sufficient in older persons, who respond better to blood pressure medications than younger people. This enhanced response is fortunate, because older people are more susceptible to the side effects of antihypertensive medications; a lower dosage minimizes the risk of side effects.

A number of different classes of drugs, taken individually or in combination, are used to treat hypertension: diuretics, beta-blockers, ACE inhibitors, angiotensin II receptor blockers, calcium channel blockers, alpha-blockers, central alpha agonists, peripheral-acting adrenergic antagonists, direct vasodilators, and aldosterone blockers (see the chart beginning on page 24). The availability of a wide variety of antihypertensive drugs, each working through a different mechanism, provides several valuable therapeutic advantages.

Although the drugs in each class are nearly equally effective in lowering blood pressure at comparable dosages, some individuals or groups of individuals respond better to one class of drugs than to another. If a drug is ineffective, switching drugs rather than adding a second one also may reduce the possibility of side effects. Moreover, people unable to tolerate the side effects of one antihypertensive drug may do better with a different medication. Finally, combinations of drugs from two different classes usually improve blood pressure control when a single drug proves inadequate.

Depending on the stage of hypertension, satisfactory control of blood pressure can be achieved with the first medication tried in about 50% of people with hypertension. Some 76% of patients will respond to either a first or a second single drug, and about 80% of patients respond to a combination of two drugs.

In patients with lipid abnormalities, the effects of antihypertensive medication on cholesterol and triglyceride levels should be considered. Thiazide diuretics and beta-blockers can have a modestly adverse effect on HDL cholesterol and triglycerides; alpha-blockers have a beneficial effect; and calcium channel blockers and ACE inhibitors have no effect on lipids.

Diuretics. Often referred to as fluid or water pills, diuretics promote water loss, a decrease in blood volume, and a fall in blood pressure by increasing the kidneys' excretion of sodium into the urine. These drugs also foster dilatation of small blood vessels. The three types of diuretics—thiazide diuretics, loop diuretics, and potassium-sparing diuretics—all produce essentially the same effect, though they act on different sites in the kidney.

Thiazide diuretics, the most commonly used type of diuretic,

NEW DEVICE APPROVAL

Breathing Device Approved for Blood Pressure Reduction

The U.S. Food and Drug Administration (FDA) has approved Resperate, a device that helps lower blood pressure through breathing exercises. The device was previously approved for stress reduction and required a prescription, but it is now available over the counter.

To use Resperate, the person puts on earphones and attaches to the torso an elastic belt that contains a respiration sensor. The device analyzes the user's breathing rate and pattern and emits two musical tones that signal when to inhale and exhale. The pace of the tones is gradually slowed until a target rate of 10 breaths per minute is reached. Slower breathing is thought to relax the muscles within the blood vessels and thus allow easier blood flow.

In a clinical trial, the device reduced blood pressure by an average of 14/9 mm Hg after eight weeks (three to four 15-minute sessions per week). The average user was 55 years old and had poorly controlled high blood pressure despite taking more than one antihypertensive medication.

No side effects were reported from using Resperate. Breathing returns to normal after each session, but the benefits of the slowed breathing may accumulate over time. Users of Resperate should not reduce their blood pressure medications without consulting their doctor.

APPROVED BY THE FDA
July 2, 2002

Antihypertensive Drugs 2003

Drug Type	Generic Name	Brand Name	Average Daily Dosage*	Wholesale Cost (Generic Cost)†
Diuretics	*Thiazide diuretics:*			
	bendroflumethiazide	Naturetin-5	2.5 to 20 mg	5 mg: $119
	chlorothiazide	Diuril	250 to 1,000 mg	250 mg: $17 ($15)
	chlorthalidone	Thalitone	25 to 100 mg	15 mg: $92 (25 mg: $17)
	hydrochlorothiazide/ triamterene	Dyazide	1 to 2 pills	25 mg/37.5 mg: $50
	hydrochlorothiazide	Ezide	25 to 100 mg	50 mg: $4
		HydroDIURIL	25 to 100 mg	25 mg: $17
	indapamide	Lozol	1.5 to 5 mg	2.5 mg: $123 ($89)
	methyclothiazide	Enduron	2.5 to 5 mg	2.5 mg: $60 (5 mg: $52)
	metolazone	Zaroxolyn	2.5 to 5 mg	5 mg: $107
	trichlormethiazide	Naqua	2 to 4 mg	4 mg: $85 ($10)
	Loop diuretics:			
	bumetanide	Bumex	0.5 to 6 mg	0.5 mg: $40 ($30)
	ethacrynic acid	Edecrin	50 to 200 mg	50 mg: $53
	furosemide	Lasix	80 mg	40 mg: $30 ($17)
	torsemide	Demadex	5 to 10 mg	5 mg: $65
	Potassium-sparing diuretics:			
	amiloride	Midamor	5 to10 mg	5 mg: $58 ($48)
	spironolactone	Aldactone	50 to 200 mg	50 mg: $98 ($82)
	triamterene	Dyrenium	200 mg	50 mg: $95
Beta-blockers	acebutolol	Sectral	400 to 800 mg	200 mg: $135 ($100)
	atenolol	Tenormin	25 to 100 mg	50 mg: $118 ($81)
	betaxolol	Kerlone	10 to 20 mg	10 mg: $106 ($88)
	bisoprolol	Zebeta	5 to 10 mg	5 mg: $131 ($118)
	bisoprolol/hydrochlorothiazide	Ziac	1 to 2 tablets	5 mg/6.25 mg: $131 ($114)
	carteolol	Cartrol	2.5 to 10 mg	5 mg: $132
	labetalol‡	Normodyne	400 to 800 mg	100 mg: $62 ($48)
	metoprolol	Lopressor	100 to 450 mg	100 mg: $121 ($76)
		Toprol XL	50 to 400 mg	100 mg: $98
	nadolol	Corgard	40 to 320 mg	80 mg: $263 ($140)
	penbutolol	Levatol	20 mg	20 mg: $154
	pindolol	—	10 to 60 mg	(10 mg: $93)
	propranolol	Inderal	80 to 160 mg	80 mg: $121 ($63)
	timolol	Blocadren	20 to 40 mg	10 mg: $66 ($34)
Calcium channel blockers (long-acting)	amlodipine	Norvasc	5 to 10 mg	5 mg: $145
	diltiazem, extended-release	Cardizem CD	240 to 360 mg	120 mg: $133 ($101)
		Dilacor XR	240 to 360 mg	120 mg: $132 ($101)
		Tiazac	120 to 540 mg	120 mg: $118 ($101)
	felodipine	Plendil	5 to 10 mg	5 mg: $113
	isradipine	DynaCirc	5 to 20 mg	5 mg: $156
	nicardipine	Cardene	60 mg	30 mg: $89 ($64)
	nifedipine, extended-release	Procardia XL	30 to 120 mg	30 mg: $152 ($116)
	nisoldipine	Sular	30 to 120 mg	30 mg: $105
	verapamil, extended-release	Calan SR	240 to 480 mg	120 mg: $129
		Covera-HS	240 to 480 mg	180 mg: $139
		Isoptin SR	240 to 480 mg	120 mg: $136 ($97)
		Verelan	240 to 480 mg	120 mg: $185

Advantages	Disadvantages
Diuretics are useful for patients with heart failure, since they help to eliminate excess fluid from the body. (ACE inhibitors also should be prescribed for heart failure patients because they lower mortality rates.) Diuretics are also the preferred drug class for treating isolated systolic hypertension. Thiazides are especially effective in older people (who may need smaller doses than younger patients). Thiazides may make other antihypertensive drugs more effective by reversing the fluid retention that some of them cause. Metolazone is helpful for people with impaired kidney function who do not respond to other thiazides. Loop diuretics sometimes are used for patients who are not helped by thiazides, especially those with impaired kidney function. Potassium-sparing diuretics can be taken alone but generally are used only in conjunction with another type of diuretic to counteract excessive potassium loss.	Thiazide diuretics may cause potassium loss, elevated triglyceride and glucose levels, decreased high density lipoprotein (HDL or "good") cholesterol levels, gout, weakness, erectile dysfunction, and dizziness on standing. Loop diuretics can cause dehydration, potassium loss, and changes in the acidity of blood. Potassium-sparing diuretics can raise potassium levels, a particular danger for people who have kidney disease. Potassium-sparing diuretics should be used cautiously, if at all, with ACE inhibitors, which can also raise potassium levels.
These drugs also are effective for patients with angina or a previous heart attack, since they help control pain and reduce the incidence of second heart attacks and total mortality.	Side effects include fatigue, vivid dreams, loss of sex drive, and erectile dysfunction. Beta-blockers may aggravate heart failure (although, in low doses, some have been shown to be beneficial). They may raise triglyceride levels and lower HDL cholesterol levels. They should not be taken by patients with asthma and are less effective in blacks and the elderly. Abruptly stopping the drug can produce serious cardiovascular problems.
Calcium channel blockers have antianginal properties. Side effects tend to be mild.	Constipation, swelling of the legs, headaches, and dizziness are possible side effects, but most people experience only mild problems, if any. Some subclasses of calcium channel blockers may aggravate heart arrhythmias and heart failure. Recent studies suggest an increased risk of heart attack in users of short-acting calcium channel blockers (see pages 30–31).

* These dosages represent an average range. The precise dosage varies from patient to patient and depends on many factors. Do not make any changes in your medication without consulting your doctor.

† Average wholesale prices to pharmacists for 100 tablets or capsules of the dosage listed. Costs to consumers are higher. If a generic version is available, the price is listed in parentheses. Source: *Red Book, 2002* (Medical Economics Data, publishers).

‡ An alpha-blocker and beta-blocker.

Antihypertensive Drugs 2003 (continued)

Drug Type	Generic Name	Brand Name	Average Daily Dosage*	Estimated Cost (Generic Cost)†
ACE inhibitors	benazepril	Lotensin	20 to 40 mg	10 mg: $94
	captopril	Capoten	100 to 150 mg	12.5 mg: $97 ($65)
	enalapril	Vasotec	10 to 40 mg	10 mg: $125 ($105)
	fosinopril	Monopril	20 to 40 mg	10 mg: $110
	lisinopril	Prinivil	20 to 40 mg	10 mg: $101
		Zestril	20 to 40 mg	10 mg: $106
	moexipril	Univasc	7.5 to 30 mg	7.5 mg: $82
	perindopril	Aceon	4 to 8 mg	8 mg: $156
	quinapril	Accupril	20 to 80 mg	10 mg: $113
	ramipril	Altace	2.5 to 20 mg	10 mg: $142
	trandolapril	Mavik	2 to 4 mg	4 mg: $88
Angiotensin II receptor blockers	candesartan	Atacand	8 to 32 mg	16 mg: $134
	irbesartan	Avapro	150 to 300 mg	150 mg: $144
	losartan	Cozaar	25 to 100 mg	25 mg: $143
	olmesartan	Benicar	20 to 40 mg	20 mg: $115
	telmisartan	Micardis	20 to 80 mg	20 mg: $141
	valsartan	Diovan	80 to 320 mg	80 mg: $140
Alpha-blockers	doxazosin	Cardura	1 to 16 mg	2 mg: $109 ($92)
	labetalol‡	Normodyne	400 to 800 mg	100 mg: $62 ($48)
	prazosin	Minipress	6 to 15 mg	2 mg: $71 ($37)
	terazosin	Hytrin	1 to 5 mg	2 mg: $204 ($161)
Central alpha agonists	clonidine	Catapres	0.2 to 0.6 mg	0.2 mg: $122 ($33)
	guanabenz	—	8 to 32 mg	(4 mg: $62)
	guanfacine	Tenex	1 to 3 mg	1 mg: $121 ($84)
	methyldopa	Aldomet	500 to 2,000 mg	250 mg: $46 ($35)
Peripheral-acting adrenergic antagonists	guanadrel	Hylorel	20 to 75 mg	10 mg: $200
	guanethidine	Ismelin	25 to 50 mg	5 mg: $63
Direct vasodilators	hydralazine	Apresoline	100 to 300 mg	50 mg: $65 ($8)
	minoxidil	Loniten	10 to 40 mg	10 mg: $175 ($129)
Aldosterone blocker	eplerenone	Inspra	50 to 100 mg	Not available

* These dosages represent an average range. The precise dosage varies from patient to patient and depends on many factors. Do not make any changes in your medication without consulting your doctor.

† Average wholesale prices to pharmacists for 100 tablets or capsules of the dosage listed. Costs to consumers are higher. If a generic version is available, the price is listed in parentheses. Source: *Red Book, 2002* (Medical Economics Data, publishers).

‡ An alpha-blocker and beta-blocker.

Advantages	Disadvantages
Cause few side effects. Some individuals report improvements in mood. Kidney damage is slowed in diabetic individuals with mild kidney disease, even if they do not have hypertension. These drugs also may slow kidney disease progression in people without diabetes. These drugs reduce mortality in people with heart failure and those who have had a heart attack. They also prevent heart failure after a heart attack.	Many individuals develop a dry cough. Skin rash may occur. Sense of taste may be altered. ACE inhibitors must be used with caution by those with severely impaired kidney function. They should not be taken by pregnant women or women in their childbearing years (unless they are using effective contraception).
These drugs are effective and cause few side effects. They need only be taken once a day.	In rare cases, these drugs may cause headache, dizziness, or fatigue. They should not be used by pregnant women or women in their childbearing years (unless they are using effective contraception).
Generally well tolerated. These drugs can reduce the symptoms of benign prostatic hyperplasia in men. Doxazosin and terazosin have the added benefit of raising HDL cholesterol.	These drugs may cause lightheadedness and even fainting in older people, especially with the first dose. They may lose effectiveness over time. When used by itself, doxazosin increases the risk of heart failure.
Side effects tend to be mild and to diminish with continued use. Clonidine is available as a transdermal patch that makes once-a-week dosing possible.	Dizziness (especially in older people), drowsiness, depression, dry mouth, sleep disturbances, or erectile dysfunction may occur. These drugs should not be stopped abruptly.
These drugs are effective for patients with severe hypertension and can be combined with other classes of antihypertensive drugs for maximum benefit. They do not cause drowsiness.	These drugs can cause diarrhea, and blood pressure may fall rapidly upon standing or with exercise when taking either of them.
Hydralazine can be very effective for patients who have severe hypertension. Minoxidil is more potent than hydralazine and is especially useful when severe hypertension accompanies kidney dysfunction. Combining these drugs with a beta-blocker and a diuretic greatly reduces side effects.	Hydralazine can cause a lupus-like syndrome at higher doses. Minoxidil may cause unwanted hair growth. Palpitations and edema are also common.
May be used alone or in combination with other antihypertensive drugs; works in a broad range of patients.	High blood potassium levels caused by poor kidney function are a rare but serious side effect. Less-serious side effects include dizziness, fatigue, flu-like symptoms, diarrhea, and cough.

have the advantage of low cost and once-a-day dosage. They provide maximal benefits at relatively small doses; higher doses, used frequently in the past, are associated with a greater incidence of side effects and little additional lowering of blood pressure. Potassium-sparing diuretics, unlike other diuretics, do not deplete the body's stores of potassium.

The Multiple Risk Factor Intervention Trial found that high doses of thiazide diuretics were associated with an increased risk of cardiac arrest. (The side effect of most concern for individuals taking diuretics is the loss of potassium, which can lead to serious cardiac risks.) These findings were confirmed by another study—the first to directly examine the effect of different dosages of thiazides on the risk of cardiac arrest. However, the study also found that low dosages of thiazides, especially when combined with potassium-sparing diuretics (but not potassium supplements), were associated with a lower risk of cardiac arrest than high-dosage thiazide therapy alone. Subjects included 114 people with hypertension who had suffered a cardiac arrest and 535 people with hypertension who had not experienced a cardiac arrest. Compared with low-dosage thiazide therapy (25 mg per day), the risk of cardiac arrest was increased 1.7-fold with a moderate dosage (50 mg per day) and 3.6-fold with a high dosage (100 mg per day). The addition of a potassium-sparing diuretic dropped the risk of cardiac arrest by 60%.

This research supports the use of low-dose thiazide therapy whenever possible and the addition of a potassium-sparing diuretic to the regimen, since thiazide and loop diuretics by themselves can cause excessive loss of potassium in the urine. People with more severe hypertension, who may need high doses of thiazides to control blood pressure, especially can benefit from the addition of a potassium-sparing diuretic, such as amiloride (Midamor), spironolactone (Aldactone), or triamterene (Dyrenium). Low blood potassium also can be prevented by taking potassium supplements. (Because potassium-sparing diuretics are relatively weak and can elevate blood potassium levels, they are generally used only in combination with thiazides.)

Other possible side effects of diuretics include weakness; fatigue; malaise; sexual dysfunction; increased blood concentrations of glucose, triglycerides, calcium, and uric acid; and reduced blood sodium and HDL cholesterol levels. Indapamide (Lozol) has fewer adverse effects on blood glucose and lipids than other diuretics.

Beta-blockers. These drugs impede the actions of epinephrine and lower blood pressure by slowing the heart rate and diminishing cardiac output (the amount of blood pumped by the heart). They offer the additional benefit of reducing oxygen consumption by the heart, thereby helping to control angina in people with CHD.

Possible side effects include the following: wheezing in people whose lungs are sensitive to various allergens and irritants or who have preexisting lung disease; fatigue; malaise; depression; erectile dysfunction or decreased libido; a rise in blood triglycerides; and a fall in HDL cholesterol. Because beta-blockers blunt the response to epinephrine, they may cause problems if low blood sugar (hypoglycemia) develops when individuals with diabetes are treated with insulin. (Epinephrine release during hypoglycemia triggers symptoms that alert patients that their blood sugar is too low.)

ACE inhibitors. ACE inhibitors decrease blood pressure by reducing the formation of angiotensin, a potent constrictor of blood vessels. These drugs are well tolerated and have no ill effects on libido or potency. A dry cough, however, occurs in about 25% of patients using ACE inhibitors, especially women. Uncommon adverse effects of ACE inhibitors are a rash and increased blood potassium levels. A study comparing two commonly used ACE inhibitors, captopril (Capoten) and enalapril (Vasotec), found that captopril therapy was associated with fewer side effects that decrease quality of life.

According to the results of a small study of 11 patients with hypertension, those taking ACE inhibitors should reduce their salt intake (as should all patients with hypertension) to minimize the need to add a thiazide diuretic to their regimen. In the study, either a low-salt diet or a diuretic produced similar reductions in blood pressure when added to ACE inhibitor therapy. Even more important, sodium reduction plus an ACE inhibitor did not affect blood potassium levels, which are critical in maintaining a normal heart rhythm and blood vessel tone. In contrast, hydrochlorothiazide (Ezide, HydroDIURIL) plus an ACE inhibitor caused a small but significant drop in blood potassium levels.

The Heart Outcomes Prevention Evaluation (HOPE) trial published in 2000 strongly suggests that ACE inhibitors may be appropriate for a wide range of patients. Researchers studied the effects of the ACE inhibitor ramipril (Altace) in more than 9,000 patients with CHD, stroke, peripheral vascular disease, or diabetes and at least one other heart disease risk factor (high blood pressure, elevated cholesterol, or smoking). After five years, 14% of the patients taking ramipril had died or suffered a heart attack or stroke, compared with 18% of the patients taking a placebo. This translates into roughly 150 fewer heart attacks or strokes for every 1,000 pa-

NEW RESEARCH

COX-2 Inhibitor Does Not Reduce Effectiveness of ACE Inhibitors

The COX-2 inhibitor celecoxib (Celebrex) does not decrease the effectiveness of the ACE inhibitor lisinopril (Prinivil, Zestril), new research shows.

Investigators randomized 178 people (average age 53) who were taking between 10 and 40 mg of lisinopril each day for high blood pressure to receive either 400 mg of celecoxib (twice the recommended daily dosage for osteoarthritis) or a placebo for four weeks.

In people who took celecoxib, 24-hour blood pressure recordings were 2.6/1.5 mm Hg higher at the end of the study than they were at the beginning. But this increase in blood pressure was not significantly different from the increase seen in the placebo group (1.0/0.3 mm Hg). The group taking celecoxib and lisinopril experienced no serious adverse effects from the drug combination.

Previous research showed that another COX-2 inhibitor—rofecoxib (Vioxx)—increased systolic blood pressure by 4.5 mm Hg in people taking ACE inhibitors to control hypertension.

HYPERTENSION
Volume 39, page 929
April 2002

tients treated with ramipril over a four-year period. The ramipril patients were also about 30% less likely to develop diabetes.

In patients with diabetes, ACE inhibitors delay or prevent the progression of kidney disease and are especially effective in those who have protein in their urine. Evidence is also emerging that ACE inhibitors may be beneficial in people without diabetes who have early kidney disease. These drugs must be used with caution, however, when kidney disease is advanced. Additionally, these drugs should not be used in women who are pregnant or plan to become pregnant.

Angiotensin II receptor blockers. Losartan (Cozaar), the first member of this class of drugs approved by the FDA, was followed by valsartan (Diovan), irbesartan (Avapro), candesartan (Atacand), telmisartan (Micardis), and olmesartan (Benicar). These drugs work by interfering with the action of angiotensin II, which raises blood pressure by constricting small blood vessels and stimulating the adrenal gland to produce the sodium-retaining hormone aldosterone. The drugs also may halt the overgrowth of smooth muscle cells in blood vessel walls. Irbesartan received FDA approval in 2001 for the treatment of kidney disease in people with hypertension and type 2 diabetes.

Side effects may include headache, digestive upset, and upper respiratory tract infection, although these occurred at about the same frequency in study participants who took a placebo. Patients who develop a cough while taking an ACE inhibitor may switch to an angiotensin II receptor blocker to eliminate this side effect. Angiotensin II receptor blockers should not be used by pregnant women or women planning a pregnancy.

Calcium channel blockers. These drugs lower blood pressure by dilating arteries and, depending on the type, by decreasing cardiac output. Like beta-blockers, calcium channel blockers help alleviate symptoms of angina. Compliance has improved with the availability of once-a-day dosages. Possible side effects include headaches, dizziness, slow or rapid heart rate with palpitations, flushing, swelling of the legs, and constipation.

Calcium channel blockers have come under fire recently because some studies suggest an increase in heart attacks and cardiac deaths in hypertensive patients treated with short-acting calcium channel blockers (for example, nifedipine). Also, compared with ACE inhibitors, certain calcium channel blockers may adversely affect kidney function. As a result, calcium channel blockers are not recommended as a first choice to treat hypertension, particularly

NEW DRUG APPROVAL

New Angiotensin II Receptor Blocker Approved by FDA

The U.S. Food and Drug Administration (FDA) recently approved a new angiotensin II receptor blocker called olmesartan (Benicar) for the treatment of hypertension.

Seven placebo-controlled trials, with data from 2,693 participants, found that 20 mg of olmesartan per day reduced blood pressure by 10/6 mm Hg compared with a placebo; a 40-mg dosage reduced blood pressure by 12/7 mm Hg relative to a placebo.

Dizziness was the only side effect experienced by more than 1% of the patients taking olmesartan, and it occurred more often with olmesartan than with a placebo (3% vs. 1%). Pregnant women should not take olmesartan because it can cause injury to or death of the fetus.

The recommended starting dose of olmesartan is 20 mg per day when used alone as a treatment for hypertension. If two weeks of olmesartan therapy do not reduce blood pressure to the desired levels, the dosage can be increased to 40 mg per day. A diuretic or other antihypertensive treatment may be added, if necessary.

APPROVED BY THE FDA
April 25, 2002

for patients with heart failure; only long-acting types should be used. Patients currently taking these drugs should not stop these medications without first talking to their doctor. More definitive answers on the relative safety of calcium channel blockers should be available after publication of the final results of the Antihypertensive and Lipid Lowering Treatment to Prevent Heart Attack Trial (ALLHAT).

Alpha-blockers. These drugs decrease blood pressure by blocking nerve impulses that constrict small arteries, thus lowering resistance to blood flow through these arteries. Alpha-blockers usually are well tolerated and have beneficial effects on blood lipid levels. They may cause lightheadedness on standing as a result of an excessive fall in blood pressure, especially in older patients, as well as weakness, fainting, headaches, and palpitations. Alpha-blockers can lose their effectiveness over time, but this problem also occurs with beta-blockers and central alpha agonists. The addition of a diuretic may overcome this loss in effectiveness, which is due to retention of water and salt in an attempt to compensate for the drop in blood pressure. However, according to early results from ALLHAT, diuretics are a better first-line therapy than alpha-blockers, which increase the risk of heart failure. Alpha-blockers also are often prescribed for the treatment of benign prostatic hyperplasia.

Central alpha agonists. Like alpha-blockers, these drugs lower blood pressure by blocking nerve impulses that constrict small arteries. Possible side effects include drowsiness, sleep disturbances, depression, dry mouth, fatigue, erectile dysfunction, and dizziness, especially in older people. These drugs should not be stopped abruptly and so should be prescribed only for individuals who are likely to adhere to their medications. Because of their high frequency of side effects, these drugs usually are used only when other medications have not controlled blood pressure.

Peripheral-acting adrenergic antagonists. Guanadrel (Hylorel) and guanethidine (Ismelin) reduce resistance to blood flow in small arteries by inhibiting the release of epinephrine and norepinephrine from nerves. During treatment with these drugs, a profound drop in blood pressure may occur when rising from a seated or reclining position or while exercising.

Direct vasodilators. These drugs act directly on the smooth muscle of small arteries, causing these arteries to widen. Concurrent treatment with both a diuretic and a beta-blocker is necessary to overcome the side effects of fluid retention and rapid heartbeat resulting from the use of either hydralazine (Apresoline) or minoxi-

NEW DRUG APPROVAL

New Type of Antihypertensive Medication Approved by FDA

The U.S. Food and Drug Administration (FDA) recently approved a new type of medication for the treatment of hypertension. Eplerenone (Inspra) works by blocking the activity of the hormone aldosterone, which plays a role in elevating blood pressure.

The effectiveness of eplerenone was evaluated in studies involving more than 3,000 people with hypertension. When taken alone in a dosage of 100 mg per day, eplerenone decreased blood pressure by 4/3 mm Hg. The blood pressure-lowering effect was evident within two to four weeks. When taken with other antihypertensive medications, eplerenone had similar blood pressure-lowering effects.

Eplerenone was well tolerated. Side effects that occurred in at least 2% of patients and were reported more often in people taking eplerenone than a placebo included dizziness, diarrhea, cough, fatigue, and flu-like symptoms. Eplerenone should not be taken by people with high blood potassium levels, patients with type 2 diabetes and microalbuminuria (small amounts of protein in the urine), those with kidney problems, or people taking potassium supplements or potassium-sparing diuretics.

The recommended starting dosage of eplerenone is 50 mg once daily. If the antihypertensive response is inadequate, the dosage can be increased to 50 mg twice daily.

APPROVED BY THE FDA
September 27, 2002

Uncontrolled Hypertension

Although effective treatments for hypertension exist, recent studies suggest that only a third of patients have their high blood pressure under control. Blood pressure is considered uncontrolled when it remains above 140/90 mm Hg despite treatment. Many factors can contribute to uncontrolled hypertension. But once the cause is identified and remedied, control of blood pressure often can be achieved. The most common reasons for uncontrolled hypertension are discussed below.

White Coat Hypertension
Some people may not appear to respond to hypertension treatment because they actually have normal blood pressure. For example, up to 20% of patients have "white coat hypertension"—their blood pressure is elevated only when they are in a doctor's office. Also, using too small a blood pressure cuff on the arm of an overweight patient can produce inaccurate readings.

White coat hypertension may be present if antihypertensive medications produce symptoms of hypotension (such as dizziness or fatigue) even though blood pressure readings are still high in the doctor's office. To confirm white coat hypertension, blood pressure readings should be taken at home or with an ambulatory blood pressure monitor, which measures blood pressure over a 24- or 48-hour period.

To avoid inaccurate readings from the use of too small a cuff, you should know the appropriate cuff size used for your measurements. You can then remind the doctor or nurse to use the correct cuff size.

Volume Overload
Volume overload, or having too much fluid in the body, is a common cause of uncontrolled hypertension. It often is due to excess salt intake (which causes the body to retain water) or to not taking a diuretic medication (which helps the excretion of excess sodium and water). In fact, many, if not most, antihypertensive drugs can cause fluid retention and should be used with a diuretic. Volume overload also can be caused by kidney disease, which can lead to retention of sodium and water.

Inadequate Treatment
Another reason why your blood pressure may not be under control is that it is not being treated aggressively enough. For example, the dose of your medication may be too low or another drug may need to be added. Some people require three or more drugs to control their blood pressure. Also, you may be taking an inappropriate combination of antihypertensive medications (for example, two medications that work in the same way, or multiple medications but not a diuretic).

Antagonizing Substances
As the name suggests, this group of medications and foods can raise blood pressure levels and counteract the effectiveness of antihypertensive medications. Patients often are not aware that these substances can affect blood pressure control and so may not think to report using them to their doctors. Antagonizing substances include:
• nonsteroidal anti-inflammatory drugs

dil (Loniten), two direct vasodilators. Excessive hair growth is an adverse side effect of minoxidil. However, this discovery led to the development of a topical form of the drug for the treatment of baldness.

Aldosterone blocker. Eplerenone (Inspra) was approved by the FDA in late 2002. It is the first aldosterone-blocker to be approved and works by selectively interfering with the sodium-retaining hormone aldosterone (see the sidebar on page 31).

Selection of Antihypertensive Medications

For patients with hypertension and no other health conditions, the JNC report recommends diuretics and beta-blockers as the first line of therapy. This recommendation was made primarily because clinical trials had found these two drug classes effective not only for reducing blood pressure but also for reducing the incidence of stroke and CHD. Recent studies show that diuretics produce signifi-

(NSAIDs), such as ibuprofen (Motrin and other brands) and naproxen (Aleve and other brands)

- over-the-counter nasal sprays, oral decongestants, and appetite suppressants
- oral contraceptives containing estrogen
- cholestyramine (Questran)
- rifampin (Rifadin)
- tricyclic antidepressants, such as amitriptyline (Elavil)
- cyclosporine (Sandimmune, Neoral)
- erythropoietin (Procrit)
- corticosteroids and anabolic steroids
- licorice
- amphetamines, cocaine, cigarettes, and excess alcohol intake (more than 24 oz. of beer, 8 oz. of wine, or 2 oz. of liquor daily)
- caffeine

Poor Compliance

An inability to control blood pressure may be due to not taking your medication as prescribed or not following lifestyle guidelines, such as reducing sodium intake or losing weight. Compliance with antihypertensive treatment is often poor because many patients experience no symptoms from their high blood pressure. Since these individuals perceive no immediate benefit from lowering their blood pressure, they may find the illness preferable to its treatment. Other factors that may contribute to noncompliance include side effects, cost, and complicated dosing schedules.

While poor compliance with medications can contribute to uncontrolled hypertension, it may not be a common cause. A recent study of 103 hypertensive patients published in the *British Medical Journal* found that noncompliance (defined as taking less than 80% of the prescribed doses) was reported in equal numbers of patients who responded and did not respond to medication.

Other Health Conditions

Health problems besides hypertension can counteract antihypertensive treatment:

- Obesity and insulin resistance (see pages 4–5) decrease the effect of antihypertensive medications.
- Sleep apnea (periodic cessation of breathing during sleep) can increase blood pressure by stimulating the sympathetic nervous system (see the sidebar on page 13).
- Anxiety or panic attacks can raise blood pressure both by constricting blood vessels and by increasing activity in the nervous system.
- Rarely, other diseases such as Cushing syndrome (excess production of corticosteroids by the pituitary or adrenal gland), primary aldosteronism (an excessive secretion of aldosterone by the adrenal gland that causes the kidneys to retain sodium and lose potassium), pheochromocytoma (a tumor of the adrenal gland that secretes epinephrine and norepinephrine, hormones that increase heart rate and blood pressure), thyroid and parathyroid disease, and renovascular hypertension (high blood pressure caused by a narrowing of the arteries that carry blood to the kidneys) may be present and can elevate blood pressure.

Treatment of the above health conditions usually results in blood pressure reduction.

cantly greater reductions in strokes and coronary events than beta-blockers, even though both classes of drugs produce equal reductions in blood pressure.

Evidence is growing that other antihypertensive drugs may be effective in disease prevention. For example, the HOPE trial, which was published after the most recent JNC report, demonstrated the cardiovascular benefits of ACE inhibitors. The HOPE trial also found that ACE inhibitors reduced the risk of diabetes and diabetes-related complications, making these drugs a first-line treatment for people with diabetes. Some of these benefits may not extend to black patients, however; a 2001 study published in *The New England Journal of Medicine* found that the ACE inhibitor enalapril reduced the risk of hospitalization for heart failure among white patients with left ventricular dysfunction but not among black patients with the same condition.

As more clinical trials are completed, additional drugs may prove to be at least as beneficial as diuretics and beta-blockers. But this is not always the case. For example, short-acting calcium channel blockers have been linked with increased heart attack risk, and alpha-blockers with heart failure. However, a recent meta-analysis of calcium channel blockers found these drugs to be roughly equivalent to diuretics and beta-blockers in terms of their ability to prevent cardiovascular events (see the sidebar on the opposite page).

In certain situations, the JNC report advises that other drugs may be more appropriate as an initial treatment. For example, a number of diseases can be beneficially or adversely affected by the different antihypertensive drugs (as was found with ACE inhibitors and diabetes).

The JNC report also pointed out that diuretics and beta-blockers are less expensive than calcium channel blockers and ACE inhibitors, which is another important reason to favor them. However, the JNC report notes that cost should be a secondary consideration if the newer antihypertensive drugs eventually prove more effective than diuretics or beta-blockers for certain patients.

Because prices differ for the various antihypertensive medications, doctors and patients may want to consider cost when selecting a drug. For example, some medications are priced the same at all doses, which could make a large difference in price for an individual taking high dosages for long periods of time. The use of combination drugs or generic formulations also may reduce costs.

Combination Therapy

In 50% to 60% of people with hypertension who need medication, a single drug is effective in controlling blood pressure. For the rest, doctors frequently prescribe an additional drug from another class. Combination therapy, as this treatment approach is known, is typically achieved by taking a separate dose of each drug.

Also available, though used less often, are a number of fixed-dose combination drugs—formulations of two different drugs combined in a single pill. Most fixed-dose combinations blend a diuretic, often a thiazide, with another type of medication, such as an ACE inhibitor or beta-blocker. The FDA recently approved three preparations that combine a calcium channel blocker and an ACE inhibitor. These preparations are amlodipine and benazepril (Lotrel), enalapril and diltiazem (Teczem), and enalapril and felodipine (Lexxel). A combination of the beta-blocker bisoprolol and the diuretic hydrochlorothiazide called Ziac is the only combination (see page 24) approved by the FDA as a first-choice treatment.

The main advantage of combining medications to treat hypertension is an enhanced blood pressure-lowering effect. Each class of antihypertensives works in a different way; the actions of drugs from two classes often complement each other and lead to greater reductions in blood pressure than can be achieved with a single agent. For example, diuretics reduce blood pressure by increasing the excretion of sodium and water by the kidneys, but in some patients this effect may stimulate the release of certain blood pressure-raising hormones (to compensate for the drop in blood volume). Adding an ACE inhibitor blocks the actions of these hormones and improves blood pressure control. By some estimates, 80% of patients have an adequate blood pressure response to two-drug therapy.

A benefit of fixed-dose combination drugs is greater convenience. Also, because combination drugs tend to contain smaller doses of individual agents than if they were taken separately, the risk of troublesome side effects may be lower. In some cases, one drug prevents the side effects of the other; for example, ACE inhibitors can reduce swelling in the legs (edema) often caused by calcium channel blockers. Moreover, combination drugs require fewer daily pills, so patients are less likely to forget or neglect to take their prescribed doses. And the cost of combination drugs is usually less than the cost of purchasing each drug separately.

However, critics point out that fixed-dose combinations reduce dosing flexibility, since doctors cannot vary the dosage of each medication separately to achieve the optimum effectiveness and tolerability (though doses of both drugs can be adjusted at their fixed proportions). Also, patients are exposed to the possible side effects of two medications rather than just one. To date, no large, long-term studies have proven that fixed-dose combinations offer any benefits over other drug therapies.

For now, fixed-dose combination drugs are most appropriate for people who have found that the combination of two drugs, taken separately at the same doses as in the combination pill, effectively controls their blood pressure.

The J-curve

A few small observational studies have suggested that patients on antihypertensive medication whose diastolic blood pressure is lowered beyond a certain point appear to have a higher risk of heart attack than hypertensive patients whose pressure is lowered to a lesser degree. This effect is called the J-curve phenomenon: If the number of deaths from heart attack in patients treated with antihy-

NEW RESEARCH

Calcium Channel Blockers May Be Effective as First-line Therapy

Calcium channel blockers help prevent cardiovascular events and deaths as well as medications currently recommended as first-line treatments for hypertension (conventional therapy), a new meta-analysis shows.

Researchers compiled data from six recent trials comparing the effects of calcium channel blockers with beta-blockers, diuretics, or ACE inhibitors in 24,322 people with hypertension.

Treatment with either calcium channel blockers or conventional therapy (beta-blockers or diuretics) resulted in the same rate of deaths from cardiovascular disease or any cause. Calcium channel blockers were associated with a 25% lower risk of nonfatal stroke but an 18% higher risk of heart attack (mainly nonfatal) compared with conventional therapy. However, in patients with both hypertension and diabetes, calcium channel blockers more than doubled the risk of heart attack (both fatal and nonfatal) compared with ACE inhibitors.

According to the authors, the increased risk of heart attack with calcium channel blockers is offset by the decreased risk of stroke, making these drugs roughly equal to beta-blockers and diuretics as a first-line therapy for hypertension.

JOURNAL OF THE AMERICAN COLLEGE OF CARDIOLOGY
Volume 39, page 315
January 16, 2002

pertensive medications is plotted against diastolic blood pressure levels on a graph, a line connecting the points shows an increase in deaths at the highest (the top of the straight part of the J) and lowest (the top of the curved part of the J) levels of diastolic pressure.

Most experts question whether a J-curve phenomenon exists. The recent Hypertension Optimal Treatment (HOT) study, which involved 18,790 hypertensive patients with diastolic blood pressures between 100 and 105 mm Hg, showed that aggressive reduction of blood pressure to 140/85 mm Hg or lower was associated with a dramatic reduction in the risk of heart attack. When blood pressure fell even further (for example, to 120/70 mm Hg), there was little additional benefit *but no significant additional risk,* thus calling into question the J-curve phenomenon.

Medical Follow-up During Treatment of Hypertension

Patients with Stage 1 hypertension and no evidence of organ damage usually are seen within one or two months of initiation of drug treatment to adjust drug doses, change medications if side effects are troublesome, and monitor and reinforce lifestyle changes that have been recommended as part of the therapy.

Patients initially require measurements of blood sodium, potassium, and creatinine levels about every three to six months to detect any adverse effects of antihypertensive drugs on these blood components and any deterioration in kidney function caused by hypertension. The frequency of subsequent doctor visits varies from patient to patient, but follow-up every three to six months often is enough once blood pressure has stabilized.

Patients with more severe hypertension and/or other medical problems need follow-up every two to four weeks until they achieve satisfactory blood pressure reduction. If the first medication proves ineffective, the next step may be to raise the dosage of the initial medication, switch to another drug, or add a second antihypertensive agent. Some patients with severe or refractory (resistant to treatment) hypertension may require three drugs to achieve reasonable blood pressure control. (The American Society of Hypertension has compiled a list of specialists to aid those patients whose hypertension does not respond to standard care. This list is available on their Web site at www.ash-us.org.) Patients should always bring their pill bottles with them to their doctors. This practice can eliminate concurrent administration of drugs that should not be taken at the same time.

It has been estimated that hypertension is poorly controlled in

30% to 40% of patients with hypertension because they do not get enough medication. Another possible reason is lack of compliance by the patient. As many as 40% to 50% of patients drop out of follow-up within one year of starting treatment. Poor compliance is understandable, considering that many patients have no symptoms from the hypertension itself yet are expected to make lifestyle changes and take medication that may be costly or cause unpleasant side effects. Nonetheless, proper compliance is crucial to prevent the severe complications that may result from high blood pressure.

Stroke

Each year, about 600,000 people in the United States suffer a new or recurrent stroke, and nearly 160,000 die. About 4.4 million Americans are stroke survivors. The actual number of stroke deaths rose from 1988 to 1998, but because the population also increased during that time, the number of strokes per 100,000 people fell by 14%. This fall is probably the result of more aggressive treatment of risk factors (such as hypertension), earlier diagnosis, and better medical management of stroke.

The news from stroke researchers is likewise encouraging. In addition to alteplase (Activase)—the first drug capable of halting a stroke in progress if administered soon enough after onset—other drugs soon may be available for emergency treatment of a stroke. Other treatments are also under investigation, as are new approaches to rehabilitation. Still, the best weapon against stroke remains prevention. More than half of all strokes could be averted if people took the appropriate preventive steps.

TYPES OF STROKE

Strokes occur when an artery supplying blood to a portion of the brain becomes blocked or ruptures, so that nerve cells (neurons) in the affected area are starved of the oxygen and nutrients normally provided by the blood. Although the brain performs no physical functions and accounts for only 2% of the body's total weight, it consumes about 25% of the oxygen and 70% of the glucose (sugar) in the bloodstream.

One reason a stroke is so dangerous is that the brain—unlike muscle or other tissues—has little or no reserve stores of energy.

NEW FINDING

Hormone Replacement Therapy Increases Risk of Stroke

Hormone replacement therapy (HRT; estrogen and progestin combined) had been theorized to reduce the risk of both coronary heart disease (CHD) and stroke. However, data from a recent large-scale, randomized study show that HRT actually increases the risk of numerous health problems, including stroke.

Investigators from the Women's Health Initiative trial randomized 16,608 postmenopausal women (age 50 to 79) to receive either a placebo pill or a tablet containing 0.625 mg of conjugated equine estrogen plus 2.5 mg of medroxyprogesterone daily.

The planned study length was 8½ years, but the main part of the study was stopped after 5 years because increased health risks were observed. One of these health risks was a 41% increased risk of stroke in women taking HRT, compared with women taking the placebo. This would result in eight additional strokes per year in every 10,000 women treated with HRT. HRT also increased the incidence of CHD, invasive breast cancer, and pulmonary embolism (blood clots in the lungs) but decreased the risk of colorectal cancer and hip fractures.

The authors of an accompanying editorial recommend that "clinicians stop prescribing [estrogen plus progestin] for long-term use."

JOURNAL OF THE AMERICAN MEDICAL ASSOCIATION
Volume 288, page 321
July 17, 2002

Consequently, when blood flow is interrupted to a part of the brain, some degree of function may be lost in as little as four minutes; after a few hours, cells cannot survive. Fortunately, the brain has some degree of natural protection against such interruptions of blood supply—a ring of blood vessels called the circle of Willis at the base of the brain. This structure helps protect neurons by connecting the brain's front and rear blood supplies and providing alternative pathways for blood flow should a major artery become blocked.

The nerve damage due to a stroke is usually permanent. But despite the death of neurons, some improvement usually occurs over time as other neurons are recruited to take over the functions of those that were lost.

The two basic types of stroke—ischemic and hemorrhagic—are described below. Even though distinctly different mechanisms are responsible for these two types of stroke, hypertension increases the risk of both. Within each of these two major categories of stroke are several subcategories. Proper diagnosis of the specific type of stroke is essential for determining the right course of treatment.

Ischemic Strokes

Approximately 75% to 80% of all strokes are ischemic (from the Greek *ischaimos,* meaning suppression of blood flow), resulting from a blocked blood vessel. Neurons are damaged not only by the lack of oxygen but also by a powerful chain of chemical reactions known as the ischemic (or glutamate) cascade, which leads to a buildup of toxins that further compounds cell destruction. The large accumulation of glutamate from injured neurons excites other neurons to release excessive amounts of nitric oxide, a neurotransmitter. The combination of high levels of both substances results in further nerve cell damage. The degree and duration of the ischemic event determine whether the brain suffers only temporary impairment, irreversible injury to a few highly vulnerable neurons, or extensive neurological damage.

Cerebral thrombosis. The most common cause of ischemic stroke is cerebral thrombosis, which accounts for approximately 40% of all strokes. Cerebral thrombosis occurs when a thrombus (blood clot) forms along the wall of one of the major arteries supplying the brain. These arteries include the carotid and vertebral arteries, which run through the front of the neck and along the vertebral column, respectively, as well as the smaller cerebral arteries within the brain itself. Clots are most likely to develop in arteries that are

The Brain's Blood Supply and How an Ischemic Stroke Occurs

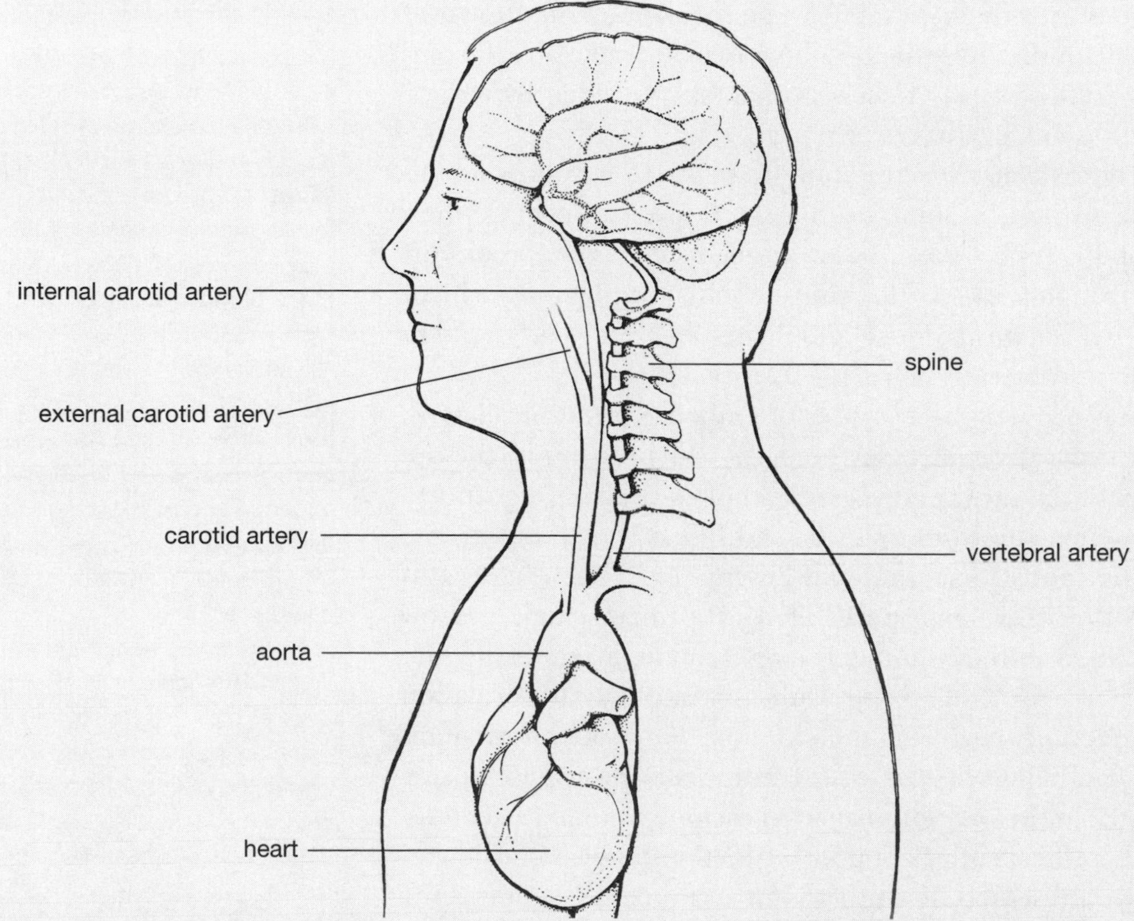

Although the brain accounts for only about 2% of a person's body weight, it receives some 20% of the oxygenated and nutrient-rich blood pumped from the heart. Two pairs of arteries—the carotid arteries and the vertebral arteries—carry this large volume of blood to the brain. The most common type of stroke, ischemic stroke, occurs when a blockage in the blood flow in one of these arteries (or the smaller arteries that branch off from them) starves the brain of the oxygen and nutrients it needs to function properly.

The left and right carotid arteries receive blood from the aorta and transport it up both sides of the front of the neck. (The pulse from these arteries can be felt on the upper part of the neck under the jaw.) As the two carotid arteries approach the top of the neck, each splits into an external carotid artery and an internal carotid artery. The external carotid arteries carry blood to the scalp, face, and neck, while the internal carotid arteries channel blood to the front two thirds of the brain and to the eyes.

The left and right vertebral arteries run up the back of the neck, parallel to the spine. (Unlike the carotid arteries, you cannot feel the pulse of the vertebral arteries because they are located deeper in the body.) At the base of the skull, the two vertebral arteries join to form the basilar artery. Branches from the vertebral and basilar arteries bring blood to the brain stem—the lower portion of the brain near the spine—and to the rear third of the brain.

The sequence of events that leads to an ischemic stroke typically begins with the formation of atherosclerotic plaques in the carotid or vertebral arteries (or their branches) that bring blood to the brain. Atherosclerosis narrows the arteries and increases the likelihood that a blood clot will form and completely block blood flow to the brain, causing an ischemic stroke. An ischemic stroke also can occur when a blood clot in one of these arteries breaks loose, lodges in one of the smaller arteries of the brain, and completely interrupts blood flow. Therapies that reduce the formation of atherosclerosis—such as blood pressure- and cholesterol-lowering drugs and cessation of cigarette smoking—may lower the risk of ischemic stroke. A surgical procedure called carotid endarterectomy also may reduce the risk of ischemic stroke.

already narrowed by a buildup of atherosclerotic plaque—the same fatty deposits that characterize CHD. The hard, rough, uneven surfaces of plaques provide ideal sites for the formation and growth of blood clots, which may eventually completely block the already narrowed artery. Ten percent of such strokes are preceded by one or more transient ischemic attacks (see page 42).

Cerebral embolism. Cerebral embolism, which accounts for up to 20% of all strokes by some estimates, most often occurs when part of a blood clot or a piece of atherosclerotic plaque breaks off and travels through the bloodstream (embolus) until it lodges in an artery supplying the brain. Most emboli are believed to originate in the heart or large arteries such as the carotid artery.

One of the most common causes of emboli is atrial fibrillation, an abnormal heart rhythm (arrhythmia) in which the atria (the upper chambers of the heart) quiver instead of contracting vigorously. The atria may not empty completely, and blood remaining in one place too long tends to stagnate and form clots. These clots can escape from the heart and travel along the increasingly narrow branches of blood vessels, ultimately lodging in an artery at any site in the body. One third of people with untreated atrial fibrillation eventually suffer a stroke during their lifetime. For more information on atrial fibrillation and stroke, see the feature on the opposite page.

Other possible sites of clot formation include injured heart muscle after a recent heart attack, a poorly functioning heart (as in cardiomyopathy), a diseased heart valve (for example, as in mitral stenosis), and, possibly, atherosclerotic plaque in the aorta (the main artery emerging from the heart). Emboli also can be composed of platelets, an air bubble, bits of fat released from the marrow of a broken bone, or calcified pieces of an arterial plaque.

Lacunes. Lacunar strokes occur when the tiny arterioles (the endmost branches of arteries) that penetrate deep into the brain become completely blocked by small emboli or atherosclerotic plaque. This typically happens at a site where a smaller vessel branches off from its larger parent artery. As a result, small areas of brain tissue degenerate, leaving behind little cavities called lacunes (lakes). Because the blood vessels involved are so small, symptoms of lacunar strokes are sometimes (but not always) mild. As a result, diagnosis may be difficult. Lacunes are often seen in older patients with high blood pressure who have had no or only minor symptoms in the past.

Other types of ischemic stroke. Global cerebral ischemia, typically caused by cardiac arrest or a life-threatening ventricular ar-

ON THE HORIZON

Device May Prevent Stroke in People With Atrial Fibrillation

More than 90% of the blood clots that cause stroke in people with atrial fibrillation (AF) form in a section of the heart called the left atrial appendage (LAA). A new device that seals off the LAA may prevent the development of these blood clots, according to a recent study.

The device is a metal cage that is placed through a catheter into the opening of the LAA. When the cage is warmed by the body, it expands and blocks blood flow into and out of the LAA. Spikes on the outside of the cage anchor it in place.

Researchers implanted the device in 15 people with AF who were at high risk for stroke and were not suitable for long-term treatment with the anticoagulant warfarin (Coumadin). Implantation was successful in all 15 patients, though one patient needed to have a second surgery to implant the device because of a complication during the first procedure. One month later, the device was still in position and no clots had formed on its surface in any of the patients.

This study is the first of many tests that the device will have to pass; larger studies are needed to prove its safety and effectiveness in preventing strokes in people with AF. Approval by the U.S. Food and Drug Administration could take several years.

CIRCULATION
Volume 105, page 1887
April 23, 2002

Atrial Fibrillation and Stroke

Atrial fibrillation (AF), the most common heart rhythm abnormality in the United States, affects approximately 2.2 million people. More common in older than younger adults, AF affects 4% of people over age 60 and 10% of people over 80. AF itself is usually not life-threatening, but it increases the likelihood of blood clots in the heart. One of these clots could then travel to the brain and cause a stroke. People with AF have a six times greater risk of having a stroke than people with a normal heart rhythm, and AF causes approximately 15% of all strokes.

In AF, the normal signal pathways that tell the heart to beat are disrupted. A normal heartbeat originates with an electrical signal from the sinus node, a bundle of cells in the right atrium (the upper right chamber of the heart). This signal causes the left and right atria to contract. The signal then travels to the atrioventricular (AV) node, a cluster of cells near the center of the heart. Here, the signal pauses briefly, allowing the atria to pump blood into the ventricles (the lower chambers of the heart). The electrical current then passes through the AV node and signals the contraction of the ventricles, which pumps blood to the lungs and through the aorta to the rest of the body. During normal activities, the heart beats 60 to 100 times per minute.

In people with AF, the heart receives signals to contract not only from the sinus node but also from other areas within the atria. Instead of contracting in a rhythmic pattern, the atria quiver (fibrillate) quickly and chaotically. Blood is not pumped effectively from the atria to the ventricles, and the ventricles begin to contract rapidly and irregularly, as well. In AF, the heart can beat up to 200 times per minute.

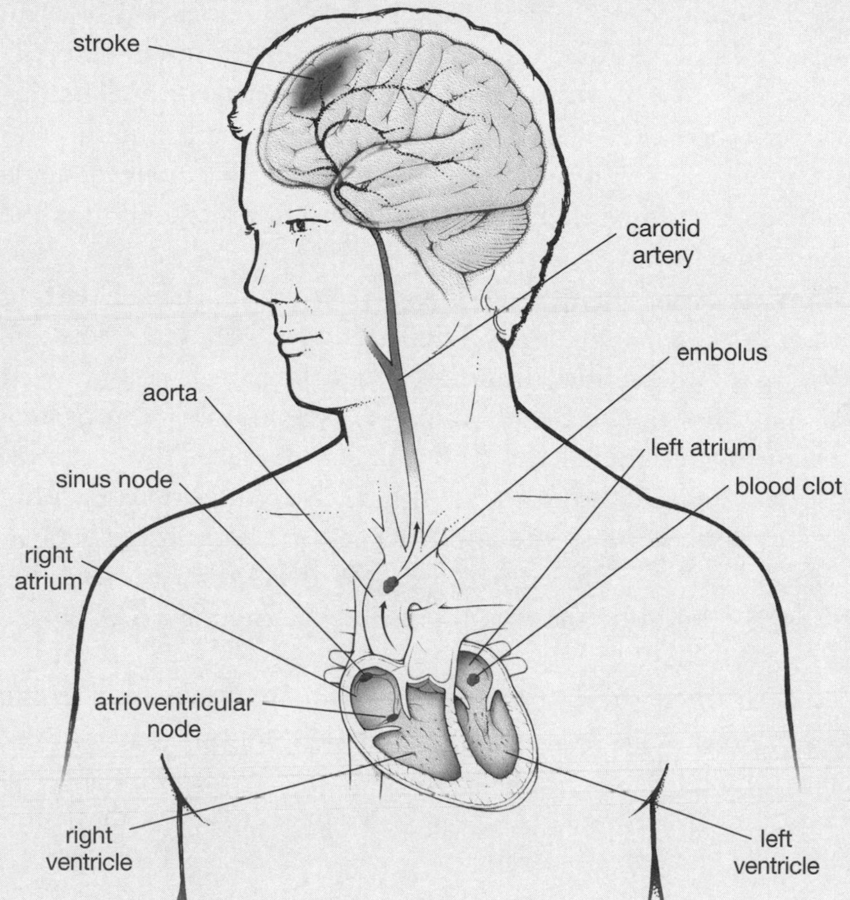

Because the atria and ventricles do not contract in a coordinated pattern, blood is not circulated efficiently to the rest of the body (although this reduced blood supply is usually still in a safe range). AF may cause weakness, lightheadedness, shortness of breath, heart palpitations, and chest pain, but many people with AF experience no symptoms.

AF can lead to a stroke because blood stagnates or pools within the atria. Clots can form when blood lingers in the atria instead of being pumped immediately to the ventricles. A piece of a clot (embolus) can break off, travel through the circulation, and block an artery supplying blood to the brain. The resulting lack of oxygen to the brain produces an ischemic stroke.

Fortunately, the risk of a stroke in people with AF can be reduced. The most common approach is to use aspirin (for people at low risk for stroke) or anticoagulant drugs such as warfarin (for people at higher risk for stroke) to help prevent the formation of blood clots. Careful monitoring of patients taking warfarin is required, however, since it can cause bleeding problems. The risk of stroke can also be reduced by treating AF with drugs that help restore normal heart rate and rhythm. Patients who do not respond to medication can be treated with cardioversion (the application of a brief electric shock to the heart) or with radiofrequency catheter ablation (the destruction of the area of the heart that is causing the abnormal signals).

rhythmia, occurs if the heart is unable to maintain a sufficient output of blood (circulatory failure). Neurons throughout the brain (as opposed to a single, localized site) are jeopardized. Unless adequate blood circulation is restored within 5 to 10 minutes, the patient is at risk for permanent brain injury.

Other causes of stroke include dissection of an artery—a tear between the inner and outer arterial layers, often caused by trauma—and coagulopathies, a group of rare blood disorders that may be inherited or result from other diseases such as cancer. The formation of blood clots within arteries and veins is a common complication of coagulopathies. Typically, dissection occurs in patients around age 40, while inherited coagulation disorders tend to affect younger patients.

Transient ischemic attacks (TIAs). TIAs are short-lived (lasting less than 24 hours) neurological deficits due to ischemia. Most episodes subside within 5 to 20 minutes, and they rarely continue for more than a few hours. By definition, TIAs do not result in permanent neurological deficits and are almost never painful. Hence, they tend to be ignored. TIAs are, however, an important warning sign of an impending stroke and thus warrant prompt medical attention. Patients may have repetitive spells of TIAs days or weeks before a stroke, and one third of those who experience a TIA have a stroke within five years.

Recognition of the cause of a TIA may help to prevent a stroke and its complications. For example, if carotid stenosis (a narrowing of one of the arteries supplying the brain) is detected, a surgical procedure called an endarterectomy (see pages 62–63) can be performed to remove the blockage.

Hemorrhagic Strokes

Accounting for approximately 20% of all strokes, hemorrhagic strokes occur when an artery in the brain suddenly bursts and blood leaks out into the surrounding tissue. The bleeding can take place either into the brain itself (intracerebral hemorrhage) or into the space between the brain and the skull (subarachnoid hemorrhage).

Damage occurs in two ways. First, the blood supply is cut off to the parts of the brain beyond the site of the arterial rupture (comparable to ischemic strokes). Second—and posing the greatest danger—the escaped blood forms a mass that, within the rigid skull, exerts excessive pressure on the brain. Blood continues to leak until it coagulates or until the pressure inside the skull is equal to the blood pressure in the ruptured artery. Massive hemorrhages are usually fatal; the death rate from an intracerebral hemorrhage is as high as 50% in some studies.

Aneurysms—blood-filled pouches that balloon out from weak spots in a blood vessel wall—cause many hemorrhagic strokes. While some aneurysms are congenital (present at birth), they may be exacerbated or even caused by hypertension. Most strokes due to a ruptured aneurysm occur between the ages of 40 and 60. Aneurysms are more common in people with polycystic kidney disease (a rare inherited condition in which the kidneys contain multiple cysts) and in those with two or more close relatives with aneurysms. Magnetic resonance angiography (see page 68) can be used to screen such people for large aneurysms before symptoms develop.

Brain hemorrhage also may result from a congenital blood vessel defect known as an arteriovenous malformation, which is characterized by a complex, tangled web of arteries and veins. The walls of these abnormal blood vessels tend to be so thin that surges in blood pressure, or simply the wear and tear of normal blood circulation, may eventually cause an arteriovenous malformation to rupture and bleed into the brain. Some people with an arteriovenous malformation experience seizures, usually during their 20s and 30s.

Intracerebral hemorrhage. Intracerebral hemorrhage accounts for about 10% of all strokes and half of hemorrhagic strokes. It is characterized by leakage of blood into tissue deep within the brain, usually the cerebrum—the part of the brain that controls higher functions such as speaking and reasoning (see pages 46–48). Hypertension is the primary cause of intracerebral hemorrhage; other causes include head injury, aneurysm, brain tumor, and the use of illicit drugs such as cocaine and amphetamines. In adults over age 80, a common cause of intracerebral hemorrhage is amyloid angiopathy—a weakening of blood vessels by deposits of amyloid, a starch-like substance.

Subarachnoid hemorrhage. Subarachnoid hemorrhage, which causes 7% to 10% of all strokes, results from bleeding into the space between the brain and the protective arachnoid membrane that lies between the brain and the skull. Most subarachnoid hemorrhages result from a ruptured aneurysm. Head injuries, arteriovenous malformations, and other blood vessel defects also may be responsible for the hemorrhage. Some 80% of subarachnoid hemorrhages occur in people 40 to 65 years old; 15%, in those age 20 to 40; and 5%, in those under 20. Women, especially during pregnancy, are at slightly higher risk for subarachnoid hemorrhage than men.

NEW RESEARCH

Osteoporosis Drug May Prevent Stroke in Women at High Risk

The osteoporosis drug raloxifene (Evista) does not increase the risk of cardiovascular disease (CVD) events (e.g., heart attack or stroke) in postmenopausal women and may even reduce the incidence in women at high risk for CVD.

Researchers randomized 7,705 postmenopausal women (average age 67) with osteoporosis to receive 60 mg of raloxifene, 120 mg of raloxifene, or a placebo daily.

After four years, women in each group had a similar rate of CVD events (between 3.2% and 3.7%). Among the 1,035 women with CVD risk factors (e.g., smoking, diabetes, high blood pressure, or high cholesterol) the rate of nonfatal CVD events was 39% and 50% lower in the 60-mg and 120-mg raloxifene groups, respectively; however, raloxifene did not lower the rate of fatal CVD events. Women taking raloxifene had significantly lower levels of total and low density lipoprotein cholesterol than those taking the placebo.

Thus, raloxifene therapy is not associated with the recently reported adverse cardiovascular risks related to other hormone replacement therapies (see the sidebar on page 37) and may provide a benefit in a select subset of patients. More research is needed to determine which groups benefit before experts can recommend raloxifene for the prevention of CVD events.

JOURNAL OF THE AMERICAN MEDICAL ASSOCIATION
Volume 287, page 847
February 20, 2002

Other Causes of Stroke

Inflammation of blood vessels (vasculitis or angiitis) in the brain can result in accumulation of blood platelets or clot formation, leading to acute cerebral ischemia and stroke. Intracranial vasculitis can complicate generalized disorders like lupus erythematosus, syphilis, or AIDS, or may occur as a primary neurological disorder; vasculitis must be considered, particularly in patients who suffer a stroke at a relatively early age. Proper diagnosis is critical because lupus and primary angiitis can be treated with vigorous use of immunosuppressive drugs.

Giant cell arteritis (also known as temporal arteritis) rarely causes a stroke but can provoke TIAs and sudden, irreversible blindness if not treated quickly with corticosteroids. This condition mainly affects people over age 60. Common symptoms include tenderness and pain over the temporal artery (found at the temples of the head), fever, weight loss, and headache. A high erythrocyte sedimentation rate (a sign of inflammation detected in a blood test) is a clue to the disorder, but definitive diagnosis requires a biopsy of the temporal artery.

About 15% of patients with sickle-cell anemia develop an ischemic stroke during a crisis in their disorder, which is due to vascular blockage by deformed, sickled red blood cells. Strokes also can result from high blood viscosity due to excessive numbers of circulating red blood cells (polycythemia), white blood cells (as in leukemia), or platelets, or to greatly elevated levels of blood proteins (such as in multiple myeloma, a form of cancer).

SYMPTOMS OF STROKE

Like a heart attack, a stroke is an emergency that requires immediate medical attention. Yet, while most people can recognize the characteristic symptoms of a heart attack, many are unaware of the symptoms of a stroke. Furthermore, symptoms of a TIA may appear suddenly and then subside just as quickly, creating the false impression that a serious problem does not exist.

But let there be no mistake about the proper course of action: *Anyone who experiences the sudden onset and persistence of any of the symptoms of stroke must call 911 or go straight to the hospital.* Rapid diagnosis and treatment may minimize damage to brain tissue and save lives. The feature on the opposite page describes in detail the symptoms of a stroke and the appropriate steps to take if these symptoms occur.

NEW RESEARCH

Dietary Folate Linked to Lower Risk of Stroke

People who consume more folate (also known as folic acid) in their diet appear to have a lower risk of stroke, according to a recent report.

Between 1971 and 1975, researchers asked 9,764 people (age 25 to 74) who did not have cardiovascular disease what they had eaten on the previous day. From this information, the researchers estimated the participants' average folate intake.

During the next 19 years, people who ate more than 300 micrograms (mcg) of folate per day had a 13% lower risk of all cardiovascular events (such as a heart attack or stroke) and a 20% lower risk of stroke than those who consumed less than 136 mcg of folate, after adjusting for factors such as diabetes, hypertension, and elevated cholesterol levels, which contribute to cardiovascular disease.

The researchers speculate that folate may reduce the risk of stroke by decreasing blood levels of homocysteine, a suspected risk factor for cardiovascular disease. The U.S. Recommended Daily Allowance for folate is 400 mcg per day, and people at risk for stroke should try to consume at least 300 mcg per day. Foods rich in folate include dark, leafy green vegetables; tomatoes; citrus fruits and juices; beans; and whole-grain or enriched pastas, breads, and cereals.

STROKE
Volume 33, page 1183
May 2002

The Warning Signs of Stroke

Like a heart attack, a stroke is an emergency that requires immediate attention. Since drug therapy is most likely to be effective within the first three hours of stroke onset, patients should go to the hospital as soon as symptoms start. Listed below are the symptoms of a stroke, as well as what to do.

Warning Signs of a Stroke

- Sudden weakness or numbness in the face, arm, or leg on one side of the body.
- Sudden loss, blurring, or dimness of vision.
- Mental confusion, loss of memory, or sudden loss of consciousness.
- Slurred speech, loss of speech, or problems understanding others.
- Sudden, severe headache with no apparent cause.
- Unexplained dizziness, drowsiness, incoordination, or falls.
- Nausea and vomiting, especially when accompanied by any of the above symptoms.

Actions To Take

- Stay calm, but ignore any tendency to downplay a symptom. It's common for people to deny the possibility of something as serious as a stroke. Don't hesitate to take prompt action.
- Call or have someone call an ambulance. (Dial 911 in most parts of the United States.) Be sure to give your name, telephone number, and exact whereabouts.
- While waiting for the ambulance, the person suffering the stroke should be made as comfortable as possible and should not drink anything other than water.
- If there is no possibility that an ambulance can arrive for an extended period of time, a family member or neighbor should drive the stroke patient to the hospital. Under no circumstances should the person experiencing the stroke symptoms drive.
- Notify the stroke patient's doctor. He or she can provide the hospital with the patient's medical history, which may be important for determining the best type of treatment.
- At the hospital, be sure to list any known medical conditions, such as high blood pressure, any allergies the patient has (particularly to medication), and any medications the patient is currently taking.

EFFECTS OF STROKE

In addition to the initial emergency symptoms, strokes generally produce lasting neurological deficits that may impair a person's senses, motor skills, behavior, language ability, memory, or thought processes, depending on which portions of the brain are damaged (as well as on the type and severity of the stroke).

At the base of the brain (at the top of the spinal cord) lies the brain stem, the most ancient part of the central nervous system, evolutionarily speaking. The brain stem maintains basic life support functions—breathing, heart rate, blood pressure, and digestion. An extensive stroke affecting the brain stem is usually fatal; when patients do survive, some sort of artificial life support is often necessary. Since the brain stem also helps maintain consciousness, many patients with a major stroke in this area fall into a coma. A coma also can result when a stroke in the cerebrum, which surrounds the brain stem, causes swelling that in turn puts pressure on the brain stem. (Many small brain-stem strokes are now detectable on MRI scans [see page 66], however, and these patients do well.)

Above the brain stem is the cerebellum, which controls coordination, balance, and posture. Early symptoms of a stroke in the cerebellum include dizziness, nausea, and vomiting. Later symptoms are clumsiness, shaking, or difficulty controlling certain muscles.

Above this part of the brain is a group of structures known as the limbic system, which we share in common with all other mammals. The limbic system is responsible for the primal urges and powerful emotions that ensure self-preservation: rage, terror, hunger, and sexual desire. Growth and reproductive cycles also are governed by the limbic system. Strokes in this area are rare, but when they do occur, basic animal drives may be severely limited or, conversely, patients may lose their natural inhibitions.

The Cerebrum

Surrounding these more primitive brain structures is the cerebrum—the largest portion of the brain in humans and a common site of strokes. Its convoluted outer layer of gray matter, known as the cortex, is the seat of conscious thought, perception, voluntary movement, and integration of all sensory input.

A unique feature of mammalian brains is the division of the cerebral cortex into two halves, or hemispheres, each responsible for a different set of duties. In most right-handed people, the right hemisphere specializes in matters of spatial relationships, color perception, visual interpretation, and musical aptitude. The left half of the brain typically oversees analytical tasks, such as mathematical computation and logical reasoning, and in right-handed people, it possesses particular regions dedicated to linguistic tasks, such as comprehending words and formulating speech. The two hemispheres constantly communicate with one another via a thick neural connecting cable known as the corpus callosum. Each hemisphere governs movement and sensory perception on the opposite side of the body. Therefore, a stroke in the left hemisphere can result in paralysis on the right side of the body. Each hemisphere of the cerebral cortex is further subdivided into four distinct sections, referred to as lobes.

Frontal lobe. The frontal lobe, as its name suggests, is situated at the front of the brain, behind the brow. Among other things, this area deals with motor function—that is, its neurons send signals that initiate muscle activity throughout the body. Damage to one side of the brain in a specific part of the frontal lobe—the motor cortex—results in weakness or paralysis somewhere on the opposite side of the body. In addition to paralysis of the limbs and torso, muscles on one side of the face or mouth may be affected, altering the person's appearance or ability to speak clearly (a condition known as dysarthria).

Expressive aphasia—difficulty in speaking, writing, or gesturing—

can result when a stroke affects the frontal lobe on the dominant side (for example, the left side of someone who is right-handed). The frontal lobe manages more abstract types of movement as well, including activities that require sequential steps. Consequently, a stroke may make it difficult or impossible to carry out a complex task, such as preparing a meal. Finally, highly abstract notions such as insight, initiative, and social inhibitions are governed by the foremost portion of the frontal lobe. A stroke here could result in uncharacteristically impulsive or uninhibited behavior. On the other hand, profound apathy, lethargy, and a lack of intentional behavior may result—a condition known as abulia.

Parietal lobe. Behind the frontal lobe, the parietal lobe is dedicated to receiving and interpreting sensory input from all parts of the body. Common problems resulting from parietal strokes are sensory loss, numbness, and visual loss to the side of the body opposite from the brain damage. Damage to the highly specialized sensory cortex may result in agnosia, wherein the stroke survivor is unable to interpret incoming visual, auditory, or tactile stimuli, even though the senses of vision, hearing, and touch are mechanically intact and function normally.

Another common consequence of a stroke involving the parietal lobe is a phenomenon known as neglect. Patients exhibiting neglect will typically stop perceiving or acknowledging events, and even sensations, on the side of their body opposite the affected cerebral hemisphere. (Patients with a stroke in the right side of the brain are particularly prone to neglect their left side.)

Temporal lobe. The temporal lobe—situated at ear level, underneath both the parietal and frontal lobes—is dedicated to hearing, auditory perception, and storage of memories. Strokes in the temporal lobe only rarely cause hearing loss; however, they do commonly result in language deficits known as aphasia—a term referring collectively to problems understanding speech, verbalizing thoughts, reading, or writing. Memory loss is also a common consequence of stroke in this brain region. However, memory deficits may be only temporary, since the temporal lobe on the other side of the brain can eventually compensate (unless, of course, both sides of the brain have been affected).

Occipital lobe. The occipital lobe lies at the rear of the cerebral cortex, in the back of the skull. It is dedicated entirely to the perception and interpretation of visual data delivered from the eyes via the optic nerves. A stroke in the right side of the occipital lobe does not cause blindness in the left eye; instead, it causes hemianopia,

NEW RESEARCH

Herbal Supplement Associated With Increased Stroke Risk

Ma huang, an herbal source of ephedrine that is often used in natural weight-loss products, may cause heart attacks and strokes, even in young people who have no history of cardiovascular disease (CVD).

Investigators collected data from the U.S. Food and Drug Administration (FDA) on the number and type of CVD events (heart attacks, strokes, and sudden cardiac deaths) that were associated with ma huang use from 1995 to 1997.

During this time, the FDA received 926 reports of possible ma huang toxicity. These included 37 serious CVD events that occurred shortly after ma huang ingestion: 10 heart attacks, 16 strokes, and 11 sudden cardiac deaths. The affected people ranged in age from 20 to 69, and only one had a history of CVD at the time of the event. Further, in all but one of the cases, ma huang was taken according to the manufacturer's instructions.

"Persons using or considering using ma huang should be informed of the possibility of associated serious adverse cardiovascular effects," the authors conclude. Although the researchers cannot conclusively say that ma huang was the cause of these CVD events, they suspect that the supplement raises blood pressure by elevating heart rate and cardiac output and constricting blood vessels, which could trigger a heart attack or stroke.

MAYO CLINIC PROCEEDINGS
Volume 77, page 12
January 2002

which leaves the victim blind to the left field of vision—or "half-blind" in both eyes, while the right field of vision remains normal in both eyes. (To a patient, this loss may be interpreted as a loss of vision in one eye only.) An occipital lobe stroke can also result in loss of the ability to recognize and interpret visual stimuli (for example, faces).

Other Consequences

In addition to the deficits described above, a stroke may produce other long-term complications, including seizures, impaired concentration, poor judgment, erratic sleep cycles, loss of libido, emotional instability, and depression. Also, immobility following a stroke may lead to aspiration pneumonia (inhalation of food and other particles into the lungs due to an inability to swallow and cough properly), bedsores, deep vein thrombosis (formation of painful blood clots in the legs, also known as thrombophlebitis), limb contractures (tightening of the muscles in the limbs), incontinence, and urinary tract infection.

RISK FACTORS FOR STROKE

A number of factors contribute to the overall chance of having a stroke. Some of them, such as age or race, obviously cannot be modified. Fortunately for people at high risk for stroke, other major risk factors can be significantly reduced through lifestyle adjustments, medical treatment, or a combination of both. One of these risk factors is hypertension, which not only accelerates the development of atherosclerosis—the arterial narrowing that accounts for two thirds of all ischemic strokes (or even more in people over 65)—but is the most important precursor of hemorrhagic stroke.

Risk Factors That Cannot Be Changed

The following important risk factors for stroke cannot be changed. Their presence, however, can alert people to their greater stroke risk and allow them to take appropriate steps.

Age. Between the ages of 55 and 85, the incidence of stroke doubles with each successive decade; only 28% of stroke victims are younger than 65.

Sex. Overall, the incidence of stroke is approximately 30% higher in men than in women, and this difference is even greater in people younger than 65. This gender difference is due to many factors, including higher cholesterol levels in men and the protective

Risk Factors for Ischemic Stroke

Many factors increase the risk of having a stroke. Some, like smoking, are modifiable; others, like family history, are not. While these factors help predict your risk of a stroke, having one (or several) of these factors does not mean that you are certain to have a stroke and having none of them does not necessarily protect you from ever having a stroke. The two graphs below show the increased risk of stroke associated with a number of nonmodifiable and modifiable risk factors. Treatment of modifiable risk factors can significantly reduce stroke risk. (Untreated sickle cell disease, not included in the graph, increases the risk of stroke by 200 to 400 times.)

Nonmodifiable Risk Factors

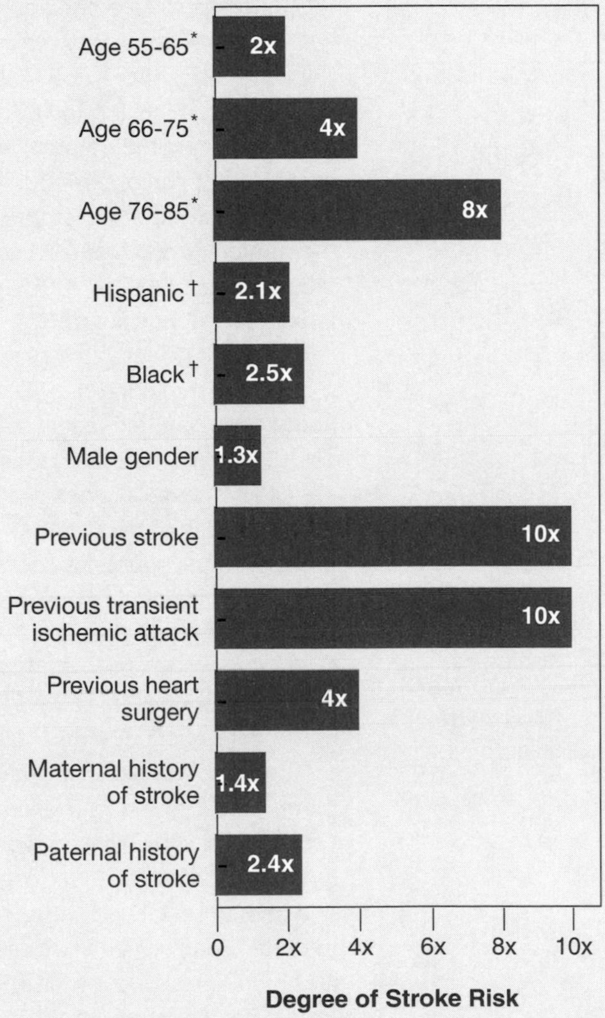

Risk factor	Degree of Stroke Risk
Age 55-65*	2x
Age 66-75*	4x
Age 76-85*	8x
Hispanic†	2.1x
Black†	2.5x
Male gender	1.3x
Previous stroke	10x
Previous transient ischemic attack	10x
Previous heart surgery	4x
Maternal history of stroke	1.4x
Paternal history of stroke	2.4x

Modifiable Risk Factors

Risk factor	Degree of Stroke Risk
High blood pressure‡	6x
Atrial fibrillation	6x
Left ventricular hypertrophy	4x
Other heart diseases	6x
Carotid stenosis	3x
Peripheral vascular disease	3x
Diabetes	3x
Smoking	2x
Total cholesterol 240–279 mg/dL	1.8x
Total cholesterol > 280 mg/dL	2.6x
Obesity	2x
Physical inactivity	2.7x
> 2 alcoholic drinks per day	1.8x

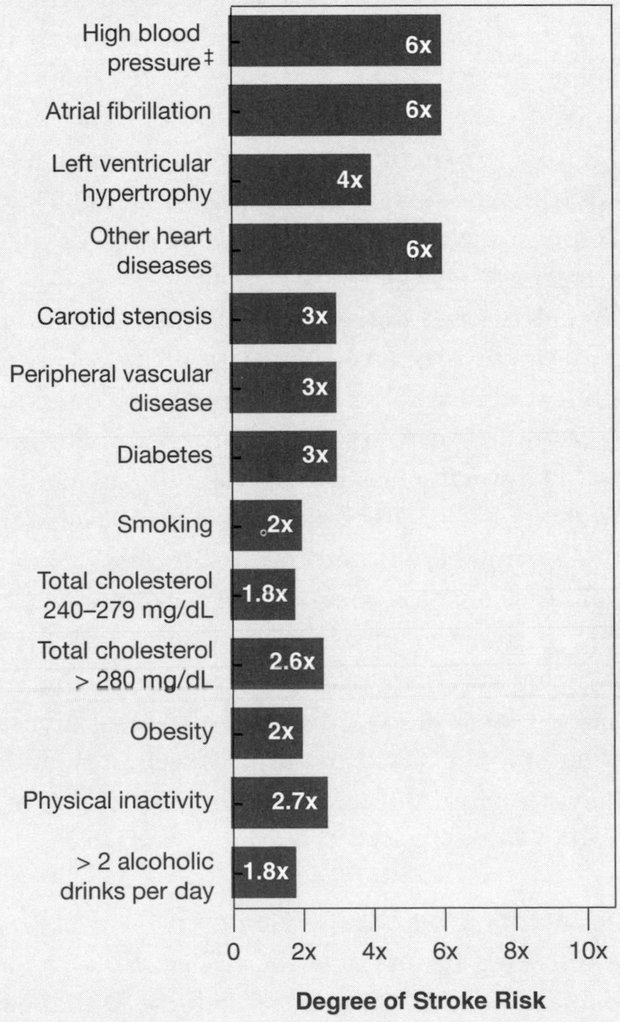

* Compared with people under age 55
† Compared with whites
‡ Consistently over 140/90 mm Hg

effect of estrogen in premenopausal women. Men also have a slightly higher mortality rate from stroke than women.

Family history. Stroke risk is greater in people whose close relatives have had a stroke.

Race. Blacks have about twice the risk of death and disability from a stroke than whites. Asian-Pacific Islanders and those of Hispanic descent also are at higher risk.

Prior history of stroke. Stroke survivors are at substantial risk for a subsequent stroke; about 13% have another one within 12 months of the initial event, and 6% have one each successive year after that.

Transient ischemic attacks. While only about 10% of strokes are preceded by these fleeting episodes, TIAs are a strong predictor of an eventual full-blown stroke. A stroke is almost 10 times more likely in someone who has experienced a TIA than in a person who has not. Eventually, about 36% of those who have had one or more TIA will have a stroke. Studies show that between 25% and 50% of TIAs result from the formation of a blood clot at a site of atherosclerosis in brain arteries. Between 11% and 30% result from emboli from the heart.

Accidents and other circumstances. Emboli may form following a bone fracture, open heart surgery, the collapse of a lung (a pneumothorax), or a too rapid ascent from deep waters. Such events may result in a cerebral embolism. A violent blow to the head may cause a hemorrhagic stroke. Subtle impairment of kidney function, as indicated by slightly elevated blood levels of creatinine (a substance normally removed by the kidneys), also may raise the risk of stroke. In one study, men with high-normal levels of creatinine had a 60% greater risk of stroke than those with lower levels. While hypertension can lead to kidney damage, in this study men with normal or elevated blood pressures were at greater risk for stroke when they had higher blood creatinine levels. A relationship between kidney dysfunction and an increased risk of stroke also has been observed in women.

Risk Factors That Can Be Changed

The following factors raise the risk of stroke, and all of them can be minimized or eliminated through lifestyle changes or medical therapy. Another treatable factor related to stroke is sleep apnea, which is characterized by periods of interrupted breathing during sleep.

Hypertension. High blood pressure, the single greatest risk factor for stroke, is estimated to play a role in about 70% of all strokes. Elevations in either systolic or diastolic blood pressure increase the risk in both sexes and in people of all ages. Indeed, stroke risk is about fourfold greater in those with blood pressures of 160/95 mm Hg or higher than in those with blood pressures of 140/90 mm Hg or be-

NEW RESEARCH

ACE Inhibitor Is Effective In Reducing Stroke Risk

The ACE inhibitor ramipril (Altace) reduces the risk of stroke in high-risk individuals, independent of its blood pressure-lowering effects, a new study shows.

Investigators randomized nearly 9,300 people (average age 66) with vascular disease or diabetes plus one other stroke risk factor to receive ramipril (up to 10 mg), 400 IU of vitamin E, ramipril and vitamin E, or placebo pills daily.

After an average of 4½ years, the ramipril group had 61% fewer fatal strokes (0.4% vs. 1.0%) and 24% fewer nonfatal strokes (3.0% vs. 3.9%) than the placebo group. The ramipril group also had a 17% reduced risk of transient ischemic attack (4.1% vs. 4.9%) and lower levels of mental impairment than the placebo group. These reductions remained significant in people who had normal blood pressure (120/70 mm Hg) or were taking aspirin to reduce stroke risk. Vitamin E did not affect stroke risk.

Regardless of patients' initial blood pressure levels, treatment with ramipril should be considered by those at high risk for stroke and should be taken in addition to other therapies, such as aspirin and blood pressure-lowering drugs, known to prevent stroke. While it is reasonable to speculate that other ACE inhibitors may also reduce the risk of stroke, limited data are available for ACE inhibitors other than ramipril.

BRITISH MEDICAL JOURNAL
Volume 324, page 1
March 23, 2002

low. A recent meta-analysis concluded that the risk of stroke was increased 10 to 12 times in people with diastolic blood pressures of 105 mm Hg or higher compared with those with diastolic pressures of less than 76 mm Hg.

Cigarette smoking. Smoking is an important contributor to both ischemic and hemorrhagic strokes. A recent meta-analysis reported that cigarette smokers have a 50% higher overall risk of stroke than nonsmokers. The more cigarettes they smoked, the greater the risk. Smoking appears to accelerate the progression of atherosclerosis as well as promote the formation of blood clots. Also, nicotine raises blood pressure briefly after each cigarette, and a buildup of carbon monoxide in the blood reduces the blood's oxygen-carrying capacity and thus the amount of oxygen available to the brain. For more information on smoking and your health, see the feature on pages 52–53.

Diabetes. Independent of other risk factors, people with diabetes have a threefold higher rate of ischemic stroke than the general population. Women with diabetes are at greater risk than men. (Diabetes, however, does not appear to increase the incidence of hemorrhagic strokes.) Diabetes is treatable, but it is not certain that controlling blood sugar lowers stroke risk.

Carotid stenosis. The carotid arteries in the neck supply blood to the brain. If a carotid artery becomes narrowed by the buildup of atherosclerotic plaque, blood rushing through it will make an abnormal sound called a bruit. A doctor can hear this sound by placing a stethoscope over the carotid arteries in the neck. When a bruit is heard, especially in patients with a history of TIAs, a duplex ultrasound (see page 68) is needed to determine the extent of the narrowing. Even without TIA symptoms, a carotid bruit suggests an increased stroke risk since it usually indicates atherosclerotic narrowing.

Coronary heart disease (CHD). Since many of the same factors contribute to both stroke and CHD, it is no surprise that the risk of stroke is doubled in those with heart problems. In addition to CHD, a number of other heart conditions can increase stroke risk by promoting the formation of emboli. These include heart attack (see the sidebar on page 55), heart failure (impaired ability of the heart to pump blood), valvular heart disease (damage to one or more of the heart's valves), and various cardiac arrhythmias (abnormal heart rhythms), especially atrial fibrillation (see page 40). Another potential risk factor is high blood levels of homocysteine, a substance thought to increase the likelihood of CHD and stroke by

NEW RESEARCH

Cardiovascular Fitness Lowers Risk of Death From Stroke

Improving cardiovascular fitness through exercise appears to reduce men's risk of dying from a stroke, according to a recent study.

Researchers studied 16,878 men (age 40 to 87), most of whom were white, who had a medical examination and an exercise stress test at one clinic between 1971 and 1994. The researchers divided the men into three groups based on their performance on the stress test. The participants also answered questions about their health habits, including alcohol use, smoking, and parental history of CHD.

An average of 10 years later, the risk of death from stroke (after adjusting for age and stroke risk factors) was 68% lower in the most-fit men and 63% lower in the moderately fit men than in the least-fit men.

The researchers hypothesize that physical activity may reduce the risk of stroke by improving blood pressure, cholesterol levels, insulin sensitivity, and blood clotting factors.

MEDICINE & SCIENCE IN SPORTS & EXERCISE
Volume 34, page 592
April 2002

Blood Vessels, Smoking, and How To Quit

Despite more than 30 years of public health warnings on the dangers of cigarettes, about a quarter of Americans still smoke. The habit results in approximately 430,000 premature deaths each year in the United States, mostly from cardiovascular disease (heart attacks and strokes), cancer, and lung disease. Quitting smoking can greatly decrease the risk of illness and death from these diseases.

The Effects of Smoking

It is not clear exactly how smoking contributes to heart attacks and stroke, probably because more than 4,000 chemicals are found in cigarette smoke. Cigarette smoking increases the risk of stroke by about 50%, and the risk is directly related to the number of cigarettes smoked. Smoking may raise stroke risk by increasing the formation of blood clots or by speeding the process of atherosclerosis. Nonetheless, the increased risk of stroke decreases after quitting; the risk returns to normal five years after smoking cessation.

The effect of smoking on blood pressure is uncertain. Some studies show that smokers have a three times greater risk of hypertension than nonsmokers, while other studies have shown that blood pressure is somewhat lower in smokers. In any case, the increased risk of heart attacks and strokes in smokers warrants aggressive efforts for smoking cessation.

Quitting Smoking

The health risks of smoking make it important for every smoker to quit. Because only about 8% of people who try to quit smoking are able to do so on their own, you can increase your chances of success by talking to your doctor or other health care provider about smoking cessation. They may be able to provide literature, advice, support, and medication to help you quit; they also may refer you to another health care professional who specializes in smoking cessation counseling.

Counseling. Individual or group counseling increases your chances of success, and the more counseling sessions you attend, the greater your likelihood of quitting will be. At these sessions, you will learn behavioral techniques, including coping skills, relapse prevention, and stress management. The sessions also will provide social support and encouragement.

Medication. Because nicotine is addictive, smoking cessation often leads to nicotine withdrawal, which can cause irritability, restlessness, food cravings, anxiety, and other symptoms. To help reduce these effects and control cravings for nicotine, your doctor may recommend or prescribe some form of nicotine replacement—either gum, skin patch, nasal spray, or inhaler. Using any of these products doubles the chances of quitting successfully. (There are no data, however, directly comparing the effectiveness of different nicotine replacement methods.) Nicotine replacement should be started on the day that you quit smoking; it appears to be safe for people who have hypertension or who have experienced a stroke.

Nicotine polacrilex gum (Nicorette) is available over the counter in doses of 2 and 4 mg. You may need between 10 and 24 pieces of gum a day to control your cravings, depending on the dose of the gum used and how much you smoked before quitting. The most effective approach may be to use the 4-mg dose for the first two weeks after cessation and then switch to the 2-mg dose. Over time, you should reduce the number of pieces you chew per day. The gum should be chewed only once or twice every few minutes and should remain between your cheek and gum the rest of the time. Side effects, including nausea and indigestion, usually are a result of chewing the gum too much and swallowing large amounts of nicotine. Ask your doctor if you need to use the gum for longer than 12 weeks.

A nicotine patch may be easier and more convenient for some people to use. Patches are available over the counter (Habitrol, Nicoderm CQ, and Nicotrol) or by prescription. Most versions come in 7-, 14-, and 21-mg doses; ask your doctor which dose you should try first. If you start at one of the higher doses, you need to taper to the lower doses after four to six weeks to wean yourself from the nicotine. The patch should be changed daily,

encouraging the formation of blood clots. It is not certain whether treatment of CHD will prevent strokes.

Alcohol abuse. Moderate alcohol consumption (two or fewer drinks per day) is associated with a reduced risk of CHD, and there appears to be a similar reduction in the risk of ischemic stroke. By contrast, even moderate alcohol use raises the risk of hemorrhagic stroke. Habitual alcohol consumption in excess of two drinks per day almost doubles the risk of stroke by producing cardiac arrhythmias,

and the recommended length of therapy is 8 to 12 weeks. If you experience minor skin irritation beneath the patch, change the area on your body where you place the patch each day. If the patch causes difficulty sleeping, try taking it off before going to bed. It is important not to smoke while on the patch. Smoking not only greatly reduces your chances of quitting but also can cause uncomfortably high levels of nicotine in your blood.

Nicotine nasal spray (Nicotrol NS) is available by prescription only. Your doctor can help you determine the exact timing and dose to use; initially, though, you should use it no more than 80 times per day. You and your doctor should work out a plan to gradually taper the number of times you use the spray each day. Side effects include nasal irritation, runny nose, throat irritation, and nausea.

Also available by prescription is a nicotine inhalation system (Nicotrol Inhaler). Patients typically use between 4 and 16 inhaler cartridges per day, with gradual tapering of the dose over a maximum of six months. Irritation of the mouth or throat is a potential adverse effect.

Bupropion (Zyban) is a prescription medication for quitting smoking that contains no nicotine but helps reduce cravings and withdrawal symptoms in some people. Researchers believe that the drug may disrupt the pleasurable feelings that cigarette smoking typically produces in the brain. (Bupropion is also sold as an antidepressant called Wellbutrin and can be a good choice for people who have a mood disorder that may make smoking cessation more difficult.) Patients begin to take bupropion a week or two before their quit date and continue to take it for up to 12 weeks afterward. People with a history of seizures, an eating disorder, or uncontrolled hypertension should not take bupropion. Side effects include trouble sleeping and dry mouth.

Combination therapy. A combination of treatments that includes counseling, nicotine replacement, and bupropion provides the highest chance of success. In one study, people who used all three therapies simultaneously had a 35% success rate.

Tips for Quitting

It is difficult for most people to stop smoking, and numerous attempts may be needed before you are successful. If you have tried to quit before without success, analyze what helped and what hindered you, and adjust your strategy accordingly. If you are concerned about weight gain after smoking cessation, remember that people usually gain fewer than 10 lbs. after they quit. Moreover, such weight gain has a much smaller impact on your health than smoking.

Here are a few general tips that may help you quit smoking. First, some people find they are more motivated if they pick a quit date that has a significant meaning—like New Year's Day or a birthday. Also, before you quit, ask for support from family, friends, and coworkers. If any of them smoke, ask them not to smoke around you.

Determine what events, situations, and other factors are cues to your smoking, and figure out ways to avoid them. For example, throw out lighters and ashtrays. If you always have a cigarette at a certain point during your drive home from work, try taking a different route. If you are used to having a cigarette with coffee after dinner, skip the coffee and do something else that distracts you. If you smoke in certain places in your house, or at certain times of the day, rearrange your furniture or your daily schedule.

Experts recommend that you avoid alcohol, or at least severely limit your intake, for the first three months after you quit. Alcohol reduces your chances of success by acting as a trigger for smoking and decreasing your inhibitions. Some people also find that deep breathing, drinking lots of liquids (preferably water, rather than soft drinks, coffee, or tea), and exercising helps them deal with cravings.

raising blood pressure, and adversely altering blood clot formation.

Oral contraceptives and estrogen. Old-fashioned, high-dose estrogen oral contraceptives increased the incidence of stroke in women who were over age 35 and smoked cigarettes, had high blood pressure, or had a history of migraine headaches. Current research still shows an association between low-dose oral contraceptives and the risk of stroke, but the risk is small.

A randomized, controlled trial called the Women's Health Initiative found that hormone replacement therapy, in which estrogen is combined with progestin, increases the risk of stroke in postmenopausal women (see the sidebar on page 37). The portion of the trial that examined this estrogen/progestin combination has been halted, but a separate part of the trial is still studying the effects of estrogen alone on the risk of stroke. Estrogen without progestin is suitable only for women who have had hysterectomies, since estrogen alone may increase the risk of uterine cancer.

Drug abuse. Stimulants such as cocaine and amphetamines can cause cardiac arrhythmias, heart attacks, and strokes (particularly intracerebral hemorrhage due to transiently high blood pressure), even in young and otherwise healthy first-time users. Also, intravenous drug use may result in cerebral embolism.

Coronary Heart Disease Risk Factors

Some risk factors affect the risk of stroke both directly and indirectly by increasing the risk of CHD:

High total and LDL ("bad") cholesterol, high triglycerides, and low HDL ("good") cholesterol. These factors contribute to atherosclerosis and CHD; though the findings have varied, evidence suggests that they are also important risks for stroke. A 21-year study of 8,586 Israeli men found that those with HDL cholesterol levels below 35 mg/dL had a 32% greater incidence of stroke than men with levels above 42.5 mg/dL. In addition, a study of about 1,500 New York City residents published in the *Journal of the American Medical Association* in 2001 found that people with HDL levels between 35 and 49 mg/dL had a 35% reduction in risk of ischemic stroke, compared with those with HDL levels below 35 mg/dL. Cholesterol reduction using statin drugs substantially reduces the risk of ischemic stroke, according to a study of 20,000 people published in *Circulation* in 2001.

Sedentary lifestyle. The few studies that have examined the effect of a sedentary lifestyle on stroke risk have consistently found that regular physical activity lowers the risk of ischemic and hemorrhagic stroke in both men and women, possibly by reducing other stroke risk factors, such as obesity and hypertension.

Obesity. Obesity increases the risk of fatal and nonfatal stroke by 50% to 100%. Although obesity is associated with other risk factors for stroke, such as hypertension and diabetes, obesity may be an independent risk factor for stroke. Abdominal obesity has an especially strong impact on diabetes and other risk factors for stroke.

PREVENTION OF STROKE

The best way to prevent a stroke is to reduce as many modifiable risk factors as possible. As noted previously, the keys to preventing hypertension—and thus stroke—are weight control, a healthy diet, a regular regimen of aerobic exercise, and, when necessary, drug therapy. Several more specific stroke prevention measures can be taken, too; these are especially important for those who have already had a stroke or a TIA or who are otherwise at high risk for having a stroke.

Antiplatelet Therapy

Drugs that reduce blood clot formation by inhibiting aggregation of blood platelets often are prescribed to prevent ischemic strokes in high-risk patients, particularly those with an asymptomatic carotid bruit, a history of TIAs, or a prior stroke.

Aspirin. Aspirin is by far the most extensively studied and widely used antiplatelet drug. A recent overview of more than 100 clinical trials concluded that aspirin therapy reduces the risk of future strokes by 25% to 30% in patients who have had TIAs or a minor stroke. (Aspirin is not advised for stroke prevention in otherwise healthy men and women over age 50 who have not had a stroke or TIA.) What is not as clear is the optimal dosage. In light of the lower incidence of side effects with smaller doses and the ease of taking a standard dose, an 81- to 325-mg tablet of aspirin a day currently is recommended by many stroke experts. People with high blood pressure should lower it before beginning aspirin therapy: A study published in 2000 found that the benefits of aspirin in people with high blood pressure are limited mainly to men whose hypertension is controlled.

Ticlopidine. Another antiplatelet drug, ticlopidine (Ticlid), is slightly more effective than aspirin in preventing stroke and is less likely to cause gastrointestinal bleeding (aspirin's primary side effect). However, ticlopidine is more costly, and 10% to 20% of patients taking it have minor reactions like diarrhea and skin rash. The most serious potential side effect is a blood disorder called thrombotic thrombocytopenic purpura, which is marked by fever, a significant decrease in the number of platelets in the blood, neurological changes, and kidney failure. Although very rare, thrombotic thrombocytopenic purpura is fatal in about 30% of cases. Ticlopidine also is associated with neutropenia (depletion of the body's infection-fighting white blood cells). Therefore, vigilant blood moni-

NEW RESEARCH

Heart Attack Substantially Increases Risk of Stroke

People who have a heart attack are at greater risk for stroke within the next six months than previously thought, according to a recent study.

Researchers studied the medical records of 111,023 Medicare beneficiaries (average age 76) who had experienced a heart attack during an eight-month period in 1994 and 1995. Over the next six months, 2,532 of the patients (2.5%) were admitted to the hospital with an ischemic stroke, suggesting a stroke rate of 5% per year. Previous estimates of stroke following a heart attack were approximately 1% per year.

Risk factors for stroke after a heart attack included being older than 75 years, black race, frailty, prior stroke, atrial fibrillation, diabetes, hypertension, and a history of peripheral vascular disease. Each of these conditions independently raised the stroke risk by 13% to 75%. Among the 20% of patients who had at least four of these eight risk factors, the risk of stroke was four times higher than among patients with none of the risk factors. Aspirin therapy at discharge was associated with a 14% lower risk of stroke.

Patients at high risk for stroke after a heart attack should receive preventive therapies, as well as education about stroke signs and symptoms to shorten any treatment delay should a stroke occur.

CIRCULATION
Volume 105, page 1082
March 5, 2002

Drugs Used To Prevent Ischemic Strokes in People at High Risk 2003

Drug Type	Generic Name	Brand Name	Average Daily Dosage*	Wholesale Cost (Generic Cost)†
Antiplatelets	aspirin	Aspir-Low	81 to 975 mg	81 mg: $3 (325 mg: $3)
		Aspirtab		325 mg: $1 ($3)
		Bayer		325 mg: $6 ($3)
		Easprin		975 mg: $59 (325 mg: $3)
		Ecotrin		325 mg: $6 ($3)
		Halfprin		81 mg: $4 (325 mg: $3)
		Norwich		325 mg: $2 ($3)
		St. Joseph		81 mg: $3 (325 mg: $3)
	buffered aspirin	Ascriptin	81 to 975 mg	325 mg: $7 ($2)
		Bufferin		325 mg: $5 ($2)
		Buffinol		325 mg: $2 ($2)
		Magnaprin		325 mg: $4 ($2)
	ticlopidine	Ticlid	500 mg	250 mg: $237 ($187)
	clopidogrel	Plavix	75 mg	75 mg: $380
	dipyridamole and aspirin	Aggrenox	400 mg dipyridamole/ 50 mg aspirin	200 mg/25 mg: $170

* These dosages represent an average range. The precise dosage varies from patient to patient and depends on many factors. Do not make any changes in your medication without consulting your doctor.

† Average wholesale prices to pharmacists for 100 tablets or capsules of the dosage listed. Costs to consumers are higher. If a generic is available, the price is listed in parentheses. Source: *Red Book,* 2002 (Medical Economics Data, publishers).

Advantages	Disadvantages
Aspirin is the most widely used and extensively studied of the antiplatelets. It reduces the risk of stroke in people at high risk for stroke, for example, those who have had a previous stroke or transient ischemic attack (TIA) and those who suffer from atrial fibrillation (a heart rhythm abnormality). Aspirin helps to prevent the formation of blood clots by inhibiting the aggregation of blood components called platelets.	Common side effects of aspirin include mild stomach pain, heartburn, indigestion, nausea, and vomiting. Serious side effects include peptic ulcers and gastrointestinal bleeding. Use of aspirin with other nonsteroidal anti-inflammatory drugs (NSAIDs) or with anticoagulant drugs such as warfarin increases the risk of these serious side effects. Contact your doctor if you experience bloody or black, tarry stools, severe stomach pain, or vomiting of blood or substances that resemble coffee grounds.
Ticlopidine reduces the risk of stroke in people who have had a previous stroke or TIA. Research shows that ticlopidine is somewhat more effective than aspirin for reducing stroke risk. Like aspirin, ticlopidine prevents platelets from aggregating.	Ticlopidine causes more side effects than aspirin, and it is generally reserved for people who cannot take aspirin or who experience strokes or TIAs while on aspirin therapy. Common side effects of ticlopidine include diarrhea, indigestion, nausea, skin rash, and mild abdominal pain. Rare but serious side effects include hepatitis and blood disorders such as thrombotic thrombocytopenic purpura (TTP) and neutropenia (a low white blood cell count). To reduce the risk of these serious side effects, blood tests are required every two weeks during the first three months of therapy. Contact your doctor immediately if you experience bruising or bleeding, particularly bleeding that is difficult to stop; fever, chills, or sore throat; sores, ulcers, or white spots in the mouth; dark or bloody urine, difficulty speaking, pale skin, pinpoint red spots on the skin, seizures, weakness, or yellow skin or eyes. Ticlopidine should be used with caution while taking other medications that reduce blood clotting. These medications include warfarin, aspirin, and other NSAIDs. Ticlopidine should not be taken by people with severe liver disease.
Clopidogrel reduces the risk of stroke in people who have had a previous stroke or heart attack or have other blood circulation problems that can lead to a stroke. Research shows that clopidogrel is somewhat more effective than aspirin for stroke prevention. Clopidogrel is preferred over ticlopidine in people who cannot take aspirin or who have strokes or TIAs while on aspirin therapy, since the risk of TTP is lower with clopidogrel. Clopidogrel prevents blood clot formation by inhibiting platelet aggregation.	Common side effects of clopidogrel include chest, abdominal, back, or joint pain, red or purple spots on the skin, upper respiratory infections, dizziness, and flu-like symptoms. Contact your doctor immediately if you experience bruising or bleeding, especially bleeding that is difficult to stop. Use of clopidogrel with aspirin or other NSAIDs can increase the risk of gastrointestinal bleeding. Clopidogrel should not be used by people with peptic ulcers.
The combination of dipyridamole and aspirin reduces the risk of stroke in people with a previous stroke or TIA. Research shows that combination therapy is more effective than aspirin alone for reducing stroke risk in people with a previous stroke; however, it is no more effective than aspirin in people who have experienced a TIA. Dipyridamole and aspirin reduces blood clot formation by inhibiting platelet aggregation.	Common side effects of dipyridamole and aspirin include abdominal pain, nausea, vomiting, diarrhea, headache, heartburn, indigestion, and muscle or joint pain. Gastrointestinal bleeding occurs more often with combination therapy than with aspirin alone. Serious bleeding can also occur when combination therapy is taken with anticoagulant drugs (such as warfarin or heparin) or with NSAIDs. Dipyridamole and aspirin should not be used by people with severe liver or kidney disease.

Drugs Used To Prevent Ischemic Strokes in People at High Risk 2003 (continued)

Drug Type	Generic Name	Brand Name	Average Daily Dosage*	Wholesale Cost (Generic Cost)†
Anticoagulant	warfarin	Coumadin	2 to 10 mg	4 mg: $71 ($63)

* These dosages represent an average range. The precise dosage varies from patient to patient and depends on many factors. Do not make any changes in your medication without consulting your doctor.

† Average wholesale prices to pharmacists for 100 tablets or capsules of the dosage listed. Costs to consumers are higher. If a generic is available, the price is listed in parentheses. Source: *Red Book,* 2002 (Medical Economics Data, publishers).

toring is necessary, especially in the first three months of treatment. Considering the risks and expense of ticlopidine, many experts recommend it mainly for patients who cannot tolerate aspirin or who continue to have TIAs or minor strokes despite aspirin therapy.

Clopidogrel. The antiplatelet drug clopidogrel (Plavix) is another option for the reduction of atherosclerotic complications. A three-year study of more than 19,000 patients who had suffered a recent stroke or heart attack or had peripheral vascular disease found that 75 mg per day of clopidogrel decreased the combined risk of future stroke, heart attack, or death from vascular disease by 34%, compared with a 25% risk reduction in patients taking 325 mg of aspirin a day. Side effects, including rash, diarrhea, and stomach discomfort, were about the same for both drugs. The risk of thrombotic thrombocytopenic purpura appears to be smaller than with ticlopidine.

Aspirin and dipyridamole. In 1999, the FDA approved a new drug for stroke prevention for people who have experienced a previous stroke or TIA. The drug (Aggrenox) contains aspirin and dipyridamole, two antiplatelet agents. In a one-year study of 6,602 patients who had suffered a stroke, a combination of aspirin and dipyridamole was twice as effective as either agent alone in preventing a second stroke, although overall mortality was unaffected. Bleeding was more common in patients taking the aspirin-dipyridamole combination than in those taking dipyridamole alone.

Advantages	Disadvantages
Warfarin reduces the risk of stroke in people with atrial fibrillation, especially those with other risk factors for stroke (for example, age 75 and over, high blood pressure, and previous TIA or stroke). In these individuals, warfarin is considerably more effective than aspirin. Warfarin also is used to prevent stroke in people with heart valve disorders and cardiomyopathy (deterioration of heart muscle). Warfarin prevents strokes by hindering the activity of substances that promote blood clot formation.	Warfarin is associated with a high risk of serious bleeding. To prevent this side effect, patients must undergo regular blood tests to ensure that they are receiving the correct dose. High doses of vitamin K (found in food or dietary supplements) can decrease the effects of warfarin. Thus, foods high in vitamin K (for example, liver, broccoli, cauliflower, and green leafy vegetables) should be eaten in moderation, and you should tell your doctor about any supplements you are taking. Many medications can increase or decrease the effects of warfarin, so be sure to tell you doctor about all the medications you are on. Contact your doctor immediately if you notice any unusual bleeding or bruising. Signs of unusual bleeding include bleeding from the gums, blood in the urine, nosebleeds, pinpoint red spots on the skin, and heavy bleeding from cuts or wounds.

Anticoagulants

Anticoagulant drugs also inhibit blood clot formation but work at a different stage in the clotting process than antiplatelets. They are the most effective agents for the prevention of embolic strokes, especially those occurring in association with atrial fibrillation (see page 40).

Patients who remain in chronic atrial fibrillation or are at high risk for recurrent episodes of atrial fibrillation are typically treated with a long-term, low-dose regimen of anticoagulant medication, usually warfarin (Coumadin). High-dose warfarin carries a greater risk of internal bleeding and intracerebral hemorrhage (see page 43) and is reserved for patients at high risk for embolism—for example, those with artificial heart valves or atrial fibrillation due to a heart valve disorder. Except for these high-risk patients, the increased chance of intracerebral hemorrhage outweighs the benefits of high-dose warfarin. However, many recent studies have indicated that *low*-dose warfarin can effectively reduce the risk of embolic stroke in people with chronic atrial fibrillation not associated with valve disease, with an acceptably low risk of intracerebral hemorrhage (though the risk of intracerebral hemorrhage still is elevated somewhat, especially in adults over age 70).

Patients taking warfarin must have regular blood tests to ensure that the dose is correct—high enough to reduce blood clotting, but not so high as to provoke bleeding. The test, called prothrombin time, measures how long it takes for blood to clot. Since prothrombin time varies according to where the test is performed and what method is used, laboratories have started to calculate a measurement called the international normalized ratio, which takes these factors into account and produces a standardized result. For most patients with atrial fibrillation, an international normalized ratio of 2 to 3 is generally recommended. In addition, tests measuring prothrombin time are now available by prescription for home use. The FDA has approved two such devices—The CoaguChek and the ProTime Microcoagulation System—which use blood obtained by a fingerstick in a manner similar to the way people with diabetes measure their blood glucose levels. Home testing allows more frequent and careful monitoring of anticoagulant therapy. However, use of these tests is not yet widespread and requires careful and detailed instruction.

Anticoagulants also are recommended to prevent stroke in patients with certain other heart problems, including cardiomyopathy (deterioration of heart muscle), evidence of heart muscle damage from a prior heart attack, presence of an artificial heart valve, other heart valve disorders, and patent foramen ovale (a hole between the left and right sides of the heart). Patients with lone atrial fibrillation—that is, atrial fibrillation with no other forms of heart disease—who are under age 60 and have no other risk factors for stroke (for example, hypertension) may benefit just as much from aspirin as from warfarin therapy. Other health problems that warrant the use of anticoagulants are intracranial arterial stenosis (clogged arteries in the brain) and hypercoagulable states (in which there is an increased propensity to form blood clots).

Patients must be aware that high doses of vitamin K from either foods or supplements can counteract anticoagulants, which work by preventing vitamin K from activating the blood factors required for clot formation. Foods high in vitamin K—such as liver, broccoli, cauliflower, kale, spinach, cabbage, and other green leafy vegetables—should be eaten in moderation. Some multivitamin supplements may contain vitamin K.

In addition, a recent study found that taking warfarin along with more than four 325-mg tablets of the pain reliever acetaminophen (Tylenol) per day for longer than a week may dangerously reduce the ability of the blood to clot and raise the risk of hemorrhagic stroke. People taking six or fewer acetaminophen tablets a week were not at elevated risk.

Carotid Endarterectomy

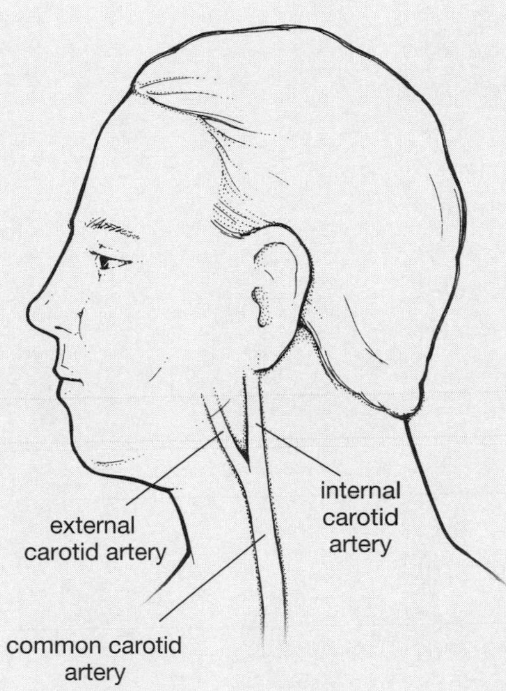

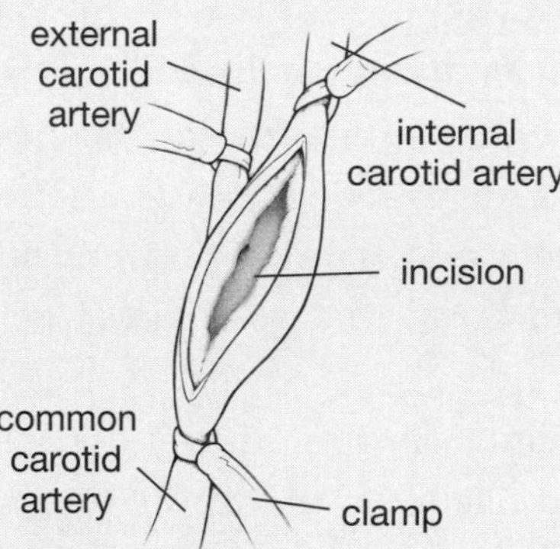

Clamps are placed on the carotid arteries to stop blood flow, and an incision is made in the area of blockage.

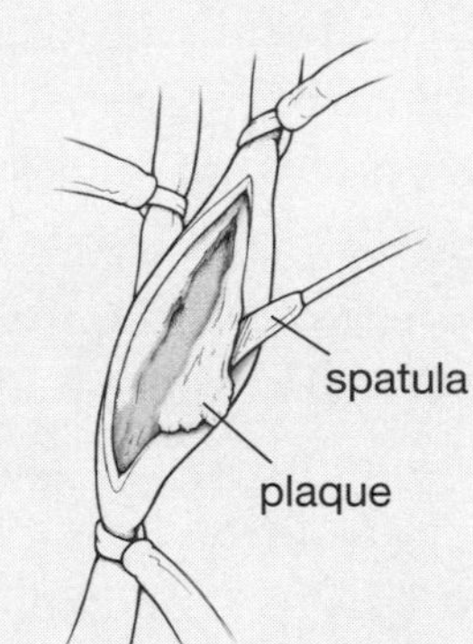

Plaque is separated from the artery using a spatula.

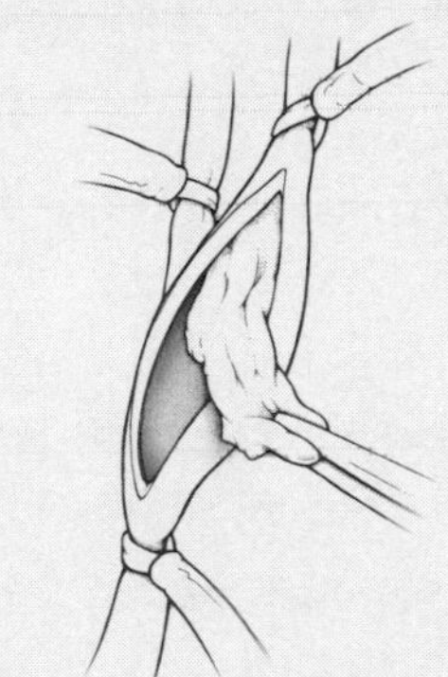

Plaque is removed with a tweezer-like instrument.

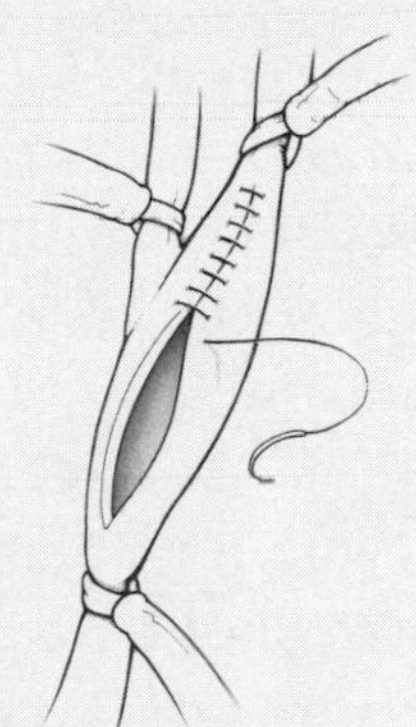

Incision is closed with stitches.

The carotid arteries are two of the major blood vessels that carry blood to the brain. If they become narrowed by atherosclerotic plaque, the risk of having a stroke increases substantially. Some patients with partially narrowed carotid arteries may be candidates for a surgical procedure called carotid endarterectomy as a way to prevent a stroke. In this procedure, doctors improve blood flow to the brain and reduce the chance of blood clot formation by removing the plaque from a carotid artery.

Carotid endarterectomy is performed using either local or general anesthesia, depending on the surgeon's preference and the patient's health status. After the anesthetic has taken effect, the surgeon makes a 4-inch-long vertical incision on one side of the neck to gain access to the carotid artery. Next, clamps are placed on the common carotid artery and the two arteries that lead from it to the brain (the external carotid artery and the internal carotid artery) to stop blood flow through the part of the artery that is being operated on.

Care must be taken to ensure that blood still reaches the brain through other arteries. If local anesthesia is used, the patient may be asked to follow basic instructions (like moving an arm or leg) so the surgical team can observe any potential problems such as altered consciousness, motor problems, or weakness that may signal a significant decrease in blood flow to the brain. For local and general anesthesia, the surgical team will observe blood flow to the brain by measuring blood pressure in the other carotid artery and electrical activity in the brain (using an electroencephalogram).

The surgical team can insert a small tube called a shunt to allow blood to bypass the clamped area of the common carotid artery. Some surgeons routinely use a shunt, while others use it only if the patient exhibits signs of decreased blood flow to the brain.

Next, the surgeon cuts open the carotid artery and separates the plaque from the artery using a device called an endarterectomy spatula. This technique allows the plaque to be removed in one piece with a tweezer-like instrument. Then the surgical team flushes the artery with a saline solution containing a combination of anticoagulant drugs to help prevent the formation of blood clots.

Once the plaque is removed, the incision is closed with either sutures (stitches) or a small patch graft, which widens the artery to allow blood to flow through it more easily.

Carotid Endarterectomy

When diagnostic imaging tests (see pages 66–69) reveal that one or both carotid arteries in the neck are substantially narrowed by atherosclerotic plaque, carotid endarterectomy can be performed to clear the arteries surgically. The procedure lasts about two hours and generally requires two to three days of hospitalization for recovery. (For more information about this procedure, see the feature on page 61.)

Carotid endarterectomy significantly reduces the risk of stroke and TIA in some patients and has been used over the past two decades. However, it is not appropriate for everyone with carotid stenosis. Long-term results are best for patients who have had a prior mild stroke or symptoms of a TIA and whose carotid arteries are severely blocked—70% or more—though completely blocked arteries cannot be reopened. Carotid endarterectomy is not recommended for patients with mild blockage (less than 30%).

For patients with moderate stenosis (between 30% and 69%) and minor stroke or TIA, carotid endarterectomy may be beneficial, but the degree of benefit is less than with higher grades of stenosis. A trial called NASCET (North American Symptomatic Carotid Endarterectomy Trial) found that patients who had carotid endarterectomy for 50% to 69% carotid stenosis had a five-year stroke rate of 16%, compared with a rate of 22% in patients treated with medical therapy alone. Men appeared to benefit more than women, and overall benefits were less in patients at high risk for complications related to the procedure itself. Decisions about carotid endarterectomy for patients with moderate carotid stenosis should be made on a case-by-case basis.

The most recent research has suggested that carotid endarterectomy also may benefit patients with no symptoms or history of stroke (that is, those with an asymptomatic carotid bruit) when blockage of the carotid artery exceeds 60%. In such cases, the risk of a first-time stroke appears to be lowered significantly in men but only minimally in women. (The reason for this difference between the sexes is probably because of higher surgical complication rates in women owing to their smaller arteries.) This reduction in risk, however, is more often for TIAs and minor strokes than for fatal or disabling strokes.

A recent review of 25 studies showed that the overall risk of death and/or stroke due to the surgery itself was significantly lower for asymptomatic patients than for those with symptoms—3.4% vs. 5.2%. Asymptomatic patients may fare better because the same factors that prevent them from having symptoms (for example, resistance to blood clots) make them less likely to have complications from carotid endarterectomy. Because the procedure only decreases the overall incidence of stroke in asymptomatic men from 10% to 5%, however, questions remain about its relative benefits and risks in such patients. These questions may be more difficult to answer for women since a recent study found that women with no history of TIA or stroke had a 5.3% risk of stroke or death during postoperative hospitalization following carotid endarterectomy, while men with the same history had only a 1.6% risk.

Medical conditions that may limit the use of carotid endarterectomy include CHD, uncontrolled diabetes or hypertension, advanced cancer, and serious deficits from a prior stroke. Advanced age, however, does *not* rule out a patient as a candidate for surgery: Studies have documented favorable results in patients in their 70s and 80s.

Carotid endarterectomy nonetheless is associated with significant risks. The rate of serious complications (such as tearing the artery or triggering a stroke or heart attack) varies with the medical center and the skill of the surgeon but ranges between 3% and 15%. By comparison, about 2% of patients have a stroke and 5% to 10% have a heart attack after bypass surgery. Experts recommend that carotid endarterectomy be done by an experienced surgeon at a medical center known to have a complication rate of no more than 3% to 4%. One study suggests that hospitals that frequently perform carotid endarterectomy (more than 21 procedures per year) have lower rates of complications. Getting a second opinion is strongly encouraged before undergoing carotid endarterectomy, especially for asymptomatic patients. Patients should be sure to discuss all these issues with their doctor.

Angioplasty and Stents

Angioplasty involves inflating a small balloon in a blocked artery to enlarge the path for blood flow. The procedure, which was first used in patients with CHD, has also been adopted to reopen partially blocked carotid arteries. Sometimes angioplasty also involves implanting a stent—a flexible metal tube placed inside a clogged artery to keep it propped open. Clinical trials are now under way to compare the results of carotid endarterectomy with those of carotid angioplasty with stenting.

During stent implantation, a radiologist threads a catheter from an artery in the groin into the narrowed portion of the carotid

NEW RESEARCH

Retinopathy and Brain Lesions Increase Risk of Stroke

Changes in cerebral white matter (brain tissue that transmits nerve impulses) are present in 27% to 87% of people age 65 and over. Now a study suggests that people with these changes (known as white matter lesions) are at an increased risk for stroke, especially if they also have retinopathy (damage to the blood vessels in the retina).

Researchers screened 1,684 people (age 51 to 72) for white matter lesions and retinopathy using cerebral magnetic resonance imaging and retinal photography, respectively. White matter lesions were more common in participants with retinopathy than in those without (23% vs. 10%).

An average of five years later, after adjusting for stroke risk factors such as high blood pressure, diabetes, and smoking, strokes were more than three times as common in people with white matter lesions as in people without these lesions. Strokes were 18 times more common in people with both retinopathy and white matter lesions than in those without either condition.

How white matter lesions and retinopathy increase stroke risk is unclear, but all three conditions may be caused by diseased blood vessels. The researchers do not recommend that people with white matter lesions be screened for retinopathy to determine stroke risk.

JOURNAL OF THE AMERICAN MEDICAL ASSOCIATION
Volume 288, page 67
July 3, 2002

artery. (The stent is initially collapsed around a deflated balloon at the tip of the catheter.) After inflating the balloon to widen the artery, the radiologist expands the stent until it locks in position. Acting as a permanent brace inside the artery, the stent helps to maintain blood flow to the brain, possibly reducing the risk of ischemic stroke.

Thus far, stent implantation has had mixed results, and some experts have raised concerns about the procedure. Of major concern are blood clots, which may be released from the carotid artery during the procedure or form on the implanted stent. Such clots may travel to an artery in the brain and cause an embolic stroke. Questions also remain about the long-term reliability and structural integrity of stents—particularly in the carotid arteries, since there is more movement in the neck than around the heart.

For now, stents may be a good option for high-risk patients with unstable heart conditions who are unable to withstand carotid endarterectomy, which is a more extensive surgical procedure. Stents also may be useful in patients who have had a prior carotid endarterectomy, neck surgery, or irradiation, which increase the risks of carotid endarterectomy. Currently under investigation is the use of mildly radioactive stents (to reduce reclosure of the blood vessel, called restenosis), as well as stents coated with anticoagulant materials or drugs. These innovations may reduce the risk of embolic stroke and eventually allow more widespread use of the technique.

DIAGNOSIS OF STROKE

When a patient arrives at an emergency room with symptoms of a stroke, time is of the essence: *Fast action can minimize neurological damage and even mean the difference between life and death.* The attending doctor must rule out other potential causes of the symptoms (such as seizure, brain tumor, diabetic coma, low blood sugar, or migraine headache) and determine the type of stroke (ischemic or hemorrhagic). It is also important to identify what caused the stroke and which part or parts of the brain are affected.

Patient History

The diagnosis of stroke is evident when there is a clear history of loss of a specific brain function or functions and when symptoms come on suddenly or become apparent on awakening, especially in a person over age 50 with vascular disease or other risk factors. Although symptoms may progress over the following few minutes to hours, the condition usually stabilizes within 12 to 24 hours.

If the apparent stroke victim is conscious and able to speak, or if a close friend or family member is present, the doctor can learn much from the answers to a few questions about the patient's medical background, including any history of TIAs, stroke, or recent head injury; when the symptoms started; how long they have lasted; and whether or not they point to a particular type of stroke. For example, language problems, incoordination, and confusion suggest ischemic stroke, while sudden, excruciating headache, vomiting, and loss of consciousness indicate hemorrhagic stroke. The patient's age, sex, race, and history of other medical conditions (such as diabetes, cardiovascular disorders, hypertension, hemophilia, or allergies) also are crucial, and the doctor must know if the patient is taking any prescription medications or illicit drugs.

Physical Examination

Along with the medical history, the doctor will conduct a general physical exam to check breathing, pulse, blood pressure, and body temperature. The doctor can listen for heart rhythm disturbances (such as atrial fibrillation) and for bruits in the carotid arteries. Close examination of the blood vessels in the eyes also is important, since it can reveal evidence of brain hemorrhage, hypertension, emboli, and other conditions related to stroke.

In addition, a bedside neurological examination is done to determine how the brain has been affected. The doctor will take a quick inventory of the patient's emotional status, memory, motor strength and skills, balance, gait, responsiveness to tactile stimuli, reflexes, vision, eye movements, and speech and language abilities. Deficits in any of these basic neurological functions determine which areas of the brain have been damaged.

Laboratory Tests

Blood tests and urine analysis can help to identify conditions—such as low blood sugar, diabetes, high red blood cell count, an infected heart valve, or syphilis—that can mimic or cause a stroke. Other blood tests that might point to a specific cause of a stroke include measurement of blood clotting, the number of platelets, and erythrocyte sedimentation rate. High cholesterol levels suggest a possible thrombotic stroke due to atherosclerosis, and an electrocardiogram (ECG or EKG) can detect a heart attack or an abnormal heart rhythm—a potential cause of an embolic stroke.

NEW RESEARCH

Subarachnoid Hemorrhage Is Partly Preventable

While genetics appears to play a role in subarachnoid hemorrhage (a type of hemorrhagic stroke), modifiable factors account for much of the risk, a new study shows.

Researchers compared the medical records of 107 patients with subarachnoid hemorrhage (not caused by trauma or tumor) with 197 control subjects matched by age, gender, and race. Information about the participants' medical history, risk factors, and family history of stroke was also obtained.

The risk of subarachnoid hemorrhage was increased 11-fold by heavy alcohol use, 4-fold by a history of hypertension, 4-fold by current smoking, and 3-fold by a family history of subarachnoid hemorrhage or brain aneurysm.

"Cigarette smoking, hypertension, and frequent alcohol use are risk factors that, if modified, could lead to reduced incidence of [subarachnoid hemorrhage]," the authors write. However, almost all heavy drinkers were also smokers, so the researchers are uncertain whether alcohol itself contributed to the increased risk.

STROKE
Volume 33, page 1321
May 2002

Brain and Blood Vessel Imaging Techniques

The most definitive ways to diagnose the type of stroke are to locate a blockage in a carotid or intracranial artery, identify the site where damage has occurred in the brain, or detect an abnormal pool of blood within brain tissue or the subarachnoid space.

Computed tomography (CT or CAT) scans. In this test, the patient lies flat on a special table while x-rays are passed through the body and sensed by a detector that rotates 360° around the patient. A computer combines all the information into a cross-sectional picture. CT scans are 10 to 20 times more sensitive than x-rays.

CT scans are best used to determine rapidly whether an intracerebral or subarachnoid hemorrhage has occurred, as well as to reveal its location and extent. Sometimes the scans can detect the presence of aneurysms or arteriovenous malformations. However, damage inflicted by even a large ischemic stroke may not show up on a CT scan until hours or days later, and evidence of small strokes (especially those deep in the brain) may not be visible at all.

Magnetic resonance imaging (MRI). This technique, which takes longer than a CT scan, requires the patient to lie still for 30 minutes or more. Magnetic fields and radio waves are used to generate a three-dimensional image of the brain. While more expensive than CT scanning and not always practical due to the time required, an MRI scan provides clearer pictures and can detect smaller injuries in all parts of the brain.

Ischemic strokes may show up on MRI scans as early as 6 to 12 hours after onset. And new developments in MRI technology may allow even earlier detection and perhaps the possibility of predicting the size, severity, and reversibility of neurological deficits. Diffusion-weighted MRI can show changes of ischemic stroke within one to two hours based on alterations in water movement in the brain. In perfusion-weighted MRI, an injection of the dye gadolinium can show changes that indicate the degree of blood flow to areas in the brain. Combining diffusion and perfusion imaging may hold the key to determining which patients might benefit from aggressive (for example, thrombolytic) therapy.

According to the most recent guidelines from the American Heart Association, imaging the brain with MRI is not justified for the routine evaluation of acute stroke and TIAs. The guidelines also state that MRI scans are not necessary to initiate emergency treatment. However, the American Heart Association recognizes the existence of special circumstances, and decisions should be made on an individual basis.

Are You a Healthy Caregiver?

About 80% of caregiving is done in the home, most often by a spouse, child, parent, or grandchild. Providing at-home care for someone who has had a debilitating stroke is inevitably a demanding role. It places great burdens on the caregiver's time, physical energy, emotional well-being, and personal finances.

The stress of caregiving can manifest itself in numerous ways. Caregivers may become depressed, begin to abuse alcohol or drugs, or neglect their own physical and mental health. As a result, caregivers have higher rates of illness and death. Distressed caregivers are also more likely to abuse or neglect the patient and to place the person in an institution prematurely. Because of these risks, it is important for caregivers to monitor their own physical and mental well-being and to seek help when they need it.

To help caregivers evaluate their level of distress, the American Medical Association has created the Caregiver Self-Assessment Questionnaire, reprinted below. It consists of 16 "Yes" or "No" questions and two questions rated on a scale of 1 to 10. Once you have completed the questionnaire, calculate your score according to the instructions. Follow the recommended next steps if the score indicates you are experiencing a high level of distress.

Caregiver Self-Assessment Questionnaire

During the past week or so, I have ...

1. Had trouble keeping my mind on what I was doing ❑ Yes ❑ No
2. Felt that I could not leave my relative alone ❑ Yes ❑ No
3. Had difficulty making decisions ❑ Yes ❑ No
4. Felt completely overwhelmed ❑ Yes ❑ No
5. Felt useful and needed ❑ Yes ❑ No
6. Felt lonely ❑ Yes ❑ No
7. Been upset that my relative has changed so much from his/her former self ❑ Yes ❑ No
8. Felt a loss of privacy and/or personal time ❑ Yes ❑ No
9. Been edgy or irritable ❑ Yes ❑ No
10. Had sleep disturbed because of caring for my relative ❑ Yes ❑ No
11. Had a crying spell(s) ❑ Yes ❑ No
12. Felt strained between work and family responsibilities ❑ Yes ❑ No
13. Had back pain ❑ Yes ❑ No
14. Felt ill (headaches, stomach problems, or common cold) ❑ Yes ❑ No
15. Been satisfied with the support my family has given me ❑ Yes ❑ No
16. Found my relative's living situation to be inconvenient or a barrier to care ❑ Yes ❑ No
17. On a scale of 1 to 10, with 1 being "not stressful" and 10 being "extremely stressful," please rate your current level of stress. ______
18. On a scale of 1 to 10, with 1 being "very healthy" and 10 being "very ill," please rate your current health compared with what it was this time last year. ______

To Determine the Score

1. Reverse score questions 5 and 15. (That is, count a "No" response as a "Yes," and a "Yes" response as a "No.")
2. Total the number of "Yes" responses.

To Interpret the Score

Chances are that you are experiencing a high degree of distress if one or more of the following is true:

- You answered "Yes" to either or both questions 4 and 11.
- Your total "Yes" score is 10 or more.
- Your score on question 17 is 6 or higher.
- Your score on question 18 is 6 or higher.

Next Steps

- Consider seeing a doctor for a check-up for yourself.
- Consider having some relief from caregiving. (Discuss with your doctor or a social worker the resources available in your community.)
- Consider joining a support group.

Valuable Resources for Caregivers

Eldercare Locator
(a national directory of community services)
☎ 800-677-1116
www.eldercare.gov

Family Caregiver Alliance
☎ 415-434-3388
www.caregiver.org

Medicaid Hotline
☎ 800-633-4227

National Alliance for Caregiving
☎ 301-718-8444
www.caregiving.org

National Family Caregivers Association
☎ 800-896-3650
www.nfcacares.org

Ultrasound scanning. Ultrasound scanning uses high-frequency sound waves to create computer-generated images of internal body structures. Because such tests are noninvasive, they pose no risk to the patient. Ultrasound is especially useful for determining the site of ischemic strokes, since it allows the doctor to visualize blockages and monitor blood flow through specific arteries.

Each of the several ultrasound techniques has its own advantage. Doppler ultrasound generally is used to measure how fast blood moves through the carotid arteries; faster flow indicates a site where atherosclerotic plaque has narrowed the blood vessel. (Color Doppler Flow Imaging is an enhancement of this technique that allows various colors to demonstrate the speed of blood flow.) B-mode imaging is another form of ultrasound. It affords a three-dimensional view of the carotid arteries and can be combined with pulsed Doppler ultrasound—a technique known as duplex scanning. This method provides the most accurate noninvasive images of the carotid arteries. Transcranial Doppler scanning may allow an assessment of circulation through the arteries within the skull.

Cerebral angiography. This procedure involves the injection of an iodine-based contrast solution into the bloodstream to produce a high-quality x-ray image of the blood vessels within the brain. Angiography provides more detailed information about blood vessels than any of the other diagnostic imaging techniques, but because of the risk of complications, it is used only when noninvasive tests prove inadequate. Possible complications include a dangerous allergic reaction to the iodine in the contrast solution, reversible neurological deficits, and stroke that causes permanent deficits. These risks occur in less than 1% of patients younger than 50 years old but rise with age and the presence of hypertension or vascular disease.

Magnetic resonance angiography (MRA). MRA can image the arteries in both the neck and the brain by manipulating the MRI scanner; the procedure adds about 15 minutes to a conventional MRI scan. MRA has not been perfected but is used increasingly as a screening test for blockage of large vessels. A normal MRA may prevent a patient from undergoing angiography. Improved images of blood vessels can be obtained by injecting a dye (gadolinium) into the veins during the MRA. The side effects of the dye are minimal, and this new technique, gadolinium-enhanced MRA, produces images that are nearly comparable to conventional angiography. Other types of dyes besides gadolinium are currently being tested.

Spiral CT scanning. Spiral CT scanning is a new method to look at blood vessels; an iodine-based dye is injected into the patient and a rapid CT scan is performed through the region of interest. Computer-based imaging software then isolates the blood vessels that fill with dye. The resulting image resembles an angiogram and can be rotated and manipulated in three dimensions to look for aneurysms or vascular narrowings. This technique cannot be used in patients allergic to iodine-containing dye or those who have compromised kidney function.

ACUTE TREATMENT OF STROKE

Immediate emergency care for a stroke requires hospitalization, where life support systems are available, if needed, to maintain breathing and heart function. Specific avenues of treatment ultimately depend on whether the stroke is ischemic or hemorrhagic. In ischemic stroke, the primary goal is to restore or at least improve blood flow to the brain; the goal in hemorrhagic stroke is to relieve pressure on the brain and arrest the bleeding.

Treatment of Ischemic Stroke

Careful monitoring and control of blood pressure are essential after a stroke. Following ischemic stroke, elevated pressure is generally acceptable, since it promotes the flow of blood through the partially blocked arteries to reach jeopardized regions of the brain. The exception is when blood pressure is so high that it is likely to damage the brain, heart, or kidneys. In such cases, it should be lowered slowly. Otherwise, efforts are aimed at preventing low blood pressure (hypotension), which can limit the amount of blood reaching the brain. If low blood pressure does occur—whether due to antihypertensive drugs, dehydration, or other causes—it can be treated with intravenous saline solutions for rehydration and blood pressure-raising drugs if needed.

Intravenous fluids containing glucose are usually avoided since excessive glucose in the brain may be detrimental in acute stroke (there is some controversy over this idea, however). Buildup of fluid in the brain (cerebral edema) also can cause damage. Cerebral edema can be treated by limiting fluid intake and raising the head of the patient's bed to a 30° angle.

Body temperature also must be carefully monitored and controlled, since fever can compound damage to the brain. A study of stroke victims found that every 2.7° F increase in body temperature more than doubled a patient's risk of a poor outcome (death or a more severe stroke). Hypothermic therapy to lower body tempera-

NEW RESEARCH

Prior Microbleeds Predict Bleeding After Ischemic Stroke

Up to 40% of people experience cerebral bleeding (bleeding into the area of the brain damaged by a stroke) within a week of an ischemic stroke. Now a study shows that people with evidence of old microbleeds (tiny spots of bleeding prior to a stroke) are at higher risk for cerebral bleeding.

French researchers looked for old microbleeds and new cerebral bleeding using magnetic resonance imaging scans and computed tomography, respectively, in 100 patients (average age 60) who had had an ischemic stroke in the previous 24 hours.

Twenty patients had evidence of old microbleeds, and 26 patients had new cerebral bleeding within a week of the stroke. Patients with old microbleeds had a sevenfold greater risk of cerebral bleeding after the stroke. Other risk factors for cerebral bleeding include diabetes, high blood pressure, thrombolytic therapy, and a severe stroke. The type of stroke therapy the patient received had no effect on cerebral bleeding, possibly due to the small number of patients in each group.

Old microbleeds are evidence of weakened blood vessels (which are more likely to bleed) or amyloid angiopathy (protein deposits in the brain's arteries). But larger studies are needed to confirm the relationship between old microbleeds and cerebral bleeding after a stroke.

STROKE
Volume 33, page 735
March 2002

ture after a stroke is being examined as a treatment option. A small study from Denmark found that stroke patients who were treated with a special cooling blanket had a 12% death rate after six months, compared with a 23% rate of death in patients who did not have their body temperature reduced.

Drug therapy. Until recently, doctors could do little to intervene while an ischemic stroke was in progress. However, with the FDA approval of the first emergency stroke drug, alteplase (Activase), doctors now have a specific course of action to follow for an ischemic stroke. Alteplase, which is also called tissue-type plasminogen activator (t-PA), is a member of a drug class known as thrombolytic ("clot-busting") agents. These agents have been used widely to treat heart attacks. Prompt administration of alteplase can dissolve a clot that is blocking blood flow to the heart muscle, thereby preventing extensive tissue damage. Some (but not all) studies have shown similar results for strokes, even though thrombolytic drugs are associated with an increased risk of cerebral hemorrhage (a side effect in about 6% of patients).

Early treatment is essential. According to American Heart Association guidelines, alteplase should be used only when treatment starts within *three hours* of the onset of an ischemic stroke. If too much time has elapsed, cerebral bleeding may be more likely, and it may be too late to prevent brain damage. Beforehand, all patients must have a neurological examination and a CT scan evaluated by an expert to ensure they are appropriate candidates. Only hospitals equipped for immediate treatment of excessive bleeding should administer t-PA. And t-PA cannot be used in certain individuals, including those who have a hemorrhagic stroke, had another stroke within the previous three months, have blood pressure greater than 185/110 mm Hg, or are currently taking the anticoagulant drugs heparin or warfarin (aspirin users are eligible if they fit all other criteria).

For embolic strokes, the anticoagulant drug heparin often is administered intravenously for several days to prevent new clots from forming and to keep existing clots from getting any larger. Heparin is also the usual immediate medical therapy for strokes due to severe atherosclerotic stenosis in the carotid, vertebral, or basilar arteries (which branch off from the vertebral arteries), although its effectiveness in these situations is not clearly established. Like all anticoagulants, heparin should not be given to patients at risk for hemorrhage, such as those with uncontrolled hypertension, gastrointestinal bleeding, or thrombocytopenia (a low number of blood platelets). The anticoagulant warfarin often is started at the same time as heparin to treat embolic stroke (and, unlike heparin, can be prescribed in pill form for long-term use), but it too should not be given to patients at high risk for hemorrhage.

Long-term use of warfarin needs careful evaluation. Although the short-term risks from this drug are small, the chance of complications accumulates over a number of years. Doctors also must consider whether patients—particularly older adults, for whom risk is higher—are likely to fall, since hitting the head could lead to serious injury.

If anticoagulants are not indicated, aspirin is the most effective therapy to reduce future risk of stroke. Patients who have not been successful with aspirin therapy or cannot tolerate it can be treated with other antiplatelet agents, such as dipyridamole and aspirin (Aggrenox), ticlopidine (Ticlid), or clopidogrel (Plavix; see pages 55–58).

Another option is the administration of a thrombolytic drug directly into an occluded artery. A study of 180 patients looked at intra-arterial administration of a thrombolytic drug called prourokinase within six hours of the onset of an acute ischemic stroke. Patients received either prourokinase plus heparin or heparin alone. After three months, 40% of the people treated with prourokinase and 25% of those in the heparin-only group were functionally independent. Prourokinase did not decrease the mortality rate, however, and people who received the drug had a higher rate of intracerebral hemorrhage.

Patients with an embolic stroke due to atrial fibrillation may be treated with antiarrhythmic medications such as amiodarone (Cordarone) and procainamide (Procan, Pronestyl, and other brands). Also, digoxin (Lanoxin), calcium channel blockers, or beta-blockers may be given to keep the heart's ventricles (lower chambers) from responding to the rapid signals from the atria. A rapid ventricular rate can lead to poor cardiac output, low blood pressure, poor blood flow through narrowed arteries in the brain, and heart failure.

There is continuing interest in an experimental group of drugs known as cytoprotective (cell-preserving) agents, some of which are designed to prevent or halt the glutamate cascade—the chain of chemical reactions that occurs with ischemic strokes (see page 38). Studies of stroke patients are currently under way throughout the United States to evaluate various cytoprotective drugs, although it likely will take years before such agents—if proven beneficial—become a standard part of stroke treatment.

Surgery. Surgery is rarely part of the immediate treatment of is-

NEW RESEARCH

Benefits of Alteplase After Stroke Are Long-Lasting

Some people given alteplase (Activase) within three hours of the onset of an ischemic stroke experience a dramatic recovery immediately after treatment. Now a study suggests that the benefits of early dramatic recovery persist 90 days later.

Researchers studied 53 patients who received alteplase within three hours of an ischemic stroke. Twelve patients (22%) experienced dramatic recovery at the end of the one-hour treatment with alteplase. This improvement persisted after 24 hours and 90 days. After 90 days, patients who had experienced a dramatic recovery were more likely to be relatively independent than those who had not experienced a dramatic recovery.

The authors conclude that dramatic recovery is a "relatively frequent occurrence" in people with ischemic strokes who are given alteplase. They write that their results emphasize the importance of early treatment.

Alteplase is also called tissue-type plasminogen activator (t-PA).

STROKE
Volume 33, page 1301
May 2002

Treating Spasticity After a Stroke

A common result of a stroke is spasticity—a persistent contraction in the muscles of the fingers, arms, or legs, which leads to tightness, rigidity, or stiffness in these areas. The condition causes pain and muscle spasms and can interfere with a patient's ability to perform basic everyday tasks like dressing, eating, and grooming. Some individuals may also experience weakness, fatigue, and a loss of dexterity.

Spasticity is caused by damage to the part of the brain that controls movement. It may improve during recovery from the stroke, but about half of patients need to undergo treatment to relieve the muscle stiffness and pain. In some cases, spasticity may serve a useful purpose. For example, a person with overall weakness or poor muscle control may benefit from leg rigidity by using the stiff leg as a brace when being moved from a bed to a wheelchair.

While no one treatment effectively addresses all aspects of spasticity, patients usually experience adequate relief through a combination of the following therapies: physical therapy, medication, and surgery.

Education and Physical Therapy

The first step in tackling spasticity is to educate the patient and the caregiver about its causes as well as the measures that can be taken to minimize its symptoms. For example, sitting improperly or lying on one's back may worsen the symptoms associated with spasticity, while correct positioning can bring some relief. Such treatment is often provided by a physical therapist.

A physical therapist also may instruct a patient in stretching and strengthening exercises to improve flexibility and reduce weakness in the limb. Casts, splints, or orthoses may be used to move the limb from its rigid position to a more normal one. In addition, physical therapists may apply cold, heat, local anesthetics, or electrical stimulation to the affected area to provide short-term relief of spasticity.

Oral Medications

The most commonly used oral medication for spasticity is the muscle relaxant baclofen (Lioresal). Taken in dosages of 40 to 100 mg daily, it helps increase range of motion while decreasing pain, tightness, and spasms. Possible side effects include drowsiness, fatigue, weakness in healthy muscle, dizziness, and confusion.

Tizanidine (Zanaflex) is one of the newer drug treatments for spasticity. Studies show that it is as effective as baclofen and is less likely to cause muscle weakness as a side effect. Potential adverse effects of tizanidine include drowsiness, dizziness, dry mouth, anxiety, constipation or diarrhea, fatigue, and depression. Tizanidine may also adversely affect liver function in a small number of patients.

Diazepam (Valium and other brands) is the oldest medication prescribed for spasticity. Taken in doses of 2 to 10 mg, two to four times per day, diazepam can increase range of motion, decrease painful spasms, and reduce other symptoms of spasticity. Its side effects include dependency, sleepiness, weakness, and confusion.

Another medication is dantrolene (Dantrium), an antispasmodic drug that helps reduce pain and tightness and improves movement by weakening spastic muscles without affecting healthy muscles. Doctors prescribe the drug in dosages of up to 400 mg per day. Common side effects in-

chemic stroke, although carotid endarterectomy (see pages 62–63) sometimes is performed to treat minor strokes and prevent additional ones in patients with severe carotid stenosis. However, in the aftermath of a large ischemic stroke, the brain should be allowed to recover before the procedure is attempted. In such cases, surgery may be postponed for as long as six weeks after the stroke. Angioplasty with or without the use of stents (see pages 63–64) is being used increasingly, especially in patients for whom standard carotid endarterectomy presents too great a risk.

Treatment of Hemorrhagic Stroke

Because hemorrhagic strokes often occur in association with excessive hypertension, doctors first attempt to lower blood pressure to

clude drowsiness, nausea, vomiting, dizziness, and diarrhea. Liver dysfunction is a potentially serious but rare complication of dantrolene, and periodic blood tests are necessary to monitor liver function. This is the least commonly used oral medication for spasticity.

Nerve Block Injections

A nerve block involves injecting a drug directly into the muscle. Nerve block injections treat spasticity by disrupting signals from nerves to muscles; the result is a reduction in muscle contraction. An example of a nerve blocking substance is botulinum toxin type A (Botox). Botulinum toxin is a poison at high doses, but when used in small amounts it is an effective treatment for spasticity. Reductions in spasticity typically begin within three days of the injection. The effects can last up to three months, although the peak effect occurs between two and six weeks after the injection. When the effect wears off, the doctor can give another injection. Side effects are uncommon but include weakness in the spastic muscle, fatigue, or pain near the site of injection.

Injections of phenol or alcohol can be used separately or in conjunction with botulinum toxin. Phenol and alcohol injections are more appropriate for large muscles (such as those in the leg), while botulinum toxin is used more often for smaller muscle groups. Improvements following phenol or alcohol injections vary in duration from one month to more than two years. Compared with botulinum toxin injections, phenol and alcohol injections cost less but are associated with a higher incidence of side effects. Their adverse effects include pain or abnormal sensations close to the injection site. The U.S. Food and Drug Administration has not approved phenol or alcohol injections for the treatment of spasticity.

Spinal Medication

If other measures are unsuccessful in treating spasticity, intrathecal baclofen may be beneficial. ("Intrathecal" refers to the space that contains the fluid surrounding the spinal cord.) This approach involves surgical implantation of a small pump containing baclofen into the abdomen. A tube extending from the pump delivers baclofen into the intrathecal space so that the medication can block the nerve signals that produce the muscle contractions that cause spasticity. Before implanting the pump, a doctor may inject baclofen by hand to see if the patient responds to the medication.

Intrathecal baclofen is much more expensive than other treatments for spasticity, and the therapy involves surgery and a hospital stay. The pump needs to be refilled every one to three months, and the whole system must be replaced when the batteries run low, usually within five years. Potential problems related to the device itself include infection, pump failure, and breaks or kinks in the tube. Adverse effects of intrathecal baclofen are similar to those of oral baclofen but occur less often, since lower dosages are used.

Surgery

If the previously mentioned treatments are ineffective, patients may require surgery to treat spasticity. Orthopedic surgery can move or cut tendons to restore some limb motion and reduce spasticity. The surgery also may involve making changes to the bone. The most drastic measure, neurosurgery, is used only as a last resort when all other treatments have failed. It involves cutting the nerves that lead from the spinal cord to the affected muscle to permanently end spasticity.

minimize the amount of bleeding from the ruptured artery. This is done carefully and conservatively, since, as with ischemic stroke, additional brain damage can occur when blood pressure is too low.

Drug therapy. Mannitol (a type of sugar) and diuretics, which counteract fluid retention by increasing sodium and water loss in the urine, can be used to reduce cerebral edema (swelling of tissues in the brain), a serious and relatively common consequence of hemorrhagic stroke. Vasospasm (spasm of cerebral blood vessels—likely to occur in the first to second week after subarachnoid hemorrhage) causes further reduction of blood flow. Occurring in about one third of patients, vasospasm is now recognized as one of the most prevalent, serious complications and a major cause of death after a subarachnoid hemorrhage. Nimodipine (Nimotop), a calcium channel blocker, may reduce brain damage due to vasospasm.

Surgery. Surgical intervention is warranted in some cases of hemorrhagic stroke, such as those associated with aneurysms or arteriovenous malformations (see pages 42–43), in which there is a high risk of rebleeding. Depending on its location in the brain, an aneurysm that has leaked or ruptured can be clipped across its neck—thus preventing any future bleeding by stopping blood flow into the aneurysm; adjacent blood vessels are then surgically repaired. A newer procedure may be tried in patients who are unable to undergo clipping: A platinum coil is fed into the aneurysm, sealing it off from blood circulation.

The risk of treating an arteriovenous malformation must be balanced against the danger of future bleeding, which is minimal in asymptomatic patients. After the first hemorrhage, patients have about a 2% to 3% annual risk of further bleeding. The mortality rate when bleeding does occur from a small arteriovenous malformation is about 15%. Therefore, the risk of intervention must be lower than these levels; if not, the arteriovenous malformation usually is monitored closely and the need for treatment reconsidered if a change occurs.

The three methods of treatment, which may be used in combination, are surgical removal, injection of a "glue" to close off the abnormal vessels from blood circulation (embolization), and radiotherapy. Which method is employed depends on the position of the arteriovenous malformation (for example, whether it is near any vital structures), its size, its accessibility, and the life expectancy of the patient. A relatively accessible arteriovenous malformation may be removed surgically, while one positioned deep within the brain might receive either radiation or embolization therapy. Radiation causes the abnormal blood vessels to be reabsorbed by the body over a period of a few years. Embolization involves passing a catheter through the arteries and into the center of the arteriovenous malformation. A "glue" then is fed slowly through the catheter so that it fills the arteriovenous malformation, solidifies, and blocks blood flow. Embolization often is done prior to surgery.

Hemorrhagic strokes often produce an intracerebral hematoma—a pool of blood within the brain that damages brain cells and can dangerously increase intracranial pressure. (Indeed, large hematomas are usually fatal.) Emergency drainage of a hematoma, known as evacuation, can relieve the excess pressure and thus minimize brain damage. Sometimes, however, the hematoma is not accessible to surgery, or the release of pressure may result in further

NEW RESEARCH

Anger After Stroke Linked To Damage to the Brain

About a third of stroke patients may experience an inability to control anger or aggression after their stroke, and these emotional outbursts may be the direct result of damage to the brain.

Korean investigators interviewed 145 stroke patients regarding their ability to control anger and aggression before and after their stroke, as well as about any poststroke depression or emotional incontinence (inappropriate crying, laughing, or both). Further, they used imaging studies to observe brain damage from the stroke.

Thirty-two percent of the patients had an inability to control anger or aggression three months to a year after their stroke. In many patients, this anger occurred spontaneously or was an inappropriate and excessive reaction to a trivial matter. Excessive anger and aggression correlated with difficulty in speaking and loss of motor skills. It was also related to the location of the brain damage from the stroke.

Because inappropriate anger or aggression was not related to patients' levels of depression, neurological deficits, or physical dependency, the authors conclude that the inability to control anger or aggression is caused directly by damage to the brain and is not secondary to physical or mental health problems.

NEUROLOGY
Volume 58, page 1106
April 9, 2002

bleeding. Blood that seeps into the subarachnoid space or into the cavities within the brain known as the ventricles eventually is reabsorbed into the body. In some patients, however, clotted blood interferes with fluid resorption from the brain, leading to an excessive accumulation of fluid (called hydrocephalus or "water on the brain"). A surgical procedure then may be needed to drain fluid through a tube.

STROKE REHABILITATION

The process of rehabilitation after a stroke starts almost immediately after admission to the hospital and often continues for at least one to two months afterward. At first, the main goal is to reduce or prevent stroke complications, such as stiffening of the limbs or deep vein thrombosis. As the patient's condition stabilizes, the focus turns toward the longer-term goals of restoring mental and physical function, adapting to disability, returning to an active life, and preventing additional strokes.

Although the exact approach depends on the specific loss of function caused by the stroke, rehabilitation typically consists of developing new strategies to overcome deficits and performing exercises designed to improve range of motion in joints, strengthen weak muscles, and restore function to the greatest extent possible. The Agency for Health Care Policy and Research has made several recommendations to help patients get the most out of rehabilitation. These include beginning rehabilitation as soon as possible, carefully selecting the most appropriate program, setting realistic goals (to avoid later frustration), frequently assessing progress, and following up during the transition back to the community (when the family plays a major role). Individuals may need to accept some degree of disability, but optimal recovery depends on a combination of crucial factors: the patient's determination to succeed, the support of family and friends, and the well-integrated efforts of specialists.

A variety of specially trained professionals are involved in the rehabilitation process. Occupational therapists teach patients new ways to perform day-to-day activities (writing, bathing, cooking, or job-related tasks) made difficult because of disability. Physical therapists provide instruction and exercises to help patients regain the ability to walk and move about independently, as well as to improve strength, flexibility, balance, and overall fitness. Social workers can provide information on the wide range of community services available to help stroke survivors and their families. Speech-language

NEW RESEARCH

Pre-and Poststroke Dementia Increase Risk of Death

People who have dementia before a stroke (prestroke dementia) and those who develop dementia after a stroke (stroke-related dementia) are at increased risk for dying, new research indicates.

Spanish investigators interviewed the relatives of 324 stroke victims to determine which patients displayed signs of dementia in the five years before their stroke. All available patients were tested three months after their stroke to determine who was displaying symptoms of dementia.

About 15% of the patients had dementia before their stroke. After an average follow-up of 16 months, 20% of patients with prestroke dementia were alive compared with 73% of those without prestroke dementia. Nearly 20% of the patients who survived to three months had dementia that was brought on by the stroke. After an average of 22 months, 58% of those with stroke-related dementia were alive compared with 95% of those without stroke-related dementia.

"Dementia seems to be one of the most important determinants of mortality in stroke patients," the authors write. Possible explanations may be that patients with dementia are less likely to adhere to their treatment after a stroke or that doctors may be less likely to prescribe anticoagulant drugs like warfarin (Coumadin) to people with dementia.

STROKE
Volume 33, page 1993
August 2002

pathologists help patients regain as much of their lost swallowing ability and language skills as possible.

The eventual goal of any rehabilitation program is to return the patient to the community, and certain steps must be taken before this transition can be made. Most patients are not yet fully independent when they first leave a rehabilitation program, so they and their families should be prepared to continue rehabilitation at home. Starting with the most basic steps, the house or apartment must be made ready by providing for any special needs. It is particularly important that patients and family members involved in care understand what to expect and what will be required of them. Doctors and therapists can offer guidance on these issues and discuss what community services are available to help.

Because continuing medical treatment after a stroke is complicated, one doctor should be selected to oversee care. This approach will ensure there are no gaps in treatment and allow frequent assessments of progress and an eventual phase out of rehabilitation when patients have progressed as far as they can. Throughout the post-stroke period, all medications must be carefully monitored. For example, anticonvulsants or benzodiazepines could affect the ability to participate in rehabilitation exercises and activities.

Stroke patients who require rehabilitation may choose from inpatient, outpatient, or home-based programs. In general, the best candidates for rehabilitation have at least one significant disability, such as paralysis or aphasia; are moderately stable medically; have the physical endurance to sit up for at least one hour; and are able to learn and participate to some extent in active rehabilitation treatments. However, rehabilitation may be either unnecessary or infeasible in some cases—for example, for patients who have no disability or, alternatively, patients who are too disabled to benefit. Patients with severe disabilities may be able to begin rehabilitation after a period of rest. ■

GLOSSARY

abulia—Reduction in speech, movement, thought, and emotional reaction.

agnosia—Loss of the ability to interpret incoming visual, auditory, or tactile stimuli, even though the senses of vision, hearing, and touch are mechanically intact and function normally.

aldosterone—A hormone released by the adrenal glands that increases blood pressure by signaling the kidneys to retain sodium, which increases the volume of blood.

aldosterone blockers—Drugs that lower blood pressure by interfering with the activity of the hormone aldosterone.

aldosteronism—An overproduction of aldosterone caused by a tumor or overgrowth of cells in the adrenal gland. Aldosteronism can lead to hypertension.

alpha-blockers—Drugs that decrease blood pressure by blocking nerve impulses that constrict small arteries.

alteplase—A drug used to treat heart attacks and strokes by dissolving blood clots. Also called tissue-type plasminogen activator (t-PA).

ambulatory blood pressure monitor—A portable device that automatically measures and records blood pressure over a 24- or 48-hour period outside of a medical setting.

aneroid blood pressure monitor—A manually operated sphygmomanometer that consists of a cuff, bulb, and gauge to register blood pressure levels.

aneurysm—A ballooning of the wall of a blood vessel caused by weakening of the wall.

angina—Episodes of chest pain caused by an inadequate supply of oxygen and blood to the heart. It occurs most often during physical activity. Also called angina pectoris.

angioplasty—A procedure in which a small balloon is inflated in a blocked artery to enlarge the path for blood flow.

angiotensin—A hormone that has two forms: angiotensin I and angiotensin II. The latter raises blood pressure by causing arteries to constrict and triggering the release of aldosterone.

angiotensin II receptor blockers—Drugs that help lower blood pressure by interfering with the action of angiotensin II, a hormone that causes arteries to constrict and triggers the release of aldosterone.

angiotensin-converting enzyme (ACE) inhibitors—Drugs commonly prescribed to lower blood pressure by preventing the formation of angiotensin II, a hormone that causes arteries to constrict and triggers the release of aldosterone. Also used to slow the progression of kidney disease in patients with diabetes.

anticoagulants—Anticlotting drugs that work by inhibiting the formation of fibrin, a protein required for blood clot development. Examples are heparin and warfarin.

antiplatelets—Anticlotting drugs that work by inhibiting the clumping of blood cells called platelets. One example is aspirin.

aphasia—Difficulty in comprehending or producing spoken or written language.

arrhythmia—An abnormal heart rhythm.

arteriovenous malformation—A congenital disorder characterized by a complex, tangled web of arteries and veins.

aspiration pneumonia—Pneumonia caused by the inhalation of food and other particles into the lungs.

atherosclerosis—The narrowing of arteries by fatty deposits and fibrous tissues, called plaques, within the walls of the arteries that can cause a reduction in blood flow.

atrial fibrillation—A common abnormal heart rhythm in which the heart contracts at a fast and chaotic rate.

atrial natriuretic factor—A hormone produced by the atria of the heart that helps regulate blood pressure by causing the kidneys to excrete more sodium and by inhibiting production of aldosterone and renin.

baroreceptors—Special nerve endings in the walls of arteries that monitor blood pressure.

beta-blockers—Drugs that impede the actions of epinephrine and norepinephrine, slow heart rate, and lower blood pressure by diminishing cardiac output.

b-mode imaging—An imaging technique that uses high-frequency sound waves to produce a three-dimensional view of the carotid arteries.

brain stem—An area located at the base of the brain and above the spinal cord that maintains basic life support functions such as breathing, heart rate, and blood pressure.

calcitriol—A hormone formed from dietary vitamin D that increases the absorption of calcium from the intestine and plays a role in the regulation of blood pressure by constricting small arteries.

calcium channel blockers—Drugs that lower blood pressure by dilating arteries and, in some cases, by decreasing cardiac output.

cardiac output—The amount of blood pumped by the heart.

carotid endarterectomy—A surgical procedure to remove plaque from the carotid arteries.

carotid stenosis—A narrowing of the carotid arteries in the neck that supply blood to the brain.

central alpha agonists—Drugs that lower blood pressure by blocking brain nerve impulses that constrict small arteries.

cerebellum—The area of the brain located above the brain stem that controls coordination, balance, and posture.

cerebral angiography—An invasive procedure involving the injection of an iodine-based contrast solution into the bloodstream to produce a high-quality x-ray image of the blood vessels within the brain.

cerebral edema—Swelling of the brain due to bleeding, trauma, a stroke, or a tumor.

cerebral embolism—A blockage of blood flow that occurs when part of a blood clot or a piece of atherosclerotic plaque breaks off and travels through the bloodstream until it lodges in an artery supplying blood to the brain.

cerebral thrombosis—A blockage of blood flow that occurs when a blood clot forms at the site of an atherosclerotic plaque within the wall of a major artery supplying the brain. The most common cause of an ischemic stroke.

cerebrum—The largest portion of the brain. It controls conscious thought, perception, voluntary movement, and integration of sensory input.

claudication—Intermittent pain in the leg muscles caused by an inadequate supply of oxygen and blood to the legs. It most often occurs with walking.

coagulopathies—A group of rare disorders of blood clotting that are inherited or result from other disorders such as cancer.

combination therapy—A treatment approach for hypertension that uses medication from two different drug classes.

computed tomography (CT) angiography—An imaging method in which an iodine-based dye is injected into the patient and a rapid CT scan is performed through the region of interest. Computer-based software then shows images of the blood vessels that fill with dye.

computed tomography (CT or CAT) scan—A test in which a patient lies flat on a table while x-rays are passed through the body and sensed by a rotating detector. A CT scan of the head will reveal strokes, hemorrhages, or tumors. May be done with or without contrast agents.

Cushing syndrome—A condition resulting from the secretion of excessive amounts of cortisone and related hormones by a tumor of the adrenal cortex (the outer portion of the adrenal gland). A potential cause of high blood pressure.

cytoprotective drugs—A class of drugs designed to protect healthy tissue, for example, during an ischemic stroke.

deep vein thrombosis—The formation of a blood clot in the legs. Also known as thrombophlebitis.

diabetes—A disorder characterized by abnormally high levels of glucose (sugar) in the blood.

diastolic blood pressure—The lower number in a blood pressure reading. Represents pressure in the arteries when the heart relaxes between beats.

digital blood pressure monitor—A battery-operated blood pressure monitor that uses a microphone to detect blood pulses in an artery.

direct vasodilators—Antihypertensive drugs that act directly on the smooth muscle of small arteries, causing them to widen.

diuretics—A class of drugs that increases loss of sodium through the kidneys, thereby increasing the production of urine and decreasing blood volume and blood pressure.

Doppler ultrasound—A technique using sound waves to measure how fast blood moves through arteries, such as the carotid arteries.

embolus—A blood clot or a piece of atherosclerotic plaque that travels through the bloodstream until it lodges in a narrowed vessel and blocks blood flow. The plural form is emboli.

endothelin—A hormone that causes blood vessels to constrict.

epinephrine—A hormone that increases blood pressure in response to stress. Also called adrenaline.

essential hypertension—See **primary hypertension**.

free radicals—Chemical compounds that can damage cells and oxidize low density lipoprotein so that it is more likely to deposit in the walls of arteries.

frontal lobe—An area at the front of the brain that deals with speech, personality, and motor function.

glomeruli—Sites in the kidneys where blood contents other than cells and proteins are filtered from the blood into the excretory tubules of the kidneys.

glutamate cascade—See **ischemic cascade**.

hematoma—A mass of clotted blood that forms as a result of a broken blood vessel.

hemianopia—A condition, often caused by a stroke, that results in blindness in one side of a person's field of vision while vision on the other side remains normal.

hemorrhagic stroke—A stroke that occurs when an artery in the brain suddenly bursts and blood leaks into the surrounding tissue.

GLOSSARY—continued

high density lipoprotein (HDL)—A particle in the blood that can protect against coronary heart disease by removing cholesterol from the body.

hypertension—High blood pressure.

hypertensive crisis—A condition characterized by extremely high blood pressure levels (diastolic pressure above 120 mm Hg). Occurs in about 1% of people with hypertension.

hypertensive encephalopathy—A brain disorder that occurs in people experiencing a hypertensive emergency. Symptoms may include intense headaches, drowsiness, seizures, loss of consciousness, blurred vision, and even blindness.

hypotension—Low blood pressure.

insulin—A hormone that controls the manufacture of glucose by the liver and permits muscle and fat cells to remove glucose from the blood. Also a medication taken by people with diabetes whose pancreas does not make enough insulin.

intracerebral hemorrhage—Leakage of blood into tissues deep within the brain.

ischemia—A lack of oxygen due to a decrease in blood supply to a body organ or tissue.

ischemic cascade—A chain of chemical reactions, occurring during an ischemic stroke, that leads to a buildup of toxins and further cell destruction. Also called glutamate cascade.

ischemic stroke—A stroke resulting from blockage of an artery supplying blood to the brain.

isolated systolic hypertension—A systolic blood pressure of 140 mm Hg or higher along with a diastolic blood pressure under 90 mm Hg. Associated with an increased risk of stroke, coronary heart disease, and kidney disease.

J-curve phenomenon—Refers to the relationship between the risk of a heart attack and blood pressure. The curve shows that those with the highest and lowest blood pressure levels are more likely to die of a heart attack than those with an intermediate blood pressure level.

kidneys—A pair of organs, located on the left and right sides of the abdomen, that remove waste products and excess water from the blood and produce urine.

lacunar stroke—A stroke that occurs when the tiny branches at the end of arteries in the brain become completely blocked by small emboli or atherosclerotic plaque.

left ventricular hypertrophy—A thickening of the muscular wall of the left ventricle that occurs when it must work harder to pump blood. Common in people with hypertension.

limb contracture—Consistent tightening of ligaments and tendons in the limbs.

limbic system—A group of structures in the brain responsible for primal urges and powerful emotions, such as hunger and terror, that help to ensure self-preservation.

low density lipoprotein (LDL)—A particle that transports cholesterol in the bloodstream. Its deposition in artery walls initiates plaque formation. A major contributor to coronary heart disease.

magnetic resonance angiography (MRA)—A technique for viewing the arteries in the neck, brain, or other organs by manipulating the scanner in a conventional MRI.

magnetic resonance imaging (MRI)—A test that employs magnetic fields and radio waves to generate a three-dimensional image of a part of the body, such as the brain.

metabolic syndrome—A group of findings, including elevated blood insulin levels, high triglycerides, low HDL cholesterol, an increased risk of diabetes and atherosclerosis, and high blood pressure, that is caused by a genetic predisposition to insulin resistance and an accumulation of fat in the abdomen. Previously called insulin resistance syndrome or syndrome X.

motor cortex—A part of the frontal lobe of the brain. Damage to this area can result in weakness or paralysis on the opposite side of the body.

nitric oxide—A substance secreted by cells lining the walls of blood vessels that causes arteries to dilate by relaxing smooth muscle cells.

norepinephrine—A hormone that increases blood pressure in response to stress.

occipital lobe—An area of the brain at the back of the skull that is dedicated to the perception and interpretation of visual data from the eyes.

orthostatic hypertension—An abrupt drop in blood pressure on standing.

parathyroid hormone—A hormone that regulates calcium metabolism. It dilates small arteries that may play a role in the control of blood pressure.

parietal lobe—An area of the brain behind the frontal lobe that receives and interprets sensory signals from all parts of the body.

peripheral-acting adrenergic antagonists—Drug that reduce resistance to blood flow in small arteries.

pheochromocytoma—A tumor in the central portion of the adrenal gland that secretes large amounts of epinephrine or norepinephrine. Can lead to hypertension.

plaque—An accumulation of cholesterol, smooth muscle cells, fibrous proteins, and calcium in artery walls.

primary hypertension—Hypertension of undetermined cause, likely related to excess weight, salt intake, or physical inactivity. Affects 90% to 95% of people with hypertension. Also called essential hypertension.

pulse pressure—The difference between systolic and diastolic blood pressures. Reflects the stiffness of arteries.

renin—An enzyme produced by cells in the kidney that converts angiotensinogen to angiotensin I.

renovascular hypertension—A type of hypertension caused by a reduction in blood flow to the kidneys.

retinopathy—Damage to the retina caused by changes in the tiny blood vessels that supply the retina. The leading cause of blindness in U.S. adults.

secondary hypertension—Hypertension caused by another heath condition or a medication. Responsible for less than 5% of cases of hypertension.

sphygmomanometer—An instrument used to measure blood pressure. Consists of an inflating bulb, inflatable cuff, and aneroid or mercury column gauge.

stent—A wire mesh tube that is inserted into an artery to help keep it open.

stroke—A sudden reduction in or loss of brain function that occurs when an artery supplying blood to a portion of the brain becomes blocked or ruptures. Neurons in the affected area are starved of oxygen and nutrients normally provided by the blood.

subarachnoid hemorrhage—Leakage of blood into the space between the brain and the arachnoid membrane, the middle of the three membranes that envelop the brain. Most commonly results from trauma or a ruptured aneurysm.

systolic blood pressure—The upper number in a blood pressure reading. Represents pressure in the arteries when the heart is pumping blood to the rest of the body.

temporal lobe—An area of the brain at ear level underneath the parietal and frontal lobes that is dedicated to hearing, auditory perception, and storage of memories.

thrombolytic drugs—Medications that breaks up blood clots.

thrombus—A blood clot. The plural form is thrombi.

transient ischemic attack (TIA)—Short-lived neurological deficits caused by insufficient blood flow to the brain. Most episodes subside within 20 minutes.

triglyceride—A lipid (fat) in the bloodstream. Elevated levels are associated with an increased risk of coronary heart disease.

vasospasm—A constriction of blood vessels in the brain that is likely to occur in the first two weeks after a subarachnoid hemorrhage.

white coat hypertension—High blood pressure readings that are only present when the patient's blood pressure is recorded by a physician or in a medical environment. Blood pressure is normal when taken at home by the patient, family members, or friends.

HEALTH INFORMATION ORGANIZATIONS AND SUPPORT GROUPS

American College of Cardiology
9111 Old Georgetown Rd.
Bethesda, MD 20814-1699
☎ 800-253-4636
301-897-5400
www.acc.org
Professional medical society that produces several publications, sponsors programs to further medical education, provides a national clinical database library, and advises on health care policy.

American Heart Association
7272 Greenville Ave.
Dallas, TX 75231
☎ 800-242-8721
www.americanheart.org
National health organization that provides information and public education programs on all aspects of heart disease. Check for local chapters.

American Occupational Therapy Association
4720 Montgomery Lane
P.O. Box 31220
Bethesda, MD 20824-1220
☎ 301-652-2682
800-377-8555 (TDD)
www.aota.org
Provides contact information for people seeking occupational therapists, and names of stroke and trauma programs from the National Institutes of Health.

American Physical Therapy Association
1111 N. Fairfax St.
Alexandria, VA 22314-1488
☎ 800-999-APTA
703-684-APTA
www.apta.org
National professional organization for physical therapists (PTs) that provides referrals to state PT associations.

American Society of Hypertension
148 Madison Ave., 5th Floor
New York, NY 10016
☎ 212-696-9099
www.ash-us.org
Largest U.S. organization dedicated exclusively to hypertension and related cardiovascular disease. Organizes and conducts educational programs to promote the development of treatment for hypertension.

American Speech-Language-Hearing Association
10801 Rockville Pike
Rockville, MD 20852
☎ 800-638-8255
www.asha.org
Toll-free help line gives information on communication disorders and referrals to speech-language pathologists and audiologists around the country.

American Stroke Association
7272 Greenville Ave.
Dallas, TX 75231
☎ 888-4-STROKE
800-553-6321 ("Warmline")
www.strokeassociation.org
A division of the American Heart Association; provides referrals to community stroke groups and information and peer counseling to survivors and caregivers. Call the "Warmline" to subscribe to their magazine, *Stroke Connection*.

HeartInfo Center for Cardiovascular Education, Inc.
P.O. Box 823
New Providence, NJ 07974-0823
www.heartinfo.org
Educational Web site backed by an international panel of cardiologists. Provides information and services for the prevention, diagnosis and treatment of cardiovascular disease.

Mended Hearts, Inc.
7272 Greenville Ave.
Dallas, TX 75231-4596
☎ 800-242-8721
214-706-1442
www.mendedhearts.org
A support group for heart disease patients and their families with 250 chapters in the United States. Call or write for information and referrals.

National Aphasia Association
156 Fifth Ave., Ste. 707
New York, NY 10010
☎ 800-922-4622
www.aphasia.org
Provides educational material, a newsletter, a directory of community support groups, and a national network of volunteers who can discuss professional and social resources in their areas.

National Heart, Lung, and Blood Institute Information Center
P.O. Box 30105
Bethesda, MD 20824-0105
☎ 800-575-WELL
301-592-8573
www.nhlbi.nih.gov/health/infoctr/index.htm
Branch of the National Institutes of Health that provides written information on all heart-related issues.

National Institute of Neurological Disorders and Stroke
P.O. Box 5801
Bethesda, MD 20824
☎ 800-352-9424
www.ninds.nih.gov
Leading supporter of neurological research in the United States. Provides list of clinical resource centers and voluntary health agencies.

National Rehabilitation Information Center
1010 Wayne Ave., Ste. 800
Silver Spring, MD 20910
☎ 800-346-2742
301-562-2400
www.naric.com
National library providing information on rehabilitation and disability, including independent living, employment, medical rehabilitation, and legislation. Makes referrals to community rehabilitation centers.

National Stroke Association
9707 E. Easter Lane
Englewood, CO 80112
☎ 800-STROKES
303-649-9299
www.stroke.org
National non-profit organization devoting 100% of its resources to stroke. Provides education, services, and community-based activities in stroke prevention, treatment, rehabilitation and recovery.

LEADING HOSPITALS

U.S. News & World Report and the National Opinion Research Center, a social-science research group at the University of Chicago, recently conducted their 13th annual nationwide survey of 1,484 physicians in 17 medical specialties. The doctors nominated up to five hospitals they consider best from among 6,045 U.S. hospitals. These are the current lists of the best hospitals for neurology and cardiology, as determined by the doctors' recommendations from 2000, 2001, and 2002; federal data on death rates; and factual data regarding quality indicators, such as the ratio of registered nurses to patients and the use of advanced technology. Since the results reflect the doctors' opinions, however, they are, to some degree, subjective. Any institution listed is considered a leading center, and the rankings do not imply that other hospitals cannot or do not deliver excellent care.

NEUROLOGY AND NEUROSURGERY HOSPITALS

1. **Mayo Clinic**
   Rochester, MN
   ☎ 507-284-2511
   www.mayoclinic.org

2. **Massachusetts General Hospital**
   Boston, MA
   ☎ 617-726-2000
   www.mgh.harvard.edu

3. **Johns Hopkins Hospital**
   Baltimore, MD
   ☎ 800-507-9952/410-955-5000
   www.hopkinsmedicine.org

4. **New York Presbyterian Hospital**
   New York, NY
   ☎ 212-305-2500
   www.nyp.org

5. **Cleveland Clinic**
   Cleveland, OH
   ☎ 800-223-2273/216-444-2200
   www.clevelandclinic.org

6. **UCSF Medical Center**
   San Francisco, CA
   ☎ 888-689-UCSF/415-476-1000
   www.ucsfhealth.org

7. **Barnes-Jewish Hospital**
   St. Louis, MO
   ☎ 314-747-3000
   www.barnesjewish.org

8. **UCLA Medical Center**
   Los Angeles, CA
   ☎ 800-825-2631/310-825-9111
   www.healthcare.ucla.edu

9. **Hospital of the University of Pennsylvania**
   Philadelphia, PA
   ☎ 800-789-PENN/215-662-4000
   www.pennhealth.com/upmc

10. **Methodist Hospital**
    Houston, TX
    ☎ 713-790-3333
    www.methodisthealth.com

CARDIOLOGY AND HEART SURGERY HOSPITALS

1. **Cleveland Clinic**
   Cleveland, OH
   ☎ 800-223-2273/216-444-2200
   www.clevelandclinic.org

2. **Mayo Clinic**
   Rochester, MN
   ☎ 507-284-2511
   www.mayoclinic.org

3. **Massachusetts General Hospital**
   Boston, MA
   ☎ 617-726-2000
   www.mgh.harvard.edu

4. **Brigham and Women's Hospital**
   Boston, MA
   ☎ 617-732-5500
   www.brighamandwomens.org

5. **Duke University Medical Center**
   Durham, NC
   ☎ 919-684-8111
   www.mc.duke.edu

6. **Johns Hopkins Hospital**
   Baltimore, MD
   ☎ 800-507-9952/410-955-5000
   www.hopkinsmedicine.org

7. **St. Luke's Episcopal Hospital**
   Houston, TX
   ☎ 713-785-8537
   www.sleh.com/sleh

8. **Emory University Hospital**
   Atlanta, GA
   ☎ 800-75-EMORY/
   404-778-7777/
   www.emory.edu/WHSC/EUH/
   euh.html

9. **Stanford University Hospital**
   Stanford, CA
   ☎ 650-723-4000
   medcenter.stanford.edu

10. **Barnes-Jewish Hospital**
    St. Louis, MO
    ☎ 314-747-3000
    www.barnesjewish.org

HYPERTENSION: EVALUATION AND TREATMENT

Hypertension is an all-too-common condition, with more than a quarter of American adults having either elevated blood pressure or receiving blood pressure-lowering treatments. Furthermore, hypertension is one of the most common reasons people visit a doctor. Yet, despite its ubiquity, there is often debate about how elevated blood pressure should be treated: Are lifestyle modifications enough? When should drug therapy be initiated? Which medications should be used?

To address these questions, George Bakris, M.D., and colleagues have presented their guidelines for the evaluation and treatment of hypertension, reprinted here from the journal *Circulation.* Based on information from randomized, controlled trials and recommendations from experts, they say that blood pressure should be maintained below 140/90 mm Hg for otherwise healthy people. To achieve this goal, lifestyle modifications—specifically weight loss for the obese, sodium restriction to 2,300 mg or less per day, and limiting alcohol intake to no more than two drinks daily—can help to lower blood pressure, particularly in the short term.

Nonetheless, many patients need treatment with medication—in addition to lifestyle modifications—to maintain optimal blood pressure over the long term. Usually, beta-blockers are tried first; ACE inhibitors should be considered in patients who are unable to tolerate beta-blockers. If beta-blockers or ACE inhibitors are ineffective or not tolerated, calcium channel blockers are the next option. Diuretics are usually the first choice for elderly patients.

Unlike otherwise healthy people, those with diabetes or kidney problems require a lower target blood pressure: 130/80 mm Hg or less. For these patients, an angiotensin II receptor blocker or ACE inhibitor should be the first treatment prescribed. If these drugs do not lower blood pressure sufficiently, a diuretic or long-acting calcium channel blocker can be added to the treatment regimen. Additional medications may be needed if blood pressure is still not adequately reduced.

The authors note that individual patient factors, such as age and whether organ damage is present, will dictate the specific therapies needed to control blood pressure and prevent cardiovascular events like heart attacks and strokes.

Clinician Update

Evaluation and Treatment of Patients With Systemic Hypertension

Jay Garg, MD; Adrian W. Messerli, MD; George L. Bakris, MD

A 65-year-old man presented for evaluation of high blood pressure found on screening at a local health fair. History and physical examination did not show any signs or symptoms suggestive of a secondary cause, nor was there evidence of target end-organ damage except for grade 1 Keith-Wagener-Barker retinopathy. The patient denied taking any prescription or over-the-counter medications.

Hypertension is the most common disease-specific reason Americans visit a physician. Despite the risks associated with an elevated blood pressure (BP), there is still woefully low achievement of recommended BP goals. From 1991 to 1994, only 27.4% of hypertensive Americans aged 18 to 74 years had a BP <140/90 mm Hg, the current stated goal for most people with hypertension, and in those with diabetes, less than half that number (11%) were controlled to the Joint National Committee on Prevention, Detection, Evaluation, and Treatment of High Blood Pressure VI (JNC VI) recommended goal of <130/85 mm Hg.[1] The present update will provide an overview of the evaluation and management of essential hypertension and help to guide clinicians in developing a management plan for a patient like the one described above.

Evaluation

Taking a proper BP is an important first step in the diagnosis of hypertension.[2] Using the proper cuff size with patients resting quietly and comfortably (with back support if seated) for at least 5 minutes before measurement, 2 or more readings separated by 2 minutes should be taken and averaged. Initial elevated BP readings should be confirmed on at least 2 subsequent visits over a period of 1 week or more. A value that is consistently ≥140/90 mm Hg is diagnostic in healthy patients; a value >130/80 mm Hg should be used for those with diabetes or kidney disease and proteinuria.

Initial evaluation of the hypertensive patient focuses on the presence or absence of target organ damage (TOD) and includes a physical examination, blood urea nitrogen/creatinine evaluation, measurement of electrolytes, urinalysis, and an ECG. Further, an assessment of cardiovascular (CV) risk factors with a thorough history and chemistry panel (glucose, cholesterol, and triglycerides) is routinely administered.[1] Although the patient in our case study did not exhibit signs or symptoms of a secondary cause of hypertension, this possibility must be entertained in every hypertensive patient.[3]

Management

Goal BP management is determined by the presence or absence of TOD, diabetes and other CV risk factors, and other comorbidities. BP goal recommendations are based on results from randomized, controlled trials and recommendations from guidelines committees (Table 1). All patients with hypertension, except those with diabetes or evidence of TOD, should reduce their BP to <140/90 mm Hg.[1] Those with diabetes mellitus or kidney disease with proteinuria (<1 g/d) should have a target BP of ≤130/80 mm Hg, and those with proteinuria >1 g/d should have a target BP of <125/75 mm Hg.[1,4,5] Achieving these BP goals requires a combination of lifestyle modifications and pharmacological treatment. Patients with JNC VI stage 2 or 3 hypertension (systolic blood pressure [SBP] ≥160 mm Hg or diastolic blood pressure [DBP] ≥100 mm Hg) and those considered to be in a high-risk group (diabetics or subjects with clinical CV disease) should be prescribed antihypertensive drug therapy.[1]

Initial lifestyle modifications include weight loss for obese hypertensive patients, modification of alcohol intake to no more than 2 drinks per day, and limiting Na^+ intake to ≤100 mmol/d. A number of trials, such as the first Trial of Hypertension Prevention (TOHP-1),[6] the follow-up Trial of Hypertension Prevention (TOHP-2),[7] the Treatment of Mild Hypertension Study (TOHMS),[8] and the Dietary Approaches to Stop Hypertension (DASH) study,[9]

From Rush University Hypertension Center, Department of Preventive Medicine, Rush Presbyterian/St Lukeís Medical Center, Chicago, Ill (J.G., G.L.B.); and Cleveland Clinic Foundation, Department of Cardiovascular Medicine, Cleveland, Ohio (A.W.M.).

Correspondence to George Bakris, MD, Rush Medical Center, 1700 W Van Buren St, Suite 470, Chicago, IL 60612. E-mail gbakris@rush.edu

(*Circulation.* 2002;105;2458-2461.)

***Circulation* is available at http://www.Circulationaha.org**
DOI: 10.1161/01.CIR.0000017143.59204.AA

TABLE 1. Recommended Target BP Goals

Guideline	Uncomplicated Hypertension	No TOD or Clinical CV Disease; at Least 1 CV Risk Factor Excluding Diabetes	Diabetes*
JNC VI	<140/90 mm Hg	<140/90 mm Hg	<130/85 mm Hg
NKF			≤130/80 mm Hg
ADA			≤130/80 mm Hg

NKF indicates National Kidney Foundation; ADA, American Diabetes Association.

*JNC VI BP goal also recommended for those with TOD or clinical CV disease.

demonstrate that lifestyle modifications, especially weight loss and a reduction in Na^+ intake, have salutary effects on BP. In the studies with a longer follow-up, there were significantly fewer CV events in the group with both pharmacological treatment and lifestyle modification.[8] High rates of recidivism were seen in the long-term studies, and drug therapy had to be resumed.[10] Thus, although lifestyle modifications can help reduce BP, it is clear that pharmacological therapy is needed to maintain the goal BP.

The primary goal of BP reduction is to reach optimal BP by the least intrusive means possible.[1] The choice of antihypertensive agent should be based on the ability of that agent to reduce morbidity and mortality, especially in the areas of cardiovascular and kidney disease. Three classes of drugs (thiazide diuretics, β-blockers, and angiotensin-converting enzyme [ACE] inhibitors) reduce CV events and mortality when used as the initial therapy for hypertension in appropriately designed and implemented clinical trials, and calcium antagonists reduce stroke mortality and morbidity in the elderly in the absence of proteinuria.[11] Thus, calcium antagonists are very useful adjuncts to help achieve BP goals because it takes an average of 3 different antihypertensive medications to achieve BP goals in high-risk individuals.[12]

Cardiovascular Disease

The process of atherosclerosis is accelerated by hypertension, increasing an individualís lifetime risk for adverse CV events ≈2- to 3-fold.[13] The optimal therapy for a hypertensive patient with known coronary artery disease should do more than simply lower blood pressure. Ideally, the drug will help prevent development of ischemia and occurrence of future cardiovascular events. For patients with angina, an additional goal is reduction of symptoms. It is important to avoid antihypertensive agents that could potentiate myocardial ischemia. Vasodilators, specifically first- and second-generation dihydropyridine calcium-channel blockers (DHCCBs) and hydralazine, cause significant vasodilation, with compensatory increases in heart rate and myocardial contractility. Once coronary blood flow supply is unable to match myocardial oxygen demand, ischemia, often manifested as angina, may result.

β-Blockers

β-Blockers without intrinsic sympathomimetic activity remain the most effective class of drugs for primary and secondary cardioprotection and are the mainstay of therapy for hypertensive patients with ischemic heart disease. They decrease heart rate and inotropy, thereby reducing myocardial oxygen demand. As primary preventive therapy, β-blockers reduce CVD and all-cause mortality in hypertensive patients.[14] In the postñmyocardial infarction setting, β-blockers limit infarct size, suppress ventricular arrhythmias, reduce the incidence of angina, reinfarction and sudden cardiac death, and improve survival.[15] Importantly, β-blockers have proven benefit regardless of the severity of left ventricular dysfunction, but they are typically withheld from heart failure patients until ACE inhibitors have been initiated and titrated.[16]

ACE Inhibitors

Initially, ACE inhibitors were recommended as standard therapy for all patients who suffered a myocardial infarction with resultant left ventricular dysfunction.[17] Given the results of the Heart Outcomes Prevention Evaluation (HOPE) study,[18] in which ramipril reduced the risk of CV events by 22% compared with placebo, however, ACE inhibitors should be considered for both primary and secondary prevention in all high-risk patients and may be considered as first-line therapy in those patients not able to tolerate β-blockers.

Calcium Antagonists

Certain calcium-channel blockers (CCBs) can be used if anginal symptoms or hypertension are not controlled with β-blockers and ACE inhibitors or if patients cannot tolerate β-blockers. Verapamil is an approved alternative if β-blockers cannot be tolerated. Caution should be exercised whenever a non-dihydropyridine CCB is combined with a β-blocker. Significant side effects, including profound hypotension, symptomatic bradycardia, and heart block, may occur in 10% to 15% of patients, predominantly those over 65 years of age or with a preexisting heart block. Long-acting DHCCBs could be used to lower BP in this setting, but they do not reduce mortality from ischemic causes of heart failure.[19,20]

Kidney Disease/Diabetes

The National Kidney Foundation and the American Diabetes Association guidelines suggest that the target BP should be

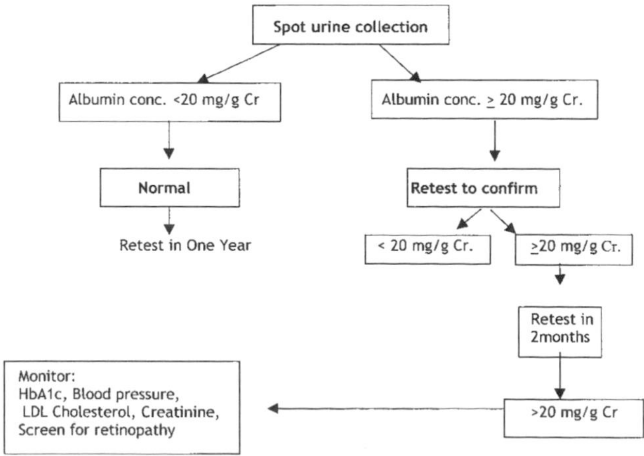

Figure 1. Recommended algorithm in screening for microalbuminuria.

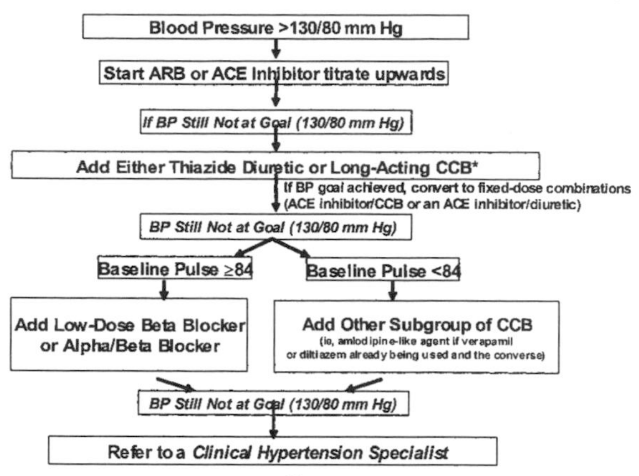

Figure 2. Algorithm for an approach to controlling hypertension in patients with type 2 diabetes mellitus.

≤130/80 mm Hg.[4,5] These recommendations were based on trials and epidemiological data that, taken together, suggested that the risk for both kidney and CV diseases starts to increase at a DBP as low as 83 mm Hg and a SBP as low as 127 mm Hg.

There is now strong evidence that drugs that inhibit the renin-angiotensin system should be a prominent part of the antihypertensive regimen for those with diabetes and/or kidney disease. In a meta-analysis using individual subject data of those with nondiabetic kidney disease, not only did ACE inhibitors reduce the risk of attaining the primary outcomes of end-stage renal disease (ESRD) or doubling of serum creatinine, they also dramatically reduced the amount of proteinuria.[21] Increased urinary albumin excretion or albuminuria is an independent risk factor for both CV and kidney disease, especially in high-risk individuals such as diabetics.[22] Because of this, it is important to evaluate all diabetics, whether hypertensive or not, for albuminuria (Figure 1). We now can use ìevidence-basedî medicine to decide which class of antihypertensive agent to use. In type 2 diabetics with gross proteinuria, only the use of an angiotensin receptor blocker (ARB) has been proven to reduce the risk of developing ESRD or doubling of serum creatinine.[23,24] Conversely, ACE inhibitors or ARBs have been shown to blunt increases in microalbuminuria and, in some cases, normalize it[25]; however, only ACE inhibitors have been shown to reduce the risk of CV events in diabetics, irrespective of whether microalbuminuria was present.[18] An algorithm to achieve BP goal in diabetics is presented in Figure 2.

It is important to note that DHCCBs should not be used in the absence of an ACE inhibitor or ARB in the treatment of hypertension in those with type 2 diabetes or kidney disease. In the Appropriate Blood Pressure Control in Diabetes (ABCD) trial, there were fewer fatal and nonfatal myocardial infarctions with enalapril versus nisoldipine ($P=0.001$).[26] In both the Irbesartan in Diabetic Nephropathy Trial (IDNT) and the African-American Study of Kidney Disease (AASK), both trials of participants with renal insufficiency and proteinuria, the amlodipine group had worse renal outcomes than the ACE inhibitor or angiotensin receptor blocker group.[23,27]

Elderly Patients

In a meta-analysis, it was found that in untreated subjects who were ≥60 years of age, the SBP was a more accurate predictor of mortality and CV events than DBP. This result may be due to the increased arterial stiffness that occurs with aging, leading to a higher SBP and lower DBP, and suggests that antihypertensive therapy in the elderly should focus on SBP rather than DBP, or even concentrate on the difference between the two, ie, pulse pressure.[28] This meta-analysis also confirmed earlier results showing that treatment of hypertension in the elderly significantly reduced the incidence of strokes and coronary heart disease, irrespective of the medication used.[28,29] JNC VI recommends that diuretics be the first-line therapy in the elderly, and there has been no evidence since its publication that has shown newer agents to be more effective. Of note, a meta-analysis published in 1998 questioned the use of β-blockers in the elderly, citing evidence that, except in subjects with coronary artery disease, they did not reduce CV morbidity or mortality.[30]

Conclusion

We presented an elderly man with probable essential hypertension. Assuming that his diagnosis of hypertension is

TABLE 2. Update and Modification of JNC VI List of Co-Morbid Conditions and Drugs That May Have Favorable Effects on Comorbid Conditions

Condition	Agent
Angina	β-blocker, calcium antagonist
Type 1 diabetes with or without proteinuria	ACE inhibitor
Type 2 diabetes with microalbuminuria	ACE inhibitor or ARB, not dihydropyridine calcium antagonist alone
Type 2 diabetes without proteinuria	ACE inhibitor or ARB, not dihydropyridine calcium antagonist alone
Type 2 diabetes with proteinuria	ARB, not dihydropyridine calcium antagonists alone
Heart failure	ACE inhibitor, ARB, β-blocker, potassium-sparing diuretic (spironolactone)
Pregnancy	Labetolol, methyldopa, calcium antagonists
Prior myocardial infarction or CAD	β-blocker and ACE inhibitors
Prostatism	α-blocker (not used alone)
Kidney insufficiency (nondiabetic)	ACE inhibitor (ARB if ACEI not tolerated)

CAD indicates coronary artery disease.

confirmed, the benefits of controlling his BP to reduce both CV and renal disease risk are clear. It is important to identify other comorbidities that he may have, such as diabetes, renal disease, or evidence of TOD, because these will impact what his goal BP should be (Table 1), as well as which antihypertensive agents should be used (Table 2). For patients with coronary heart disease, β-blockers and ACE inhibitors are the first-line therapy, with the option of using a non-dihydropyridine CCB. For patients with nondiabetic renal disease, ACE inhibitors are the initial agent of choice. For patients with type 2 diabetes mellitus, ACE inhibitors reduce cardiovascular risk and ARBs reduce the risk of progression of renal disease in those with overt nephropathy. DHCCBs should not be used in these patients without the concomitant administration of either an ACE inhibitor or an ARB.

References

1. The Sixth Report of the Joint National Committee on Prevention, Detection, Evaluation, and Treatment of High Blood Pressure (JNC VI). *Arch Intern Med.* 1997;157:2413ñ2446.
2. Perloff D, Grim C, Flack J, et al. Human blood pressure determination by sphygmomanometry. *Circulation.* 1993;88:2460ñ2470.
3. Black H, Bakris G, Elliott W. Hypertension: epidemiology, pathophysiology, diagnosis, and treatment. In: Fuster V, Alexander R, OíRourke R, eds. *Hurst's the Heart.* New York, NY: McGraw-Hill; 2001:1553ñ1606.
4. American Diabetes Association: clinical practice recommendations 2002. *Diabetes Care.* 2002;25(suppl 1):S1ñS147.
5. Bakris GL, Williams M, Dworkin L, et al. Preserving renal function in adults with hypertension and diabetes: a consensus approach. National Kidney Foundation Hypertension and Diabetes Executive Committees Working Group. *Am J Kidney Dis.* 2000;36:646ñ661.
6. The Trials of Hypertension Prevention Collaborative Research Group. The effects of nonpharmacologic interventions on blood pressure of persons with high normal levels: results of the Trials of Hypertension Prevention, phase I. *JAMA.* 1992;267:1213ñ1220.
7. The Trials of Hypertension Prevention Collaborative Research Group. Effects of weight loss and sodium reduction intervention on blood pressure and hypertension incidence in overweight people with high-normal blood pressure: results of the Trials of Hypertension Prevention, phase II. *Arch Intern Med.* 1997;157:657ñ667.
8. Neaton JD, Grimm RH Jr, Prineas RJ, et al. Treatment of Mild Hypertension Study: final results. Treatment of Mild Hypertension Study Research Group. *JAMA.* 1993;270:713ñ724.
9. Sacks FM, Svetkey LP, Vollmer WM, et al. Effects on blood pressure of reduced dietary sodium and the Dietary Approaches to Stop Hypertension (DASH) diet. DASH-Sodium Collaborative Research Group. *N Engl J Med.* 2001;344:3ñ10.
10. Whelton PK, Appel LJ, Espeland MA, et al. Sodium reduction and weight loss in the treatment of hypertension in older persons: a randomized controlled trial of nonpharmacologic interventions in the elderly (TONE). TONE Collaborative Research Group. *JAMA.* 1998;279:839ñ846.
11. Staessen JA, Wang JG, Thijs L. Cardiovascular protection and blood pressure reduction: a meta-analysis. *Lancet.* 2001;358:1305ñ1315.
12. Bakris GL. Maximizing cardiorenal benefit in the management of hypertension: achieve blood pressure goals. *J Clin Hypertens (Greenwich).* 1999;1:141ñ147.
13. Multiple risk factor intervention trial: multiple risk factors changes and mortality results. Multiple Risk Factor Intervention Trial Group. *JAMA.* 1982;248:1465ñ1477.
14. Wikstrand J, Warnold I, Olsson G, et al. Primary prevention with metoprolol in patients with hypertension. Mortality results from the MAPHY study. *JAMA.* 1988;259:1976ñ1982.
15. Antman EM, Lau J, Kupelnick B, et al. A comparison of results of meta-analyses of randomized control trials and recommendations of clinical experts: treatments for myocardial infarction. *JAMA.* 1992;268: 240ñ248.
16. Packer M, Bristow MR, Cohn JN, et al. The effect of carvedilol on morbidity and mortality in patients with chronic heart failure. US Carvedilol Heart Failure Study Group. *N Engl J Med.* 1996;334: 1349ñ1355.
17. Pfeffer MA, Braunwald E, Moye LA, et al. Effect of captopril on mortality and morbidity in patients with left ventricular dysfunction after myocardial infarction: results of the survival and ventricular enlargement trial. The SAVE Investigators. *N Engl J Med.* 1992;327:669ñ677.
18. Yusuf S, Sleight P, Pogue J, et al. Effects of an angiotensin-converting-enzyme inhibitor, ramipril, on cardiovascular events in high-risk patients: the Heart Outcomes Prevention Evaluation Study Investigators. *N Engl J Med.* 2000;342:145ñ153.
19. Packer M, OíConnor CM, Ghali JK, et al. Effect of amlodipine on morbidity and mortality in severe chronic heart failure: Prospective Randomized Amlodipine Survival Evaluation Study Group. *N Engl J Med.* 1996;335:1107ñ1114.
20. OíConnor CM, Carson PE, Miller AB, et al. Effect of amlodipine on mode of death among patients with advanced heart failure in the PRAISE trial: Prospective Randomized Amlodipine Survival Evaluation. *Am J Cardiol.* 1998;82:881ñ887.
21. Jafar TH, Schmid CH, Landa M, et al. Angiotensin-converting enzyme inhibitors and progression of nondiabetic renal disease: a meta-analysis of patient-level data. *Ann Intern Med.* 2001;135:73ñ87.
22. Keane WF, Eknoyan G, Proteinuria, albuminuria, risk, assessment, detection, elimination (PARADE): a position paper of the National Kidney Foundation. *Am J Kidney Dis.* 1999;33:1004ñ1010.
23. Lewis EJ, Hunsicker LG, Clarke WR, et al. Renoprotective effect of the angiotensin-receptor antagonist irbesartan in patients with nephropathy due to type 2 diabetes. *N Engl J Med.* 2001;345:851ñ860.
24. Brenner BM, Cooper ME, de Zeeuw D, et al. Effects of losartan on renal and cardiovascular outcomes in patients with type 2 diabetes and nephropathy. *N Engl J Med.* 2001;345:861ñ869.
25. Bakris GL. Microalbuminuria. what is it? Why is it important? What should be done about it? *J Clin Hypertens (Greenwich).* 2001;3:99ñ102.
26. Estacio RO, Jeffers BW, Hiatt WR, et al. The effect of nisoldipine as compared with enalapril on cardiovascular outcomes in patients with non-insulin-dependent diabetes and hypertension. *N Engl J Med.* 1998; 338:645ñ652.
27. Agodoa LY, Appel L, Bakris GL, et al. Effect of ramipril vs amlodipine on renal outcomes in hypertensive nephrosclerosis: a randomized controlled trial. *JAMA.* 2001;285:2719ñ2728.
28. Staessen JA, Gasowski J, Wang JG, et al. Risks of untreated and treated isolated systolic hypertension in the elderly: meta-analysis of outcome trials. *Lancet.* 2000;355:865ñ872.
29. Insua JT, Sacks HS, Lau TS, et al. Drug treatment of hypertension in the elderly: a meta-analysis. *Ann Intern Med.* 1994;121:355ñ362.
30. Messerli F, Grossman E, Goldbourt U. Are beta-blockers efficacious as first-line therapy for hypertension in the elderly? *JAMA.* 1998;279: 1903ñ1907.

KEY WORDS: drugs ■ diabetes mellitus ■ coronary disease ■ kidney ■ aging

NOTES

The information contained in this White Paper is not intended as a substitute for the advice of a physician. Readers who suspect they may have specific medical problems should consult a physician about any suggestions made.

Please address inquiries on bulk subscriptions and permission to reproduce selections from this White Paper to Medletter Associates, Inc., 632 Broadway, 11th Floor, New York, NY 10012. The editors are interested in receiving your comments at the above address but regret that they cannot answer letters of any sort personally.

ISBN 0-929661-56-7
ISSN 1542-1724
Fourth Printing
Printed in the United States of America

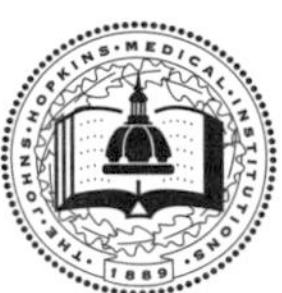

The Johns Hopkins White Papers are published yearly by Medletter Associates, Inc.

LUNG DISORDERS

Simeon Margolis, M.D., Ph.D.

and

Edward F. Haponik, M.D.

2003

LUNG DISORDERS

The ability to breathe is possibly the most fundamental and important function of the body and is required to sustain life. Therefore, any disorder that compromises breathing has the potential to have a considerable impact on health, quality of life, and life span. In this White Paper, we discuss both the common and uncommon types of lung disorders—including asthma, chronic obstructive pulmonary disease, sleep apnea, interstitial lung disease, lung cancer, pulmonary embolism, and infection. The causes, symptoms, effects, and treatments of these conditions are addressed, as well as the best ways to prevent them. Also, we provide numerous practical tips to help in the day-to-day life of someone coping with a lung disorder.

■ ■ ■

Highlights:

■ ■ ■

www.HopkinsAfter50.com
Visit us for the latest news on lung disorders and other information that will complement your Johns Hopkins White Paper.

THE AUTHORS

▪ ▪ ▪

Simeon Margolis, M.D., Ph.D., received his B.A., M.D., and Ph.D. from the Johns Hopkins University School of Medicine and performed his internship and residency at Johns Hopkins Hospital. He is currently a professor of medicine and biological chemistry at the Johns Hopkins University School of Medicine and medical editor of *The Johns Hopkins Medical Letter, Health After 50.* He has served on various committees for the Department of Health, Education, and Welfare, including the National Diabetes Advisory Board and the Arteriosclerosis Specialized Centers of Research Review Committees. In addition, he has acted as a member of the Endocrinology and Metabolism Panel of the U.S. Food and Drug Administration.

A former weekly columnist for the *Baltimore Sun,* Dr. Margolis lectures regularly to medical students, physicians, and the general public on a wide variety of topics, such as the prevention of coronary heart disease, the control of cholesterol levels, the treatment of diabetes, and the use of alternative medicine.

Edward F. Haponik, M.D., is a professor of medicine and director of clinical operations in the Division of Pulmonary and Critical Care Medicine at the Johns Hopkins University School of Medicine.

Peter B. Terry, M.D., also contributed to this White Paper. Dr. Terry is a professor of medicine in the Division of Pulmonary and Critical Care Medicine at the Johns Hopkins University School of Medicine. He is also an associate professor in the Department of Anesthesiology/Critical Care Medicine at Johns Hopkins Hospital and an associate professor in the Department of Environmental Health Sciences at the Johns Hopkins School of Public Health.

CONTENTS

LUNG DISORDERS

Disorders of breathing (respiration) are common in the United States and are expected to increase in prevalence with the aging of the population. Close to 361,000 Americans die of lung disease every year, and more than 25 million are now living with chronic lung disease. Fortunately, technological advances are producing unprecedented opportunities to prevent, diagnose, and treat respiratory disease. The result is considerable improvements in the life spans and quality of life of people who have with these diseases. The topics covered in this White Paper include the following:

Asthma. Asthma is an inflammatory lung disease characterized by shortness of breath, wheezing, coughing, and tightness in the chest. It is considered an obstructive lung disease because it causes narrowing of the airways, but proper treatment can reverse the obstruction.

Chronic obstructive pulmonary disease. Chronic obstructive pulmonary disease (COPD) includes chronic bronchitis and emphysema. Like asthma, COPD is an obstructive lung disease. But the obstruction is more difficult to reverse in COPD, and there is evidence of permanent damage to the lungs.

Sleep apnea. Sleep apnea refers to temporary, recurrent breathing interruptions during sleep.

Interstitial lung disease. Interstitial lung disease refers to a group of conditions that cause extensive scarring of the tissue (called the interstitium) between the air sacs in the lungs.

Lung cancer. Lung cancer, which is most often caused by cigarette smoking, is the leading cause of cancer death in the United States.

Pulmonary embolism. A pulmonary embolism usually occurs when a blood clot from a deep vein breaks loose and blocks an artery that leads to the lungs.

Infections. Common lung infections include acute bronchitis, influenza, bacterial pneumonia, and tuberculosis.

The purpose of this White Paper is to provide people with knowledge about the prevention and treatment of a number of common lung disorders so that they can work closely and effectively with their doctors and other health care professionals.

SYMPTOMS OF RESPIRATORY DISORDERS

Many lung disorders produce similar symptoms, which can occur alone or in combination and may worsen gradually or rapidly.

Respiratory disorders can be acute (with a short and relatively severe course) or chronic (persisting over a long time). Pneumonia and pulmonary embolism are acute lung disorders; asthma, COPD, and interstitial lung disease are chronic. Lung conditions may wax and wane in severity and may worsen rapidly if a secondary problem, such as a lung infection, occurs.

Common symptoms of lung disorders include shortness of breath, coughing, noisy breathing, and chest pain. However, some people with lung disorders have only mild symptoms or none at all. In these individuals, the disorder may be detected on a chest x-ray or by a pulmonary function test during medical evaluation to rule out a pulmonary problem.

Shortness of breath. Shortness of breath (dyspnea) can dramatically compromise quality of life. The underlying cause of dyspnea is usually a mechanical problem that makes breathing more difficult. Examples of mechanical problems are airway obstruction (as with asthma, COPD, and lung cancer), increased stiffness of the lungs (as with interstitial lung disease, pneumonia, and heart failure), severe spine and rib cage abnormalities, and obesity. If left untreated, shortness of breath can lead to severe weakness that may profoundly limit activities. In turn, weakness related to deconditioning (being out of shape) or musculoskeletal disease may worsen shortness of breath.

Coughing. Coughing up phlegm, infectious agents, and foreign matter is one of the ways in which the lungs protect themselves. Severe coughing, however, may signal a respiratory disease. Obstructive diseases of the lungs (asthma and COPD) and lung cancer often cause a person to cough up phlegm. Yellow or green phlegm may signal an infection. Coughing up blood (hemoptysis) may suggest a benign problem such as bronchitis or a potentially life-threatening disease such as lung cancer or pulmonary embolism. Hemoptysis is a serious sign, especially in a current or former cigarette smoker. Chronic cough in an adult with a normal chest x-ray is most often the result of postnasal drip, asthma, or gastroesophageal reflux (in which stomach acid flows back into the esophagus), alone or in combination. Interstitial lung disease, bronchiectasis (persistent dilation of the bronchi or bronchioles), and pneumonia, all of which produce inflammation or scarring of the lungs, also cause coughing.

Noisy breathing. Noisy breathing is an especially common sign of respiratory disease. The noise may originate from problems at any level of the airway. Abnormal sounds range from a high-pitched

The Respiratory System

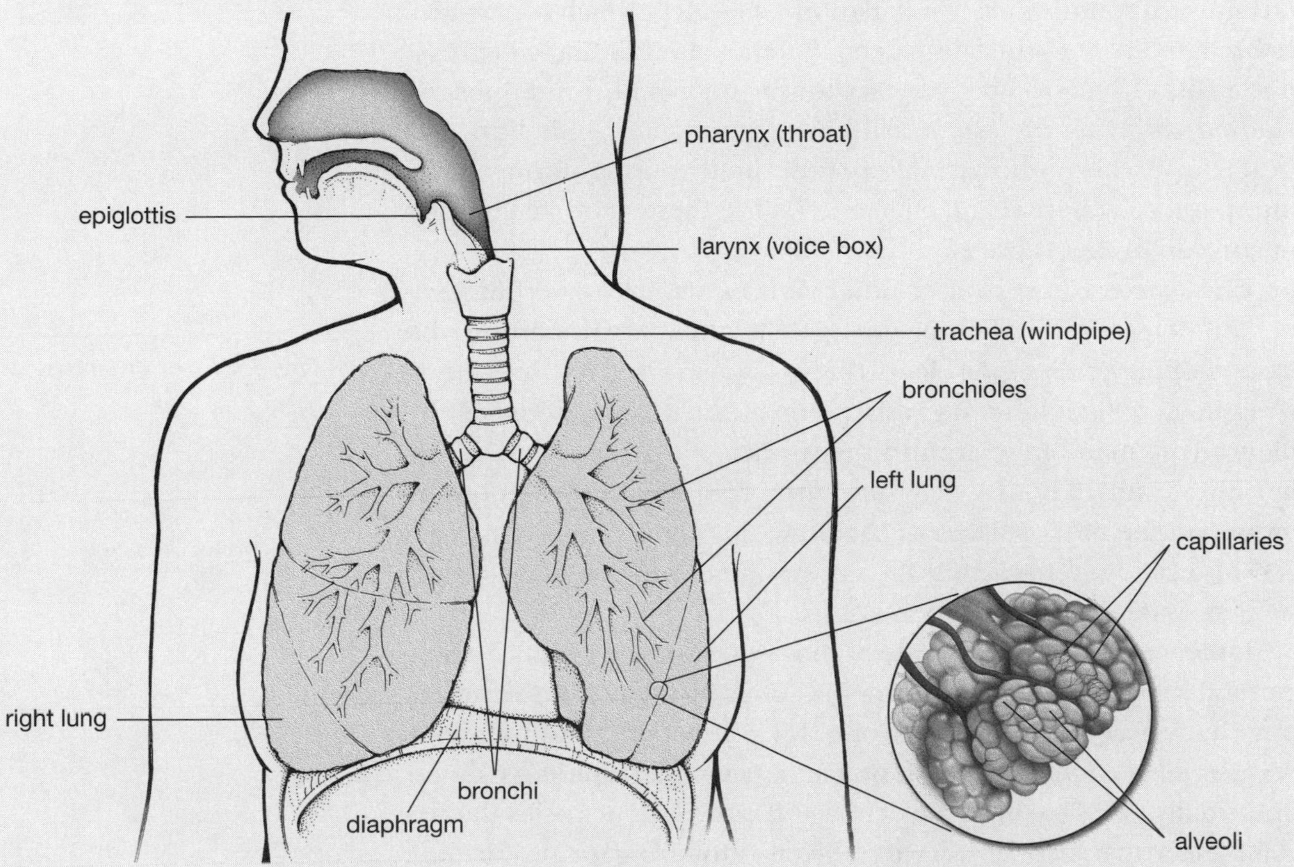

Most people take nearly 25,000 breaths a day and inhale more than 10,000 L of air. Air enters the body through the nose and mouth, passes down the pharynx (throat), through the larynx (voice box) and into the trachea (windpipe), the largest airway. The entrance to the larynx is covered by a flap of cartilage called the epiglottis that prevents food from entering the trachea. The trachea divides into two smaller airways (bronchi) that supply air to the lungs. The bronchi eventually branch into smaller airways called bronchioles.

Movement of air into the lungs is facilitated by the diaphragm, a strong muscle that separates the chest cavity from the abdominal cavity. When the diaphragm contracts, it moves downward and creates a partial vacuum in the chest, which pulls air through the trachea into the lungs.

The lungs are pinkish, sponge-like organs that are located in the chest cavity and extend from the trachea to the diaphragm. They are divided into sections called lobes; the right lung is slightly larger and has three lobes, while the left lung has two.

The lungs are protected by the rib cage and by a slippery membrane called the pleura, which encases them. The pleura has two thin layers, one that surrounds the lungs (visceral pleura) and one that lines the inside of the chest cavity (parietal pleura). The two membranes glide over each other as the lungs expand and contract with each breath.

The lungs have the job of supplying oxygen to the body while removing carbon dioxide from the blood. This process, called gas exchange, occurs in the alveoli, small air-filled sacs that cluster by the dozens at the end of each bronchiole. Each of the millions of alveoli in the lungs is surrounded by a thin layer of tiny blood vessels called capillaries. Oxygen from inhaled air travels through the thin walls of the alveoli and into the bloodstream via the capillaries. At the same time, carbon dioxide (a waste product that accumulates in the blood) moves from the capillaries to the alveoli and is exhaled through the nose and mouth.

In addition to gas exchange, the lungs also defend against viruses, bacteria, and other foreign matter. Cells in the membranes lining the airways secrete mucus to trap dust and germs. Cilia, small "hairs" that line the bronchial tubes, move the mucus in a wavelike motion, up through the bronchioles and into the throat. Once in the throat, the dust and germs are removed by sneezing, coughing, or swallowing.

crowing during inhalation (stridor, which occurs with croup, inflammation of the epiglottis, or tumors in the upper airway) to continuous musical sounds during exhalation (wheezing, which occurs with asthma and some other disorders). The maxim "all that wheezes is not asthma" underscores the fact that many health conditions, including laryngeal disease, heart failure, pulmonary embolism, and COPD, can cause wheezing. Repetitive loud snoring during sleep, interrupted by periods of silence in which there is no airflow, is a major sign of sleep apnea.

Chest pain. Chest pain or other discomfort has numerous causes, and determining whether the cause is a heart or respiratory disease is often challenging. Pain that worsens with deep breathing, coughing, or laughing suggests pleurisy, an inflammation of the pleura (the membrane around the surface of the lungs and the inner chest wall). Pleurisy may be caused by a viral infection, pneumonia on the outer surface of the lung, pulmonary embolism, cancer, or a systemic (affecting the entire body) inflammatory disease such as systemic lupus erythematosus.

Other symptoms. Respiratory illnesses also can produce some general symptoms. For example, low levels of oxygen in the blood, fragmented sleep patterns, chronic lung infections, and lung cancer can all lead to fatigue. Many patients whose respiratory illness limits daily activities have particular difficulty with activities that involve the arms, such as carrying objects, showering, or performing other grooming tasks. These tasks are often more difficult than walking.

GENERAL EVALUATION OF RESPIRATORY SYMPTOMS

The first steps in the evaluation of respiratory problems involve providing a medical history and having a physical examination. These will help the doctor determine which tests, chest imaging techniques, and other studies are required.

Medical History

The doctor will ask a number of questions about current symptoms, past behaviors, occupations, toxic exposures (for example, to cigarette smoke, silica [fine dust from quartz], or asbestos), and family medical history. The presence of infections such as influenza and tuberculosis in the family or community also will be taken into account.

For example, the doctor will want to know if you have ever smoked cigarettes and whether you have inhaled any other potentially injurious agents, such as asbestos. You also will need to give information about any previously diagnosed respiratory illnesses in yourself and your family. Your doctor also will ask about any allergies you may have and any medications you take. Sometimes calcium channel blockers, diet pills, amiodarone (Cordarone; used to treat an irregular heart rhythm), or other medications can contribute to lung disease.

In some people, problems that seem unrelated to the lungs—such as skin rash, joint pain, and visual changes—are symptoms of a more generalized inflammatory disease with respiratory difficulty as one of its symptoms. In addition, a disease such as lung cancer can cause symptoms elsewhere in the body if it spreads (metastasizes).

Physical Examination

The physical examination for a possible lung disease includes a check of breathing rate and pattern and an assessment of how the torso moves during breathing. The way the torso moves is important because some people with lung disease use extra muscles in their abdomen, neck, and rib cage to aid in breathing. Also, reduced movement in one side of the chest might suggest disease localized to that lung. Finally, abnormalities in the structure of the chest could be the cause of breathing difficulty.

In addition, the doctor will use his or her senses of touch and hearing to evaluate the condition. Palpating (touching) the chest wall may reveal rib fractures or other sources of chest pain. Percussion (tapping to generate sound) of the chest will help the doctor determine how far the diaphragm moves and how much the lungs inflate during respiration. A hollow sound is normal, but accentuated hollowness suggests either overinflation of the lung, as occurs in emphysema, or leakage of air into the space around the lung (pneumothorax). A dull or flat sound suggests reduced inflation of the lung (atelectasis), disease within the airspaces (such as pneumonia), or fluid within the pleural space (pleural effusion).

The doctor also will listen to breath sounds using a stethoscope, a technique called auscultation. The intensity of breath sounds is diminished in people with obstructive lung diseases, pneumonia, or pleural effusion. Wheezing and prolonged exhalation also are associated with obstructive lung diseases. Lower-pitched sounds (rhonchi) may suggest secretions within the airways. Velcro-like sounds (crackles, formerly called rales) suggest pneumonia, heart failure, or interstitial lung disease. A harsh "leathery" sound (rub) occasionally is heard with pneumonia or pulmonary embolism.

NEW RESEARCH

Respiratory Disease Associated With More Panic Attacks

Adults with lung disorders are at an increased risk for panic attacks, a new study shows.

To study this link, researchers interviewed more than 3,000 people and asked them if they had suffered from any physical illness in the past 12 months. Participants also were asked about symptoms of mental disorders experienced in the past year.

Thirteen percent of the participants reported having some type of lung disorder. Compared with people who had no lung disorders, those with asthma or chronic obstructive pulmonary disease (COPD) were 70% more likely to have panic attacks, and those who had lung disorders other than asthma or COPD were more than twice as likely to have panics attacks. People who had either asthma or COPD plus another lung disease were about four times more likely to suffer from panic attacks and five times more likely to have symptoms of generalized anxiety disorder than people without lung disorders.

While there appears to be a clear relationship between panic attacks and lung disorders, the researchers cannot ascertain from these data whether panic attacks lead to lung disorders, or vice versa. Alternately, a third factor, such as cigarette smoking or low socioeconomic status, may contribute to both lung disorders and panic attacks.

CHEST
Volume 122, page 645
August 2002

Examination of the hands may reveal discoloration of the nail beds or clubbing of the fingers (a thickening of the fingertips and increased curvature of the fingernails). Blue nail beds suggest low levels of oxygen in the blood, while clubbing suggests lung cancer, interstitial lung disease, bronchiectasis, or other problems. Swelling of the legs and feet suggests that a heart problem may be the cause of symptoms. Heart failure can cause difficulty breathing, as can heart disease caused by resistance to the passage of blood through the lungs (cor pulmonale). Swelling in one leg suggests a blood clot, which could potentially lead to pulmonary embolism.

Laboratory Tests

Other tests can provide complementary information and are obtained on an individual basis according to the doctor's suspicions. Routine blood tests may show a low hemoglobin level (anemia), which might help explain a patient's shortness of breath or suggest a chronic condition (such as lung cancer). An elevated hemoglobin level might suggest chronically low oxygen levels for which the body has attempted to compensate. Elevated white blood cell counts might suggest lung infection or noninfectious inflammatory disease. Blood chemistry measurements describing the functions of other organs (such as the liver or kidney) or specialized tests for rheumatic disease might clarify widespread disease that also involves the lung. Samples of phlegm, when examined in a timely way by a laboratory, may reveal organisms causing lung infection or, in patients with lung cancer, malignant cells.

Chest imaging and pulmonary function tests are two diagnostic tools that are commonly used in people suspected of having a lung disorder. Chest imaging provides information primarily about the structure of the lungs and chest, while pulmonary function tests provide objective measures of lung function. The two tests complement each other.

Chest imaging. A chest x-ray may reveal an abnormality that clearly explains the respiratory problem or identifies areas for further evaluation. Lung tumors, pneumonia, most tuberculosis, occupational lung diseases, emphysema, interstitial lung diseases, and collections of fluid all can be seen on a chest x-ray. The current availability of computed chest tomography (CT) scans is a major advance, allowing a more detailed assessment of abnormalities found on the chest x-ray. Comparing current chest images with previous images is very important and can help to differentiate a new disease from a known condition and to see the progression of a disease over time.

Pulmonary function tests. Pulmonary function tests measure lung capacity and reveal patterns characteristic of particular diseases. A person's measurements are compared with those expected for a healthy person of the same age, height, and gender. Just as people with hypertension or diabetes need measurements of blood pressure and blood glucose, respectively, people with respiratory diseases need tests of their pulmonary function. Commonly performed pulmonary function tests include spirometry, lung volume tests, and diffusion capacity tests. Spirometry (see the feature on page 8) measures the volume of air that can be exhaled, lung volume tests measure the amount of air in the lungs, and diffusion capacity testing measures how well gas moves across the membranes in the lungs. These tests can help characterize the lung abnormality as primarily obstructive (in which the airways are narrowed) or restrictive (in which the ability of the lungs to expand is impaired), or a combination of the two. They also determine whether the functional deficit is mild, moderate, or severe. People with suspected asthma may need to be tested before and after inhaling medication to see if lung function is improved.

Exercise testing. Exercise testing using a treadmill or stationary bicycle also can be used to evaluate shortness of breath and to determine whether it is caused by a lung problem, heart disease, or deconditioning.

Blood gases. If the lungs are not functioning properly, the amount of oxygen and carbon dioxide in the blood (blood gases) may be affected. Blood gases can be measured by taking a sample of blood from an artery. Alternatively, pulse oximetry provides a noninvasive way to measure hemoglobin oxygen saturation (the level of oxygen in the blood). In pulse oximetry, a sensor that directs a beam of light through the tissue is placed on the fingertip or earlobe. The sensor monitors oxygen saturation by measuring the amount of light absorbed by oxygenated hemoglobin (the oxygen-carrying pigment in red blood cells).

Sleep studies. Sleep studies (polysomnography) can be used to monitor certain body functions during sleep. Polysomnography involves electrocardiography to monitor heart rate and rhythm; electroencephalography to monitor brain waves; electromyography to monitor muscle activity; pulse oximetry to measure oxygen saturation; and measures of airflow and movements of the chest and abdomen. These studies detect the presence, pattern, and severity of sleep-related breathing disorders such as sleep apnea and typically are performed in sleep laboratories.

NEW RESEARCH

Quitting Smoking at Any Age Increases Life Span

The earlier in life one quits smoking, the greater the impact on life expectancy. But even older people who quit smoking add years to their life, a new study shows.

Beginning in 1982, researchers collected information on the smoking habits of 877,243 adults. Participants were followed through 1996.

Compared with people who continued to smoke, men who quit smoking at age 35 added as much as 8.5 years to their life; women who quit smoking at this age added up to 7.7 years to their life. Men who quit at age 65 extended their life by 2 years, and women who quit at this age extended their life by 3.7 years.

"These findings reinforce the urgency of emphasizing smoking cessation to all smokers, irrespective of age, and the importance of never assuming that a smoker is 'too far gone,'" the researchers write.

AMERICAN JOURNAL OF PUBLIC HEALTH
Volume 92, page 990
June 2002

Spirometry

Just as doctors use a sphygmomanometer to measure blood pressure, they use a spirometer to measure lung function. A spirometer is similar to a peak flow meter, a portable device that people with asthma use to evaluate their lung function at home (see pages 12–13). But a spirometer is more sophisticated, is generally used only in a doctor's office or a hospital, and provides results that are more accurate.

Spirometry has a number of functions. First, it is used to help diagnose respiratory diseases, such as asthma and chronic obstructive pulmonary disease (COPD). If these diseases are caught early enough, interventions such as quitting smoking can slow the decline in lung function. Second, spirometry can help assess changes in lung function in people diagnosed with lung disorders. Third, doctors also use spirometry to see how medications like bronchodilators affect a patient's lung function.

Experts recommend that smokers over age 45 and anyone with a chronic cough, excess mucus production, shortness of breath, or wheezing be evaluated with spirometry.

How It Works

The first step in using a spirometer is to inhale deeply to fill your lungs as much as possible. The next step is to exhale as rapidly as you can into a mouthpiece that is connected by a flexible tube to a spirometer. You need to exhale forcefully until your lungs are completely empty, which can take 6 seconds in a healthy person but up to 15 seconds in someone with a lung obstruction. The test is usually repeated two or three times to get the most accurate reading.

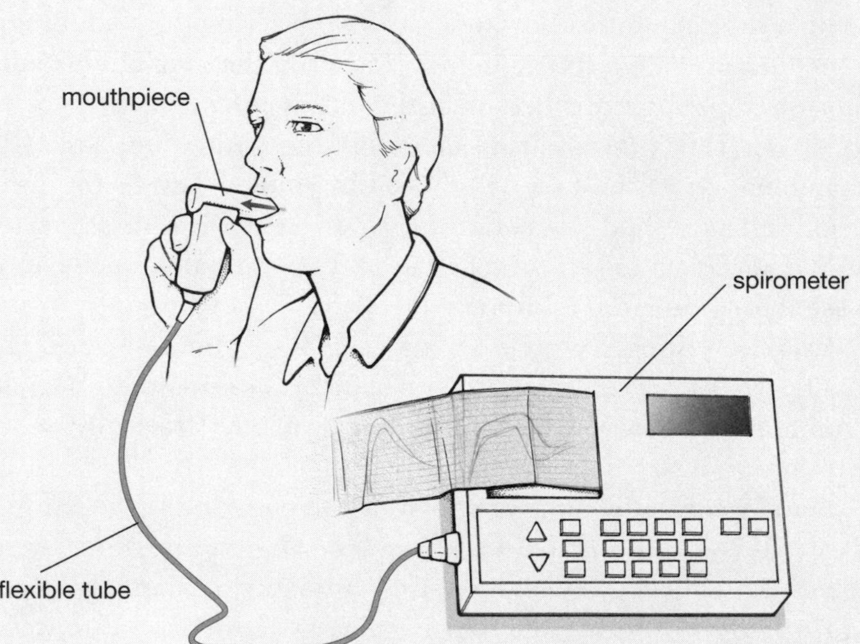

The Results

The two most important values that spirometry measures are forced expiratory volume in one second (FEV_1) and forced vital capacity (FVC). FEV_1 measures the amount of air expelled from the lungs in the first second of a forced exhalation, while FVC is a measure of the total volume of air exhaled. These values are calculated automatically by the spirometer, along with the ratio comparing the amount of air exhaled in the first second with the total amount of air exhaled: FEV_1/FVC.

People with normal lung function usually exhale about 70% to 85% of their capacity in the first second of forced expiration (that is, an FEV_1/FVC of 0.70 to 0.85) This value tends to vary, however, depending on a person's age, height, gender, and ethnicity. (For example, lung function gradually decreases with age, and values considered normal for an 80-year-old are lower than those considered normal for a 50-year-old.) Your FEV_1/FVC ratio is compared with the expected value for your personal characteristics.

If your FEV_1/FVC ratio is less than 70% of your expected value, you likely have some form of obstructive lung disease, like asthma or COPD, and may be at risk for experiencing a high rate of lung-function loss. You may be asked to repeat the test after using a bronchodilator; someone whose FEV_1 improves at least 12% after using a bronchodilator probably has asthma. Your doctor likely will perform further evaluations of lung function to determine what type of lung disease you have, what stage of the disease you are in, and how reversible the condition is.

How Often Spirometry Is Performed

Older smokers and people with chronic lung disease will need to undergo spirometry periodically to monitor their lung function. In patients whose conditions are stable, doctors usually perform spirometry every one to two years. However, more frequent spirometry may be necessary if symptoms suddenly worsen or if the lung condition becomes unstable.

GENERAL APPROACHES TO MANAGEMENT

Usually, the general evaluation just described provides enough information to diagnose a lung disorder and devise a management plan. Sometimes, however, the initial evaluation does not provide a definitive diagnosis. If this is the case, invasive procedures to obtain biopsy samples of lung fluids, cells, and tissues may be necessary. For example, when fluid collects in the space around the lung, it may be sampled ("tapped") with a needle (a procedure called thoracentesis). Analysis of the fluid may aid in diagnosis and treatment, while removal of the fluid might help relieve shortness of breath.

Treating someone with a respiratory illness involves weighing the risks and benefits of each treatment option and taking the patient's personal preferences into account. In some instances, the problem is self-limiting and clears on its own or with treatment. A cure is available for some lung disorders, including many caused by infections. But for most lung disorders, the goal of treatment is to relieve symptoms.

OBSTRUCTIVE DISEASES OF THE LUNGS

Asthma and chronic obstructive pulmonary disease (COPD) are obstructive lung diseases. Obstructive lung diseases are characterized by a reduction in the diameter of the airways that obstructs airflow during exhalation. The obstruction tends to be intermittent and reversible in asthma but unremitting and less responsive to medication in COPD.

Asthma

Asthma is a chronic inflammatory disorder of the airways. It is the eighth most common chronic condition in the United States, affecting nearly 18 million adults. Asthma can be life threatening without proper management and prompt treatment of attacks. In the year 2000, 4,487 people—mostly elderly—died of asthma. Asthma is becoming more commonly recognized in people over the age of 65, who account for about 10% of all people with asthma. Proper care of asthma is especially important in older individuals, who tend to have other health problems and more frequent asthmatic symptoms.

Causes. Asthma is caused by an immune abnormality that appears to have genetic and environmental components. The three

NEW RESEARCH

Asthma Often Undertreated In Older Women

Many older women with asthma do not follow the appropriate treatment guidelines for their condition, a new study shows.

Researchers studied data from 5,107 women in the Nurses' Health Study (average age 63) who had been diagnosed with asthma. Participants were asked about the extent of their symptoms, their use of medication, and related factors.

Only 55% of women treated their asthma adequately, according to the National Asthma Education and Prevention Program guidelines. While 57% of women with mild asthma and 55% of those with moderate asthma took the recommended amount of medication, the number fell to 32% for women with severe asthma. Low adherence rates for women with severe asthma mainly resulted from underuse of oral and inhaled corticosteroids and long-acting bronchodilators. Older age, cigarette smoking, lower socioeconomic status, onset of asthma early in life, and presence of additional medical conditions were factors associated with poorer adherence to asthma guidelines.

The authors conclude that physicians should make a greater effort to evaluate asthma severity and to prescribe more effective therapy when appropriate.

ARCHIVES OF INTERNAL MEDICINE
Volume 162, page 1761
August 12/26, 2002

Minimizing Allergens in the Home

The quality of outdoor air undergoes a great deal of scrutiny, even being rated daily by the U.S. Environmental Protection Agency. When people hear that the air outside is "unhealthy," they may decide to stay home. But indoor air also can be unhealthy if it contains high levels of allergens—substances such as dust mites, pet dander, and mold that can trigger allergic reactions and breathing difficulties in susceptible people.

Assessing the quality of air in the home is especially important for older adults and for those with lung disorders. Allergens cannot be completely eliminated from the home, but they can be kept to a minimum. In addition, no one should smoke in the home of someone with a lung disorder because smoke from cigarettes and other tobacco products can exacerbate allergies and cause breathing problems.

Dust Mites

Dust mites are found in every home and are the most common cause of allergies and breathing difficulties. These microscopic eight-legged creatures live mainly in fabrics, such as carpets, upholstery, bedding, curtains, and stuffed animals. Dust mites feed on human dander (dead skin flakes) and thrive in humid areas of the house. The allergen is actually a protein in the feces of the dust mites. People allergic to dust mites often experience a stuffy or runny nose, sneezing (especially in the morning), itchy or watery eyes, coughing, or wheezing.

To reduce the concentration of dust mites in your home:

• Keep the humidity below 50%. (A small instrument called a hygrometer, available at hardware stores, can be used to measure the humidity level.) A dehumidifier or air conditioner may be needed to control humidity.

• Dust often with a damp cloth, and vacuum carpets and upholstered furniture weekly. (Anyone with a lung disorder should not be in the room while it is being vacuumed.) A central vacuum or a vacuum cleaner with a high-efficiency particulate air (HEPA) filter is most effective.

• Wash sheets and blankets once a week in hot water.

• Down pillows and cotton comforters should be replaced with synthetic materials or encased in plastic or allergen-impermeable covers. Mattresses also should be placed in covers.

If these measures do not help relieve your allergy symptoms or improve breathing, you may need to take further steps to reduce dust mites in your home:

• Wall-to-wall carpeting may need to be replaced with hardwood, tile, or linoleum, which are easier to clean. Throw rugs are fine, as long as they can be dry cleaned or washed regularly in hot water.

• Keep your belongings in closed cabinets or drawers, rather than on top of a dresser or counter where they can collect dust.

Animal Dander

Many people have allergies to pets. Pet allergies are caused by a protein in the saliva, dander, or urine of animals with fur. The protein is carried through the air on microscopic particles that can land on a person's eyelids or be inhaled. Animal allergies can cause sneezing, an itchy or runny nose, or itchy or swollen eyes and throat. All breeds of cats and dogs produce the protein and so can trigger an allergic reaction—or an asthma attack—in a susceptible person.

The most effective way to reduce pet allergies is not to have a pet with

characteristic features of asthma are airway inflammation, airflow obstruction, and hyperreactivity of the airways. Airway inflammation involves swelling of the bronchial lining and excessive production of mucus. These problems can be worsened by a respiratory infection such as sinusitis, influenza, or a cold. Airflow obstruction involves a narrowing of the airways as a result of smooth muscle contraction, swelling of the bronchial lining of the airway, and/or accumulation of excessive mucus. Hyperreactive airways tend to "twitch" when exposed to allergens and other irritants. Although asthma is characterized by repeated asthma attacks (in which symptoms worsen, requiring the use of medication), the inflammation persists even when symptoms are absent and usually requires treatment with medication.

fur or feathers. Keeping a pet outdoors can help, but allergens will still be present in the house. If an animal has been removed, the house must be thoroughly cleaned, especially the areas where the animal spent time. Bedding and carpeting should be replaced if they contain animal dander. People with allergies may still experience symptoms for up to a year or more after the animal is removed from the home.

If you already have a pet that you cannot give away or keep outside:

- Minimize contact between the pet and the person with allergies. Make sure the animal does not go into the bedroom or other rooms where the person with allergies spends a lot of time.
- Washing cats and dogs weekly may reduce the amount of allergens released into the air, but this practice may dry out the animal's skin, so first check with your veterinarian.
- Keep all mattresses and cushions in plastic covers.
- Allergens can sink into the lower levels of carpeting from which they cannot be removed by vacuuming, so hardwood, tile, or linoleum floors are preferable.

Mold

Mold is another common household pollutant that can aggravate allergies and trigger symptoms in people with asthma or chronic obstructive pulmonary disease. Mold starts out as microscopic spores that are present in both indoor and outdoor air. Mold spores begin to grow when they land on wet surfaces, and they thrive in moisture-rich environments. Houses (particularly newer ones) that contain more insulation to prevent drafts often provide ideal conditions for mold growth by trapping excess moisture inside.

A house or apartment may be prone to mold growth if it smells musty, is overly humid, or has condensation on the walls or windows, buckling walls or ceilings, sweaty-looking pipes, or cracking or peeling paint. Mold appears on household surfaces as a white, orange, green, brown, or black discoloration. Inhaling or touching mold can cause breathing problems in susceptible people. Symptoms of mold allergy are similar to those of hay fever and include sneezing, runny nose, red eyes, and skin rash. Mold also can irritate the eyes, skin, nose, throat and lungs of people without mold allergies.

Mold spores cannot be eliminated, but without moisture they cannot grow and become a problem. To eliminate mold growth:

- Make sure your house is well ventilated. Use the bathroom fan or open the window when showering. In the kitchen, use exhaust fans or open the windows when cooking or using the dishwasher.
- Fix any leaking pipes or faucets.
- Keep the humidity between 30% and 50%, using air conditioners or dehumidifiers if necessary.
- To prevent water from entering the house, make sure that the drainage system outside is intact and that the gutters are clean.
- Clean areas where mold is likely to grow: pans under refrigerators or air conditioners, old flowerpots, humidifiers, shower curtains, bathrooms, kitchens, and basements.
- Do not carpet concrete or damp floors, and do not keep clothes or papers in damp places.
- If you find mold on hard surfaces, wash it off using a solution of 5% bleach. Be sure to dry the surface completely.
- Any absorbent surfaces such as carpets or ceiling tiles may need to be replaced if they become moldy.

Depending on the factors that trigger an attack, asthma sometimes is considered either extrinsic or intrinsic. However, the distinction between the two types is not always clear, and some people have both types. In people with extrinsic asthma, which usually begins before age 30, acute episodes are initiated by exposure to a specific environmental irritant. Cigarette smoke, industrial fumes, pollen, molds, dust, animal dander or saliva, and perfumes are common environmental irritants in people with extrinsic asthma. Constriction of smooth muscles in the bronchi when exposed to such irritants can trigger an asthma attack by narrowing the airways and plugging them with sticky mucus. Intrinsic asthma, the most common form in people who develop asthma after age 30, often is characterized by the absence of any identifiable trigger for worsening of symptoms. However,

Using Your Peak Flow Meter

Peak flow meters are handheld devices that measure the rate of airflow expelled from the lungs (the peak expiratory flow rate). They are generally used by people with moderate to severe asthma; people with chronic obstructive pulmonary disease (COPD) usually require spirometry (see the feature on page 8), which provides much more specific information on lung function. Peak flow meters can help determine the severity of the lung condition, monitor the effectiveness of treatments, detect deterioration or improvement in lung function, and identify triggers for attacks. They are a convenient and inexpensive way for patients to monitor lung function on their own on a day-to-day basis.

How To Use a Peak Flow Meter

To use a peak flow meter, you should be standing; sitting upright is acceptable if you have a disability that prevents you from standing. To begin, make sure that the marker is at the bottom of the numerical scale. Breathe in deeply, then tightly close your lips around the mouthpiece, and blow out as hard as possible for a second or two. Avoid pressing your tongue against the hole of the mouthpiece. The marker will denote, in liters per minute, how rapidly you expelled air from your lungs. Record this number, and repeat the process two more times. The highest of the three readings is your peak flow number.

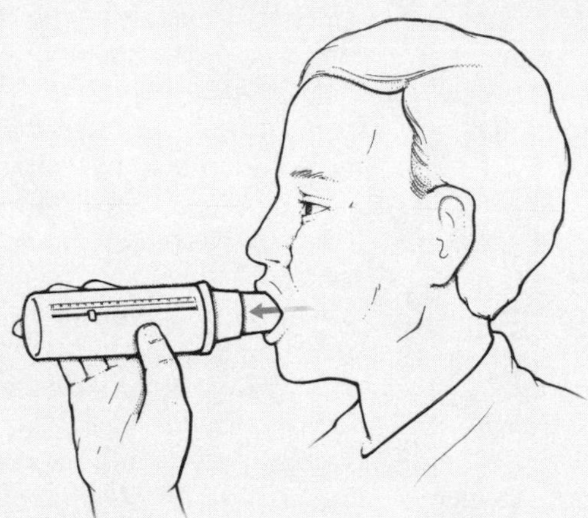

Personal Best Number

To determine how well your asthma is controlled, you will need to compare each peak flow number you obtain to your personal best reading, which is the highest peak flow number you can reach. To determine your personal best peak flow reading, record your peak flow numbers every day for up to three weeks. This process should be done during a time period when your asthma is well controlled. Take the readings at midday (preferably between noon and 2 P.M.), after using an inhaled bronchodilator to relieve symptoms, and whenever else your physician recommends. Record each number. The highest reading you obtain during this three-week period is considered your personal best peak flow number. (As your treatments or condition changes, you may need to determine a new personal best reading.)

exercise, cold or dry air, emotional stress, and gastroesophageal reflux may trigger attacks in people with intrinsic asthma.

Symptoms. The onset of an asthma attack may be gradual or sudden. Some attacks resolve on their own, but most require medication.

During severe attacks, extreme shortness of breath is accompanied by wheezing, tightness in the chest, coughing up thick phlegm, sweating, an elevated respiratory rate, and a rapid pulse. Symptoms may last for only a few minutes, particularly if treated promptly, or may persist for hours or even days despite treatment with medication. Coughing can continue for a week or longer after other acute symptoms disappear.

Milder attacks are more common. They usually begin with tightness in the chest and a cough. Wheezing may be heard with breathing. Restlessness and difficulty sleeping may accompany these

When To Use Your Meter

Once you have established a personal best peak flow number, you and your doctor will need to determine how often you should use your peak flow meter. Many people check their peak flow each morning on awakening, before taking any asthma medication. Many also take readings before and after using an inhaled bronchodilator for symptom relief to see how well the medication is working. If your asthma is severe, you may need to take readings many times a day. When your asthma is under control, you may only need to obtain peak flow readings if your symptoms worsen. Keep a record of your peak flow readings and bring them with you when you see your doctor.

Interpreting Peak Flow Readings

When comparing your peak flow number with your personal best reading, many experts recommend that you categorize the reading into one of three peak flow zones (green, yellow, or red, corresponding to the colors of traffic lights) to determine the status of your asthma and whether you should take actions to get it under control. In general, the peak flow zones and the actions to be taken for each are defined as follows (your doctor may have different recommendations):

Green zone: The peak flow number is between 80% and 100% of your personal best reading. When your peak flow reading falls within the green zone, your condition is well controlled. Continue taking any long-term medications your doctor has prescribed. If your readings are consistently in the green zone, your doctor may consider reducing the amount of your medication.

Yellow zone: The peak flow number is 50% to 79% of your personal best. A reading that falls in this zone indicates that your condition is worsening. You may need to use an inhaled bronchodilator for immediate relief of your symptoms. If you regularly obtain readings in the yellow zone, your doctor will likely increase the amount or dosage of your long-term medications.

Red zone: The peak flow number is lower than 50% of your personal best. A score in this zone indicates the need for immediate action. Use your inhaled bronchodilator for quick relief of your symptoms. If this action does not bring your peak flow number to at least 50% of your personal best, you should contact your doctor or seek immediate medical treatment. Scoring in the red zone indicates that your long-term medications need to be increased to control your symptoms better or that you have an infection.

Buying and Caring for Your Peak Flow Meter

While you can purchase a peak flow meter at a drug store without a prescription for about $20 to $30, you should choose one recommended by your physician. He or she will likely recommend a specific type of peak flow meter, since there are numerous varieties to choose from. Note that "low range" meters are designed for small children; older children and adults should use a "standard range" peak flow meter.

Be sure to keep your peak flow meter clean to obtain the most accurate readings. (Dirt, mucus, and germs can easily accumulate in them.) Generally, they can be cleaned with a mild soap and hot water, but be sure to check the cleaning instructions that come with the meter.

symptoms. Sometimes these mild attacks seem to improve, only to be followed by the reappearance of persistent symptoms that may require treatment in a hospital.

Diagnosis. Diagnosis during an attack usually is apparent from the symptoms, especially if the person has a history of asthma attacks. In older individuals, asthma must be distinguished from COPD and cardiac conditions like heart failure or a heart attack. These conditions can cause fluid to accumulate in the lungs, producing some of the same symptoms as asthma.

Between asthma attacks, a diagnosis may require pulmonary function tests to measure airway obstruction, an examination of mucus from the nose and lungs, and, possibly, allergy tests.

Prevention. People with asthma should avoid asthma triggers whenever possible or take preventive medications as described on

Commonly Used Anti-Inflammatory Drugs 2003

Drug Type	Drug Class	Generic Name	Brand Name	Average Daily Dosage*
Inhaled	Corticosteroids, long-acting	beclomethasone, standard aerosol	Beclovent	2 puffs 3 or 4 times a day
			Vanceril	
		budesonide, powder	Pulmicort Turbuhaler	1 or 2 puffs 2 times a day
		flunisolide, standard aerosol	AeroBid	2 puffs 2 times a day
		flunisolide, menthol	AeroBid-M	2 puffs 2 times a day
		fluticasone, powder	Flovent	1 to 2 puffs 2 times a day
		fluticasone, rotadisk	Flovent Rotadisk	1 to 2 puffs 2 times a day
		triamcinolone, powder	Azmacort	2 puffs 3 or 4 times a day or 4 puffs 2 times a day
	Respiratory inhalers, nonsteroidal	cromolyn, standard aerosol	Intal	2 puffs 4 times a day
		nedocromil, standard aerosol	Tilade	2 puffs 4 times a day
Oral	Corticosteroids, short-acting	methylprednisolone	Medrol	4 to 160 mg
		prednisone	Deltasone	5 to 100 mg
			Meticorten	
			Sterapred	
	Leukotriene modifiers, nonsteroidal	montelukast	Singulair	10 mg
		zafirlukast	Accolate	40 mg
		zileuton	Zyflo	2,400 mg

* These dosages represent an average range for the treatment of asthma and chronic obstructive pulmonary disease. The precise effective dosage varies from patient to patient and depends on many factors. Do not make any changes in your medication without consulting your doctor.

† Average wholesale prices to pharmacists for one device or 100 tablets or capsules of the dosage strength listed. Costs to consumers are higher. Source: *Red Book, 2002* (Medical Economics Data, publishers).

pages 18–22. A handheld device called a peak flow meter measures how well air flows out of the lungs. Taking peak flow meter measurements at home is a simple and accurate way to detect worsening of lung function prior to the onset of symptoms. A person with

Wholesale Cost (Generic Cost)†	Possible Side Effects
16.8-g inhaler: $44.94	Common side effects include sore throat, white patches in the mouth or throat, and hoarseness.
16.8-g inhaler: $46.52	
1 turbuhaler: $129.43	
7-g inhaler: $67.01	
7-g inhaler: $67.01	
7.9-g inhaler: $38.09	
60-dose rotadisk: $37.91	
20-g inhaler: $68.58	
8.1-g inhaler: $53.59	Common side effects include throat irritation and dryness. Rare but serious side effects include difficulty swallowing; hives; itching; swelling of the face, lips, or eyelids; rash; and nosebleeds.
16.2-g inhaler: $42.72	There are no common side effects. Rare but serious side effects include increased wheezing, tightness or pain in the chest, and difficulty breathing.
4 mg: $90.97	Common side effects include increased appetite, indigestion, nervousness, insomnia, greater susceptibility to infections, increased blood pressure, slowed wound healing, weight gain, easy bruising, and fluid retention. Rare but serious side effects include vision problems, frequent urination, increased thirst, rectal bleeding, blistering skin, confusion, hallucinations, paranoia, euphoria, depression, and mood swings.
5 mg: $5.46	
1 mg: $20.70	
5 mg: $42.05	
10 mg: $264.19	Common side effects include headache. Rare but serious side effects include skin rash (indicating potentially life-threatening allergic reaction) and gastroenteritis (causing loss of appetite, nausea, vomiting, stomach upset, fever, and diarrhea).
10 mg: $118.10	Common side effects include headache. Rare but serious side effects include burning or prickling sensation, skin rash, and liver dysfunction (symptoms include abdominal pain, nausea, fatigue, lethargy, itching, yellow discoloration of the eyes or skin, and flu-like symptoms).
600 mg: $85.99	Common side effects include headache, general pain, abdominal pain, nausea, indigestion, muscle soreness, and weakness. Rare but serious side effects include liver problems causing nausea, fatigue, lethargy, skin rash or itching, yellow discoloration of the eyes or skin, flu-like symptoms, and urine that is unusually dark.

asthma determines a "personal best" level of function; decreases from this level signal the need for more aggressive use of medications. For more information on how to use a peak flow meter, see the feature on pages 12–13.

Commonly Used Bronchodilators 2003

Drug Type	Drug Class	Generic Name	Brand Name	Average Daily Dosage*
Inhaled	Anticholinergics, short-acting	ipratropium, standard aerosol	Atrovent	2 puffs every 4 to 6 hours
	$Beta_2$ agonists, short-acting	albuterol, standard aerosol	Proventil Ventolin	2 puffs every 4 to 6 hours
		albuterol, non-CFC propellant	Proventil HFA Ventolin HFA	2 puffs every 4 to 6 hours
		metaproterenol, standard inhaler	Alupent	2 or 3 puffs every 3 to 4 hours
		pirbuterol, standard aerosol	Maxair	1 to 2 puffs every 4 to 6 hours
	$Beta_2$ agonists, long-acting	salmeterol, diskus	Serevent Diskus	1 puff 2 times a day
		formoterol, capsule	Foradil Aerolizer	1 or 2 puffs 2 times a day
	Combination agents	albuterol and ipratropium	Combivent	2 puffs 4 times a day
		albuterol and ipratropium, nebulizer	DuoNeb	1 vial 4 to 6 times a day
		salmeterol and fluticasone, diskus	Advair Diskus	1 puff 2 times a day

* These dosages represent an average range for the treatment of asthma and chronic obstructive pulmonary disease. The precise effective dosage varies from patient to patient and depends on many factors. Do not make any changes in your medication without consulting your doctor.

† Average wholesale prices to pharmacists for one device or 100 tablets or capsules of the dosage strength listed. Costs to consumers are higher. Source: *Red Book, 2002* (Medical Economics Data, publishers).

Wholesale Cost (Generic Cost)†	Possible Side Effects
14-g inhaler: $44.56	Common side effects include dry mouth, cough, and unpleasant taste. Rare but serious side effects include persistent constipation, lower abdominal pain or bloating, wheezing or difficulty breathing, tightness in chest, severe eye pain, skin rash or hives, and swelling of the face, lips, or eyelids.
17-g inhaler: $35.17 17-g inhaler: $35.06 6.7-g inhaler: $33.88 18-g inhaler: $35.06	Common side effects include nervousness, tremor, dizziness, headache, and insomnia. Rare but serious side effects include severe breathing difficulty (signs include persistent wheezing, coughing, shortness of breath, confusion, bluish color to lips or fingernails, and inability to speak).
14-g inhaler: $29.59	Common side effects include trouble sleeping, dry mouth, sore throat, nervousness, and restlessness. Rare but serious side effects include severe breathing difficulty (signs include persistent wheezing, coughing, shortness of breath, confusion, bluish color to lips or fingernails, and inability to speak).
14-g inhaler: $63.78	Common side effects include sleeping difficulty, dry mouth, sore throat, nervousness, excitability, and restlessness. Rare but serious side effects include severe breathing difficulty (signs include persistent wheezing, coughing, shortness of breath, confusion, bluish color to lips or fingernails, and inability to speak), chest pain or heaviness, irregular heartbeat, light-headedness, fainting, severe weakness, and severe headaches.
28-dose diskus: $49.40	Common side effects include headache, sore throat, and runny or stuffy nose. Rare but serious side effects include severe breathing difficulty (signs include persistent wheezing, coughing, shortness of breath, confusion, bluish color to lips or fingernails, and inability to speak), chest pain or heaviness, irregular heartbeat, light-headedness, fainting, severe weakness, and severe headache.
12-dose aerolizer: $22.20	Common side effects include fast heartbeat, headache, nervousness, and trembling. Rare but serious side effects include shortness of breath, difficulty breathing, tightness in the chest, increased wheezing, swelling of the face or eyelids, and skin rash or hives.
14.7-g inhaler: $47.56	Common side effects include coughing, headache, and nausea. Rare but serious side effects include increased wheezing, shortness of breath, chest pain, irregular heartbeat, skin rash or hives, and swelling of the face, lips, eyelids, mouth, or throat.
60 mL: $60.00	There are no common side effects. Rare but serious side effects include swelling of the face, lips, eyelids, mouth, or throat, shortness of breath, increased wheezing, chest pain or discomfort, irregular heartbeat, skin rash or hives, coughing, headache, and nausea.
60-dose 100/50 diskus: $107.06	Common side effects include a high-pitched noise while breathing, body aches, runny or stuffy nose, coughing, dry or sore throat, fever, hoarseness, swollen glands, trouble swallowing, voice changes, and sneezing. Rare but serious side effects include difficulty breathing; shortness of breath; tightness in the chest; increased wheezing; black, tarry stools; chest pain; chills; painful or difficult urination; ulcers; white spots on lips or mouth; fatigue; burning, tingling, or numb sensation in hands and feet; abdominal pain; loss of appetite; nausea; and flu-like symptoms.

Commonly Used Bronchodilators 2003—continued

Drug Type	Drug Class	Generic Name	Brand Name	Average Daily Dosage*
Oral	Methylxanthine derivatives	theophylline, extended-release capsule, 24 hr	Theo-24	300 to 600 mg
		theophylline, extended-release tablet, 12 hr	Theo-Dur	300 to 600 mg
		theophylline, extended-release tablet, 24 hr	Uniphyl	300 to 600 mg

* These dosages represent an average range for the treatment of asthma and chronic obstructive pulmonary disease. The precise effective dosage varies from patient to patient and depends on many factors. Do not make any changes in your medication without consulting your doctor.

† Average wholesale prices to pharmacists for one device or 100 tablets or capsules of the dosage strength listed. Costs to consumers are higher. Source: *Red Book, 2002* (Medical Economics Data, publishers).

Treatment. People with asthma must have a plan of action in case of an attack. They should always have inhaled medication available for self-treatment. A severe attack requires taking medication immediately and quickly getting to a doctor's office or emergency room. A milder attack may require a call or visit to the doctor if symptoms persist longer than usual after using medication. Drug therapy includes the use of bronchodilators and anti-inflammatory drugs. Bronchodilators reduce the constriction of bronchial muscles, while anti-inflammatories help to overcome bronchial inflammation or excessive sensitivity to irritants.

Bronchodilators. Bronchodilators, which promptly open airways by relaxing bronchial smooth muscles, are the most rapidly effective treatment for asthma attacks. They can be taken by mouth (in tablet or capsule form), but inhaled sprays usually are preferred because oral forms take longer to act and produce more side effects. Bronchodilators can be used before activities (such as exercise or exposure to cold air) that are known to trigger asthma. This step may help to prevent an attack or make it less severe and improve a person's ability to perform the activity.

The three types of bronchodilators are beta$_2$ agonists, anticholinergics, and methylxanthine derivatives. Beta$_2$ agonists are the most commonly used type of bronchodilator because they work the fastest and may keep airways open for many hours. The short-acting beta$_2$ agents—albuterol (Proventil, Ventolin), metaproterenol (Alupent), and pirbuterol (Maxair)—begin to act in about 10 minutes and last for 4 to 6 hours. Longer-acting beta$_2$ agents—salmeterol

Wholesale Cost (Generic Cost)†	Possible Side Effects
100 mg: $43.55	Common side effects include restlessness, insomnia, loss of appetite, nervousness, irritability, and nausea. Rare but serious side effects include vomiting; trembling; confusion; rapid, irregular, or pounding pulse; chest pain; dizziness; convulsions; and skin rash.
100 mg: $22.77	
400 mg: $101.83	

(Serevent) and formoterol (Foradil)—act within 15 to 30 minutes and continue to work for up to 12 hours. If symptoms do not improve adequately, people may add the anticholinergic ipratropium (Atrovent), which takes effect in 15 to 30 minutes and lasts for 4 to 6 hours. Combivent, a combination of the beta$_2$ agonist albuterol and the anticholinergic ipratropium, also is available. When used excessively, beta$_2$ agonists can cause tremors and heart palpitations. They also become less effective when overused. People who cannot tolerate beta$_2$ agonists or anticholinergics or who experience asthma symptoms at night may use one of the extended-release oral forms of the methylxanthine derivative theophylline (Theo-24, Theo-Dur, Uniphyl). Side effects of theophylline include nausea and insomnia.

Anti-inflammatory medications. Continuous use of anti-inflammatory drugs to control chronic inflammation is a critical aspect of asthma therapy. The first choice of medications to counter inflammation in adults is inhaled corticosteroids, which include beclomethasone (Beclovent, Vanceril), budesonide (Pulmicort), flunisolide (AeroBid), and fluticasone (Flovent). A combination of the corticosteroid fluticasone and the long-acting beta$_2$ agonist salmeterol is also available (Advair). The most frequent side effects of inhaled corticosteroids are irritation of the throat and a yeast infection of the mouth and throat. These side effects can be reduced by rinsing the mouth and cleaning the inhaler after each use.

Corticosteroids also can cause osteoporosis, high blood pressure, roundness of the face, weight gain, diabetes, cataracts, and

Using a Metered Dose Inhaler

For people with asthma or chronic obstructive pulmonary disease (COPD), using an inhaler is the fastest method of delivering medication to the lungs. It is also the safest; the risk of side effects is lower than with tablets or capsules because inhaled medications act primarily on the lungs.

Inhaled medications may be delivered three ways—the most common is using a metered dose inhaler (MDI), a pressurized canister that releases an aerosol spray. Dry powder inhalers (such as Diskhaler and Turbuhaler) and nebulizers are the other two options for delivering inhaled medications to the lungs.

An inhaler can be difficult to use because it requires coordination between releasing the medication and breathing in. Even when an inhaler is used correctly, most of the medication sticks to the back of the throat and no more than 10% to 20% reaches the lungs. The key to getting the most from your inhaler is to use the proper technique. If you follow these steps on how to use an MDI, more of the medicine will reach your lungs. In addition, your doctor can observe you using your inhaler to make sure that you are using it properly.

Using a Metered Dose Inhaler

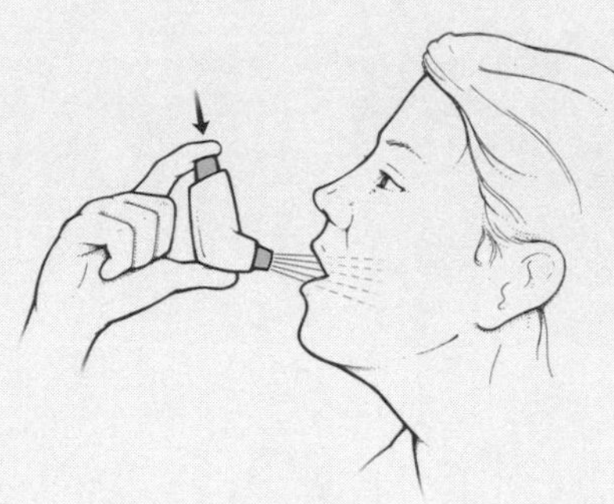

1. Place the metal canister into the plastic mouthpiece.

2. Remove the cap from the mouthpiece and shake the inhaler for 5 to 10 seconds.

3. Breathe out to the end of a normal breath (but don't force air out).

4. Hold the mouthpiece of the inhaler 1 to 2 inches (about two finger widths) from your mouth, tilt your head back slightly, and open your mouth wide. Start to breathe in slowly as you press down once on the metal canister to release a puff of medication.

5. Continue to inhale until your lungs are full (for about five seconds). Inhaling too quickly will increase the amount of medication that sticks to the back of the throat.

6. Hold your breath for 10 seconds, or for as long as is comfortable.

7. Before exhaling, move the inhaler away from your mouth and release your finger from the canister.

8. Replace the cap on the mouthpiece to avoid contamination by dust and other particles.

9. For an additional dose, wait one minute and repeat steps 2 through 8.

10. Clean the plastic mouthpiece once a week by removing the metal canister and rinsing the plastic portion in warm water; allow it to air dry. Replace the metal canister and the cap on the mouthpiece.

When Using a Spacer

A spacer (also called a holding chamber) holds the medication for a few seconds after it has been released from the inhaler. This delay can be helpful for people who have difficulty coordinating their breathing with the use of an inhaler. People on inhaled corticosteroids also may benefit from spacers, since they help reduce side effects such as sore throat and hoarse voice that are caused by medication sticking to the back of the throat. Spacers are simple to use, can be fitted to most inhalers, and can either be rigid or collapsible. Here are guidelines for using both types of spacers:

thinning of the skin when used for long periods of time, but these side effects are rare with inhaled corticosteroids because little of the medication is absorbed into the bloodstream. Oral corticosteroids can provide rapid and dramatic relief of symptoms during a severe attack, but they must be used at the lowest effective dose and for the shortest possible time to avoid the side effects listed above. Also, using corticosteroids for more than several weeks suppresses the adrenal gland. Consequently, the medication must be discontinued slowly to allow recovery of adrenal function.

Nonsteroidal anti-inflammatory inhaled medications also are used in people with asthma. Cromolyn (Intal) and nedocromil (Tilade), which act to prevent the release of histamine, are inhaled drugs used only for long-term prevention of asthma symptoms (not

Using a Rigid Spacer

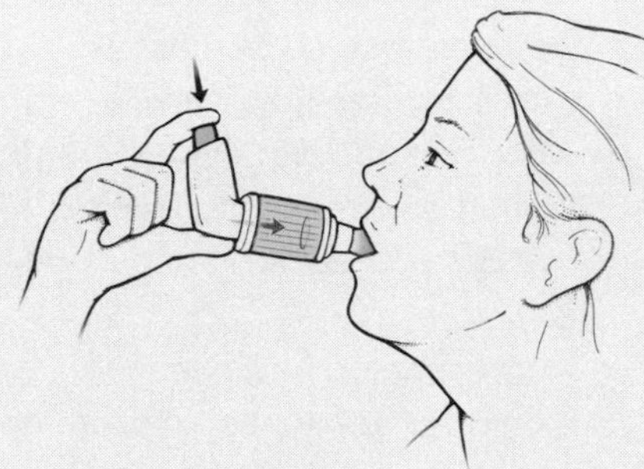

Press down on the metal canister so that the spacer fills with medication.

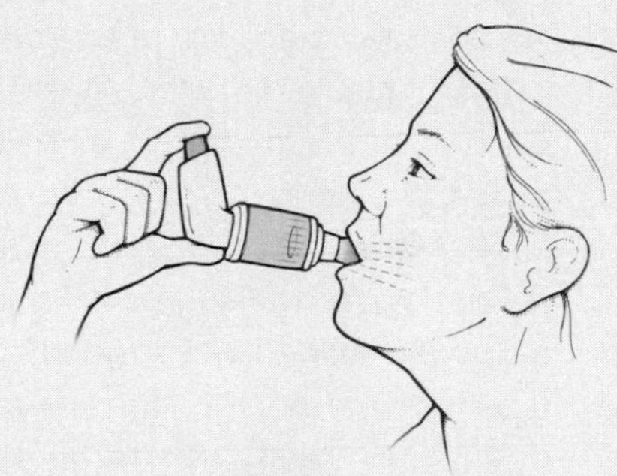

Breathe in slowly for about five seconds.

1. Remove the cap from the mouthpiece of the inhaler and insert the mouthpiece into the large opening of the rigid spacer. For a collapsible spacer, insert the mouthpiece of the spacer into the opening of the reservoir bag. Align the locking tabs and twist to lock. Then, untwist the reservoir bag until it is entirely open.

2. For a rigid spacer, hold the spacer and inhaler together and shake for 5 to 10 seconds. For a collapsible spacer, shake the metal canister separately for five seconds before inserting it into the adapter port of the spacer's mouthpiece.

3. Breathe out, then put the mouthpiece in your mouth, closing your lips around it.

4. Press the metal canister down.

5. Breathe in slowly for about five seconds.

6. Hold your breath for about 10 seconds or as long as is comfortable.

7. If your spacer is rigid, slowly exhale through your mouth or nose (not into the spacer), then take another breath through the mouthpiece to ensure you receive the full amount of medication released by the inhaler. If you have a collapsible spacer, slowly exhale into the spacer. Breathe in and out a second time (steps 5 and 6) with your lips around the mouthpiece.

8. Repeat steps 2 through 7 for each puff that your doctor prescribes, waiting a full minute between each.

Using a Collapsible Spacer

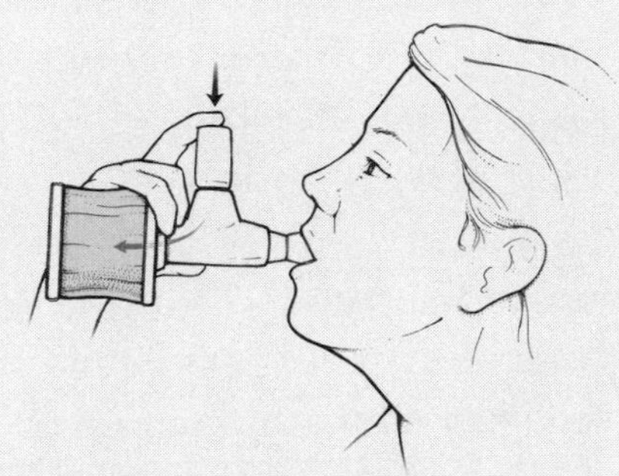

Press down on the metal canister so that the spacer fills with medication.

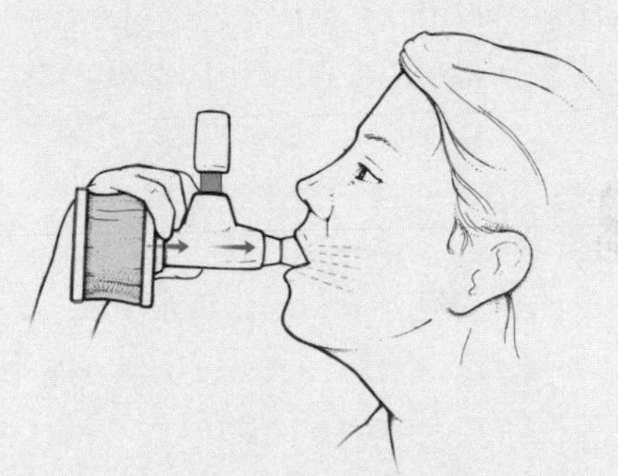

Breathe in slowly for about five seconds.

9. To ensure that your spacer is clean, run warm water through the large opening and allow it to air dry. If your spacer is collapsible you should replace it once or twice each month.

for immediate relief). The leukotriene modifiers montelukast (Singulair), zafirlukast (Accolate), and zileuton (Zyflo), which counter the actions of leukotrienes (hormones that narrow bronchi and stimulate the production of mucus), may prevent exercise-induced asthma and can enhance the action of inhaled corticosteroids. The effectiveness of these medications varies considerably from person to person.

Inhaled medications usually are administered through a device called a metered dose inhaler (MDI). An MDI delivers a highly concentrated amount of medication directly to the bronchi. Inhaled medications are less likely to produce systemic side effects than oral medications. But proper technique (see the feature above) is important, and most people use their MDI incorrectly. People who find it difficult to use an MDI can choose a spacer, an attachment that eliminates the need to release the medication and inhale simultaneously. Many people experience considerable improvement in their condition after adding a spacer. Another option is to use a device called a nebulizer, which vaporizes liquid medication into a fine mist that can be inhaled easily.

Chronic Obstructive Pulmonary Disease (COPD)

Chronic obstructive pulmonary disease is a term that encompasses chronic bronchitis and emphysema. The symptoms of COPD develop slowly over several years and include wheezing, chronic cough with production of phlegm, and progressive shortness of breath. COPD is the fourth leading cause of death in the United States.

Emphysema is a disorder characterized by destruction of lung tissue, including its elastic fibers. By reducing the elasticity of the lungs and destroying the walls between the alveoli, emphysema leads to airway collapse and reduced airflow. More than 1 million Americans have emphysema, and nearly 17,000 people die of it each year. Emphysema rates are highest for men age 65 and older.

Chronic bronchitis is a recurrent problem defined by coughing up phlegm nearly every day for at least three months of the year (for example, every winter) for two or more consecutive years (assuming there is no other underlying cause of these symptoms). The condition reduces the diameter of the airways through a combination of bronchial inflammation and overproduction of mucus. There are nearly 9 million cases of chronic bronchitis a year in the United States and more than 1,000 deaths. Chronic bronchitis is more prevalent in women than in men.

Causes. Cigarette smoking causes the vast majority of COPD cases. Cigarette smoking is thought to release proteases, enzymes that damage a protein called elastin that makes the lungs elastic. Smoking also is believed to inactivate alpha$_1$-antitrypsin, a protein produced by the liver that protects elastin from the action of proteases.

About 1 in 2,500 white people have a genetic mutation that prevents the secretion of alpha$_1$-antitrypsin by the liver and increases the risk of developing premature emphysema, especially in smokers. Other factors that increase the likelihood of emphysema include a family history of COPD, male gender, and respiratory illnesses in childhood.

Symptoms. People with COPD typically began smoking at an early age and have a long history of a morning cough that produces phlegm. Their lung function often declines slowly over a period of

NEW RESEARCH

Nitrogen Dioxide, Ozone Raise Death Risk With Severe Asthma

New research shows that people with severe asthma have an elevated risk of dying of their condition on days with high levels of two pollutants: nitrogen dioxide and ozone.

Investigators reviewed the records of 1,078 people over age 14 with severe asthma who died between 1985 and 1995 in Barcelona, Spain. The researchers analyzed the levels of air pollution (particulate matter, nitrogen dioxide, ozone, and black smoke), pollen, and spores on the days of each death.

For people with severe asthma (i.e., more than one emergency room visit for asthma), the risk of death from any cause was 50% higher on days with the highest nitrogen dioxide levels than on days with the lowest levels. During the spring and summer, the risk of death was 90% higher on days with the highest ozone levels than on days with low ozone. Pollen, spores, and particulate matter were not related to the risk of death.

Some previous research had linked air pollutants to worsening asthma symptoms, although the link is much stronger for chronic obstructive pulmonary disease. This is the first study to demonstrate that nitrogen dioxide and ozone are associated with increased death rates in people with severe asthma.

THORAX
Volume 57, page 687
August 2002

many years before they seek medical advice, usually after age 50 and after noting significant shortness of breath on exertion. As COPD worsens over time, breathlessness begins to severely limit activities. The slow decrease in function often is punctuated by acute episodes of worsening symptoms, usually due to a viral infection with or without a bacterial infection. These acute episodes are marked by increased shortness of breath, wheezing, and a cough that produces greater-than-usual amounts of phlegm. Though acute episodes may be severe enough to be life threatening, they do not necessarily speed the rate of disease progression. COPD also may cause low levels of oxygen in the blood, which can lead to a rise in pressure in the arteries to the lungs (pulmonary hypertension). Pulmonary hypertension increases the workload of the right ventricle of the heart, causing it to enlarge. At advanced stages of COPD, patients often are thin because they find eating to be tiring.

Diagnosis. People with COPD have abnormal results on spirometry testing (see the feature on page 8). Spirometry not only indicates the presence and severity of the disorder but also predicts the prognosis.

People with COPD may appear breathless at rest and may grunt or wheeze with each exhalation, and the chest often is enlarged from overinflation of the lungs. Chronic bronchitis often is accompanied by raspy breath sounds that can be heard with a stethoscope. Emphysema is characterized by a hyperinflated chest and diminished breath sound intensity. Patients who develop cor pulmonale may have enlarged neck veins, swelling of the legs (edema), and a loud pulmonic second heart sound found during a heart examination, suggesting pulmonary hypertension.

A chest x-ray may show increased volume of air in the lungs and enlargement of the pulmonary arteries. Sometimes, changes also can be seen on an electrocardiogram, depending on the stage of the disease. Seeking a genetic cause by measuring levels of alpha$_1$-antitrypsin may be useful when COPD occurs in a young person or nonsmoker.

Prevention. Avoidance of cigarette smoking is the most obvious and effective way to prevent COPD. People with a deficiency of alpha$_1$-antitrypsin may receive some protection from weekly intravenous injections of the substance, but such treatments are expensive and inconvenient.

Treatment. Only about half of people with COPD survive for 10 years or more after the diagnosis is made. The goals of COPD treatment are to prolong life, maintain independence, and make people

NEW RESEARCH

Inhaled Corticosteroids Reduce Risk of Death from Asthma

Use of inhaled corticosteroids may lower the risk of death from asthma, a new study indicates. By contrast, excessive use of short-acting beta$_2$ agonist inhalers is linked to a greater chance of dying of asthma.

Researchers analyzed data from 96,258 people (age 10 to 78) with asthma who were in the United Kingdom's General Research Database between 1994 and 1998. Each of the 43 people who died from asthma was matched by age and gender to 20 people with asthma who had not died.

Compared with people who needed fewer than 3 prescriptions for short-acting beta$_2$ agonist inhalers in a year, those who obtained 7 to 12 prescriptions were 16 times more likely to die of asthma, and those who obtained 13 or more prescriptions were 52 times more likely to die of asthma. In people who needed 13 or more prescriptions of short-acting beta$_2$ agonists, the risk of death decreased by 60% if they also received 7 or more prescriptions of inhaled corticosteroids.

"Evidence is mounting to suggest that inhaled steroids prevent asthma death," the authors write. However, the lack of effect of short-acting beta$_2$ agonists is "disconcerting," they conclude.

THORAX
Volume 57, page 683
August 2002

Eating Well With COPD

A healthy diet may be especially helpful for people with chronic obstructive pulmonary disease (COPD). Some studies show that COPD patients who eat a well-balanced diet are less likely to experience worsening symptoms and to die of COPD. This is because good nutrition is required for the proper functioning of the lungs and of the muscles involved in breathing. Good nutrition also may reduce the risk of respiratory infections, which are often the cause of death in COPD patients.

Despite the potential benefits of a healthy diet, experts estimate that between 20% and 60% of people with COPD do not get enough calories and nutrients from their diet. The reasons are multifold. People with COPD have increased energy demands and need to consume more calories than people with healthy lungs. At the same time, COPD can make it difficult to get those extra calories. Shortness of breath and fatigue can make preparing food arduous and eating it unenjoyable. In addition, some of the medications used to manage COPD can cause gastrointestinal upset or sore throat, making people less likely to want to eat. The result is that many COPD patients lose weight and their condition worsens.

A Healthy Diet

People with COPD may need to make an extra effort to eat well.

Get enough calories. Weight loss is common in people with COPD, particularly those with emphysema. Weight loss occurs when energy expenditure exceeds the amount of energy received from food.

People with COPD use 20% to 50% more energy than healthy people, mainly because their breathing requires more work. Infection and medications such as bronchodilators also may be contributing factors. As a result, COPD patients need to consume more calories. But they often do not feel well enough to eat properly, so they lose weight.

Weight loss leads to loss of muscle mass, including the muscles used for breathing. When these respiratory muscles atrophy and weaken, the ability of the lungs to do their job may be impaired and symptoms can worsen. Some studies show that underweight COPD patients are more likely to have their symptoms worsen and are at higher risk for death from COPD. But research also shows that increasing calorie intake can strengthen the respiratory muscles and may improve lung function.

You can determine whether you are underweight by calculating your body mass index (BMI). First, multiply your weight in pounds by 704. Second, multiply your height in inches by itself. Then, divide the first number by the second. If your BMI is less than 20, you are considered underweight and should talk to a doctor or dietitian about increasing your calorie intake. You can gain weight by eating more food or by adding liquid nutritional supplements to your diet. Tips on increasing your calorie intake are described at right.

Eat a variety of foods. Not unlike healthy people, those with COPD need to eat foods from each of the five basic food groups (fruits; vegetables; cereals and grains; dairy products; and protein [meat, poultry, fish, legumes, nuts, and eggs]) to make sure they are getting adequate nutrients. The U.S. Department of Agriculture's Food Guide Pyramid recommends that adults eat 2 to 4 servings of fruit, 3 to 5 servings of vegetables,

more comfortable. These goals are achieved through a combination of lifestyle measures, medications, vaccinations, oxygen therapy, and, rarely, surgical procedures.

Lifestyle measures. Two interventions associated with improved survival in people with COPD are smoking cessation and (in patients with low oxygen levels) pulmonary rehabilitation. Of utmost importance is smoking cessation, the sooner the better. Even people with advanced COPD can increase their life expectancy if they stop smoking. (For tips on quitting smoking, see the feature on pages 44–45). People with COPD should avoid exposure to other airborne toxins (including secondhand cigarette smoke), exercise as much as possible, and follow an adequate diet (see the feature above). People who find eating to be tiring may prefer to eat several

6 to 11 servings of cereals and grains, 2 to 3 servings of dairy products, and 2 to 3 servings of protein each day. To learn more about the Food Guide Pyramid and what constitutes a serving, visit www.nal.usda.gov:8001/py/pmap.htm.

Certain nutrients are of particular importance to people with COPD, because some studies show that they may improve lung function and reduce symptoms. One such group of nutrients is the antioxidant vitamins, which include vitamin C, vitamin E, and beta-carotene. These nutrients are thought to protect the airways against damage from free radicals and inhaled oxidants, which may cause or worsen COPD. Deep green and yellow-orange fruits and vegetables are rich sources of antioxidants. Beta-carotene supplements are not recommended as a source of antioxidants because they increase the risk of lung cancer in people who smoke.

Some studies also have shown that high intakes of fish and whole grains are associated with better lung function and less severe symptoms in people with COPD. Fish contains omega-3 fatty acids, a type of fat that may help prevent lung damage by reducing inflammation. Whole grains, like fruits and vegetables, contain antioxidants.

Limit salt, caffeine, and alcohol. These compounds may negatively affect COPD. Excess salt intake can cause fluid retention, which can interfere with breathing. Caffeine can interact adversely with certain COPD medications and can make you feel nervous. And alcohol in excessive amounts can exacerbate the symptoms of COPD.

Avoid foods that cause gas or bloating. Gas and abdominal bloating can be a problem for people with COPD because it makes breathing more difficult. Foods that can cause gas and bloating include apples, melons, cabbage, broccoli, cauliflower, onions, legumes, nuts, and carbonated beverages. These foods should be avoided if they cause problems.

Tips for Increasing Calorie Intake

Here are some tips to help you add more calories to your diet:

- Eat five to six small meals per day instead of three large ones. Eating small meals uses up less oxygen and produces less carbon dioxide. In addition, a full stomach puts pressure on your diaphragm, which can make breathing more difficult.
- Choose calorie-dense foods such as peanut butter, cheese, and eggs.
- Choose foods that are soft in texture. They are easier to eat when you are short of breath.
- Use convenience and prepared foods (but read the labels to make sure they are not high in salt).
- Use an exhaust fan or open a window while cooking. Cooking odors and heat can make breathing difficult.
- If you use supplemental oxygen, wear your cannula while eating and after meals. Eating and digestion require extra oxygen.
- Prepare extra servings of your favorite dishes when you're not feeling tired. Then store them in the freezer for later use.
- Some groups provide meals for people either free or at a small charge. Check with government agencies or religious organizations in your area.
- Ask your doctor whether you may benefit from a high-fat diet. In addition to boosting calorie intake, a high-fat diet may reduce the need to breathe by decreasing production of carbon dioxide. The danger of a high-fat diet is that it may contribute to cardiovascular disease, so the benefits and risks must be weighed carefully.

small meals a day rather than a few large ones. Adding a liquid protein supplement to the daily diet may improve overall nutrition and help prevent weight loss. It is also important to drink plenty of fluids to avoid dehydration. People with COPD should be careful to rest when they get tired and should avoid exerting themselves when it is too hot, cold, or humid, or when air quality is poor.

Recent observations have underscored the benefits of pulmonary rehabilitation programs for people with COPD. While maintaining general strength through regular aerobic exercise is beneficial, lung exercises to strengthen the muscles used for breathing are particularly important. Breath training helps to control breathing rate, decrease the amount of energy required for breathing, and improve the position and function of the respiratory muscles. A respiratory therapist can help people with COPD practice the following techniques:

• Pursed-lip breathing. Inhale through your nose, and then exhale with your lips pursed in a whistling or kissing position. Each inhalation should take about four seconds, and each exhalation about six seconds. It is not clear how pursed-lip breathing brings symptom relief, but it may work by keeping the airways open.

• Diaphragmatic breathing. The diaphragm is the main muscle used in normal breathing. People with COPD, however, may use the muscles in the rib cage, neck, and abdomen to aid in breathing. This method is less efficient than using the diaphragm. To practice using the diaphragm, lie on your back, place your hand on your abdomen, and breathe. Your hand should rise on inhalation and fall on exhalation. Practice for 20 minutes twice daily. Once you have mastered this skill while lying down, try to do it while sitting up.

• Forward-bending posture. Breathing while bending slightly forward from the waist relieves symptoms for some people with severe COPD, possibly because the diaphragm has more room to expand.

Medications. Despite their fixed obstruction, many people with COPD do have some response to bronchodilators. Most commonly used are the $beta_2$ agonists, which are described on page 18. Theophylline derivatives are less effective than $beta_2$ agonists, but they may ease symptoms in about 20% of people with COPD. If bronchodilators fail to relieve airway obstruction adequately, corticosteroids (described on page 19) may diminish inflammation. But corticosteroids are less effective for COPD than for asthma, and their side effects may be heightened in older patients. Because of the difficulty in predicting who will respond to corticosteroid therapy, a carefully monitored two- to three-week trial period of oral corticosteroids is often tried. Oral corticosteroids are discontinued promptly in people who do not benefit from them and are tapered to the lowest effective dose in people who do benefit. Inhaled corticosteroids may be helpful in selected patients, and their role in the treatment of COPD continues to be assessed.

Expectorants (such as guaifenesin, found in Robitussin and other medications) may help to loosen mucus secretions in the airways. Antibiotics, such as tetracycline, ampicillin, erythromycin, and combinations of trimethoprim and sulfamethoxazole, are given when increased production of yellow or green phlegm signals a respiratory infection that can worsen COPD. Although moderate exacerbations can be treated at home, severe episodes require hospitalization.

Vaccinations. Patients with COPD should receive the pneumo-

NEW RESEARCH

Exercise Improves Shortness Of Breath With COPD

Engaging in a regular program of exercise training can help improve symptoms of dyspnea (shortness of breath) in patients with chronic obstructive pulmonary disease (COPD), a recent report shows.

Researchers randomized 103 people over age 40 who had COPD to either a mild exercise group (walking 20 minutes a day, four times a week), a moderate exercise group (walking plus a 30-minute supervised treadmill exercise session every other week), or a high exercise group (walking plus treadmill exercise three times a week).

Though all groups reported less dyspnea after eight weeks, the more exercise patients performed, the more their dyspnea symptom scores dropped. Patients in the high exercise group had much less dyspnea than those in the moderate and mild exercise groups during an incremental treadmill test, an endurance treadmill test, and a six-minute walk. Patients in the high exercise group also felt that they had more energy and were in better control of their condition.

By relieving dyspnea, exercise training may be an important way to improve quality of life in patients with COPD.

JOURNAL OF CARDIOPULMONARY REHABILITATION
Volume 22, page 109
March/April 2002

coccal vaccine and have annual influenza vaccinations to minimize the risk of acute exacerbations of their symptoms (see the feature on pages 52–53).

Oxygen therapy. Supplemental oxygen can improve function and survival for people whose severely impaired lung function is due to abnormally low concentrations of oxygen in the blood. Home oxygen therapy typically improves sleep and mood, increases mental alertness and stamina, allows patients to carry out normal functions more efficiently, and may prevent the development of cor pulmonale.

A variety of oxygen delivery systems and oxygen conservation devices are available. Home oxygen is available as compressed gas or as a liquid, or it can be extracted from room air. Gas and liquid oxygen must be purchased from a supplier and stored in steel or aluminum canisters. Larger canisters usually are kept in the bedroom; smaller ones are used when away from home. Liquid oxygen often is preferred by active people. It is more portable than compressed gas because larger amounts can be stored in smaller containers, but it has a limited shelf life and is more expensive.

An electric device called an oxygen concentrator can be used to extract oxygen from room air, which is about 20% oxygen. Oxygen concentrators are easier to maintain than other forms of oxygen therapy, but they are not suitable for everyone. They are not portable, some emit heat and are noisy, and the concentration of oxygen is lower than that in purchased gas or liquid oxygen. In addition, a backup source of oxygen is necessary in case of power failure.

All forms of oxygen therapy are expensive; costs may be several hundred dollars a month, depending on the type of system. Oxygen concentrators are the least costly.

Lung volume reduction surgery. Some people whose emphysema is associated with large bullae (balloon-like spaces in the lung) may benefit from surgery to remove diseased lung tissue, called lung volume reduction surgery. Removing diseased lung tissue is believed to create more space in the chest cavity for the good lung tissue to expand. Lung volume reduction surgery is experimental and is available only as part of a clinical trial.

Lung transplantation. Another option for people with emphysema is lung transplantation. About 1,250 lung transplants are performed annually worldwide. About 60% of these involve a single lung (unilateral), and 40% involve both lungs (bilateral). Unilateral transplants are used for emphysema and pulmonary fibrosis (chronic inflammation and progressive scarring of the walls of the alveoli);

NEW RESEARCH

Tiotropium Beats Salmeterol for COPD

Tiotropium (Spiriva), an investigational dry-powder inhaled medication, is better than salmeterol (Serevent) for treating many aspects of chronic obstructive pulmonary disease (COPD), a new study indicates.

Researchers randomized 623 people (age 40 and older) who had COPD to take 8 micrograms (mcg) of tiotropium once daily, 50 mcg of salmeterol twice daily, or a placebo.

After six months, the tiotropium group showed greater benefits than the salmeterol group on a test of forced expiratory volume in one second (FEV_1) in the morning before the medication was taken (137 mL vs. 85 mL improvement over the placebo). While both groups showed improvements in FEV_1 during the 12-hour period after a dose of drugs, tiotropium provided greater improvements than salmeterol (215 mL vs. 138 mL). Tiotropium improved shortness of breath significantly better than the placebo, while salmeterol did not. Both medications improved health-related quality of life, but more patients had significant improvements with tiotropium.

"Tiotropium can be considered as an appropriate first-line therapy for patients experiencing symptomatic COPD," the authors say. Tiotropium is not approved for use in the United States.

CHEST
Volume 122, page 47
July 2002

Ozone and Your Health

Ozone is a popular topic in the news: In the summertime, we hear about ozone alerts, and throughout the year, we hear about depletion of the ozone layer. So just what is ozone, and how does it affect your health, specifically your lungs?

What Is Ozone?

Ozone is a compound similar to oxygen. But whereas oxygen (O_2) is composed of two oxygen atoms, ozone (O_3) is made up of three oxygen atoms. Ozone occurs naturally in the upper atmosphere, 10 to 30 miles above the earth, where it helps filter out the sun's ultraviolet rays. This "good" type of ozone is damaged by chlorofluorocarbons and other pollutants that have created holes in the ozone layer in the upper atmosphere. These holes permit ultraviolet light to reach the earth's surface, leading to health problems (such as skin cancer) and environmental damage.

Ozone is harmful when it is located closer to the earth, in the air that we breathe. This "bad" ozone is formed, in part, from nitrogen dioxide (NO_2), a by-product of burning fuel from automobiles, utility plants, and factories. On hot, sunny days, the heat and strong sunlight break NO_2 into two parts: nitric oxide (NO) and an oxygen atom (O). This single oxygen atom can then combine with oxygen (O_2) in the air to form ozone (O_3). On cooler days, ozone readily turns back into oxygen.

Ozone: Where and When?

Ground-level ozone is mostly a problem in large urban and suburban centers, where pollution levels from cars and industrial plants are high. Rural areas typically, but not always, have lower ozone levels. Ozone carried by the wind for hundreds of miles from urban centers can linger in rural areas; factories and utility plants in rural areas also can contribute to high ozone levels there.

Ozone levels tend to be highest in the hotter months, owing to the roles of sunlight and heat in ozone formation. In the southern and southwestern United States, which tend to be hot year-round, ozone problems can last all year. In addition, ozone levels tend to be highest during the day and lowest at night.

How Ozone Affects the Lungs

When ozone is inhaled, it can inflame and damage the bronchioles (the smaller air passages that branch off from the larger bronchi) and the alveoli (the sacs that branch off from the bronchioles and pass oxygen into the bloodstream). Symptoms of ozone exposure include throat irritation, an uncomfortable feeling in the chest, and coughing. Ozone can also temporarily reduce lung capacity and make physical activity difficult. Extended exposure to high amounts of ozone over months or years can, in some cases, result in permanent lung damage. While ozone exposure has been shown to make people more vulnerable to bacterial pneumonia, it has not been linked to any form of cancer.

Who Is Most Affected?

Three types of people are most likely to be adversely affected by ground-level ozone. A small number of people are inherently sensitive to ozone exposure for reasons that are unclear. Healthy people who spend a lot of time exercising outdoors also are susceptible to ozone damage.

The final group of people who are highly vulnerable to the effects of ozone are those with a lung disease such as asthma or chronic obstructive pulmonary disease. For people with such conditions, ozone exposure can make breathing difficult and

bilateral transplants are used for cystic fibrosis (an inherited disease in infants, children, and young adults) and bronchiectasis.

The scarcity of donor lungs and the risks of the procedure make it necessary to carry out extensive evaluations to select the most suitable candidates for lung transplantation. Candidates must meet disease-specific criteria for severe (end-stage) lung disease and yet be able to survive the wait for one or both donor lungs and the rigors of the operation and postoperative period. In 1998, international guidelines established an upper age limit of 64 for unilateral and 59 for bilateral transplants. Transplants cannot be performed in people with major abnormalities in other organs; human immunodeficiency virus (HIV); malignancies (other than basal or squamous cell skin cancers) diagnosed within the prior

aggravate symptoms. For example, people with asthma are more likely to have asthma attacks on days when ozone levels are high.

Limiting Ozone Exposure
Although the symptoms of ozone exposure may diminish with extended exposure, damage to the lungs still occurs. Therefore, all people, but especially those with a lung disease, need to take precautions to limit their ozone exposure.

The first step is to find out what the ozone levels will be in your area each day. Many news outlets print or broadcast an Air Quality Index daily (see the box at right).

If you have a lung disease and ozone levels are predicted to exceed 100 for the day, or an ozone alert is declared, you should avoid spending long periods of time outdoors and severely limit any outdoor physical exertion. (The amount of ozone you inhale is directly related to the amount of time you are exposed to it and how much you exert yourself during this time.)

If you plan to perform activities outdoors on a day when the ozone levels are high, do them either in the morning or in the evening when ozone levels are lower.

Air Quality Index
When news organizations report the air quality for a given day, they use the Air Quality Index, a scale developed by the U.S. Environmental Protection Agency (see the table below). When ozone levels are predicted to be particularly high, officials may declare an "Ozone Alert" or an "Ozone Action Day." (Rather than using numbers to depict ozone levels, many organizations use the color-coded alerts listed in the table below.) If your local news does not provide ozone information, go to www.epa.gov/airnow for detailed information on ozone and other pollutants in your area. Alternatively, visit the Web site www.weather.com, and under "Health," click on "Air Quality Forecast." Select your state to find out the ozone levels for cities in your area.

Air Quality Index	Air Quality	Precautions for People With Lung Disease
0-50	Good (green)	Outdoor activity is safest.
51-100	Moderate (yellow)	People highly sensitive to ozone should limit exertion outdoors, but conditions should otherwise be safe for those with a lung disease.
101-150	Unhealthy for sensitive groups (orange)	Limit extended periods of exertion outdoors.
151-200	Unhealthy (red)	Avoid prolonged exertion outdoors.
201+	Very unhealthy (purple)	Avoid all outdoor exertion.

two years; positive tests for hepatitis B antigen; or hepatitis C infection with liver disease. The procedure may not be suitable for people who have severe osteoporosis or are extremely overweight.

Like those who receive transplants of other solid organs, lung transplant patients are required to take medications for the rest of their life to suppress the immune system and prevent it from rejecting the transplanted lung(s). After successful transplantation, patients may have some limitations in exercise tolerance but usually not enough to interfere with normal daily activities or adversely affect their quality of life. The two-year survival rate following lung transplantation (approximately 62%) is highest in those treated for underlying emphysema and lowest in those with idiopathic pulmonary fibrosis (progressive scarring of the lungs in which the cause is unknown) or pulmonary hypertension. The most common cause of rejection, and the most dangerous complication of transplantation, is a condition called bronchiolitis obliterans, in which the bronchioles become blocked. Other common complications are infections and the side effects of the immunosuppressive drugs.

SLEEP APNEA

Sleep apnea is a disorder characterized by repeated episodes of breathing cessation (apnea) during sleep. Episodes last from 10 seconds to several minutes, occur throughout the night, and worsen sleep quality. Periods of apnea end with a brief awakening that may disrupt sleep hundreds of times a night. The resulting daytime sleepiness was made famous by Charles Dickens's description of an overweight boy in *The Pickwick Papers* who was affected by the condition. Sleep apnea is more common in men, but women (particularly postmenopausal women) also suffer from the disorder. According to epidemiological studies, sleep apnea is common, affecting 2% of women and 4% of men in the United States. An estimated 20 million Americans have clinically significant obstructive sleep apnea, and 95% of individuals with this condition remain undiagnosed and untreated.

Causes

Sleep apnea results from either a collapse and blockage of the upper airway during sleep or a central nervous system abnormality that interferes with the drive to breathe. Some people have an anatomical abnormality (such as large tonsils, excess fat in the tissues around the throat, or an enlarged tongue) that narrows the upper airway. A large neck or collar size (more than 17 inches in men or 16 inches in women) is strongly associated with sleep apnea. Obesity, older age, weakness of the airway muscles, hypothyroidism (insufficient production of thyroid hormone), and cigarette smoking are additional risk factors. Consuming alcohol or sedatives before sleeping can further reduce the activity of the airway muscles and blunt the normal increases in breathing after the fall in oxygen concentration associated with apnea.

Symptoms

The most pervasive and troublesome symptom of sleep apnea is excessive daytime sleepiness caused by poor sleep. People with mild sleep apnea may fall asleep during the day while reading or even

NEW RESEARCH

Mucus Clearance Device Improves Response to Inhaled Drugs

Using a mucus clearance device before an inhaled bronchodilator can improve lung function and exercise capacity while decreasing shortness of breath (dyspnea) in patients with chronic obstructive pulmonary disease (COPD), a new study from Canada shows. Such devices create vibrations in the chest that loosen mucus and may allow medication to penetrate the lungs more easily.

On two different days, 23 people with severe COPD used a mucus clearance device or a sham device (in which part of the device was removed to prevent vibrations) prior to taking four puffs from a bronchodilator inhaler; each puff contained 20 micrograms (mcg) of ipratropium (Atrovent) and 120 mcg of salbutamol (not available in the United States). Patients underwent lung function tests before use of the device and after administration of the bronchodilators.

Forced expiratory volume in one second (FEV_1) and forced vital capacity (FVC) improved after bronchodilator use, regardless of which device the patients used, but these improvements were greater when the active device was used. Also, the distance patients could walk and their symptoms of dyspnea improved more with use of the active device. Patients with a history of coughing up phlegm benefitted most.

CHEST
Volume 121, page 702
March 2002

Should You Use a Humidifier?

The amount of humidity in your home can affect your breathing. Air that is too dry can irritate the airways, especially in people with respiratory problems or even just a cold. Humidifiers can make breathing easier by adding moisture to the air. But if not used properly, humidifiers can cause problems. A humidifier that is not kept clean can harbor bacteria and spread them into the air, along with mold and dust mites, making breathing more difficult. Too much humidity in the air also promotes the growth of these microorganisms.

How To Keep Your Humidifier Clean

For portable humidifiers:

- Always unplug the unit before cleaning it.
- Empty the tank every day. Wipe all surfaces dry before refilling.
- Every third day, clean the humidifier. Empty the tank and clean it with a brush or scrubber. Remove any scale or film from the sides of the tank or on other interior surfaces, then wipe dry before refilling.
- Follow the manufacturer's instructions on using cleaning products or disinfectants. If no instructions are given, clean any surface that comes into contact with water with a 3% solution of hydrogen peroxide. Scale can be removed with a solution of equal parts vinegar and water. After using any chemical product, rinse the tank thoroughly several times before refilling.
- When storing the humidifier for an extended time, clean as directed. Make sure all the parts are dry, and throw out any used demineralization cartridges, cassettes, or filters. Store the humidifier in a dry place. Before using again, clean it and remove any dust from the outside of the unit.

For console and central humidifiers:

- Follow the manufacturer's directions for cleaning. If the humidifier contains a tank, keep the water clean and do not allow it to stand for long periods of time.

Types of Humidifiers

Humidifiers used in the home come in three varieties: console (encased in a cabinet and set on the floor), central (built into heating and air-conditioning systems), and portable. There are four types of portable humidifiers. Ultrasonic models emit a cool mist using sound vibrations. Impeller humidifiers, the most common type, produce a cool mist using a high-speed rotating disk. Evaporative models add moisture to the air with a fan that blows air through a moistened material such as a wick or filter. Steam vaporizers use electrical heating elements to warm water; some models cool the steam before it enters the air.

No evidence has shown that one type of humidifier is more effective than another, but their safety does differ. The warm mist of a steam vaporizer can cause burns if people or pets get too close. Ultrasonic and impeller models are more likely than evaporative and steam models to introduce microorganisms into the air.

Proper Use of a Humidifier

Used improperly, a humidifier (particularly an ultrasonic or impeller model) could make your breathing worse by releasing microorganisms and minerals into the air. One way to prevent this is to keep your humidifier clean (see the inset box above). Another way is to use distilled water instead of tap water in your humidifier. Tap water contains minerals that can be released into the air and leave a white dust on furniture and other surfaces. Although this white dust is not considered a health risk, some people are bothered by it. More important, minerals in tap water can also leave crusty deposits, called scale, in your humidifier. Scale is fertile ground for the growth of microorganisms, which can then be sent into the air.

Most bottled water is not distilled: "spring," "artesian," and "mineral" water all contain minerals. Demineralization cartridges, filters, or cassettes can be used in some humidifiers, but they may be less effective and more expensive than using distilled water.

Overhumidifying a room is also a problem. Excess moisture can lead to the growth of mold and dust mites, which can trigger allergic reactions or breathing difficulties in some people. The optimal range for room humidity is between 30% and 50%.

Some humidifiers have a built-in humidistat that can be set to control the moisture level automatically. For humidifiers that do not have a humidistat, a hygrometer, available at hardware stores, can be used to test the amount of moisture in a room. If you notice water condensing on windows, walls, or pictures, you need to change the position of the humidifier, lower the humidistat setting, or use the humidifier less frequently. In addition, do not point the humidifier at carpets, drapes, or tablecloths, which could become damp and moldy. You also may want to consider using a humidifier only during the winter or when you or someone else has a cold or the flu.

If you begin to have breathing problems that you think are associated with using a humidifier, even if you are cleaning and maintaining it properly, stop using it and call your doctor.

while driving, so there is a major risk of motor accidents. People with sleep apnea also may suffer from memory loss and personality changes. Although loud snoring is a common manifestation of sleep apnea, snoring itself does not indicate obstructive sleep apnea.

More than half of those with sleep apnea also have high blood pressure, and their blood pressure levels do not fall during sleep as they do in most people. In fact, sleep apnea has been shown to be an independent, treatable cause of high blood pressure. Heart rate tends to slow dramatically during periods of apnea and then rise rapidly when breathing resumes. Some evidence suggests that periods of apnea and low blood oxygen levels, along with persistently high blood pressure, increase the risk of coronary heart disease. This association is being studied.

Diagnosis

Obtaining a sleep history is key to recognizing this common respiratory disorder. Seeking input from a person's bed partner is especially important, because the bed partner is likely to notice snoring associated with frequent periods of apnea. A definitive diagnosis usually requires the patient to spend a night in a hospital sleep laboratory for sleep studies (polysomnography). Polysomnography involves monitoring brain waves to determine which stages of sleep are associated with episodes of apnea, as well as observing heart rhythms, airflow and breathing patterns, eye and leg movements, and blood oxygen levels. Expensive sleep lab studies can be replaced in some people by using a pulse oximeter to record blood oxygen levels while sleeping at home. A pulse oximeter test that shows low blood oxygen levels during sleep can aid in the diagnosis, but a normal result does not rule out the possibility of sleep apnea.

Treatment

Lifestyle measures that may reduce sleep apnea include losing weight (for overweight and obese people), avoiding alcohol and sedatives at bedtime, quitting smoking, and sleeping sideways or in a more upright position. If hypothyroidism is present, treating it may help reduce the apnea.

If these measures are unsuccessful, continuous positive airway pressure (CPAP) may be necessary. This technique, which involves wearing a nasal mask that delivers a steady stream of air to maintain airway pressure and keep the airways open, is effective in 80% to 90% of people. However, many people discontinue CPAP because they find the mask cumbersome or experience nasal dryness or congestion or skin irritation. Use of a humidifier or a properly fitting mask can alleviate some of these problems. Also, people may be more likely to use devices that gradually increase pressure as they fall asleep or provide different levels of air pressure during inhalation and exhalation.

Some people benefit from a dental appliance that helps maintain an open airway by keeping the jaw and tongue in a forward position during sleep. Carefully selected people who cannot tolerate CPAP may benefit from uvulopalatopharyngoplasty, a surgical procedure that increases the size of the upper airway by removing the uvula (the tag-like structure that hangs down from the back of the throat) and any excessive soft tissue surrounding it. This procedure is successful in only 40% to 50% of people, typically persons with mild disease. Tonsillectomy, surgical treatment of other upper airway obstructions, and facial reconstructive procedures are helpful in some cases.

INTERSTITIAL LUNG DISEASE

Interstitial lung disease (ILD) refers to a group of more than 200 chronic disorders that are characterized by overgrowth of cells of the interstitium (the tissue between the alveoli), varying degrees of inflammation, and scarring (fibrosis). Though many of the disorders are uncommon, taken together ILD is a frequent cause of respiratory problems and accounts for 15% of all cases seen by pulmonologists (lung specialists).

The lung scarring associated with ILD leads to stiffness that makes breathing more difficult. Changes in the normal relationships between airspaces and capillaries limit the transfer of oxygen. The pace and severity of this process vary greatly from person to person.

Interstitial lung disease comprises several different disorders, including pulmonary sarcoidosis, bronchiolitis obliterans organizing pneumonia, asbestosis, and silicosis. Pulmonary sarcoidosis is an inflammatory disease in which cell overgrowth occurs in the lungs. Bronchiolitis obliterans organizing pneumonia refers to inflammation with blockage of the bronchioles. Asbestosis and silicosis refer to damage caused by exposure to dust from asbestos or silica, respectively. Idiopathic pulmonary fibrosis is another important condition in which progressive scarring of the lung markedly compromises day-to-day function.

NEW RESEARCH

Sleep Apnea Treatment Decreases Risk of Heart Attack, Stroke

People with sleep apnea are at increased risk for cardiovascular disease (CVD), but effective treatment for sleep apnea negates this excess risk, a new study shows.

Swedish researchers studied 182 men (age 30 to 69) without CVD (i.e., no high blood pressure, angina, heart failure, or history of heart attack or stroke) who were referred to a sleep laboratory because of snoring or suspected sleep apnea. The men who were diagnosed with sleep apnea during monitoring in an overnight sleep clinic were offered treatment for the apnea (surgery, continuous positive airway pressure, or an oral appliance).

One third of the men were diagnosed with sleep apnea. Men with sleep apnea were nearly five times more likely to develop CVD during the seven-year follow-up than those without sleep apnea. Men whose sleep apnea was ineffectively treated had an 11-fold increased risk of CVD, while the 15 men whose apnea was successfully treated were not at increased risk for CVD.

The study's authors conclude that all people with sleep apnea should consider treatment, even if their condition is mild.

AMERICAN JOURNAL OF RESPIRATORY AND CRITICAL CARE MEDICINE
Volume 166, page 159
July 15, 2002

Causes

A variety of factors can injure the alveoli and result in ILD. Possible causes of ILD include:

- certain illegal and prescription drugs (including chemotherapy agents and cardiovascular medications);
- exposure to environmental toxins;
- infectious agents (such as viruses, bacteria, or fungi);
- substances that trigger allergic or hypersensitivity reactions;
- connective tissue diseases such as scleroderma, rheumatoid arthritis, and systemic lupus erythematosus, all of which can cause inflammation and scarring of organs (including the lungs); and
- the spread of cancer to the lungs from other parts of the body.

In many cases, the cause of lung injury is unknown (idiopathic).

Symptoms

People with ILD usually become short of breath when they exert themselves and have a persistent cough that does not produce phlegm. As the disease progresses, they may experience fatigue, loss of appetite, and weight loss. Less frequent symptoms are wheezing, chest pain, hemoptysis (coughing up blood), and fever. The course of the disease can last for several weeks, but more often the disease follows a chronic course that persists for months or years.

Diagnosis

Abnormalities on a chest x-ray may be the first evidence of ILD, but the changes often are not specific to a particular disorder. Pulmonary function tests typically show a decrease in total lung capacity (the amount of air in the lungs after a deep inhalation). Measurements of arterial oxygen and carbon dioxide levels at rest may not be helpful for diagnosis, but the effects of exercise on these blood gases may be useful in following the progression of the disease or its response to treatment. A common abnormality in people with ILD is a decrease in diffusion capacity (a pulmonary function test that measures how well gas moves across the membranes in the lungs). Like chest x-rays, however, this abnormality does not distinguish among the various underlying causes of ILD. In people suspected of having ILD, the results of high-resolution chest CT scans may be helpful. For example, such a scan showing changes in which the severely damaged lung resembles a honeycomb may eliminate the need for a lung biopsy. In some cases, a specific diagnosis can be made from the examination of lung fluids obtained using bronchoalveolar lavage (washing out the lungs with a saline solution) during bronchoscopy (in which a thin, hollow, flexible tube is passed through the mouth and into the windpipe to allow viewing of the main bronchial passages).

Because different ILDs may have similar x-ray features and decreases in lung capacity, a lung biopsy may be necessary to make a definitive diagnosis and determine the activity of the disease. Least invasive is a biopsy done through a bronchoscope. This procedure can be done on an outpatient basis, but the small size of the tissue sample is often insufficient for diagnosis. If this approach is inconclusive, an open surgical biopsy in a hospital may be necessary.

Prevention

Avoidance of potential triggers of ILD is important. In this regard, wearing appropriate masks and monitoring inhalational exposures in work environments are worthwhile interventions.

Treatment

In several of the disorders, notably sarcoidosis and hypersensitivity reactions, the lung disorder resolves on its own or responds to corticosteroids. Treatment of responsible infections or avoidance of toxins or allergen exposures may be quite beneficial. Unfortunately, for other causes of ILD, there is no specific treatment to slow disease progression or reverse the damage that has already occurred. Further inflammation and scarring of lung tissue lead to worsening respiratory function and right heart failure (heart failure that mainly affects the right side of the heart, slowing the movement of blood to the heart). Corticosteroid treatment, which speeds the resolution of sarcoidosis, may be prescribed for symptomatic people with other forms of ILD, but it often is unsuccessful. Chemotherapy drugs such as cyclophosphamide (Cytoxan, Neosar) or azathioprine (Imuran), antifibrotic agents such as colchicine (available only in a generic form), and interferon (Infergen) have been tried in people with idiopathic pulmonary fibrosis, but an effective treatment remains elusive for this debilitating and progressive condition. Supportive care includes supplemental oxygen, adequate nutrition, pulmonary rehabilitation programs to remain as active as possible, and treatment of right heart failure. In some cases, a single or double lung transplant can be performed (see page 27).

NEW RESEARCH

Early Exposure to Dogs, Cats Lowers Allergy Risk

Children who are exposed to at least two dogs or cats in their first year of life are less likely to have allergies at age six or seven than children who have one pet or no pets, a new study shows.

The study included data from 474 children living near Detroit, Michigan. When their child was one year old, parents were asked how many dogs and cats were living in their residence. Up to six years later, children were given skin prick and blood tests for six common allergies (dogs, cats, short ragweed, blue grass, and two types of dust mites).

After adjusting for factors such as parental asthma, children exposed to two or more cats or dogs at age one were 77% less likely to test positive for allergies on the skin prick test and 67% less likely to test positive on the blood test than those who had not been exposed to a dog or cat at that age. Being exposed to one dog or cat at age one had no effect on allergies at age six or seven.

According to an accompanying editorial, avoiding pets in the home is not a good way to prevent future allergies but, rather, may increase a child's risk.

JOURNAL OF THE AMERICAN MEDICAL ASSOCIATION
Volume 288, pages 963 and 1012
August 28, 2002

Traveling With Supplemental Oxygen

Thanks to portable oxygen equipment, people with chronic obstructive pulmonary disease (COPD) are able to travel—by car, bus, train, boat, and even plane. With careful planning, few destinations are off-limits. You should bear in mind, however, that trips to some destinations (such as a developing country) will be extremely expensive to arrange, and the type of oxygen equipment you are familiar with may not be available. One of the best choices for vacationers on oxygen therapy is a cruise, because your oxygen equipment can be delivered directly to the ship.

Air Travel

Traveling by air can be a good choice for people with COPD because it is the most efficient way to cover long distances. Some people with COPD need oxygen only while in the air. Those who require continuous supplemental oxygen will need to consider their oxygen requirements at the airport and at their final destination.

To make your trip faster and easier, try to arrange for a nonstop flight. Even if the airfare costs more than for a connecting flight, you will avoid the costs of oxygen during a layover. Another option is a direct flight that makes one or more stops but does not require you to leave the plane.

On the plane. Air travel is considered safe for people with COPD as long as they receive the oxygen they need. Because there is less oxygen at high altitudes than at sea level, people usually need more supplemental oxygen when flying than they do on the ground.

Federal regulations bar travelers from bringing their own oxygen aboard an airplane, although most airlines permit you to check in empty oxygen tanks that can be filled when you arrive at your destination. Be sure to inform the airline of what you are shipping. Oxygen is sometimes available for a fee, but only on jet planes (not smaller propeller planes).

To arrange for oxygen, you will need to call the airline anywhere from two or three days to a month in advance, depending on the carrier, and provide documentation of your oxygen needs. Some airlines require a written prescription or a phone call from your doctor, while others require your doctor to fill out and submit a special airline form. The prescription should indicate the flow rate you will need during the flight; this is usually 1½ times the rate used at sea level.

You should be aware that not all airlines provide adjustable flow rates; the oxygen may simply be "on." Some provide masks or nasal cannulas, but it is a good idea to bring your own as a precaution.

The cost of oxygen varies greatly among carriers. A 1999 study published in the journal *Chest* examined the cost of oxygen for a six-hour, round-trip flight. Most of the airlines charged between $100 and $250, but a few charged nothing and two charged more than $1,000. Be sure to find out the charge and how it is determined before your flight; most airlines charge according to how many segments there are to the flight.

At the airport. Because most airlines do not provide supplemental oxygen while you are on the ground, you will need to make separate arrangements for oxygen at the airport before and after the flight and during layovers.

You will be permitted to bring your oxygen canisters beyond the screener checkpoint after they have gone through inspection. If you need assistance, the check-in desk will issue a special pass to allow one person through the security checkpoint without a ticket. You also will need to arrange for someone to meet you at the plane with oxygen when you arrive at your destination.

If you cannot avoid a layover, contact your oxygen provider and see if it has a branch office that can deliver a portable oxygen unit to you at the airport. Another possibility is to hire an oxygen service such as Advanced Aeromedical (800-346-3556 or www.aeromedic.com) to meet you at the plane with oxygen and wait with you until you board your next flight.

LUNG CANCER

Lung cancer was rare before the beginning of the 20th century, but it is now the most common cause of death from cancer in both men and women in the United States; an estimated 154,900 Americans died of lung and bronchial cancer in 2002. Death rates from lung cancer are high because lung cancer is difficult to treat and usually is not detected until it has already spread (metastasized). Most cases occur in people between the ages of 45 and 75 who have had years

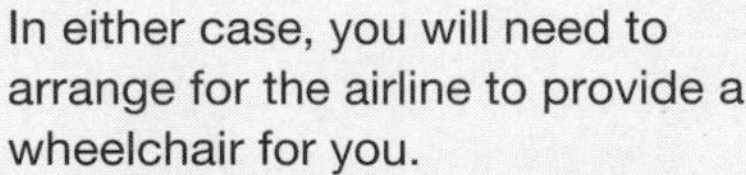

In either case, you will need to arrange for the airline to provide a wheelchair for you.

At your destination. A local oxygen provider can deliver oxygen to your hotel so that it will be there when you arrive.

Ground Travel

Traveling by train, bus, or car sometimes can be more convenient because you often can use your own equipment. These methods of travel still require advance planning, however. For example, if you are traveling to a higher altitude, your oxygen needs may increase. Before your trip, find out the altitudes of your route and destination by checking with your auto club, local library, or the Internet.

Train. Amtrak will allow you to bring up to two 75-lb. or six 20-lb. tanks on board; the tanks must be UL or FM listed. After boarding, be sure to remove any wheels fastened to the tanks so they cannot roll.

Equipment that requires the use of on-board electrical power must have a backup supply of at least 12 hours of oxygen to allow for power interruptions. To cover possible delays, be sure to bring at least 20% more oxygen than you think you will need. If you are not able to bring an adequate supply, you should arrange for an oxygen supply company to resupply you at a scheduled stop.

Let the reservation agent know that you will be traveling with oxygen when you make your reservation, preferably at least one day before your trip (800-USA-RAIL). Amtrak does not require you to bring medical documentation. Other railways may have different requirements, so be sure to check in advance.

Bus. Greyhound will allow you to bring up to four oxygen tanks; these can be up to 4½ inches in diameter and 26 inches in length. One or two can be carried on board with you; the others should be well padded for transportation in the luggage compartment. Be sure to call Greyhound's Disabilities Line (800-752-4841) at least one or two days in advance.

National Home Oxygen Patients Association
☎ 888-NHOPA-44
888-646-7244
www.homeoxygen.org
An organization for people who use supplementary oxygen. The $15 membership includes a monthly newsletter, a booklet on oxygen therapy, and a pamphlet on airline travel with oxygen.

Breathin' Easy Travel Guide
☎ 888-699-4360
www.breathineasy.com
Publishes a travel guide for people with lung disorders for $28.60. Also provides travel information on their Web site.

Cruising

Many cruise lines accept people who use supplemental oxygen, but passengers are responsible for making their own arrangements. Selecting a cruise that departs from and returns to the same location will greatly simplify this task.

You can either bring on your own oxygen or arrange for an oxygen provider to deliver oxygen tanks to the cruise ship. Some cruise lines can refer you to local contractors who arrange for oxygen delivery.

As with airplane travel, the cruise ship will require specific health information from your doctor. Contact the cruise line at least one to two months in advance to see whether they accept passengers who use oxygen and what the requirements are.

Final Advice

Whatever plans you make, be sure to factor in the cost of oxygen. Many people are surprised to discover that charges for transporting or purchasing oxygen can be higher than their travel ticket. It is also important to start planning early, confirm your travel arrangements two or three days in advance, and allow plenty of extra time to deal with unexpected problems. And finally, because your health is more fragile than that of someone who does not require supplemental oxygen, always purchase travel insurance that allows you to cancel for preexisting conditions.

of exposure to cigarette smoke or other pollutants. Tragically, only about 10% to 15% of people with lung cancer are alive five years after diagnosis.

Lung cancer may be primary or secondary. Primary lung cancer, which originates in the lungs, is grouped into two broad categories: small cell carcinoma (about 20% of cases) and non-small cell carcinoma (about 80%). Because small cell carcinoma spreads especially quickly and is more difficult to treat, most people with this type die within a year of diagnosis. Primary lung cancer can spread to nearly any organ. Cancer also may spread to the lungs from other sites in the body (secondary lung cancer). Such tumors usually are incurable, in which case palliative treatments are used. Palliative treatments are aimed at delaying the progression of disease, relieving pain, and limiting disease complications, rather than curing the disease.

Causes

Smoking causes more than 90% of cases of primary lung cancer. Nonsmokers have only a small risk, and smokers who quit (even after smoking for years) greatly reduce their risk. One recent study provided some of the first direct evidence of how cigarette smoking leads to lung cancer. Researchers found that the body converts a substance in cigarette smoke, called benzo[a] pyrene diol epoxide (BPDE), into a potent carcinogen.

Air pollution, traffic fumes, and smokestack emissions also may contribute to lung cancer. Several comprehensive reports also have concluded that passive smoking (inhaling the smoke from cigarettes smoked by others) can cause lung cancer in nonsmokers. This conclusion is based on the presence of carcinogens in the smoke coming from the end of a burning cigarette (sidestream smoke), the presence of cigarette smoke particles in the homes of smokers, detection of tobacco-smoke components in the body fluids of nonsmokers, and the increased incidence of lung cancer in the nonsmoking spouses of smokers. Some data suggest that passive smoking is one of the leading causes of preventable deaths in this country, if projected deaths from lung cancer and cardiovascular disease are counted together.

Exposure to toxic substances such as asbestos and radon also may cause lung cancer. Asbestos is a fibrous mineral that was used in building materials until the 1980s. Chronic exposure to asbestos can cause both lung cancer and mesothelioma, a cancer involving the pleura (the membranes that cover the lungs). The combination of asbestos exposure with cigarette smoking is especially dangerous. Radon is a colorless, odorless gas formed from radium during the decay of naturally occurring uranium in rocks and soil. Radon in the soil can pollute the air of a home by entering through cracks or other openings, usually in the basement. The amount of radon in the ground varies widely from one part of the country to another, and even from one home to another in the same neighborhood. The level of lifetime exposure determines the degree of risk, which is greatly increased in cigarette smokers. The incidence of lung cancer caused by radon is highest among miners of uranium and certain other substances who are exposed to high levels of radon.

Symptoms

Lung cancer produces no symptoms in its early stages. Later, lung cancer patients often note symptoms of fatigue, poor appetite, and unexplained weight loss that are common to many forms of cancer. Symptoms also can result from cancer growth within the lungs or from its spread to adjacent or distant sites. Lung symptoms may include coughing up red or rust-colored phlegm, wheezing, and shortness of breath. Infection behind an obstructed bronchus may produce a fever, and invasion of cancerous cells into the pleura or other nearby structures can produce pain in the chest, shoulders, or arms. If the cancer spreads to surrounding structures, it also can lead to hoarseness resulting from enlarged lymph nodes in the chest or neck or involvement of various nerves, such as the recurrent laryngeal nerve; difficulty swallowing, due to narrowing of the esophagus; and swelling of the neck and face from blockage of blood returning from these sites to the heart. In about 30% of patients, lung cancer causes clubbing of the fingers (a thickening of the fingertips and increased curvature of the fingernails).

Lung cancer often spreads to the liver and bone marrow, where it can interfere with the formation of blood cells. Spread to the bones causes pain and fractures, while spread to the brain produces neurological symptoms such as seizures. Small cell tumors may secrete hormones such as corticotropin or antidiuretic hormone. Overproduction of corticotropin stimulates excessive release of corticosteroids by the adrenal gland, leading to Cushing syndrome. This syndrome produces such complications as osteoporosis, high blood pressure, and roundness of the face. Release of antidiuretic hormone results in fluid retention. Other lung cancer cell types secrete parathyroid hormone (PTH) or a PTH-like hormone. Spread of cancer to the bone and/or the PTH-like hormone trigger the release of calcium from the bone, which can lead to excessive blood levels of calcium (hypercalcemia). Hypercalcemia may cause fatigue, muscle weakness, confusion, drowsiness, and coma.

Diagnosis

About 10% of lung cancers are discovered in people with no symptoms, usually when a chest x-ray is performed for another reason. However, the majority of lung cancers are diagnosed after a doctor requests testing for cancer based on a patient's medical history and the results of a physical examination.

Doctors usually do not recommend general screening for lung cancer in at-risk individuals (for example, smokers and former smokers). A standard chest x-ray is not sensitive enough to locate small tumors, and studies have shown that two screening methods—regular chest x-rays and phlegm examinations—do not decrease the number of deaths from lung cancer.

However, a recently developed technology called low-radiation-dose spiral computed tomography (spiral CT) may provide a much-needed breakthrough in the early detection and treatment of lung cancer. What makes this technique so promising as a screening tool is that it is relatively inexpensive, provides clear images, and can be performed in about 20 seconds. Spiral CT generates a series of cross-sectional images of the lungs that are used to create a three-dimensional image.

Preliminary evidence suggests that spiral CT screening for lung cancer may particularly benefit smokers and former smokers over age 60. The majority of lung cancers detected by spiral CT appear to be in the earliest, most treatable stage. In one study of 1,000 asymptomatic smokers and former smokers, the scan detected 23 early-stage cancers; standard chest x-rays missed 83% of them. Spiral CT outperformed chest x-rays on all fronts, uncovering three times as many suspicious nodules and four times as many cancerous tumors. Of the 27 cancerous tumors found by spiral CT scans in the study, 26 were successfully removed. Although this approach may detect tumors at earlier stages and allow for a surgical cure, such scans also identify far more lung nodules that are benign (that is, false positives for cancer) and might lead to unnecessary follow-up tests.

Radiation exposure from a spiral CT scan is slightly higher than that from a regular chest x-ray, but its benefits may outweigh this risk. Both the speed and lower cost (about $300 for a spiral CT scan, compared with $150 for the less accurate chest x-ray and $2,000 for the time-consuming positron emission tomography [PET] and magnetic resonance imaging [MRI] scans) may encourage high-risk individuals to undergo earlier and regular screening. Since spiral CT scans detect both benign and malignant (cancerous) tumors, accurate distinction between the two is necessary before people undergo needless and risky lung biopsies. Further research is needed to enable this distinction. A multicenter study of spiral CT is under way to assess the rate of false-positive results and the test's impact on long-term lung cancer cure rates.

A biopsy of cancerous tissue is essential to make the diagnosis of lung cancer and to guide treatment decisions by determining the type of cancer. A biopsy sample can be obtained from the suspicious area using bronchoscopy, in which a thin, hollow, flexible tube is passed through the mouth and into the windpipe to allow viewing of the main bronchial passages. Tissue is obtained either directly from a bronchus or by passing a needle through a bronchus into adjacent tumor tissue. Alternately, a CT-scan-guided needle biopsy through the chest wall may be used to obtain tissue from a suspicious growth within the lung. In patients with suspected lung cancers, a positive result for cancer generally is reliable. A negative result does not necessarily exclude cancer, and other testing usually is necessary. Sites of cancer spread—such as the lymph nodes, bone marrow, and pleura—also are suitable areas for biopsy.

Formal staging of cancer—including characteristics such as tumor size, involvement of particular lymph nodes within the chest, and presence of metastatic disease at other sites—is important for determining prognosis and selecting treatment options. Imaging procedures (for example, CT or MRI scans) are important components of this evaluation, and the recent availability of PET scans has been a major advance. While CT scans provide worthwhile anatomical information, PET scanning—in which a radioactive form of glucose (sugar) is administered to the patient—provides a metabolic assessment. Because growing tumors have high energy needs, detection of increased glucose uptake by the tumor may clarify the extent of cancer spread more accurately than CT scanning alone. An MRI provides more detailed evaluation of brain metastases.

Prevention

The best ways to prevent lung cancer are to avoid smoking and limit exposure to certain pollutants.

Smoking. Cigarette smoking is unquestionably the single greatest, readily controllable risk factor for lung cancer and the most common preventable cause of all premature deaths. Half of all smokers die prematurely from diseases related to smoking. While smoking cigars and pipes greatly increases the danger of cancers of the mouth, pharynx, larynx, and esophagus, the risk of lung cancer is not as high as with cigarette smoking because smoke from pipes and cigars usually is not inhaled as deeply or as frequently as cigarette smoke. The risk of lung cancer is greatest in those who start smoking at an early age and smoke the most cigarettes daily.

Because the risk of lung and other cancers gradually diminishes with time after smoking is discontinued, smokers can benefit from quitting at any age. (For help on quitting smoking, see the feature on pages 44–45.) This benefit of smoking cessation becomes evident after about five years. The risk of developing lung cancer continues to decrease as the period without smoking lengthens but does not return completely to that of people who never smoked.

Radon. Many studies have examined the risk of lung cancer posed by radon in the home. Data from miners suggest that household levels of radon might account for about 15% of lung cancer deaths, an estimate supported by studies that directly measured the risk of indoor radon. The U.S. Environmental Protection Agency (EPA) has recommended measuring radon levels in homes and reducing the levels when they exceed 4 picocuries per liter (pCi/L) over a year, a level estimated to be present in about 5% of American homes. Some critics have disagreed with this EPA recommendation, arguing that these levels of radon do not pose a significant risk and that attention should be focused on finding the homes with the highest levels. Recently, researchers estimated that reducing radon levels in all homes with readings higher than 4 pCi/L would result in 2% to 4% fewer lung cancer deaths.

To determine whether radon levels are high in your area, call your local EPA office. Taking a radon measurement in an individual house is the only way to definitively know the radon level, and several inexpensive kits are available in most hardware stores. Etched-track or electret detectors are both good choices; the best of these kits take measurements over at least a three-month period. The label on the kit should say that it meets EPA requirements or is certified by the state. A state-certified contractor, or one who has passed the EPA Radon Contractor Proficiency Program, should be used if it is necessary to reduce radon levels in a home.

Dietary measures. Since damage of DNA by free radicals is considered one of the causes of many types of cancer, it was hoped that antioxidant supplements or an increased intake of antioxidant-rich foods might reduce the risk of lung cancer. A Scandinavian study, however, found that the antioxidant beta-carotene increased the risk of lung cancer in cigarette smokers. Currently, no dietary measures are known to diminish the risk of lung cancer.

Treatment

The three options for treating lung cancer—surgery, chemotherapy, and radiation therapy—may be used alone or in combination. The choice of treatment depends on a number of factors, including the size and location of the tumor; whether the cancer is small cell or non-small cell; the physical condition of the patient; and whether the cancer has spread to lymph nodes or further. Because of the complexity involved in choosing a treatment option, people with lung cancer are best served by discussing their options with a multidisciplinary team of experts, which includes a pulmonologist, thoracic surgeon, medical and radiation oncologists, and other health professionals.

Surgery. An evaluation for possible surgery is essential because it is the most effective treatment for non-small cell cancer. In this regard, resectability and operability are major considerations in evaluation of the patient. A resectable tumor is one that can be removed in its entirety. If the tumor has spread extensively or is too close to vital structures such as the heart or major blood vessels, it is no longer resectable. The decision that a tumor is not resectable is usually based on biopsy information, rather than scan abnormalities alone. A tumor is considered operable if the patient is able to undergo the surgical procedure safely and can tolerate the extent of resection necessary for a cure. The patient's lung function and the presence of other diseases are key factors in determining operability.

Surgery may involve removal of a lobe (lobectomy) or an entire lung (pneumonectomy), and a hospital stay of one to two weeks usually is required. People with otherwise healthy lungs often can resume normal activities after a period of recuperation that varies based on their health status before surgery.

Chemotherapy. Chemotherapy is individualized for each patient and may involve administration of a combination of several drugs which are given in four to six cycles, each consisting of a three- to four-week treatment period followed by a rest period. Possible side effects of chemotherapy include nausea and vomiting, loss of appetite, and hair loss. Reduced formation of red blood cells, white blood cells, and platelets owing to bone marrow effects of these drugs can result in anemia, an increased risk of infection, and bleeding.

Radiation. External radiation may be the main form of treatment for people unable to tolerate surgery and for those whose cancer has spread beyond the reach of surgical removal. Radiation is administered five days a week for four to eight weeks. Radiation also may be directed to areas of cancer in the lung that cannot be removed with surgery or used to treat cancer that has spread to the brain or bones or that compresses the spinal cord. Side effects of external radiation include nausea and vomiting, local skin irritation, and fatigue.

The Lungs, Smoking, and How To Quit

Despite more than 30 years of public health warnings on the dangers of cigarettes, about a quarter of Americans still smoke. The habit results in approximately 430,000 premature deaths every year in the United States, mostly from heart attacks, strokes, cancer, and lung disease. Quitting smoking can greatly decrease the risk of illness and death from these diseases.

The Effects of Smoking

While cigarette smoking affects many parts of the body, it most directly damages the respiratory system. In fact, smoking is known to cause or aggravate nearly every lung disorder. It is not clear why this is the case, but it is known that cigarette smoking damages the cells in the lungs, destroys the alveoli, and causes other changes that make the lungs less able to function properly.

Studies show that, compared with nonsmokers, smokers have roughly twice the rate of (and significantly more severe) colds and are about 78% more likely to die of influenza. Smoking also raises the risk of bacterial pneumonia by allowing bacteria to grow more easily in the respiratory tract. In addition, tuberculosis infections are more common in smokers.

While cigarette smoking has not been shown to cause asthma in adults, adult smokers with asthma tend to have higher-than-normal rates of worsening lung function as they age and higher rates of asthma-related death. Up to 90% of chronic obstructive pulmonary disease (chronic bronchitis and emphysema) cases are directly related to cigarette smoking.

But possibly the most devastating consequence of smoking is lung and bronchial cancer, which—accounting for an estimated 154,900 deaths in 2002—kills more than three times as many people as any other cancer. About 90% of lung cancers are the direct result of smoking.

Quitting Smoking

Since quitting smoking can reduce the risk or impact of nearly all lung diseases, it is especially important for every smoker to stop smoking. Only about 8% of people who try to quit smoking are able to do so on their own, but you can increase your chances of success by talking with your doctor or health care provider about smoking cessation. These health professionals may be able to provide literature, advice, support, and medication to help you quit; they may also refer you to another health care professional who specializes in counseling for smoking cessation.

Counseling. Attendance at individual or group counseling sessions increases your chances of success. In fact, the more sessions you attend, the greater your likelihood of quitting. At these sessions, you will learn behavioral techniques, including coping skills, relapse prevention, and stress management. Counseling sessions also provide social support and encouragement.

Medication. Because nicotine is addictive, smoking cessation often leads to nicotine withdrawal, which can cause irritability, restlessness, food cravings, anxiety, and other symptoms. To help reduce these effects and control cravings for nicotine, your doctor may recommend or prescribe some form of nicotine replacement—either gum, skin patch, nasal spray, or inhaler. Using any of these products doubles the chances of quitting successfully. (There are no data, however, directly comparing the effectiveness of one method of nicotine replacement with another.) Nicotine replacement should be started on the day that you quit smoking.

Nicotine polacrilex gum (Nicorette) is available over the counter in doses of 2 and 4 mg. You may need between 10 and 24 pieces of gum a day to control your cravings, depending on the dose of the gum and how much you smoked. It may be most effective to use the 4-mg dose for the first two weeks of cessation and then switch to the 2-mg dose. Over time, you should reduce the number of pieces you chew per day. The gum should be chewed only once or twice every few minutes and remain between your cheek and gum the rest of the time. Side effects, including nausea and indigestion, usually result from chewing the gum too much and swallowing large amounts of nicotine. Ask your doctor if you need to use the gum for longer than 12 weeks.

Some people may find a nicotine patch easier and more convenient to use. Patches are available over the

PULMONARY EMBOLISM

A pulmonary embolus is a blockage in one or more of the arteries leading to the lungs. In almost all cases, it occurs when a blood clot (thrombus) originating in a deep vein in the extremities or pelvis breaks loose and travels to the lungs. Depending on its size, the

counter (Habitrol, Nicoderm CQ, and Nicotrol) or by prescription. Most versions come in 7-, 14-, and 21-mg doses; ask your doctor which dose you should try first. If you start at one of the higher doses, you will need to taper to the lower levels after four to six weeks to wean yourself from the nicotine. The recommended length of use of this therapy is 8 to 12 weeks, and the patch should be changed daily. If you experience minor skin irritation beneath the patch, change the area on your body where you place the patch each day. If the patch causes difficulty sleeping, try taking it off before going to bed. It Is important not to smoke while on the patch. Smoking not only greatly reduces your chances of quitting but also can cause uncomfortably high levels of nicotine in your blood.

Nicotine nasal spray (Nicotrol NS) is available by prescription only. Your doctor can help determine the exact timing and dose, but you should initially use it no more than 80 times per day. Work out a plan to gradually reduce the number of times the spray is used each day. Side effects include nasal irritation, runny nose, throat irritation, and nausea.

Also available by prescription is a nicotine inhalation system (Nicotrol Inhaler). Patients typically use between 4 and 16 inhaler cartridges per day and gradually taper the dosage over a maximum of six months. Irritation of the mouth and throat are two potential adverse effects.

Bupropion (Zyban) is a prescription medication for quitting smoking that contains no nicotine but helps reduce cravings and withdrawal symptoms in some people. Researchers believe that the drug may disrupt the pleasurable feelings that cigarette smoking typically produces in the brain. (Bupropion is also sold as an antidepressant called Wellbutrin and can be a good choice for people who have a mood disorder that may make smoking cessation more difficult.) Smokers begin to take bupropion a week or two before their quit date and continue to take it for up to 12 weeks afterward. People with a history of seizures, an eating disorder, or uncontrolled high blood pressure should not take bupropion. Common side effects include trouble sleeping and dry mouth.

Combination therapy. A combination of treatments that includes counseling, nicotine replacement, and bupropion provides the highest chance of success. In one study, people who used all three therapies at once had a 35% success rate.

Tips for Quitting

It is difficult for most people to stop smoking, and numerous attempts may be needed before you are successful. If you have tried to quit before without success, analyze what helped and what hindered you, and adjust your strategy accordingly. If you are concerned about weight gain after smoking cessation, remember that people usually gain no more than 10 lbs. after they quit; such weight gain has a much smaller impact on your health than smoking.

Here are a few general tips that may help if you are trying to quit smoking. First, some people find that their motivation is helped by picking a quit date that has a significant meaning—like New Year's Day or a birthday. Also, before you quit, ask for support from family, friends, and coworkers. If any of them smoke, ask them not to smoke around you.

Determine what events, situations, and other factors are cues to your smoking, and figure out ways to avoid them. For example, throw out lighters and ashtrays. If you always have a cigarette at a certain point during your drive home from work, try taking a different route. If you are used to having a cigarette with coffee after dinner, skip the coffee and do something else that distracts you. If you smoke in certain places in your house, or at certain times of the day, rearrange your furniture or your daily schedule.

Experts recommend that you avoid alcohol, or at least severely limit your intake, for the first three months after you quit. Alcohol may act as a trigger for smoking and reduces your chances of success by decreasing your inhibitions. Some people also find that deep breathing, drinking lots of liquids (preferably water, rather than soft drinks, coffee, or tea), and exercising can help deal with cravings.

embolus (usually a thrombus that has broken loose) obstructs a large or small pulmonary artery within the lungs and blocks the flow of blood through that vessel. Estimates suggest that about 500,000 people in the United States suffer a pulmonary embolus each year, and about 10% of cases are fatal. Fortunately, steps can be taken to prevent pulmonary emboli.

Pulmonary emboli may vary in their severity and effects. Most dangerous is an acute, massive blood clot that blocks a main pulmonary artery and/or one of its branches. Another acute manifestation results when a small blood clot blocks a peripheral pulmonary artery (one near the surface of the lung). Some people have multiple, asymptomatic clots that block many small pulmonary arteries and, over time, lead to chronic complications. The network of blood vessels in the lungs is large enough to tolerate considerable amounts of obstruction, but such extensive blockage can increase the resistance to blood flow through the pulmonary arteries and eventually produce pulmonary hypertension (high blood pressure in the pulmonary artery). Pulmonary hypertension places excessive stress on the heart's right ventricle, which pumps blood into the pulmonary arteries, potentially leading to right heart failure.

Causes

Fat released from a broken bone, air, or amniotic fluid may travel to a pulmonary artery and cause a pulmonary embolism. But the vast majority of pulmonary emboli are caused by blood clots from a deep vein in the leg, pelvis, or arm (deep vein thrombosis, or DVT). An estimated 5 million people in the United States suffer an episode of DVT annually. The condition is most common among women and older people.

A common cause of DVT is stagnation of blood flow due to immobility in bedridden patients or in healthy people who sit still for an extended period, such as on a long trip. Women taking oral contraceptives or hormone replacement therapy after menopause are at increased risk for DVT. Patients are at high risk for DVT after any major surgery, but especially after knee- or hip-replacement surgery.

A tendency for the blood to coagulate excessively (hypercoagulability) can predispose a person to DVT. The most frequent genetic abnormality that leads to hypercoagulability (present in about 5% of whites) is called factor V Leiden, which is due to a mutation in the gene for coagulation factor V. Having cancer also can cause the blood to coagulate excessively. In addition, injury to blood vessels caused by trauma, intravenous catheters or needles, or certain medications can cause blood clots.

Symptoms

Pulmonary emboli may produce sudden, severe shortness of breath, rapid breathing, and chest pain. Massive emboli, which often result in death within a short period of time, also may be accompanied by a feeling of impending doom, profuse sweating, loss of consciousness, a fall in blood pressure (shock), and cyanosis (a bluish color in the lips and fingertips). Peripheral emboli, which also occur abruptly and without warning, are associated with chest pain and coughing up blood (hemoptysis). People with multiple small emboli may have no symptoms for many months until they develop right heart failure with symptoms of fatigue, swelling of the ankles, weight loss, and shortness of breath.

Deep vein thrombosis can cause pain and swelling in the affected body part, and the area may be tender and feel hot to the touch. But because the condition occurs deep within the body, about half the time there are no signs or symptoms. Often, DVT is discovered only when a physician looks for it in someone at high risk for the condition.

Diagnosis

Although a pulmonary embolus is suspected when typical symptoms occur in a person with typical findings of DVT, often there is no evidence of DVT. Large pulmonary emboli may be associated with changes that can be identified with an electrocardiogram. Measurements of arterial blood gases (oxygen and carbon dioxide) may aid in making a diagnosis, but the results are not definitive.

Probably the most effective noninvasive test is a pulmonary isotope ventilation/perfusion (V/Q) scan. The test involves the intravenous injection of particles labeled with a radioactive substance. The particles become trapped in the small pulmonary blood vessels, and an external detector is used to locate the radioactivity. Radioactivity is evenly distributed throughout the lungs in a normal scan but is not seen in an area of the lung that has its blood supply blocked by a blood clot. The diagnosis of a pulmonary embolus is highly unlikely when the V/Q scan is normal.

Spiral CT scanning of the chest (see page 40) is being increasingly used to assess people with suspected pulmonary embolism. Studies to define its optimal applications in this setting are under way.

The most definitive diagnostic test is an angiogram of the pulmonary arteries—an x-ray following the injection of a contrast material into the pulmonary artery. An angiogram is an invasive procedure and is performed only when the results of other tests are insufficient to guide therapy.

Prevention

The only effective ways to prevent pulmonary emboli are to take measures to prevent the development of DVT and to recognize and treat DVT vigorously when it occurs. Steps to prevent DVT include taking frequent walks on long trips, getting out of bed as soon as possible after surgery, and using anticoagulants and other therapies (for example, pneumatic compression stockings) when possible in bedridden patients and people who have had surgical procedures. People with a family history of frequent DVT should take special precautions, since they may have inherited an abnormal tendency for their blood to clot. People who have had DVT in the past also are at increased risk for a recurrence.

Treatment

During diagnostic evaluation, supportive treatment for someone with a large pulmonary embolus includes pain relief, oxygen, and psychological support. Administration of "clot-busting" drugs (thrombolytic agents) may dissolve the clot and restore blood flow through the blocked artery. Surgical removal of the blood clot may be required if a patient has a large life-threatening clot and if his or her condition deteriorates during medical treatment. Thrombolytic therapy and surgery generally are reserved for people with massive clots and hemodynamic instability (shock). Most of the time, however, people with any type of pulmonary embolus are treated with anticoagulants—heparin and warfarin (Coumadin)—in both the short and long term. Intravenous heparin is started at once and continued for at least five days, and oral warfarin is continued for three to six months, with close patient monitoring.

Anticoagulants are ineffective for preventing further emboli in some people and can be dangerous in people who are at high risk for bleeding in the skull (such as people with an aneurysm or a vascular malformation) or have active gastrointestinal bleeding. In these instances, a sieve-like filtering device may be placed in the inferior vena cava (the vein that returns blood from the lower body to the heart) to prevent blood clots from entering the heart and lungs. Filters also are useful for people who have had recurrent bouts of pulmonary emboli. These devices become obstructed over time, but the flow of blood is not significantly affected because blood can be carried back to the heart through smaller blood vessels that develop around the obstruction (collateral vessels). Continued use of anticoagulants is needed because clots can still reach the lungs through these new blood vessels.

INFECTIONS

The respiratory tract has a remarkable defense system to protect against the numerous microorganisms we breathe in each day. But sometimes bacteria, viruses, or other microorganisms overwhelm this defense system and cause a respiratory infection. There are many different types of respiratory infections, but this White Paper focuses on acute bronchitis, influenza, bacterial pneumonia, and tuberculosis.

The signs and symptoms of a lung infection may overlap with those of a noninfectious lung disease and make diagnosis difficult. In fact, people with noninfectious lung diseases are at increased risk for respiratory infections, either from the lung disease itself, its treatment (for example, with corticosteroids), or a combination of both. Conversely, a respiratory infection may cause scarring of the lungs and worsening lung function that set the stage for future, recurrent episodes of lung infection.

Acute Bronchitis

Acute bronchitis refers to inflammation of the bronchi. When the bronchi are infected, they become inflamed and plugged with mucus. This can cause wheezing, coughing up of phlegm, and breathing difficulties.

Causes. Bronchitis usually is caused by a viral infection, typically a cold virus. It also can be triggered by exposure to chemical fumes, dust, smoke, or other air pollutants. Cigarette smokers and people with obstructive lung disease (such as asthma or COPD) or heart failure are at increased risk for acute bronchitis.

Symptoms. The predominant symptom of acute bronchitis is a persistent cough that may produce gray, green, or yellowish phlegm. The cough may be preceded by a headache, fever, sore throat, or other symptoms typical of the common cold. Severe coughing bouts may produce chest pain. In healthy adults, the symptoms of bronchitis generally disappear on their own in a few days.

Diagnosis. A diagnosis is based on the signs and symptoms. A chest x-ray may be needed to rule out other lung disorders, but bronchitis does not produce any abnormalities on an x-ray.

Prevention. The most important thing you can do to prevent bronchitis is not to smoke. In addition, you can reduce your chances of picking up a cold virus by avoiding exposure to people with respiratory infections.

Treatment. Usually, no treatment other than smoking cessation

NEW RESEARCH

New Bacterial Strain May Worsen Chronic Bronchitis

For patients with chronic bronchitis, infection with a new strain of bacterium can increase the risk of worsening symptoms, a new study indicates.

The study included 81 patients (average age 67) with chronic bronchitis. For over four years, researchers took phlegm samples from the patients once a month, as well as any time they had symptoms indicative of an exacerbation of bronchitis. The investigators then analyzed the phlegm to determine if the person had been infected with a new strain of bacterium since the previous visits.

Infection with new bacterial strains increased the risk of symptom exacerbation more than twofold: In the 270 clinic visits when patients were infected with a new strain of bacterium, 33% of patients had worsening of symptoms; in the 1,385 visits at which no new strain was detected, 15% of patients had symptom exacerbations. *Haemophilus influenzae*, *Moraxella catarrhalis*, and *Streptococcus pneumoniae* were the three bacteria linked to an increased risk of exacerbations.

These results indicate that patients may develop protective immune responses to bacteria that have caused prior infections. The authors conclude that new strains, even of the same species, may make a person susceptible to an exacerbation of symptoms.

THE NEW ENGLAND JOURNAL OF MEDICINE
Volume 347, page 465
August 15, 2002

is necessary for acute bronchitis. Antibiotics and antihistamines appear to have no effect. However, in people with chronic pulmonary disease, such as asthma, COPD, cystic fibrosis, or interstitial lung disease, a viral infection that destroys the protective layer of cells that lines the trachea and bronchi may lead to a superimposed bacterial infection that can worsen the underlying lung disease or lead to pneumonia. In such people, an attack of acute bronchitis usually is treated with antibiotics.

Influenza

Influenza is an acute infection usually involving the upper respiratory tract. Outbreaks of influenza occur each winter and last for two to three months, producing infection in 10% to 20% of the general population. Influenza can worsen the symptoms of COPD and asthma. Influenza can make a person more prone to a bacterial infection that causes pneumonia, or the influenza virus itself can cause pneumonia.

Causes. The cause of influenza is a viral infection. Influenza A virus is responsible for most of the outbreaks, causing more severe disease and more deaths than influenza B or C.

Symptoms. Influenza produces the well-recognized symptoms of the flu—headache, fever, and muscle aches that may be accompanied by chills, cough, sore throat, and weakness. Acute symptoms usually last for two to five days.

Diagnosis. A diagnosis of influenza can be made when an influenza outbreak is present in the community and a person's complaints fit the current pattern of symptoms.

Prevention. The Centers for Disease Control and Prevention (CDC) recommends annual flu vaccinations for certain individuals to prevent or ameliorate influenza (see the feature on pages 52–53). In addition, the antiviral drugs amantadine (Symmetrel) and rimantadine (Flumadine) are 70% to 100% effective in preventing influenza during an outbreak when given to high-risk people who did not receive the flu vaccine. Another antiviral drug, oseltamivir (Tamiflu), was recently approved for prevention of influenza in adults and adolescents; it has been shown to protect close contacts of people with influenza from becoming infected.

Treatment. Although antibiotics may be helpful when influenza is complicated by a superimposed bacterial infection, these drugs have no impact on the influenza virus itself. Symptoms of the flu may be alleviated by acetaminophen (Tylenol). Amantadine and rimantadine can reduce symptoms by about half if administered

NEW RESEARCH

Antibiotic Is Ineffective For Acute Bronchitis

Although doctors frequently prescribe the antibiotic azithromycin (Zithromax) for acute bronchitis, a new study indicates that it might be no more effective than vitamin C for treating the condition.

Researchers randomly assigned 220 adults with acute bronchitis but no underlying lung disease to take either azithromycin or 250 mg of vitamin C daily for five days. (Vitamin C is not known to be effective in treating acute bronchitis.) All participants also received dextromethorphan syrup and an albuterol inhaler, treatments with known benefit for acute bronchitis.

Both groups improved at the same rate. There were no significant differences between the groups' health-related quality of life on day three or day seven. Eighty-nine percent of people in both groups were able to return to their normal daily activities by day seven. About 20% in each group reported at least one treatment-related side effect. The most common adverse effects of azithromycin and vitamin C were diarrhea and nausea.

For patients with acute bronchitis, "azithromycin is ineffective and should not be prescribed," the authors conclude. One reason for the ineffectiveness of the antibiotic may be that acute bronchitis is usually caused by a virus (which is unaffected by antibiotics).

THE LANCET
Volume 359, page 1648
May 11, 2002

within 48 hours of the onset of influenza. About 10% of people have central nervous system side effects, such as anxiety and jitters, when treated with amantadine. These problems are less common with rimantadine. Because of the side effects and inconsistent effectiveness of these drugs, the recent availability of two other antiviral therapies, oseltamivir and zanamivir (Relenza), has been an important development for patients with influenza. Oseltamivir is an oral medication; zanamivir is an inhaled medication. Use of these drugs early in the illness (within the first two days of onset of symptoms) has been associated with symptomatic improvement and a milder course of infection.

Bacterial Pneumonia

Pneumonia is an infection of the air spaces (alveoli) and surrounding (interstitial) tissue. It is the sixth leading cause of death and the primary cause of death from infectious disease in the United States, claiming the lives of about 40,000 Americans annually. Most fatalities occur in people over the age of 65, who often have underlying disorders that increase their susceptibility to infection. Others at high risk for pneumonia include people with lung cancer or a suppressed immune system (for example, people with HIV or those who take immunosuppressive medications). Based on x-ray findings, the types of pneumonia often are divided into those that affect an entire lobe of one lung (lobar pneumonia) and those that occur as patches in several lobes (multilobar pneumonia). In addition, pneumonia may involve either one lung (unilateral) or both lungs (bilateral).

Causes. Hundreds of different microorganisms can infect the lungs. The most common infectious agents that cause acute pneumonia are viruses and bacteria, but other organisms (such as *Mycobacterium tuberculosis*, fungi, and the parasite *Pneumocystis carinii*) may be responsible, especially if a person's immune defenses are compromised. Environmental exposure and the setting in which pneumonia occurs (for example, in a community, nursing home, or hospital) are major determinants of the type of pneumonia and the type of microorganism that most likely caused it.

The most common type of bacterial pneumonia, pneumococcal pneumonia, is caused by *Streptococcus pneumoniae*, which frequently is present in the throats of healthy people. It can spread from person to person (for example, by coughing) when people are in close contact with others, for example, in military barracks, prisons, and nursing homes. Most people who develop pneumococcal pneumonia

NEW RESEARCH

Influenza Vaccine Is Effective, Underused

Nearly half of all hospitalizations for pneumonia and influenza and deaths from all causes can be prevented by giving the influenza vaccine each year to people 65 and older, a new report shows. However, less than two thirds of people in this age group get the vaccine in a given year.

Researchers analyzed data from people age 65 and older during the flu seasons of 1996 to 1997 (122,974 people) and 1997 to 1998 (158,454 people). The rate of vaccination was roughly 58% during both seasons.

During the first season, the rate of hospitalization for pneumonia or influenza or overall death among unvaccinated people was 8 of every 1,000 healthy persons and 38 of every 1,000 high-risk persons; this rate dropped to 29 of 1,000 high-risk persons the following season. Vaccination reduced the risk of hospitalization for pneumonia or influenza or death by 48% in the first season and 31% in the second season.

"The data are clear," writes the author of an accompanying editorial. "Vaccination of elderly persons, whether they are healthy or have high-risk, chronic medical conditions, saves lives and decreases hospitalization rates." He adds that, given the benefits of the vaccine, all older people should consider influenza vaccination every year.

CLINICAL INFECTIOUS DISEASES
Volume 35, pages 370 and 378
August 15, 2002

Vaccines You Should Consider If You Have a Lung Disorder

Influenza and pneumonia are major causes of illness and death; they result in thousands of hospitalizations and premature deaths every year. These diseases can be especially dangerous for people with chronic lung conditions such as asthma or chronic obstructive pulmonary disease (COPD). For people with asthma, for example, the flu can decrease lung function and increase the risk of airway constriction.

Older people with a chronic lung condition are at even greater danger because increased age also contributes to the potential severity of influenza or pneumonia. Specifically, older people with a chronic lung disease are two to seven times more likely to be hospitalized for pneumonia than older people without a lung disorder. Therefore, numerous health associations recommend that people age 65 and older and those with chronic health conditions—particularly lung diseases such as COPD—obtain an influenza vaccine (or flu shot) every year and a pneumonia vaccine at least once in their lifetime. (The pneumonia vaccine only protects against pneumococcal pneumonia, which is caused by the bacterium *Streptococcus pneumoniae*. This organism is only one of many causes of bacterial pneumonia.)

Despite the serious risks posed by influenza and pneumonia, about 35% of the older population is not regularly vaccinated for influenza, and more than 50% has not been vaccinated for pneumonia. Moreover, people with chronic lung diseases appear no more inclined than others to get these vaccinations. According to some studies, only 10% of people with asthma are regularly vaccinated against influenza.

It is unclear why older people and those with a chronic lung disease have low rates of immunization. Possibly to blame are some uncertainties or misconceptions about the effectiveness of these vaccines in people with chronic lung diseases. However, both vaccines are safe and effective for people with respiratory conditions.

The Evidence

To evaluate the effectiveness of the influenza vaccine, researchers from Minnesota studied 1,898 people, age 65 and older, with chronic lung diseases such as asthma and COPD. Each year during the study, roughly three quarters of the participants elected to be vaccinated against influenza. Between 1993 and 1996, people who chose to be vaccinated against influenza had 52% fewer hospitalizations for influenza and pneumonia and were 70% less likely to die of any cause during the influenza season. Vaccinated participants were also less likely to visit a doctor for any respiratory problems.

Among this same group of people, those who received a pneumococcal vaccination (about two thirds of the participants) had a 43% reduction in pneumonia hospitalizations and 29% fewer deaths from any cause. Receiving both the influenza and pneumococcal vaccinations had an additive effect: a 72%

have some underlying disease. It may be an acute infection like influenza, but more often it is a chronic condition such as diabetes, alcoholism, cirrhosis, lung diseases like COPD, AIDS, and blood disorders like leukemia. Also at increased risk are cigarette smokers and individuals who are chronically malnourished or debilitated. Pneumococcal pneumonia is far more common in elderly than in young people. For example, the number of cases per 100,000 people ranges from 20 in young adults to 280 in people over the age of 75.

Other common causes of bacterial pneumonia include *Haemophilus influenzae* (not to be confused with the influenza virus), *Legionella pneumophila* (the cause of Legionnaires' disease), *Staphylococcus aureus* (staph), and gram-negative organisms like *Klebsiella pneumoniae, Pseudomonas aeruginosa,* and *Proteus.* Staph and gram-negative pneumonias often are acquired during hospitalization and are associated with a high risk of death.

Symptoms. Bacterial pneumonia typically has an abrupt onset of symptoms including a cough that produces yellow phlegm, high

reduction in hospitalizations for both influenza and pneumonia, and 82% fewer deaths from any cause compared with those who received neither vaccination.

Also, the vaccines are not known to worsen symptoms in people with lung disorders. For example, a study of 2,032 people with asthma showed that exacerbations in asthma symptoms occurred equally among people given the influenza vaccine and those given a placebo.

The Vaccinations

The influenza vaccine is recommended once a year for high-risk people, including people age 65 and older, those with lung diseases (such as asthma and COPD), and people with certain chronic illnesses. The vaccine must be given annually because the properties of the influenza virus tend to change from year to year. Because the flu season usually peaks from January to March and the shot takes about two weeks to take effect, you should get the influenza vaccine between the months of October and December.

People who are allergic to eggs should talk to their doctor before getting the flu shot, because the vaccine is grown in chicken eggs. People with Guillain-Barré syndrome (a disease affecting the peripheral nervous system) also should consult their doctor before getting the vaccine. Vaccination should be postponed by those who have a fever or severe cold on the day they intend to get the shot.

Side effects of the influenza vaccine include swelling, redness, and soreness at the injection site. Some people may experience mild aches and fever for a day or two after the injection. However, you cannot get the flu from the vaccine because the viruses in the vaccine are not active—they have been killed in the preparation of the vaccine. Rare side effects include difficulty breathing, dizziness, a high fever, and hives. These symptoms indicate an allergic reaction and require immediate medical attention.

Since pneumonia is often a complication of influenza, getting a flu shot is one good way to prevent pneumonia. However, pneumonia caused by *S. pneumoniae* can also be prevented by getting the pneumonia vaccine. The shot is recommended for those at high risk for pneumonia, such as people age 65 and older and those with lung diseases. Doctors used to recommend that the vaccine be given only once, but experts now recommend that anyone who received the vaccine before age 65 get a booster shot once every five years. For younger people with asthma and no other risk factors, the pneumococcal vaccine is not necessary, according to the Centers for Disease Control and Prevention.

Like the influenza vaccine, side effects can include soreness at the injection site and mild fever. Similarly, allergic reactions may occur in a small number of people, and they require medical attention. People should delay getting the pneumonia vaccine if they have a fever or severe cold.

Medicare covers both the influenza and the pneumonia vaccines.

fever, chills, sharp chest pain precipitated by breathing or coughing, and shortness of breath. Young patients usually have increased respiratory and heart rates and appear acutely ill. Many older adults have fewer symptoms, often have no fever, and instead experience lethargy and confusion.

Diagnosis. The diagnosis of pneumonia is made from the patient's medical history, physical examination, and chest x-ray, which may show a variety of abnormalities. The bacteria responsible for the pneumonia may be determined by examining phlegm under a microscope. Culture of phlegm may conclusively identify the bacteria and allow testing for their sensitivity to various antibiotics. It is important to obtain a phlegm specimen that is derived from the lungs, rather than one containing mostly saliva. Ideally, phlegm should be obtained before treatment with any antibiotic, but treatment should not be delayed.

Other routine laboratory tests in people with suspected pneumonia include a blood cell count, measurement of serum electrolytes, urinalysis, and liver function tests. In bacterial pneumonia, the white blood cell count typically is high and shows many young polymorphonuclear cells (a type of white blood cell). In contrast, the white cell count usually is low or normal in people with viral or mycoplasma pneumonia but may also be low in people with severe bacterial pneumonia.

Prevention. Although most types of bacterial pneumonia cannot be prevented, influenza vaccination and vigorous treatment of chronic lung diseases may prevent some cases of pneumonia. Pneumococcal vaccine is effective against 88% of the bacterial strains of *S. pneumoniae* and is effective in preventing 60% to 70% of cases of pneumococcal pneumonia.

Experts estimate that at least half of the deaths related to pneumococcal pneumonia could be averted if everyone followed the guidelines from the CDC. The CDC recommends vaccination against pneumococcal pneumonia for the following people: anyone age 65 or older; people with chronic cardiovascular or lung disorders (but not those with uncomplicated asthma); people with diabetes or chronic liver or kidney disease; and those with immune suppression due to cancer chemotherapy or to conditions such as leukemia, multiple myeloma, or HIV. Even people who have already had pneumococcal pneumonia should get the pneumococcal vaccine; an *S. pneumoniae* infection may confer natural immunity to one particular strain of the bacterium, but an infection with another strain is still possible. While the vaccine was given only once in the past, a booster is now recommended every five years for people who were first vaccinated before age 65.

Treatment. Antibiotics are the mainstay of treatment for bacterial pneumonia, and early treatment produces the best outcomes. The antibiotic of choice depends on the type of pneumonia. Because of practical difficulties in obtaining satisfactory phlegm specimens and delays in obtaining results, antibiotic treatment often is empiric, meaning that it is based on the patient's characteristics, where he or she likely became infected, and the physician's suspicions about the most likely causative organism.

The severity of pneumonia, the patient's general medical status, and the availability of family and other caregivers at home determine whether treatment requires hospitalization. *S. pneumoniae* at one time was highly sensitive to penicillin, but penicillin-resistant strains have become more common, and newer antibiotics may be needed to treat highly resistant strains. In addition, because mycoplasmas and other atypical microorganisms also may cause pneumonia and their symptoms may overlap with those of pneumonia caused by *S. pneumoniae*, combinations of antibiotics (including macrolides) or treatment with drugs called quinolones generally are used.

With treatment, clinical improvement usually is rapid, and the speed at which it occurs depends on the patient's previous health status. For hospitalized patients, an early switch from intravenous to oral antibiotics as clinical improvement occurs has been found to be safe and effective and allows earlier discharge. The clearing of chest x-ray abnormalities typically lags behind clinical improvement, especially in older people with multilobar pneumonia, COPD, or alcoholism.

Tuberculosis

Worldwide there are more deaths from tuberculosis (TB) than from any other single infectious disease. Recent studies show that TB is responsible for 7% of all deaths and 26% of all preventable deaths. About 95% of these deaths (and 95% of the estimated 8 million new cases of TB in 1997) occurred in developing countries. New TB cases in the United States declined steadily between 1950 and the mid-1980s, then began to increase, and reached a peak in 1992. Most new cases occur in ethnic and racial minorities. Compared with non-Hispanic whites, the incidence of new cases is 10 times greater in blacks and 5 times greater in Hispanics and Native Americans. The number of TB cases is three times higher in urban than in rural areas and is increased in the elderly and in people with diabetes.

One probable cause for the rise in TB in recent years is the epidemic of HIV and AIDS, which greatly increases the chance that an inactive TB infection will become activated and produce clinical disease and symptoms. The rise in U.S. cases of TB also is attributable to increasing numbers of immigrants, homeless people, and drug users, all of whom are at increased risk for TB. Another major problem is the development of TB organisms that are resistant to the drugs used to treat the disease. Over the last 30 years, the prevalence of multidrug-resistant organisms has risen from 2% to 9% and is especially high in certain urban areas.

Causes. Tuberculosis infections are caused by *Mycobacterium tuberculosis*, which usually infects the lungs, but about one third of infections also involve other organs. Most often, people become infected by inhaling TB-containing microdroplets released into the air from the upper airway of a person infected with pulmonary TB.

NEW RESEARCH

Pneumonia Risk Decreased By Good Oral Hygiene

Nursing home residents who receive thorough, regular oral care have a reduced risk of pneumonia, researchers report.

Japanese investigators randomized 417 residents of nursing homes to receive either thorough oral care (tooth brushing after every meal performed by a caregiver, weekly cleanings by a dentist or dental hygienist, and, in some cases, regular use of a dental rinse) or usual oral care. (Many of the residents were very frail and only a few of them brushed their teeth.)

Over the next two years, significantly fewer people in the thorough oral care group experienced fevers compared with those in the usual care group (15% vs. 29%). More important, significantly fewer people in the thorough oral care group were diagnosed with pneumonia (11% vs. 19%). In addition, among the people who did develop pneumonia, those in the thorough oral care group were much less likely to die of pneumonia than those in the usual oral care group (7% vs. 16%).

One cause of bacterial pneumonia may be the inhalation of bacteria from oral secretions into the lungs. Oral care may reduce the number of these bacteria, and therefore, the risk of bacterial pneumonia, the authors speculate.

JOURNAL OF THE AMERICAN GERIATRICS SOCIETY
Volume 50, page 430
March 2002

These microdroplets are released when the infected person coughs, sneezes, or speaks. Once a person becomes infected, the development of an immune response to the organism, which occurs over a 4- to 10-week period, normally reduces the extent of inflammation and causes the bacteria to become dormant. However, the organisms remain alive and can become reactivated at any time.

Symptoms. Most people have no symptoms during the stage of a TB infection when the bacteria are dormant, but some may notice a low-grade fever, sweats, and cough for a short period. In about 10% of people with a TB infection, the bacteria become reactivated and symptoms of active TB appear. The likelihood of developing active disease is greatest in the first year or two after infection and diminishes with the length of time following the infection. The risk of activation is especially high for those with diminished immunity due to older age, HIV or other chronic viral infections, Hodgkin disease, leukemia, malnutrition, or treatment with immunosuppressive agents for an organ transplant or with corticosteroids for other medical problems. The risk of activation also is increased in people with silicosis, chronic kidney failure that requires dialysis, hemophilia, and diabetes. In about one third of cases, active disease results from reinfection rather than activation of latent disease. Symptoms of active disease include fever, night sweats, weight loss, and fatigue. Other manifestations depend on whether the disease remains localized to the lungs or spreads to other sites. While TB can spread to almost any site of the body, the most common sites, in decreasing order of frequency, are the lymph nodes, urogenital system, bones and joints, and linings of the brain (meninges), abdominal cavity (peritoneum), and heart (pericardium).

In the lung, the disease is most commonly located in the upper lobes, but it often affects the lower lobes in the elderly, in immunosuppressed people, and in those with diabetes. Progression of the disease in the lungs may cause cough, production of bloody phlegm, and shortness of breath. Spread of TB through the bloodstream may produce myriad tiny lesions throughout both lungs—a condition known as miliary tuberculosis, because the 1- to 2-mm, yellow lung lesions resemble millet seeds. Spread to the pleura is common and may produce chest pain, fever, and pleural effusion that, if large, can cause shortness of breath.

Diagnosis. During the early infectious stage, before the onset of active disease but after the development of immunity, the presence of TB infection can be confirmed by a positive skin test, which involves injecting PPD (a purified protein from the tuberculosis bacterium) into the skin of the forearm. Most infected people will show an area of skin thickening (induration) at the injection site 48 to 72 hours later. The response to the PPD test often is blunted in people who are immunosuppressed. The PPD skin test is not useful for the diagnosis of active disease: It is negative in about 20% of such people because of immunosuppression or severe disease, while a positive test may only indicate a prior infection that is not active.

Once infection has progressed to active disease, the diagnosis can be strongly suspected from a chest x-ray that shows the typical upper lobe location of changes in the lungs, often with lesions that have a central cavity. The x-ray also may show enlargement of lymph nodes. The diagnosis is confirmed by finding the TB organism in phlegm examined under a microscope. Definitive diagnosis requires growing the organism, obtained from phlegm or other sites, in culture. These cultured bacteria are tested for their sensitivity to various drugs. Because the TB bacteria grow so slowly, conventional culturing techniques require four to eight weeks to obtain a result; newer culture methods allow growth in two to three weeks. Tuberculosis requires microscopic identification and culture of bacteria from the affected site(s).

Prevention. People with active TB need to be treated so that they will not spread the infection. People in contact with TB patients can reduce their risk of contracting the infection by using masks and special lamps that kill the bacteria with ultraviolet light. Isoniazid (Laniazid, Nydrazid), also known as INH, may be used to prevent TB in people at high risk, such as those with HIV or other causes of immunosuppression and those living in a crowded household with an infected individual. Studies also have shown a highly significant decrease in the development of active TB when people with latent infection, indicated by a positive PPD test, are treated for 6 to 12 months with daily INH.

Vaccination with an weakened strain of a bovine form of mycobacterium (BCG) once was widely advocated as a way to raise immunity to TB bacteria. Though still used in the United States in special circumstances (for example, in highly exposed health care workers), BCG vaccination is not recommended for the general population because of questions about its effectiveness.

Treatment. More than half of untreated people die within five years, yet TB can be cured in almost all people infected with a TB organism that is sensitive to drugs. Treatment of TB typically involves

NEW RESEARCH

Vitamin E May Exacerbate Respiratory Infections

Vitamin E supplements appear to increase the severity of acute respiratory tract infections in older people, a new study indicates.

Dutch investigators randomized 652 people (age 60 and older) to receive either a multivitamin (containing 100% of the U.S. Recommended Daily Allowance of vitamins and 25% to 50% of the recommended levels of minerals), a multivitamin plus 200 mg of vitamin E, 200 mg of vitamin E, or a placebo each day.

During an average of about 15 months, people who took the multivitamin were just as likely to have an acute respiratory infection as those who did not take a multivitamin, and symptoms were no less severe. People who took vitamin E had the same number of respiratory infections as those who did not take vitamin E, but symptoms tended to be more severe in vitamin E users. Their infections lasted longer (19 vs. 14 days on average) and were more likely to be accompanied by fever, symptoms were more numerous, and activities were more likely to be restricted.

The researchers suggest that a balanced mixture of antioxidant vitamins may be the most important factor for optimal health and that long-term supplementation with vitamin E may upset this balance.

JOURNAL OF THE AMERICAN MEDICAL ASSOCIATION
Volume 288, page 715
August 14, 2002

the simultaneous use of two or more drugs to avoid the emergence of resistant strains. Before treatment is started, a complete blood count is performed and baseline tests are carried out to measure liver and kidney function. Standard treatment now involves triple drug therapy—most commonly, a combination of INH, rifampin (Rifadin, Rimactane), and pyrazinamide (available only in a generic form), either daily or three times a week, for two months. This period is followed by a four-month course of INH plus rifampin given two or three times weekly. Because INH interferes with the action of pyridoxine (vitamin B_6), supplements of the vitamin are given to people at high risk for vitamin deficiency. Ethambutol (Myambutol) or streptomycin may be added when a resistant strain is suspected. Treatment should continue for at least nine months in people whose disease has spread beyond the lungs. People who do not follow their medication regimens may be required to take their medication under observation.

During treatment, people with phlegm that contains the TB organism have regular phlegm cultures; repeat chest x-rays are not required in all patients. Phlegm cultures no longer contain the TB organism in about 80% of patients after two months of treatment and in virtually all patients with drug-sensitive organisms after three months. Persistence of organisms at three months is considered a treatment failure. Most people with pulmonary TB become noninfectious to others after about two weeks of treatment.

Although INH is included in nearly all regimens for the treatment of TB, about 5% of patients have an adverse reaction to the medication. Of greatest concern is life-threatening liver toxicity, manifested by loss of appetite, nausea and vomiting, fatigue, weakness, jaundice, and dark urine. The risk of liver toxicity increases in older patients and in people taking rifampin. Blood tests to check for liver disease are not obtained regularly during treatment but are done if the patient develops one or more of the signs of liver toxicity mentioned above. The drug INH also can cause skin rash and peripheral neuropathy (nerve damage in the hands and feet) with paresthesias (tingling sensations). Side effects of rifampin include hepatitis and gastrointestinal symptoms. Blood uric acid is measured before and during treatment in people taking pyrazinamide, which can elevate uric acid levels and cause joint pain or gout. Visual acuity is assessed before starting ethambutol, which can cause optic neuritis (inflammation of the optic nerve in the eye). Streptomycin, which must be given by injection, can cause dizziness, difficulty walking, or hearing loss. ■

GLOSSARY

acute—Having a short and relatively severe course.

alpha$_1$-antitrypsin—A naturally occurring substance in the body that protects against damage to the walls of the alveoli by blocking the action of enzymes that break down proteins. A deficiency in this substance is one cause of emphysema.

alveoli—Tiny air sacs in the lungs. The walls of the alveoli contain capillaries, which absorb inhaled oxygen into the bloodstream and release carbon dioxide from the bloodstream to the lungs to be exhaled.

apnea—Cessation of breathing.

arterial blood gases—A measurement of the oxygen, carbon dioxide, and acidity of blood taken from an artery.

asthma—A disease characterized by inflammation and narrowing of the bronchi, making breathing difficult.

atelectasis—Reduced inflation of the lung, often related to blockage of a bronchus by mucus, a tumor, or a foreign body.

blood pressure—Pressure of blood against the walls of an artery.

bronchi—Large airways in the lungs that branch from the trachea.

bronchiectasis—Persistent dilation of the bronchi or bronchioles as the result of another disease, such as a lung infection, tumor, or cystic fibrosis.

bronchioles—Small airways in the lungs that branch from the bronchi.

bronchiolitis obliterans—Restrictive inflammation of the bronchioles.

bronchoscopy—Passage of a thin, hollow, flexible tube through the mouth and windpipe to allow viewing of the main bronchial passages.

catheter—A thin, flexible tube.

chronic—Persisting over a long period.

chronic obstructive pulmonary disease (COPD)—A group of lung diseases, mainly emphysema and chronic bronchitis, characterized by an obstruction of airflow during exhalation.

cilia—Small hairs that line the bronchioles and move mucus out of the lungs with a wavelike motion.

cor pulmonale—Heart disease due to resistance of the passage of blood through the lungs; it often leads to right heart failure.

corticosteroid—Medication that reduces inflammation, for example, in the airways.

cyanosis—Bluish color of the skin as a result of insufficient oxygen in the blood.

diaphragm—The muscular structure that separates the chest cavity from the abdomen. The diaphragm plays an important role in breathing.

diffusion capacity—A measurement of how well gas passes across the membranes in the lungs.

dyspnea—Sensation of shortness of breath or difficulty in breathing.

emphysema—A disease in which damage to the alveoli causes the lungs to lose their elasticity. People with emphysema are unable to move adequate quantities of fresh air through their lungs.

epiglottis—A flap of cartilage in the back of the throat that prevents food from entering the trachea.

expiration—Exhalation.

fibrosis—A process by which inflamed tissue becomes scarred. Scarring in the lungs is called pulmonary fibrosis.

hemoptysis—Coughing up blood.

hypoxemia—Inadequate oxygen in the blood.

inspiration—Inhalation.

interstitial lung disease—A group of lung disorders that affect the supporting matrix of the lungs.

interstitium—The supporting matrix of the lungs, as opposed to the airways and air sacs.

larynx—Voice box.

lobe—A section of the lung; the right lung has three lobes, while the left lung has two.

lobectomy—Removal of an entire lobe of the lung.

lung volume—The amount of air in the lungs.

lung volume reduction surgery (LVRS)—A surgical procedure in which lung tissue affected by emphysema is removed.

lung volume tests—Tests to measure the amount of air in the lungs.

pharynx—Throat.

pleura—The membranes that cover the outside of the lungs and the inside wall of the chest cavity.

pleural effusion—Fluid within the pleural space.

pneumonectomy—Removal of an entire lung.

pneumonia—An infection in the lungs.

pneumothorax—Leakage of air into the space around the lung.

pulmonary artery—The blood vessel that delivers oxygen-poor blood from the right ventricle to the lungs.

pulmonary embolism—A blood clot that travels from a vein in the leg, pelvis, or arm and lodges in the pulmonary artery.

pulmonary fibrosis—Chronic inflammation and progressive scarring of the walls of the alveoli. When the cause is unknown, it is called idiopathic pulmonary fibrosis.

pulmonary function tests—A group of procedures used to evaluate the status of the lungs and to confirm the presence of certain lung disorders.

pulmonary hypertension—Abnormally high blood pressure in the arteries of the lungs.

respiration—The process of breathing; also defined as gas exchange from air to the blood and from the blood to the body's cells.

sleep apnea—Temporary cessation of breathing during sleep, often leading to daytime sleepiness.

spirometer—An instrument used in a pulmonary function test; it records the total volume and rate of air being breathed out. This test helps to diagnose or assess a lung disorder or to monitor its treatment.

spirometry—Measurement of the volume of air forcefully exhaled by the lungs as a function of time.

systemic—Affecting the body as a whole.

total lung capacity—The amount of air in the lungs after maximal inspiration.

trachea—Windpipe.

vasodilator—An agent that widens blood vessels.

ventilation—Movement of air (gases) in and out of the lungs.

x-ray—A procedure that uses invisible electromagnetic energy to produce images of bones, organs, and internal tissues.

HEALTH INFORMATION ORGANIZATIONS AND SUPPORT GROUPS

American Academy of Allergy, Asthma & Immunology
611 East Wells St.
Milwaukee, WI 53202
☎ 800-822-2762
414-272-6071
www.aaaai.org
Offers public education on allergies and asthma through children's books, tips brochures, videos, newsletters, and a Web site. Offers referrals for allergists and immunologists. Supports asthma and allergy research through grants to medical training programs.

American Association for Respiratory Care
11030 Ables Ln.
Dallas, TX 75229
☎ 972-243-2272
www.aarc.org
Society of respiratory health professionals. Web site supplies respiratory health tips, quizzes, and links to other organizations.

American Lung Association
61 Broadway, 6th Floor
New York, NY 10006
☎ 212-315-8700
www.lungusa.org
Oldest voluntary health organization in the United States. Funds and conducts research on all lung disorders, with a special emphasis on asthma. Institutes school and workplace educational programs; provides information on air quality and tobacco dangers.

American Thoracic Society
61 Broadway
New York, NY 10006
☎ (212) 315-8600
www.thoracic.org
International organization that funds research and education programs to improve patient care. Offers referrals to support groups and information on respiratory disorders. Provides educational materials and classes.

COPD-Support, Inc.
PMB 127
1940 Kings Hwy, Ste. 4
Port Charlotte, FL 33980
www.copd-support.com
On-line group offering e-mail lists, chat rooms, forums, and a newsletter for people involved with COPD. Dedicated to providing patients and caregivers with support, education, and a way to share ideas and solutions for dealing with this disorder.

The Canadian Lung Association
3 Raymond St., Ste. 300
Ottawa, ON K1R 1A3
Canada
☎ 613-569-6411
www.lung.ca
Canadian national not-for-profit health association funds medical research, provides health education and programs with a focus on lung diseases (such as asthma and COPD), tobacco, and clean air. Ten provincial Lung Associations offer programs for the one in five Canadians living with lung disease.

The National Emphysema Foundation
15 Stevens St.
Norwalk, CT 06850
☎ 203-299-0723
www.emphysemafoundation.org
Nonprofit organization that supplies information on emphysema and other lung diseases. Web site provides articles and tips on quitting smoking. Affiliated with the Norwalk Hospital in Connecticut.

National Heart, Lung, and Blood Institute
P.O. Box 30105
Bethesda, MD 20824-0105
☎ 301-592-8573
www.nhlbi.nih.gov
Lead component of the National Institutes of Health for lung disease research; provides written information on noncancerous lung disorders (e.g., asthma, COPD, and cystic fibrosis).

National Lung Health Education Program (NLHEP)
HealthONE Center
1850 High St.
Denver, CO 80218
☎ 303-839-6755
www.nlhep.org
The mission of the NLHEP is to promote the early diagnosis of COPD and related disorders through the widespread use of spirometry. "Test Your Lungs, Know Your Numbers" is the motto of the NLHEP.

LEADING HOSPITALS FOR LUNG DISORDERS

U.S. News & World Report and the National Opinion Research Center, a social-science research group at the University of Chicago, recently conducted their 13th annual nationwide survey of 1,484 physicians in 17 medical specialties. The doctors nominated up to five hospitals they consider best from among 6,045 U.S. hospitals. This is the current list of the best hospitals for lung disorders, as determined by the doctors' recommendations from 2000, 2001, and 2002; federal data on death rates; and factual data regarding quality indicators, such as the ratio of registered nurses to patients and the use of advanced technology. Since the results reflect the doctors' opinions, however, they are, to some degree, subjective. Any institution listed is considered a leading center, and the rankings do not imply that other hospitals cannot or do not deliver excellent care.

1. **National Jewish Medical and Research Center**
   Denver, CO
   ☎ 800-222-LUNG (5864)
   www.njc.org
2. **Mayo Clinic**
   Rochester, MN
   ☎ 507-284-2511
   www.mayoclinic.org
3. **Johns Hopkins Hospital**
   Baltimore, MD
   ☎ 410-955-5000
   www.hopkinsmedicine.org
4. **Barnes-Jewish Hospital**
   St. Louis, MO
   ☎ 314-747-3000
   www.barnesjewish.org
5. **Massachusetts General Hospital**
   Boston, MA
   ☎ 617-726-2000
   www.mgh.harvard.edu
6. **UCSF Medical Center**
   San Francisco, CA
   ☎ 888-689-UCSF/415-476-1000
   www.ucsfhealth.org
7. **University of Colorado Hospital**
   Denver, CO
   ☎ 800-621-7621/303-372-2929
   uch.uchsc.edu
8. **Cleveland Clinic**
   Cleveland, OH
   ☎ 800-223-2273/216-444-2200
   www.clevelandclinic.org
9. **UCSD Medical Center**
   San Diego, CA
   ☎ 800-926-UCSD (8273)
   www.health.ucsd.edu
10. **University of Michigan Medical Center**
   Ann Arbor, MI
   ☎ 800-211-8181/734-936-4000
   www.med.umich.edu

INHALED CORTICOSTEROIDS FOR COPD

Chronic obstructive pulmonary disease (COPD) has become an increasingly common condition. While doctors frequently prescribe inhaled corticosteroids for the treatment of COPD, far less is known about their effects in people with COPD than in people with asthma.

To help fill this gap in knowledge, Canadian researchers led by Abdullah Alsaeedi, M.D., pooled data from nine studies that looked at the effects of inhaled corticosteroids in 3,976 COPD patients. All of these studies were randomized and placebo controlled and lasted at least six months.

On average, patients who used inhaled corticosteroids, regardless of whether they were also taking oral corticosteroids, had 30% fewer exacerbations of COPD than patients who were assigned to receive a placebo. However, the definition of an exacerbation varied greatly among the studies, ranging from more cough and phlegm than usual to hospitalizations for respiratory symptoms. And while patients taking inhaled corticosteroids had a slightly reduced risk of death from any cause in the five studies that evaluated mortality, this reduction was not statistically significant and could have been a chance occurrence.

The risk of two common adverse reactions to inhaled corticosteroids—oropharyngeal candidiasis (a yeast infection commonly called thrush) and skin bruising—was more than doubled in patients taking inhaled corticosteroids compared with those taking a placebo. Other possible side effects of inhaled corticosteroids, including low bone mineral density, fractures, cataracts, and adrenal insufficiency, did not occur, probably because the studies were of relatively short duration.

While the authors note that these studies indicate inhaled corticosteroids help to reduce the number and rate of COPD exacerbations, they write that more studies are needed to determine whether they reduce death rates and to identify their long-term side effects.

REVIEW

The Effects of Inhaled Corticosteroids in Chronic Obstructive Pulmonary Disease: A Systematic Review of Randomized Placebo-Controlled Trials

Abdullah Alsaeedi, MD, Don D. Sin, MD, MPH, Finlay A. McAlister, MD, MSc

PURPOSE: Although inhaled corticosteroids are commonly used to treat patients with chronic obstructive pulmonary disease (COPD), their effect on clinical outcomes such as exacerbation and mortality is unknown. This systematic review was conducted to determine whether inhaled corticosteroids improve clinical outcomes for patients with stable COPD.

SUBJECTS AND METHODS: All placebo-controlled randomized trials of inhaled corticosteroids given for at least 6 months for stable COPD were identified by searching MEDLINE (1966–2000), EMBASE (1980–2001), CINAHL (1982–2000), SIGLE (1980–2000), the Cochrane Controlled Trial Registry, and the bibliographies of published studies. We independently extracted data from each of the studies using a specified protocol, and determined the summary risk ratios (RRs) and 95% confidence intervals (CIs) for exacerbations and deaths.

RESULTS: Nine randomized trials (3976 patients with COPD), including four with a systemic steroid run-in phase, were identified. Use of inhaled corticosteroid therapy reduced the rate of exacerbations (RR = 0.70; 95% CI: 0.58 to 0.84), with similar benefits in those who were and were not pretreated with systemic steroids. Inhaled corticosteroid therapy was also associated with increased rates of oropharyngeal candidiasis (RR = 2.1; 95% CI: 1.5 to 3.1), skin bruising (RR = 2.1; 95% CI: 1.6 to 2.8), and lower mean cortisol levels. No effects were seen on all-cause mortality (RR = 0.84; 95% CI: 0.60 to 1.18) in the five trials that measured this outcome.

CONCLUSION: This systematic review demonstrates a beneficial effect of inhaled corticosteroids in reducing rates of COPD exacerbation. Further research is required to define the long-term effects of these medications and the benefit/risk ratio for patients with COPD. **Am J Med. 2002;113:59–65.** ©2002 by Excerpta Medica, Inc.

Approximately 14 million people in the United States have chronic obstructive pulmonary disease (COPD), and its prevalence has risen by 41% since 1982 (1). Age-adjusted mortality increased by 17% between 1966 and 1982, in contrast with the decline in age-adjusted rates from all other major causes of mortality during that time (1). The World Health Organization predicts that COPD will be the fifth most prevalent disease (currently 12th) and the third most common cause of death (currently sixth) by 2020 (2).

Airway inflammation is a prominent feature of COPD. Although the benefits of inhaled corticosteroids are well established in asthma, there remains controversy about their effects in patients with COPD (3,4). A recent meta-analysis suggested that high, but not medium or low, doses were beneficial in COPD (5). However, this study's primary outcome was the rate of decline in forced expiratory volume in 1 second (FEV_1). Previous studies suggest that physiologic outcomes are only loosely associated with clinically important endpoints such as rates of COPD exacerbation or mortality (6). Thus, we conducted a systematic review of placebo-controlled randomized trials to evaluate the long-term effects of inhaled corticosteroid therapy in patients with COPD on clinically important outcomes such as death and exacerbation.

METHODS

Searching for Relevant Studies

MEDLINE (1966–2000), EMBASE (1980–2001), CINAHL (1982–2000), SIGLE (1980–2000), and the Cochrane Controlled Trial Registry were searched for placebo-controlled randomized clinical trials evaluating the effect of inhaled corticosteroids in COPD. The search was restricted to human studies, but no language restrictions were applied. Subject headings used in the search included *COPD, chronic airflow obstruction, chronic obstructive pulmonary disease, chronic bronchitis, emphysema, glucocorticosteroids, corticosteroids, inhalation therapy, beclomethasone, budesonide, fluticasone*, and *triamcinolone*. Bibliographies of identified studies were hand searched, and content experts were contacted to identify any studies missed by the electronic searches.

From the Divisions of Pulmonary Medicine (AA, DDS) and General Internal Medicine (FAM), University of Alberta, Edmonton, Canada.

Requests for reprints should be addressed to Don D. Sin, MD, MPH, 2E4.29 Walter C. Mackenzie Centre, University of Alberta, Edmonton, Alberta T6G 2B7, Canada, or don.sin@ualberta.ca

Manuscript submitted October 31, 2001, and accepted in revised form March 8, 2002.

0002-9343/02/$–see front matter
PII S0002-9343(02)01143-9

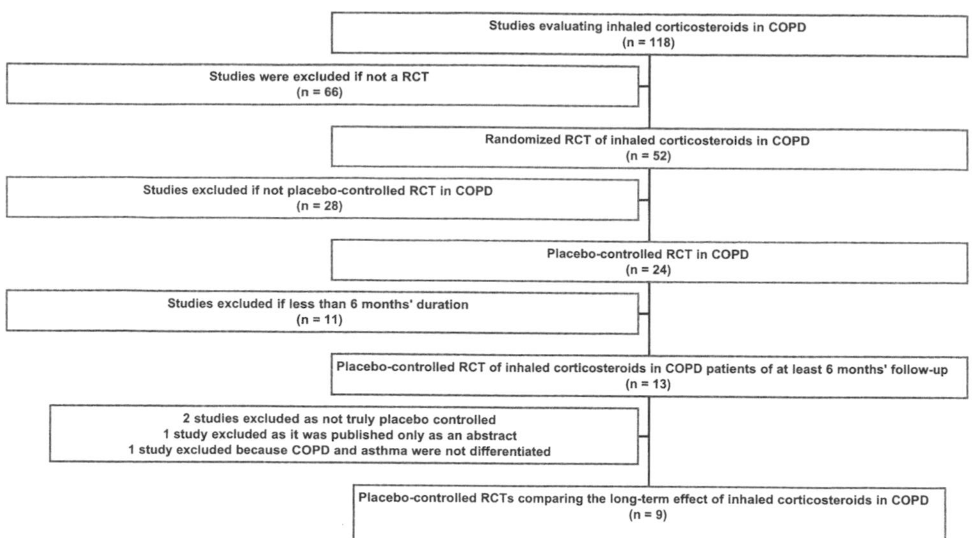

Figure 1. Study selection process. COPD = chronic obstructive pulmonary disease; RCT = randomized controlled trial.

Study Selection and Data Abstraction

We independently reviewed the results of the search strategy and selected all placebo-controlled randomized trials of the long-term effects (at least 6 months) of inhaled corticosteroids in patients with stable COPD. The primary outcome of this systematic review was to compare the frequency (risk) of respiratory exacerbations between patients treated or not treated with inhaled corticosteroids. Secondary outcomes included the rate of decline in FEV_1 and all-cause mortality. Trials that included both patients with COPD and patients with asthma were excluded if they did not report the results for the COPD patients separately.

Data were abstracted from each trial using a standardized abstraction form. Discrepancies were resolved by iteration and consensus. The definitions for each outcome (including exacerbation) were those used by the investigators in the original studies. In trials that did not define exacerbation (e.g., the Lung Health Study), we assumed that an exacerbation was a hospitalization for a respiratory condition. One investigator was contacted to clarify published data. Trial quality was assessed independently using the Jadad scale by two of the authors (AA, DDS) (7).

Statistical Analysis

Analyses were performed using Meta-Analyst 0.998 software (J. Lau, New England Medical Center, Boston, Massachusetts). Because the outcomes of interest were common, risk ratios (RRs) and 95% confidence intervals (CIs) were determined for all-cause mortality and for COPD exacerbations. The data on FEV_1 could not be combined across studies, but the summary data from each trial were noted. We examined the number of patients who had at least one COPD exacerbation, but this was reported only in four trials. Because we were interested in assessing whether inhaled corticosteroids reduced recurrent exacerbations as well as first-time exacerbations, we analyzed the total COPD exacerbation rate using a previously published method (8). We assumed that the frequency of COPD exacerbations followed a Poisson distribution and calculated the frequency of COPD exacerbations per patient-month of treatment (9). Thus, a patient suffering three exacerbations during the course of follow-up would contribute three events to whichever treatment to which they had been assigned. Data on all-cause mortality and COPD exacerbations were combined using the DerSimonian-Laird random-effects models and the Mantel-Haenszel-Peto fixed-effects models. Only the random-effects results are reported.

RESULTS

Of the 118 citations identified in our search, 13 were retrieved for detailed evaluation (Figure 1). Four of these studies were excluded: two were not truly placebo controlled (10,11), one was published only as an abstract and the author did not answer requests for clarification of the data (12), and one did not distinguish between patients with COPD and those with asthma when outcomes were reported (13). Thus, nine studies (n = 3976 patients) were eligible for inclusion (Table 1) (14–22). In all of these trials, the control groups received usual care. Four trials had a systemic steroid run-in phase (varying from 1.5 to 2.0 weeks) (19–22). The definitions of "COPD exacerbation" varied among trials (Table 1).

Beneficial Effects of Inhaled Corticosteroids

Four trials reported the number of patients suffering at least one exacerbation, and six reported the total number

Table 1. Description of Studies Included

Study (reference)	No. of Subjects	Study Sample	Mean Age (years)	Current Smoker (number [%])	Baseline FEV_1 (L) (mean ± SD)	Comparison	Duration (months)	Definition of Exacerbation
Studies with systemic steroid run-in phase								
Vestbo et al. (22)	290	COPD, aged 30–70 years, community survey program, Denmark	59	222 (77)	2.37 ± 0.82	Budesonide (867 μg/d) vs. placebo	36	Cough and phlegm, more than usual
Senderovitz et al. (21)	26	COPD, aged 18–75 years, outpatient, five centers in Denmark	54	Not reported	1.49*	Budesonide (800 μg/d) vs. placebo	6	Not specified
Bourbeau et al. (20)	79	COPD, aged >40 years, university-affiliated hospital, Canada	66	31 (39)	0.95 ± 0.33	Budesonide (1600 μg/d) vs. placebo	6	Use of oral steroids for worsening of symptoms
Burge et al. (19)	751	COPD, aged 40–75 years, outpatient, 18 countries	64	284 (38)	1.24 ± 0.45	Fluticasone (1000 μg/d) vs. placebo	36	Use of oral steroids or antibiotics for worsening of symptoms
Studies without systemic steroid run-in phase								
Lung Health Study (18)	1116	COPD, screened for Lung Health Study trial of smoking cessation, aged 40–69 years, 10 centers in the U.S. and Canada	56	998 (90)	2.13 ± 0.63	Triamcinolone (1200 μg/d) vs. placebo	40	Hospitalization for respiratory conditions
Renkema et al. (17)	58	COPD, aged <70 years, outpatient men. The Netherlands	56	26 (45)	1.98 ± 0.61	Budesonide (1600 μg/d) vs. placebo	24	Not specified
Pauwels et al. (16)	1277	COPD, aged 30–65 years, population based, nine European countries	52	1277 (100)	2.54 ± 0.64	Budesonide (800 μg/d) vs. placebo	36	Not reported
Weir et al. (15)	98	COPD, United Kingdom	66	38 (39)	1.10 ± 0.07	Beclomethasone (1500–2000 μg/d) vs. placebo	24	Worsening of symptoms (leading to study withdrawal in some cases)
Paggiaro et al. (14)	281	COPD, aged 50–70 years, 13 centers, Europe	63	138 (49)	1.57 ± 0.60	Fluticasone (1000 μg/d) vs. placebo	6	Worsening of symptoms requiring changes to normal treatment

* Median.
COPD = chronic obstructive pulmonary disease; FEV_1 = forced expiratory volume in 1 second.

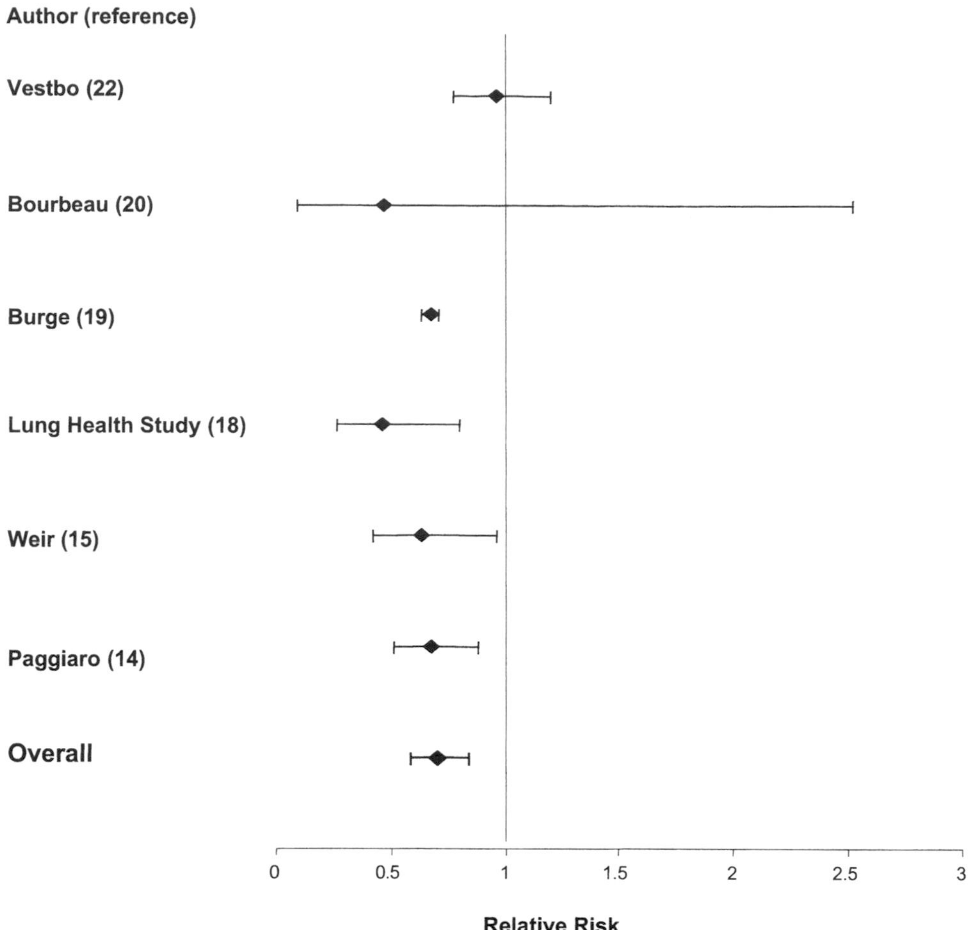

Figure 2. Relative risk of exacerbations in patients with chronic obstructive pulmonary disease treated with inhaled corticosteroids compared with placebo. **Horizontal bars** represent 95% confidence intervals.

of COPD exacerbations in each treatment arm (14,15,18–20,22). When the total number of COPD exacerbations was considered, use of inhaled corticosteroids led to about a 30% reduction in exacerbations (RR = 0.70; 95% CI: 0.58 to 0.84; Figure 2). The benefits of inhaled corticosteroids were similar in patients who were (RR = 0.77) and were not (RR = 0.63) receiving systemic corticosteroids during the run-in phase (Table 2). Analysis of the proportion of patients suffering one or more exacerbations was very similar (RR = 0.77; 95% CI: 0.66 to 0.90) and supported a beneficial effect of inhaled corticosteroids in reducing COPD exacerbations.

The test for heterogeneity was significant ($P = 0.03$), indicating that the effects of corticosteroids on exacerbations varied among the studies. This appeared to be driven largely by the discrepant results of the Copenhagen City Lung Study (RR = 0.96; 95% CI: 0.77 to 1.20) (22). The most likely explanation for this discrepancy is the investigators' definition of a COPD exacerbation, which relied on patient recall and defined an exacerbation as an affirmative answer to the question "have you since your last visit experienced more cough and phlegm than usual?" (22). This less rigorous definition may have led to misclassification of clinical outcomes, potentially obscuring any beneficial effects of inhaled corticosteroids. The frequency of more definite clinical endpoints was substantially reduced with inhaled corticosteroid therapy in that study. For example, 16 diagnoses of "pneumonia" were recorded in the active treatment arm versus 24 cases in the placebo arm. In an analysis that excluded the Copenhagen City Lung Study, the summary estimate for the efficacy of inhaled corticosteroids in preventing COPD exacerbations was a relative risk of 0.67 (95% CI: 0.63 to 0.71), with no evidence of heterogeneity ($P = 0.79$).

In a further sensitivity analysis, we examined differences in treatment efficacy by dosage of inhaled corticosteroids. However, the doses were generally similar (and almost uniformly high), and no dose-response effect was demonstrated. Sensitivity analysis by trial quality was not possible because all but one of the six trials that reported COPD exacerbation rates were assigned scores of five on the Jadad scale; the other trial (15) was assigned a score of three out of five.

Table 2. Effect of Interventions on Pulmonary Function Tests, All-Cause Mortality, and Total COPD Exacerbation Rates

	Change in FEV_1 (95% confidence interval)		All-cause mortality (no. of patients)			All COPD exacerbations (no. of patient-months)		
Study	Treatment	Placebo	Treatment	Placebo	Relative risk (95% confidence interval)	Treatment	Placebo	Relative risk (95% confidence interval)
Studies with systemic steroid run-in phase								
Vestbo et al.*	−45 mL/yr	−42 mL/yr	4 (145)	5 (145)	0.80 (0.22–2.92)	155 (5220)	161 (5220)	0.96 (0.77–1.20)
Senderovitz et al.*	−20 mL	−125 mL	Not reported	Not reported	Not reported	Not reported	Not reported	Not reported
Bourbeau et al.	−8 mL (−68 to +51 mL)	−12 mL (−85 to +61 mL)	Not reported	Not reported	Not reported	2 (225)	4 (210)	0.47 (0.09–2.52)
Burge et al.	−50 mL (−42 to −58 mL)	−59 mL (−50 to −57 mL)	32 (376)	36 (375)	0.89 (0.56–1.40)	1596 (8826)	2109 (7821)	0.67 (0.63–0.71)
Subtotal	—	—	36 (521)	41 (520)	0.88 (0.57–1.35)	1753 (14271)	2274 (13251)	0.77 (0.56–1.09)
Studies without systemic steroid run-in phase								
Lung Health Study	−44 mL (−39 to −50 mL)	−47 mL (−41 to −53 mL)	15 (559)	19 (557)	0.79 (0.40–1.53)	18 (22360)	39 (22280)	0.46 (0.26–0.80)
Renkema et al.*	−34 mL/yr	−60 mL/yr	0 (21)	0 (18)	Not reported	Not reported	Not reported	Not reported
Pauwels et al.*	−140 mL	−180 mL†	8 (634)	10 (643)	0.81 (0.32–2.04)	Not reported	Not reported	Not reported
Weir et al.	−12 mL/yr (−42 to +17 mL/yr)	−45 mL/yr (−18 to −73 mL/yr)	Not reported	Not reported	Not reported	35 (816)	56 (828)	0.63 (0.42–0.96)
Paggiaro et al.	+110 mL (+40 to +160 mL)	−40 mL (−110 to +10 mL)	Not reported	Not reported	Not reported	76 (852)	111 (834)	0.67 (0.51–0.88)
Subtotal	—	—	23 (1214)	0.80 (0.47–1.36)	129 (24028)	206 (23942)	0.63 (0.51–0.77)	
Total			59 (1735)	70 (1738)	0.84 (0.60–1.18)	1882 (38299)	2480 (37193)	0.70 (0.58–0.84)

* Standard deviation for FEV_1 decline not reported.

† Statistically significant difference between experimental and control arms.

COPD = chronic obstructive pulmonary disease; FEV_1 = forced expiratory volume in 1 second; not reported = not reported in the trial or not calculable from the available data.

Five trials evaluated all-cause mortality (16–19,22), with a nonsignificant summary relative risk of 0.84 (95% CI: 0.60 to 1.18) in favor of inhaled corticosteroids. The test for heterogeneity was not significant ($P = 0.99$); and the relative risks were identical under the random- and fixed-effects models.

The effects of corticosteroids on pulmonary function tests were variable. A statistically significant difference between treatment and placebo groups was achieved in only two trials.

We were unable to examine the relation between the efficacy of inhaled corticosteroids and smoking status or lung function at baseline, or to perform analyses by cause of death or other clinical outcomes.

Adverse Effects of Inhaled Corticosteroids

The definitions of adverse events were not uniform among the trials. Although the frequency of oropharyngeal candidiasis (RR = 2.1; 95% CI: 1.5 to 3.1) and skin bruising (RR = 2.1; 95% CI: 1.6 to 2.8) were increased in patients treated with inhaled corticosteroids, the effects on bone mineral density were variable. Whereas the Lung Health Study (18) reported significantly lower bone density measurements in the lumber spine and femur in patients treated with inhaled corticosteroids (both P values <0.01), the European Respiratory Society Study on Chronic Obstructive Pulmonary Disease (16) reported no difference between study arms. Furthermore, whereas the Inhaled Steroid in Obstructive Lung Disease study investigators (17) and the International COPD Study Group (14) reported statistically significant but probably clinically irrelevant decreases in mean cortisol concentrations with inhaled corticosteroid therapy, no appreciable differences were detected in mean cortisol concentrations in another study (16). No differences in the rates of cataract or fracture were seen in these trials, although the duration of follow-up was generally short.

DISCUSSION

The findings of this systematic review suggest that inhaled corticosteroids improve patient outcomes in COPD. Regular use of inhaled corticosteroids in the doses employed in these trials reduced the chance of an exacerbation, and the total exacerbation rate, by almost one third. Although the summary relative risk of the trials was consistent with a small survival benefit, the effect was not statistically significant. Thus, the effects of chronic inhaled corticosteroid therapy on all-cause mortality remain uncertain. As expected, inhaled corticosteroids increased the frequency of oropharyngeal candidiasis and skin bruising. The trials were too short to demonstrate clear adverse effects on bone density, fractures, risk of cataracts, or clinically apparent adrenal insufficiency.

Previous reviews have concluded that long-term use of inhaled corticosteroids leads to a slower deceleration in disease-specific health status than does placebo (19), which was associated with better symptom control, as well as improved exercise tolerance and fewer pulmonary symptoms (14). We extend these findings by showing that inhaled corticosteroid therapy is associated with reductions in the rate of exacerbations of COPD.

How inhaled corticosteroids affect patient outcomes in COPD is not known. Airway inflammation and hyper-responsiveness are important in COPD (23). Indeed, airway hyper-responsiveness is associated with increased mortality independent of FEV_1 (24). Whereas short-term studies have shown inconsistent results (25), long-term use of inhaled corticosteroids (i.e., longer than 8 weeks) appears to mitigate airway inflammation and to improve patient symptoms in COPD, without significantly altering expiratory lung volumes (26,27).

Although some may criticize our choice of endpoints as being too broad, we believe that it is most appropriate to look at outcomes that are relevant to patients, such as all-cause mortality or COPD exacerbations, rather than surrogate measurements (6). Although the heterogeneity among the six trials that examined total COPD exacerbation rates may raise concern, this heterogeneity was attributable to one trial that had a less rigorous definition of COPD exacerbations. To be conservative in our interpretation of the data, we chose to report the results using a random-effects model.

This study has several potential limitations, including the relatively small sample size and our inability to identify unpublished studies. These may lead to an overestimation of treatment effects (28) and emphasize the need for further studies with clinically important outcomes such as all-cause mortality. In addition, the trials did not provide adequate data on potential adverse effects of chronic inhaled corticosteroid therapy. However, several observational studies suggest that inhaled corticosteroid therapy increases the risk of cataracts (29,30), adrenal suppression (31), and osteoporosis (32) in a dose-dependent fashion. There were also differences in the follow-up period among the reported trials (range, 6 to 40 months). However, the beneficial effects of inhaled steroids were seen in long (e.g., the Lung Health Study) as well as in short trials (e.g., Paggiaro et al.). Although these trials demonstrated substantial reductions in COPD exacerbation rates, we cannot comment on the cost-effectiveness and economic effects of inhaled corticosteroids. Finally, because the mean FEV_1 among patients in the trials that was included in this systematic review was usually between 1.0 and 2.0 L, our findings may not apply to patients with very mild or very severe COPD.

Chronic obstructive pulmonary disease is an emerging epidemic in the United States and elsewhere (1). Unlike other major illnesses, COPD-related morbidity and mortality will continue to rise for the next 30 years (2). Despite our increased understanding of COPD and its pathophysiology, there has been little progress in developing new and effective therapies for patients (33). Our findings suggest that inhaled corticosteroids are beneficial in this disease. However, additional studies are needed to clarify the effects of inhaled corticosteroids on mortality and to define their long-term adverse effects.

ACKNOWLEDGMENT

The authors thank Ms. Casandra Higgs-Carey for her editorial assistance.

REFERENCES

1. Hurd S. The impact of COPD on lung health worldwide: Epidemiology and incidence. *Chest.* 2000;117(Suppl 2):1S–4S.
2. Murray CJ, Lopez AD. Global mortality, disability, and the contribution of risk factors: Global Burden of Disease Study. *Lancet.* 1997; 349:1436–1442.
3. British Thoracic Society, British Pediatric Association, Royal College of Physicians of London, The King's Fund Center, National Asthma Campaign, et al. The British guidelines on asthma management 1995 review and position statement. *Thorax.* 1997;52(Suppl 1):1–21.
4. National Asthma Education and Prevention Program. Expert panel report II: Guidelines for the diagnosis and management of asthma. Bethesda, MD: National Institutes of Health; 1997. Publication 97-4051.
5. van Grunsven PM, van Schayck CP, Derenne JP, et al. Long term effects of inhaled corticosteroids in chronic obstructive pulmonary disease: A meta-analysis. *Thorax.* 1999;54:7–14.
6. Bucher HC, Guyatt GH, Cook DJ, et al. Users' guides to the medical literature. XIX. Applying clinical trial results. A: How to use an article measuring the effect of an intervention on surrogate end points. *JAMA.* 1999;282:771–778.
7. Jadad AR, Moore RA, Carroll D, et al. Assessing the quality of reports of randomized controlled trials: Is blinding necessary? *Control Clin Trials.* 1996;17:1–12.
8. Le Saux N, Pham B, Moher D. Evaluating the benefits of antimicrobial prophylaxis to prevent urinary tract infections in children: A systematic review. *CMAJ.* 2000;163:523–529.
9. Hasselblad V, McCrory DC. Meta-analytic tools for medical decision making: A practical guide. *Med Decis Making.* 1995;15:81–96.
10. van Schayck CP, Dompeling E, Rutten MP, et al. The influence of inhaled steroid on quality of life in patients with asthma or COPD. *Chest.* 1995;107:1199–1205.
11. Rutten-van Molken MP, van Doorslaer EK, Jansen MC, et al. Costs and effects of inhaled corticosteroids and bronchodilators in asthma and chronic obstructive pulmonary disease. *Am J Respir Crit Care Med.* 1995;151:975–982.
12. Derenne JP. Effects of high dose inhaled beclomethasone in the rate of decline in FEV_1 in patients with chronic obstructive pulmonary disease: Results of 2 years prospective multicenter study. *Am J Respir Crit Care Med.* 1995;151:A463.
13. Kerstjens HA, Brand PL, Hughes MD, et al. A comparison of bronchodilator therapy with or without inhaled corticosteroid therapy for obstructive airways disease. *N Engl J Med.* 1992;327:1413–1419.
14. Paggiaro PL, Dahle R, Bakran I, et al. Multicentre randomised placebo-controlled trial of inhaled fluticasone propionate in patients with chronic obstructive pulmonary disease. *Lancet.* 1998;351:773–780.
15. Weir DC, Bale GA, Bright P, Burge P. A double-blind placebo-controlled study of the effect of inhaled beclomethasone dipropionate for 2 years in patients with non-asthmatic chronic obstructive pulmonary disease. *Clin Exp Allergy.* 1999;29(Suppl 2):125–128.
16. Pauwels A, Lofdahl CG, Laitinen LA, et al. Long-term treatment with inhaled budesonide in persons with mild chronic obstructive pulmonary disease who continue smoking. European Respiratory Society Study on Chronic Obstructive Pulmonary Disease. *N Engl J Med.* 1999;340:1948–1953.
17. Renkema TE, Schouten JP, Koeter GH, Postma DS. Effects of long-term treatment with corticosteroids in COPD. *Chest.* 1996;109: 1156–1162.
18. The Lung Health Study Research Group. Effects of inhaled triamcinolone on the decline in pulmonary function in chronic obstructive pulmonary disease. *N Engl J Med.* 2000;343:1902–1909.
19. Burge PS, Calverley PM, Jones PW, et al. Randomised double blinded placebo-controlled study of fluticasone propionate in patients with moderate to severe chronic obstructive pulmonary disease: The ISOLDE trial. *BMJ.* 2000;320:1297–1303.
20. Bourbeau J, Rouleau MY, Boucher S. Randomised controlled trial of inhaled corticosteroids in patients with chronic obstructive pulmonary disease. *Thorax.* 1998;53:477–482.
21. Senderovitz T, Vestbo J, Frandsen J, et al. Steroid reversibility test followed by inhaled budesonide or placebo in outpatients with stable chronic obstructive pulmonary disease. *Respir Med.* 1999;93: 715–718.
22. Vestbo J, Sorensen T, Lange P, et al. Long-term effect of inhaled budesonide in mild and moderate chronic obstructive pulmonary disease: A randomised controlled trial. *Lancet.* 1999;353:1819–1823.
23. Hill A, Gompertz S, Stockley R. Factors influencing airway inflammation in chronic obstructive pulmonary disease. *Thorax.* 2000;55: 970–977.
24. Hospers JJ, Postma DS, Rijckin B, et al. Histamine airway hyper-responsiveness and mortality from chronic obstructive pulmonary disease: A cohort study. *Lancet.* 2000;356:1313–1317.
25. Postma DS, Kerstjens HA. Are inhaled glucocorticosteroids effective in chronic obstructive pulmonary disease? *Am J Respir Crit Care Med.* 1999;160(Suppl 5):S66–S71.
26. Llewellyn-Jones CG, Harris TA, Stockley RA. Effects of fluticasone propionate on sputum of patients with chronic bronchitis and emphysema. *Am J Respir Crit Care Med.* 1996;153:616–621.
27. Confalonieri M, Mainardi E, Della Porta R, et al. Inhaled corticosteroids reduce neutrophilic bronchial inflammation in patients with chronic obstructive pulmonary disease. *Thorax.* 1998;53:583–585.
28. Schulz KF, Chalmers I, Hayes RJ, Altman DG. Empirical evidence of bias. Dimensions of methodological quality associated with estimates of treatment effects in controlled trials. *JAMA.* 1995;273: 408–412.
29. Garbe E, Suissa S, LeLorier J. Association of inhaled corticosteroid use with cataract extraction in elderly patents. *JAMA.* 1998;280: 539–543.
30. Cumming RG, Mitchell P, Leeder SR. Use of inhaled corticosteroids and the risk of cataracts. *N Engl J Med.* 1997;337:8–14.
31. Lipworth BJ. Systemic adverse effects of inhaled corticosteroid therapy: A systematic review and meta-analysis. *Arch Intern Med.* 1999;159:941–955.
32. Wong CA, Walsh LJ, Smith CJ, et al. Inhaled corticosteroid use and bone-mineral density in patients with asthma. *Lancet.* 2000;355: 1399–1403.
33. Bach PB, Brown C, Gelfend SE, McCrory DC. Management of acute exacerbation of chronic obstructive pulmonary disease: a summary and appraisal of published evidence. *Ann Intern Med.* 2001;134: 600–620.

NOTES

NOTES

NOTES

NOTES

NOTES

NOTES

ISBN 0-929661-81-8
ISSN 1542-1961
First Printing
Printed in the United States of America

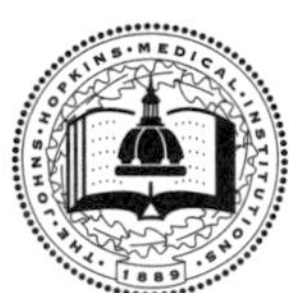

The Johns Hopkins White Papers are published yearly by Medletter Associates, Inc.

MEMORY

Peter V. Rabins, M.D., M.P.H.

and

Simeon Margolis, M.D., Ph.D.

2 0 0 3

MEMORY

As the number of older people in the United States continues to grow, so does the number of people with dementia-causing illnesses such as Alzheimer disease. The prospect of a potential public health crisis has led to a spate of research on dementia. In this year's White Paper, we sort through the facts and provide the latest information on which therapies are promising and which are proven effective. Also, this year we present more practical tips for people who are caring for someone with dementia.

▪ ▪ ▪

Highlights:

▪ ▪ ▪

THE AUTHORS

Peter V. Rabins, M.D., M.P.H., received his M.D. from the Tulane University School of Medicine and his M.P.H. from the Tulane University School of Public Health. He completed his residency in psychiatry at the University of Oregon. Currently, he is codirector of the Division of Geriatric and Neuropsychiatry at the Johns Hopkins School of Medicine, as well as a professor of psychiatry with a joint appointment in the Department of Internal Medicine and School of Hygiene and Public Health. Dr. Rabins is serving as the principal investigator on a National Institute of Mental Health study of Alzheimer disease in the community and a National Institute of Neurological Disorders and Stroke study of late-stage care for Alzheimer disease patients.

Dr. Rabins has spent his career studying psychiatric disorders in the elderly. His current research includes the development of scales to measure impairment in people with severe dementia and the study of visual hallucinations in a variety of psychiatric and neurological conditions. He has published extensively in such journals as the *American Journal of Psychiatry,* the *Journal of the American Geriatrics Society,* and the *Journal of Mental Health.*

■ ■ ■

Simeon Margolis, M.D., Ph.D., received his B.A., M.D., and Ph.D. from the Johns Hopkins University School of Medicine and performed his internship and residency at Johns Hopkins Hospital. He is currently a professor of medicine and biological chemistry at the Johns Hopkins University School of Medicine and medical editor of *The Johns Hopkins Medical Letter, Health After 50.* He has served on various committees for the Department of Health, Education and Welfare, including the National Diabetes Advisory Board and the Arteriosclerosis Specialized Centers of Research Review Committees. In addition, he has acted as a member of the Endocrinology and Metabolism Panel of the U.S. Food and Drug Administration.

A former weekly columnist for the *Baltimore Sun,* Dr. Margolis lectures regularly to medical students, physicians, and the general public on a wide variety of topics, such as the prevention of coronary heart disease, the control of cholesterol levels, the treatment of diabetes, and the use of alternative medicine.

CONTENTS

MEMORY

Shakespeare called memory "the warder of the brain," charged with keeping watch over an individual's personal account of being. Should this sentry begin to fail, a person's own record of self can become endangered. This is a frightening prospect for most people.

Memory loss ranges from age-associated memory impairment, which is a normal degree of forgetfulness, to dementias such as Alzheimer disease (AD) that can profoundly affect a person's ability to function. AD, the most common form of dementia, affects 4 million Americans. According to the American Academy of Neurology, 10% of people older than age 65 and 50% of people age 85 and older suffer from AD. The National Institutes of Health estimates that there will be 8.5 million Americans with AD by the year 2030.

Although AD is irreversible, memory impairment resulting from other causes, such as depression or thyroid problems, can be improved with treatment. As for AD, recent research advances should lead to improved treatments and, someday, a cure.

THE BIOLOGY OF MEMORY

Deep within the brain lies a small, S-shaped structure known as the hippocampus (Greek for "seahorse," which it resembles). This relatively small region of the brain plays a major role in the process of forging memories: It instantly evaluates incoming data from the five senses and determines whether to store or discard this new information.

But memories cannot be said to reside in the hippocampus or, for that matter, in any other specific site in the brain. Instead, memories are stored throughout the brain, especially in the cerebral cortex—the convoluted outer layer of gray matter that constitutes the "thinking" portion of the brain—as well as in the cerebellum (the fist-sized structure, located at the base of the brain beneath the cortex, that coordinates movement and balance).

For the nervous system to function, the body's billions of neurons (nerve cells) must be able to communicate with one another over a vast and highly complex network of nerve fibers. Any one neuron can have hundreds—or even thousands—of connections with other neurons. Messages are relayed between individual neurons via specialized chemicals called neurotransmitters. The sum of the interactions among the brain and the rest of the nervous system

NEW RESEARCH

Healthy Diet Helps Maintain Mental Functions

Older people who eat a healthy diet are more likely to maintain their cognitive abilities than those who eat less healthful diets, researchers from Italy say.

Investigators studied 1,651 men and women, age 65 and older. They found that people who ate a diet low in fat and sugar and high in fruits, vegetables, and complex carbohydrates were moderately—but significantly—less likely to have cognitive dysfunction than those who ate a less healthy diet. No single component of the diet contributed significantly to the results, suggesting that a combination of factors in a healthy diet contribute to the maintenance of cognitive function. The researchers also found that people who drank up to three alcoholic drinks per day were 25% less likely to have cognitive dysfunction than abstainers or heavy drinkers.

Other studies have shown that diets rich in beta-carotene, vitamin C, vitamin E, and omega-3 fatty acids may help prevent cognitive decline. The researchers concluded that more research is needed to examine in detail which factors in a healthy diet play a role in maintaining mental function.

EUROPEAN JOURNAL OF CLINICAL NUTRITION
Volume 55, page 1053
December 2001

is what is referred to as the mind.

During that fleeting period when the mind recognizes what the senses perceive and determines which details are important, the incoming information is said to dwell in the realm of the sensory memory. From there, data are transferred to short-term memory to be processed for immediate use and then either discarded or retained. Also known as working memory, short-term memory is sometimes equated with consciousness.

Long-term memory holds information that was learned as recently as a few minutes ago and as long ago as early childhood. For example, your name and address, what you ate for dinner last night, and the multiplication tables are all stored in long-term memory. Intentional memorization and studying can promote the transfer of information from short-term to long-term memory.

Furthermore, items that have a particular emotional impact are especially likely to earn a niche in long-term memory. (For example, nearly all people who were alive at the time remember where they were when they first heard of President Kennedy's assassination.) Indeed, it appears that the mind's ability to associate new information with other relevant information contained in long-term memory is key to both the storage of new data and the ability to recall previously stored information. The conceptual links between new and old information serve as retrieval cues; the more numerous the links and the more powerful the associations, the stronger the memory is.

Information may be difficult to recall for several reasons: It may get only as far as short-term memory and then be forgotten; it may be too similar to—or too different from—information that has already been stored; or the proper cues for retrieval may be unavailable. For example, eating similar cereals at breakfast each morning may lead people to forget which particular brand they had that day. Or remembering a person's face may not be possible until some associated fact (such as where you last saw the person) provides the necessary cue.

AGE-ASSOCIATED MEMORY IMPAIRMENT

A certain amount of forgetfulness is to be expected with age. Most people have more difficulty recalling names and words as they get older, so this is by no means symptomatic of dementia. An adage can serve to reassure those who are occasionally forgetful: "You need not worry if you forget where you put your car keys; you only

Memory and the Brain

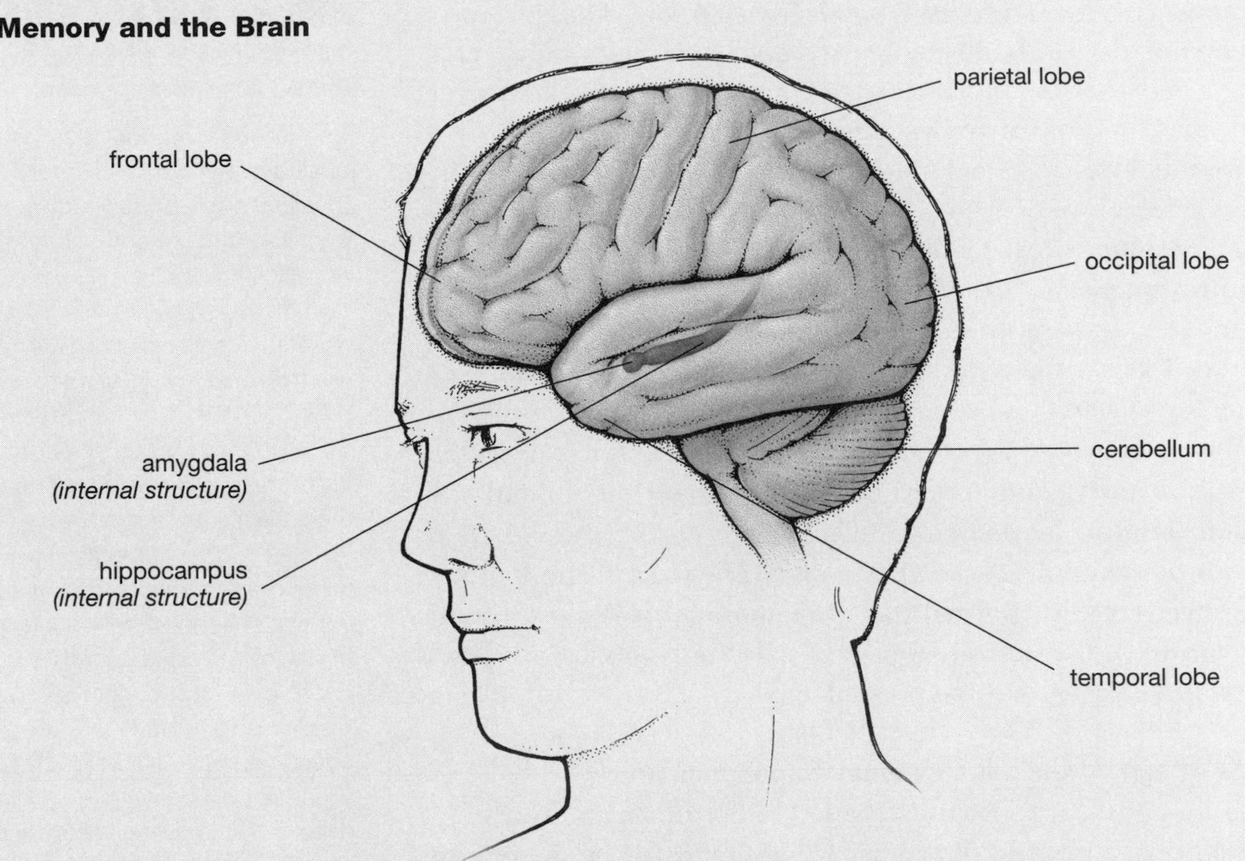

Memory can be divided into two components: the recall of facts (declarative memory) and the recall of motor skills (procedural memory). Dementia-causing diseases such as Alzheimer disease (AD) impair memory for facts (such as a name or face) much earlier than memory for motor skills (for example, skating or crocheting). This pattern occurs because the memory-robbing effects of dementia damage those areas of the brain involved in declarative memory while generally sparing the parts involved in procedural memory. However, the brain has no single "memory center." Almost the whole organ is involved in memory.

One of the most important brain areas involved in the processing of new memories is the temporal lobes (located near the ears), which contain a group of structures called the hippocampal complex. The hippocampal complex—which includes the hippocampus and amygdala—controls the processing of new factual memories, like learning new words and faces. However, it does not deal with older, previously learned information. Because the hippocampal complex is one of the first areas damaged in AD, people with this disease often cannot recall recent events but may still have accurate memories of things that occurred decades earlier.

The outer part of the temporal lobes generally governs older autobiographical memories (for example, one's first kiss), the recognition of familiar items and people, and the memory of language (such as the recall of nouns).

The frontal lobes, located at the front of the brain, help integrate factual memory and emotion. Because this brain area allows a person to recall the outcomes and consequences of various behaviors, it helps govern a person's judgment and ability to interact socially. The frontal lobes also control "remembering in the future" (for example, remembering to shut off the stove in 10 minutes), and the ability to judge how long ago events took place.

The parietal lobes, located above the temporal lobes on the top of the brain, receive sensory information from the five senses (touch, taste, smell, hearing, and sight) and play a role in the recall of items relating to touch and pain. As AD advances, the damage tends to spread from the temporal lobes to the frontal and parietal lobes, leading to an inability to recognize familiar objects and places.

The back part of the brain behind the temporal lobes—an area called the occipital lobes—primarily deals with vision and the visual components of long-term memories, such as shape, form, and color. This area is less affected by AD, but it is not entirely spared. The cerebellum, an area in the lower back of the brain below the occipital lobes, helps a person to recall and perform motor skills (procedural memory) and is generally not damaged in conditions like AD.

need to worry if you forget what they're used for." The difference between normal forgetfulness that increases with age—known clinically as age-associated memory impairment—and serious dementia is that the former is frustrating but not disabling.

The memory lapses associated with age-associated memory impairment are more likely to occur when a person is tired, sick, distracted, or under stress. Under less stressful circumstances, the same person is usually able to remember the necessary information with ease. Indeed, studies repeatedly show that older people who do poorly on timed tests actually do as well as or better than their college-age counterparts when they are permitted to work at their own pace.

People who worry about memory loss are unlikely to suffer from a serious memory condition, while people with serious memory impairment tend to be unaware of their lapses, do not worry about them, or attribute them to other causes. However, if the memory lapses interfere with normal daily functioning, or if close friends and relatives of the individual believe that the lapses are serious, a more complex cause may be present.

Causes of Age-Associated Memory Impairment

The brain contains approximately 100 billion neurons, and it is a common misconception that tens of thousands of brain neurons die each day. In fact, few neurons die over a person's lifetime. However, neurons do shrink, and this may explain some of the slowing of mental functioning that occurs in middle and old age. Serious memory problems occur from cell death when whole clusters of neurons are destroyed by major disorders such as a stroke or AD.

In addition to neuronal shrinkage, the brain begins producing smaller quantities of many neurotransmitters starting in middle age. Brain blood flow is also reduced 15% to 20% from age 30 to 70, although this may be accounted for by neuronal shrinkage (less tissue needs less blood flow).

Other issues, such as cultural attitudes, can also contribute to the increasing frequency of memory lapses as people age. In one study, researchers compared the memory skills of two groups known for having few old-age-related stereotypes (natives of China and deaf Americans) with a third group that has numerous preconceptions about age (hearing Americans). Among these preconceptions is the notion that aging causes an inevitable decline in memory skills. The results of the study suggested a strong link between culture and memory: The first two groups were less forgetful than the third, and older Chinese participants performed as well as the younger subjects

NEW RESEARCH

Moderate Alcohol Intake May Prevent Cognitive Impairment

Consuming a moderate amount of alcohol each day may decrease the risk of developing cognitive impairment, according to a recent report.

In the study, 15,807 hospitalized Italians were asked about their daily intake of alcohol. The participants' cognitive function was also tested. If patients had cognitive impairment, caregivers reported the patient's alcohol intake.

Overall, 29% of people who never drank alcohol had cognitive impairment compared with 19% of drinkers, a significant difference. The risk of cognitive impairment was reduced in men who consumed up to a liter (34 oz.) of wine per day; drinking more than a liter a day increased the rate of cognitive impairment. Among the women, drinking up to half a liter (17 oz.) of wine was associated with decreased rates of cognitive impairment, while consuming more increased the risk.

Alcohol may reduce the risk of atherosclerosis (the buildup of fatty plaques in the arteries), which contributes to Alzheimer disease and vascular dementia. Most U.S. experts recommend no more than two drinks a day for men and one for women. A drink equals 12 oz. of beer, 5 oz. of wine, or 1.5 oz. of spirits. While several other studies have reported similar results, some studies have found no association between alcohol use and dementia.

ALCOHOLISM: CLINICAL AND EXPERIMENTAL RESEARCH
Volume 25, page 1743
December 2001

in each of these groups.

Other research demonstrates that the ability to remember newly acquired information depends on the same faculties used to retrieve memories from long ago—something most older people do with great ease. The implication is that a person who can still remember past events and tell interesting stories about his or her life has the faculties necessary to do the same for more recent events. This has suggested to some researchers that occasional memory lapses suggest a failure to pay attention rather than an inability to learn. Forging new memories thus depends heavily on staying interested, active, and alert.

Methods To Assist Memory

Although age-associated memory impairment is common and is not a sign of a serious neurological disorder, it can be frustrating and socially embarrassing. While there is no way to eliminate completely the minor memory lapses that occur with age-associated memory impairment, a number of strategies can improve overall memory ability at any age.

Stay mentally active. When some people retire, they no longer regularly engage in activities that challenge and stimulate the mind. But staying mentally active is a key part of maintaining memory, as well as other cognitive skills. Experts recommend such activities as doing crossword puzzles, playing Scrabble, studying a foreign language, learning to play a musical instrument, starting a new career or hobby, reading, volunteering at a hospital, and maintaining regular social interactions.

Stay physically active. An adequate blood supply to the brain is necessary for all mental functions, including memory. Regular physical exercise helps get more blood to the brain and therefore facilitates better mental functioning. Exercising for 20 to 30 minutes most days of the week is recommended.

Rule out other causes of memory loss. If you suspect you have memory difficulties, consult your doctor. Many medical conditions and other factors can cause reversible memory problems; these include depression, hearing or vision loss, thyroid dysfunction, certain medications, vitamin deficiencies, and stress. Treating these problems may improve memory.

Do not smoke. Smokers are at greater risk for mental decline than nonsmokers, and smoking cessation may reduce this risk. One study showed that current smokers over age 65 were 3.7 times more likely to experience mental decline over a one-year period than

NEW RESEARCH

Mental Activity May Protect Against AD

Engaging in mentally stimulating activities may prevent some people from developing Alzheimer disease (AD), according to new research.

Investigators interviewed 801 Catholic nuns, priests, and brothers, age 65 and older, without dementia to determine their level of cognitive ability and how frequently they engaged in cognitively stimulating activities. Participants were reinterviewed each year for an average of four-and-a-half years.

People who engaged in the highest rates of cognitively stimulating activities at the beginning of the study were 47% less likely to be diagnosed with AD at the end of the study than those reporting the lowest rates of mental activity. Low levels of cognitive stimulation were also associated with a faster rate of mental decline.

There are four possible explanations for this association: The repeated use of cognitive skills makes them more resistant to decline; cognitive stimulation strengthens other mental faculties that compensate for AD-related mental decline; low levels of cognitive activity are characteristic of early AD; or AD is already affecting behavior before there is any other manifestation that can be recognized by doctors or loved ones.

JOURNAL OF THE AMERICAN MEDICAL ASSOCIATION
Volume 287, page 742
February 13, 2002

Can a Pill Protect Against Dementia?

In addition to searching for ways to treat dementia, researchers are investigating whether currently available medications, vitamins, and herbal supplements might help prevent or delay the onset of dementia in people at high risk. Most of the early evidence for these preventive therapies has come from retrospective studies—reviews of medical records or interviews with patients. This type of research has helped experts identify the factors most likely to contribute to the development or prevention of dementia. However, the conclusions from retrospective studies need to be confirmed by clinical trials that specifically examine the effect of preventive therapies.

The following are some of the more promising preventive therapies for dementia, although more research is needed to prove their benefits.

Statins

Some (but not all) studies suggest that people who take statin drugs for high cholesterol have reduced rates of dementia. In one nonrandomized study of 60,000 people, those who took pravastatin (Pravachol) or lovastatin (Mevacor), but not simvastatin (Zocor), were 70% less likely to develop Alzheimer disease (AD) than people in the study as a whole. In another study, people who took any type of statin drug, including simvastatin, also had a 70% lower rate of dementia than those who did not take statins. A third recent study of 1,315 people found that the people who took statins or other cholesterol-lowering medications had a 74% lower risk of AD than those who did not use these drugs, but only if they were under the age of 80.

High cholesterol levels are thought to increase the risk of AD and other dementias by contributing to atherosclerosis (which may impair blood flow to the brain) or damaging neurons in the brain. Researchers are unclear whether statins lower the risk of dementia through their cholesterol-lowering properties or through some other effect, such as reducing inflammation in the brain. Statins and other cholesterol-lowering medications can have serious side effects, and there is not enough evidence yet to recommend them solely for the prevention of dementia.

Antihypertensives

High blood pressure can lead to vascular dementia (see page 14) and, like high cholesterol, may increase the risk of developing AD. In one study of 1,449 people, those whose systolic blood pressure was 160 mm Hg or higher had a 2.3-fold greater chance of developing AD 20 years later than people whose systolic pressure was 140 mm Hg or lower.

In another study, 2,418 people over age 60 with a systolic blood pressure of 140 mm Hg or above received either an antihypertensive medication or a placebo. People taking the placebo were two times more likely to develop vascular dementia than those taking the medication. Other studies, however, have found no evidence that high blood pressure is associated with an increased risk of dementia.

people who did not smoke or smoked only in the past. Smoking may impair mental function by damaging the blood vessels that supply nutrients to the brain.

Limit alcohol consumption. Heavy alcohol consumption can interfere with proper memory function, but people who drink moderately have a smaller risk of mental decline than either heavy drinkers or nondrinkers. Although no optimal level of alcohol consumption has been established, experts recommend no more than two drinks per day for men and one drink per day for women. (One drink equals 12 oz. of beer, 4 oz. of wine, or 1.5 oz. of 80 proof liquor.)

Place commonly lost items in the same spot. If you are prone to losing items, such as keys or eyeglasses, choose a place to leave them, and always put them in that spot when not using them.

Write things down. If you have trouble remembering phone numbers or appointments, write them down and place the list in a conspicuous spot. Making a daily "to do" list can serve as a re-

Nonsteroidal Anti-Inflammatory Drugs

Nonsteroidal anti-inflammatory drugs (NSAIDs) such as ibuprofen (Advil and others) may hold the most promise as a preventive strategy against AD. Many studies show that people who take NSAIDs for other conditions, such as arthritis, have a lower risk of AD than people who do not take NSAIDs. In addition, recent research suggests that patients can benefit even from low doses of NSAIDs.

How NSAIDs may protect against AD is not understood. Originally, researchers thought the benefit came from the drugs' anti-inflammatory properties; inflammation occurs in the brains of people with AD. However, a recent study found that AD patients who took NSAIDs performed better on neuropsychological tests despite having about the same amount of inflammatory plaques and tangles as AD patients who did not take NSAIDs.

Despite this promising evidence, NSAIDs are not recommended for the prevention of AD. One reason is that side effects such as gastrointestinal bleeding and ulcers occur frequently with long-term use. More research is being done to examine how NSAIDs may protect against AD.

Vitamin E and Other Antioxidants

A few studies have suggested that vitamin E and other antioxidants may help prevent AD and other forms of dementia. In one study, people with moderately severe AD who took vitamin E supplements, selegiline (a medication used to treat Parkinson disease that may have antioxidant properties), or both were less likely than patients taking a placebo to die, be institutionalized, lose basic function, or develop severe dementia. Another study suggested that vitamin E is related to memory performance but did not conclude that low levels of vitamin E lead to memory loss.

Some research suggests that vitamins C and E may protect against vascular dementia. In one study of 3,385 Japanese-Americans in Hawaii, those who took both vitamin supplements had an 88% lower risk of vascular dementia. They also had a 69% lower risk of mixed or other types of dementia but showed no change in the risk of AD compared with men who did not take the supplements.

It is too soon to recommend that people take antioxidant supplements to prevent dementia. But the Memory Impairment Study, a randomized, placebo-controlled trial of vitamin E and the cholinesterase inhibitor donepezil (Aricept) is now underway and will help determine whether vitamin E can prevent AD in people with mild cognitive impairment.

Ginkgo Biloba

Ginkgo biloba may have antioxidant and anti-inflammatory effects on the brain, and much research has focused on its potential to treat dementia. In one study, ginkgo biloba appeared to slow the rate of cognitive decline in people with dementia. However, no research has shown that ginkgo biloba has any protective effect against AD or other forms of dementia. In fact, a recent study (see the reprint on page 48) shows that ginkgo does not improve cognitive function in people without memory impairment. Ginkgo biloba may cause bleeding in people taking aspirin.

minder of important tasks and obligations. In fact, the mere act of writing notes and making lists reinforces memory.

Say words out loud. Saying, "I've turned off the stove," after shutting off the stove will give you an extra verbal reminder when you later try to recall whether it is still on. Incorporating someone's name into the conversation just after you have met him or her will serve the same purpose. For example, saying, "Very nice to meet you, Jennifer," will help consolidate the memory of this name.

Use memory aids. Use a pocket notepad, personal digital assistant, wristwatch alarm, voice recorder, or other aids to help remember what you have to do or to keep track of information.

Use visual images. When learning new information, such as someone's name, create a visual image in your mind to make the information more vivid and, therefore, more memorable. For example, if you have just been introduced to a Mr. Hackman, imagine him hacking his way through a dense jungle with a machete.

Group items using memory games. When memorizing lists, names, addresses, etc., try alphabetizing them, grouping them using an acronym (a word made from the first letters of a series of words, e.g., NATO), or creating a story that connects each element. The more compact the acronym or the more meaningful the story, the easier it will be to remember the information.

Concentrate and relax. Many environmental stimuli compete for your attention at any given time. To remember something, you need to concentrate on the items to be remembered. Pay close attention to new information that you need to remember and try to avoid or block out distractions. Have you ever forgotten information during a test that you know you learned well beforehand? Anxiety and stress can inhibit recall, so slow down and relax when trying to remember information. Learning a relaxation technique, such as deep breathing or muscle-relaxing exercises, may help.

MILD COGNITIVE IMPAIRMENT

Mild cognitive impairment falls somewhere between age-associated memory impairment and early dementia. People with mild cognitive impairment forget more than is normal for their age, but do not experience other cognitive problems associated with dementia, such as becoming disoriented or confused about routine activities. They are generally able to live independently, but may be less active socially.

Many experts believe that mild cognitive impairment may be an early warning sign for memory disorders later in life. In fact, studies show that 10% to 15% of people with mild cognitive impairment progress to AD each year, compared with a rate of 1% to 2% a year for the general population. And large-scale studies are currently under way to test whether therapies can halt or slow the conversion from mild cognitive impairment to AD. By intervening at the first signs of memory trouble, researchers hope to delay AD or prevent it altogether.

DEMENTIA

Dementia refers to a significant intellectual decline or impairment that persists over time (often diagnosed months or even years after its onset) and affects several areas of cognition (thinking). Memory loss is a universal feature of dementia, but other functions are impaired as well—for example, abstract thinking and language.

NEW RESEARCH

Functional Problems Predict AD in People With MCI

People with mild cognitive impairment (MCI) who lack awareness of the problems they have with everyday activities are at increased risk for developing Alzheimer disease (AD), a new report demonstrates.

Investigators asked 107 people with MCI (average age 68) about their ability to perform daily living activities important for independent functioning (e.g., paying bills, preparing meals, shopping, and remembering appointments). The investigators also obtained information about each participant's daily living skills from an "informant," usually the participant's spouse or an adult child, who could provide a more objective perspective on the person's skills.

MCI patients who lacked awareness of their functional deficits (i.e., those who reported fewer problems than their informants) were eight times more likely to develop AD within two years than patients whose reporting of deficits was similar to that of the informants.

These findings indicate that it may be beneficial for doctors to obtain information about cognitive function from both the patient and a family member or close friend. The authors conclude that patients who overestimate their cognitive abilities compared with the ratings of family or friends may be at increased risk for AD or in the early stages of the disease.

NEUROLOGY
Volume 58, page 758
March 12, 2002

Approximately 1% of dementia cases are reversible. In these instances, patients may have a physical or psychological condition that can be cured with treatment, such as an operable brain tumor, vitamin B_{12} deficiency, thyroid disease, alcoholism, or depression. The most common cause of reversible dementia is a toxic reaction to prescription or over-the-counter medications.

Diagnosis of Dementia

According to guidelines published by the Agency for Health Care Policy and Research, a person who has difficulty with one or more of the following activities should be evaluated for dementia:

Learning and retaining new information. The person regularly misplaces objects, has trouble remembering appointments or recent conversations, or is repetitive in conversation.

Handling complex tasks. The individual has trouble with previously familiar activities, like balancing a checkbook, cooking a meal, or other tasks that involve a complex train of thought.

Ability to reason. The person finds it difficult to respond appropriately to everyday problems, such as a flat tire. Or a previously responsible, well-adjusted person may display poor social or financial judgment.

Spatial ability and orientation. Driving and finding one's way in familiar surroundings become difficult or impossible, and the person may have problems recognizing known objects and landmarks.

Language. The ability to speak or comprehend seems impaired, and the person may have problems following or participating in conversations.

Behavior. Personality changes emerge. For example, the person appears more passive and less responsive than usual, or more suspicious and irritable. Visual or auditory stimuli may be misinterpreted.

Differentiating between age-associated memory impairment and dementia due to a medical condition involves a process of systematic elimination. Doctors often start by looking for conditions that are most readily correctable. If these possibilities can be eliminated, then more serious, irreversible dementias—such as AD—are considered. In addition, the presence of reversible disorders can complicate the irreversible forms of dementia. In these cases, diagnosing and treating concurrent depression, for example, make it possible to gain a clearer view of any conditions that may persist.

The first step in diagnosis is a thorough medical history and physical examination to identify any vision, hearing, cardiovascular, or other disorders. While checking for these conditions might seem

NEW FINDING

Oxidative Stress Linked to AD, Mild Cognitive Impairment

A biological marker of oxidative damage in the brain is elevated in people with Alzheimer disease (AD) and mild cognitive impairment (MCI) but not in healthy older people, a new study reveals.

Researchers selected 50 people with AD, 33 with MCI, and 40 with normal cognition (all of similar age) and measured levels of a specific type of isoprostane in the participants' urine, blood, and cerebrospinal fluid. Isoprostanes are modified fatty acids that are formed when free radicals, a normal by-product of the use of oxygen by cells, cause oxidative damage. Oxidative damage may contribute to AD.

Patients with AD had the highest levels of isoprostane in their urine, blood, and cerebrospinal fluid. While the MCI patients had lower levels of isoprostane than the AD patients, their levels were significantly higher than levels in those participants with normal cognition.

This is the first study to demonstrate increased oxidative damage in people with MCI. The results suggest that doctors may one day be able to diagnose MCI or AD with a simple blood or urine test for isoprostane. Identifying patients with MCI will become more important if researchers develop strategies to help prevent MCI from progressing to AD. Currently, nearly half of people with MCI develop AD within four years.

ARCHIVES OF NEUROLOGY
Volume 59, page 972
June 2002

unnecessary, they often go unrecognized in older adults and can have an important effect on memory.

For example, heart failure (a decreased ability of the heart to pump blood) may impede mental function by reducing the amount of blood circulating to the brain. Recovering from cardiac arrest or heart bypass surgery can also affect memory. A study published in *The New England Journal of Medicine* in 2001 found that about 50% of people who undergo heart bypass surgery experience a decline in cognitive function. A complete medical history is also necessary to account for any preexisting conditions, such as psychiatric disorders, head trauma, or alcohol abuse.

Tests of mental status—for example, the Mini-Mental State Examination, the Short Test of Mental Status, or the Cognitive Capacity Screening Examination—are also given to check for any basic cognitive impairment. These tests, which take 5 to 15 minutes to complete, offer a baseline for comparison should further testing be necessary.

A history should also include an interview with a family member or close friend. Such an interview can be crucial, since someone close to the patient knows the patient's former level of functioning and therefore is able to help the physician determine whether deterioration has occurred.

The American Academy of Neurology recently issued guidelines on dementia. They recommend the following tests in the routine evaluation of a patient with dementia:

- complete blood cell count;
- serum electrolytes (potassium, sodium, and chloride);
- blood glucose (sugar), blood urea nitrogen, and creatinine;
- serum vitamin B_{12} levels;
- depression screening;
- liver function tests and thyroid function tests; and
- a brain scan such as computed tomography (CT) or magnetic resonance imaging (MRI).

A routine evaluation would not include single-photon emission computer tomography (SPECT), genetic testing, or apolipoprotein E (APOE) genotyping. Screening for syphilis and lumbar puncture should be performed only in special circumstances.

The usefulness of positron emission tomography (PET), other genetic markers for AD, markers for AD in cerebrospinal fluid, and AD gene mutations in patients with frontotemporal dementia is unknown at this time, according to the American Academy of Neurology.

NEW FINDING

New Bypass Method Does Not Prevent Long-Term Cognitive Decline

Some patients experience cognitive decline after undergoing traditional heart bypass surgery. Researchers thought that a newer bypass technique, in which the heart is not stopped, would result in fewer cases of cognitive problems, but a recent study from the Netherlands suggests that this may not be true.

The investigators randomized 281 people with coronary heart disease who were scheduled for bypass surgery to undergo traditional bypass surgery, in which the heart is stopped and a heart-lung machine is used, or to a newer "off-pump" bypass procedure, in which the heart continues to beat.

After three months, 29% of patients who underwent the traditional bypass procedure experienced cognitive decline compared with 21% of the off-pump patients, a statistically nonsignificant difference. By one year, 34% of traditional bypass surgery patients had cognitive decline, as did 31% in the off-pump group; again, this was not statistically significant.

Keeping the heart beating "may not be enough to have a brain-safe [bypass] surgery," according to an accompanying editorial. Other factors, such as the physical trauma of bypass surgery, may contribute more to cognitive decline. However, the study was too small to reach definitive conclusions about all the potential benefits and risks of the off-pump procedure.

JOURNAL OF THE AMERICAN MEDICAL ASSOCIATION
Volume 287, page 1405
March 20, 2002

Tests for Measuring Dementia Symptoms

Although the Mini-Mental State Examination (MMSE) is one of the standard tests used by physicians to screen people for dementia, it has several drawbacks. The test is time-consuming, taking about 15 minutes to administer. In addition, the results can be affected by the patient's educational level and do not always correlate with function in the real world. For these reasons, doctors have developed several simple alternatives. The most widely studied are the Clock Drawing Test and the Time and Change Test. These brief tests do not provide a definitive diagnosis, but they can help determine who needs a thorough evaluation for dementia.

Clock Drawing Test

The Clock Drawing Test examines how well a person can represent time. The person is instructed to draw a clock with all the numbers on it and is then told to add hands to the clock to make it read a specific time—for example, 2:45, 11:10, or 3:40.

The clocks shown below (all drawn by patients with Alzheimer disease) are from a study of 67 patients with AD and a control group of 83 people without AD. Six different scorers rated each drawing from 1 to 10 (1 being the worst to 10 being the best representation of a clock and the designated time). Patients with AD had an average score of 4.9; the control group averaged 8.7. The scorers did not know which patients had AD. Scoring involved looking for disorganization, incompleteness, and the tendency to stay in one area of the drawing—all of which can indicate impairments in the ability to think or reason spatially.

Several studies have shown that the Clock Test can identify patients with known dementia and is especially helpful for identifying patients with AD. Unlike the MMSE, the Clock Test is not affected by a person's education level. It is also inexpensive, brief, and easy to administer. It does not appear to be useful in distinguishing between mild AD and normal aging, however.

Time and Change Test

Another type of screening test for dementia assesses a person's ability to tell time and perform simple math. First, a picture of a large clock reading "11:10" is held 14 inches from the patient's face. The person is asked to say what time the clock is showing. If the answer is incorrect, the person gets a second try. The time limit for this portion of the test is 60 seconds. In the second portion of the test, three quarters, seven dimes, and seven nickels are placed on a well-lighted table. The person is asked to give $1 in change to the tester. Two tries are allowed in a three-minute period. For both portions of the test, the tester records the time, the result, and any physical limitations (such as vision problems, tremor, weakness, and pain) that may affect the person's ability to perform the test.

Correct responses within 3 seconds for the time test and 10 seconds for the change test are thought to rule out dementia. The test is less accurate for identifying people in the early stages of dementia, who may still be able to tell time and make change. An incorrect response on either test suggests dementia and means that the patient requires further evaluation. Like the Clock Drawing Test, the Time and Change Test is brief, inexpensive, and less affected by the patient's education level than the MMSE.

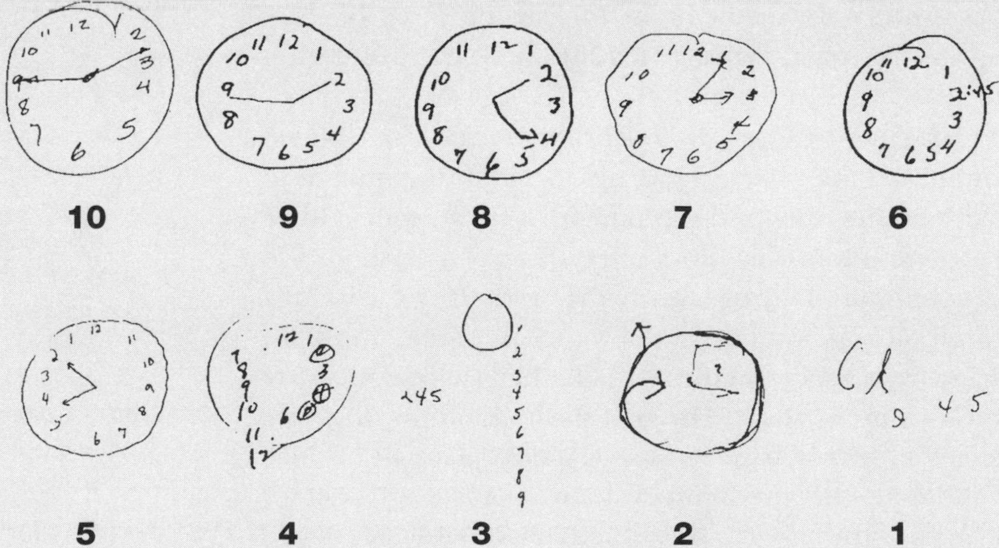

Source: *Journal of the American Geriatrics Society,* August 1989.

MEMORY AND REVERSIBLE DEMENTIA

Memory loss can often result from things that can be controlled by the patient or physician. Medication side effects, depression, and certain medical conditions are important concerns.

Memory Loss Due to Medication

Although older adults make up only 12% of the population, they receive about 30% of all prescriptions written in the United States. Unfortunately, as people age, natural changes within the body make adverse effects more likely from medication: The kidneys may not remove drugs from the bloodstream as quickly as in younger adults; drug metabolism in the liver may be slowed; and a greater ratio of fat to muscle increases the time it takes to eliminate some drugs from the body. More important, however, is the fact that older adults take an average of more than five prescription drugs and three over-the-counter drugs at the same time. In geriatric clinics, about 5% to 10% of the patients seen for memory impairment have reversible dementia due to medication.

Some of the medications that may cause memory impairment include the anti-inflammatory drug prednisone (Deltasone, for example); heartburn drugs such as cimetidine (Tagamet), famotidine (Pepcid), and ranitidine (Zantac); antianxiety/sedative drugs such as triazolam (Halcion), alprazolam (Xanax), or diazepam (Valium); or even insulin—too high a dose can cause low blood sugar (hypoglycemia), leading to abnormal mental function. Other possibilities are certain medications for cancer, heart disease, high blood pressure, pain, nausea, Parkinson disease, allergies, and colds.

Memory impairment caused by medications can often be reversed or minimized by changing drugs or lowering the dose (which should be done only under a doctor's supervision). Other strategies to prevent adverse memory effects from medications are to avoid the use of multiple drugs, verify that each drug is carefully monitored (preferably by a single primary care physician), and use drug-free periods as a way to determine whether adverse memory effects are due to a medication. The best way to monitor drug use with a doctor is the "brown bag" review—patients place all of their prescription and nonprescription medications in a bag and bring it to the doctor's office. In this way, the patient eliminates the chance of forgetting to mention any of the drugs or of confusing drug names and doses.

Alcohol is the most prevalent intoxicant implicated in dementia. Fortunately, as is often the case with other drugs, the negative effects of alcohol on intellectual abilities can be reversed with abstinence, though chronic abuse may lead to permanent damage.

Memory Loss Due to Depression

Because the cognitive changes of dementia—impairment of memory, learning, attention, and concentration—can occur in people who are depressed, the diagnosis of dementia can be more difficult. In fact, depression and cognitive decline often occur together.

A person is more likely to be suffering from depression than dementia if there is a history of psychiatric illness, a sudden onset of cognitive symptoms, difficulties with sleep, or a rapid decline in the ability to perform everyday activities. In addition, depressed patients often complain that they are unable to concentrate or remember things, while individuals with dementia are generally unaware of any mental problems. For example, when depressed persons are asked a question, they are likely to say "I don't know the answer." By contrast, someone with AD might attempt to answer but be unable to do so correctly. Because depression and dementia are difficult to distinguish, it may be necessary to start antidepressant therapy and later reassess the patient for the presence of dementia.

Memory Loss Due to Medical Conditions

A number of medical conditions can lead to memory problems, and in some cases treatment of the underlying illness can reverse or reduce the memory deficit. These conditions include hormonal imbalances due to thyroid disease or Cushing disease (overproduction of steroid hormones by the adrenal gland); infectious diseases including AIDS, neurosyphilis, and chronic meningitis resulting from fungal infections or tuberculosis; tumors of the frontal or temporal lobe of the cerebral cortex; subdural hematomas (a collection of blood between the skull and the brain); normal pressure hydrocephalus (caused by excess fluid in the brain); and vitamin deficiencies (vitamin B_{12}).

MEMORY AND IRREVERSIBLE DEMENTIA

After eliminating other causes of memory loss, physicians will consider irreversible dementias as possible diagnoses. These include AD, vascular dementia, dementia with Lewy bodies, frontotemporal

NEW FINDING

Low HDL Cholesterol Linked To Cognitive Impairment

Older people with low levels of high density lipoprotein (HDL) cholesterol are at increased risk for cognitive impairment, according to a study from the Netherlands. HDL, or "good," cholesterol protects against coronary heart disease (CHD), while high levels of total cholesterol and low density lipoprotein (LDL, or "bad") cholesterol contribute to CHD.

Researchers took blood samples from 561 85-year-old people to determine levels of triglycerides and total, LDL, and HDL cholesterol. The volunteers also underwent cognitive testing with the Mini-Mental State Examination to assess cognitive function.

Overall, people with higher levels of HDL cholesterol (average 30 mg/dL) did better on the exam than those with lower levels (average 17 mg/dL). The effects of HDL cholesterol on cognition were unrelated to a history of cardiovascular disease or stroke, indicating that its effects on cognition were not caused only by the presence of overt cardiovascular disease. Levels of the other blood lipids did not affect cognitive performance.

HDL cholesterol may reduce the risk of cognitive impairment by preventing the buildup of beta-amyloid in the brain or by reducing inflammation, the authors write. The National Cholesterol Education Program guidelines have concluded that an HDL cholesterol level of less than 40 mg/dL increases the risk of CHD.

ANNALS OF NEUROLOGY
Volume 51, page 716
June 2002

dementia (for example, Pick disease), Parkinson disease, and Huntington disease. Other causes include infectious diseases such as Creutzfeldt-Jakob disease and AIDS.

Vascular Dementia

After AD, the most common cause of memory loss is vascular dementia—a disorder often resulting from a series of tiny strokes (known as infarcts) that destroy brain cells. Each infarct may be so small that it is inconsequential alone; however, the cumulative effect of many infarcts can destroy enough brain tissue to impair memory, language, and other intellectual abilities. Symptoms often develop suddenly and involve other brain functions: Loss of bladder or bowel control (incontinence), a mask-like facial expression, and weakness or paralysis on one side of the body are thought to be noncognitive hallmarks of vascular dementia. Vascular causes account for 10% to 20% of dementia cases.

Other causes of vascular dementia include lupus erythematosus and other collagen-vascular diseases (these may be at least partially reversible), as well as a major stroke. Many people suffer from vascular dementia owing to chronic high blood pressure, diabetes, or coronary heart disease (a narrowing of the coronary arteries that jeopardizes the supply of blood to the heart). Patients who survive a cardiac arrest can also suffer from memory deficits.

Preventive measures can help forestall the development of dementia and prevent further deterioration. For example, weight control, exercise, and a low-salt diet can reduce blood pressure, while a low-fat diet can decrease the risk of coronary heart disease. Medications can be taken to lower blood pressure or cholesterol when necessary, and a daily aspirin may be prescribed to prevent blood clots from forming in the arteries feeding the brain or heart. In some cases, a procedure known as a carotid endarterectomy may be performed to remove a blockage from one of the main arteries that lead to the brain. People can reduce their risk of developing diabetes by controlling their weight with diet and exercise.

According to results from what is referred to as the Nun Study, the same measures used to lower stroke risk may also reduce the risk of dementia related to AD. In this study, 102 elderly nuns (average age 83) were evaluated for Alzheimer- and stroke-related symptoms while they were alive, and careful examinations of their brains were made after death. Among the nuns who had the brain lesions of AD, those who also had evidence of infarcts due to vascular dis-

Causes of Dementia

Dementia can be caused by a number of diseases that affect the brain. The most common cause is Alzheimer disease, which is responsible for 60% to 70% of dementia cases. Another common cause is vascular dementia. In this type of dementia, areas of the brain die because of an interruption of blood flow. Damage to nerve cells in these areas causes impaired cognition (thinking). In a small number of people, dementia is due to potentially treatable causes and is therefore considered reversible. Reversible dementias include those caused by depression, alcohol abuse, vitamin B_{12} deficiency, thyroid disease, and side effects of medication.

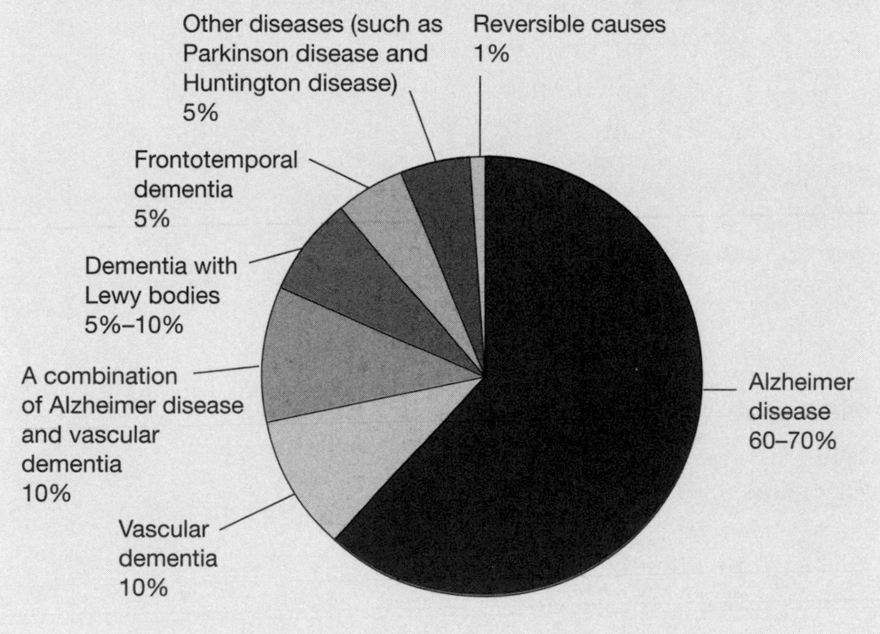

ease were 11 times more likely to have shown signs of dementia when they were alive.

Dementia with Lewy Bodies

Dementia with Lewy bodies, which sometimes occurs simultaneously with AD or Parkinson disease, accounts for 5% to 10% of cases of dementia. An individual with this form of dementia experiences episodes of confusion, falls, and repetitive hallucinations (such as always seeing the same person sitting on a particular chair), and also has signs of parkinsonism (such as shuffling gait; rigid, stooped posture; poor balance; and slowness) early in the disease. At autopsy, examination of the brain reveals cortical Lewy bodies—abnormal structures within brain cells that are distributed throughout the brain. Lewy body dementia progresses over several years. Risk factors for developing the disease have yet to be identified. While there are no current treatments for slowing the progression of the

NEW RESEARCH

High Blood Pressure Linked To Vascular Dementia

New research shows that older people with high blood pressure may not be at increased risk for developing Alzheimer disease (AD), but they may be more likely to develop vascular dementia, particularly if they also have heart disease or diabetes.

In the study, researchers obtained medical histories from 1,259 Manhattan residents, age 65 and older, who did not have dementia. The participants were tested periodically for dementia over a seven-year period.

By the end of the study, almost 13% of the participants had AD and 4% had vascular dementia. People with a history of high blood pressure (>140/90 mm Hg) had no increased risk of developing AD but were nearly two times more likely to develop vascular dementia than people without a history of high blood pressure. The risk of vascular dementia was threefold higher in those with a history of both high blood pressure and heart disease and sixfold higher in people with high blood pressure and diabetes, compared with those with no history of high blood pressure, heart disease, or diabetes.

The authors note that the association between high blood pressure and vascular dementia is small and that much of the link may be attributed to heart disease and diabetes, which are common in people with high blood pressure.

NEUROLOGY
Volume 58, page 1175
April 23, 2002

disease, a study published in *The Lancet* in 2000 found that rivastigmine (Exelon) appeared to improve symptoms such as apathy, anxiousness, delusions, and hallucinations.

Frontotemporal Dementia

Frontotemporal dementia is much less common than AD and accounts for 5% of cases of dementia. It has several forms and probably several causes. Personality changes or problems with language are usually the earliest symptoms. Pick disease is responsible for approximately one third of cases of frontotemporal dementia. Symptoms associated with Pick disease include impaired initiation of plans and goal setting, personality changes, unawareness of any loss of mental function, and language difficulties (aphasia). Palilalia—compulsive repetition of a word or phrase with increasing rapidity—sometimes occurs later in the illness. The course of the disease can vary from 2 to 10 years, but its final result is death.

Huntington Disease

Huntington disease is a rare hereditary disorder of the central nervous system characterized by uncontrollable movement and dementia. (In the past, the disease was called Huntington's chorea, from the Greek word meaning "dance.") The illness begins gradually, usually between the ages of 30 and 40, and can last for up to 20 years. Early signs of Huntington disease include changes in behavior and unusual, fidgety movements. Symptoms may be mild enough for the disease to go unnoticed for several years. Eventually, however, twisting and jerking movements that spread to the entire body are followed by memory loss, confusion, and hallucinations.

Huntington disease directly affects the parts of the brain that control coordination. Studies have shown a striking decrease in brain levels of the neurotransmitter gamma-aminobutyric acid (GABA), but it is unclear whether this change plays a role in the disease. In 1993, scientists identified the gene defect believed to cause Huntington disease. The gene is dominant, meaning that children with a parent who carries the defective gene have a 50% chance of developing Huntington disease. The discovery raises the possibility that a therapy may be developed to correct the defective gene, though currently no treatment is available. The genetic test is 100% accurate.

Personal Care: Dressing and Bathing

In the early stages of dementia, a person can usually perform everyday tasks of personal care and hygiene, such as dressing and bathing. These activities become more difficult, however, as the disease progresses. People with dementia may be unable to recall the last time they changed their clothes or took a bath, and they may become apathetic about their hygiene. Also, tasks like dressing and bathing involve many steps and may become too complicated for people in the advanced stages of dementia. Therefore, it is important for caregivers to understand and anticipate the problems that people with dementia may have with personal care so that these problems can be addressed quickly and with as little resistance as possible.

Dressing

Getting dressed can present a number of problems for people with dementia. In addition to being overwhelmed with the number of choices, they may lack the ability to tell colors apart and the coordination to execute the movements involved in dressing. Despite these difficulties, many people with dementia still enjoy being dressed well and receiving compliments on their appearance.

To make the task of dressing go more smoothly, choose what the person will wear or give the person a limited number of choices. When buying clothes or choosing them in the morning, keep in mind the person's tastes. Try to select clothes with plain colors or simple patterns, since complex designs may cause confusion. (To avoid adding to your workload, choose clothing that is easy to wash and requires no ironing.) Clothes and other items that the person rarely wears or are out of season should be put in storage to lessen the chances for confusion.

Set out the clothes in the order the person should put them on. Alternatively, hand the person the clothing items one by one with brief instructions on what to do with each. Determine if the person would benefit from a mirror. Some people with dementia enjoy seeing what they look like when fully dressed; others may be disturbed by or not recognize their reflection.

Shirts and sweaters with simple buttons in the front may be easier for the person to handle than clothing that needs to be pulled over the head. However, many people with dementia have trouble with buttons as well as zippers and snaps. Try replacing these with Velcro. Tube socks (which have no designated heel) may be easier to put on than regular socks. Shoes with Velcro are easier to put on and take off than shoes with laces.

Some people with dementia prefer to wear the same clothes every day. If this is the case, buy several of the person's favorite shirts, pants, etc., so he or she can wear a set of clean clothes each day. If the person insists on wearing oddly matched clothes or an unusual outfit, it may be best to allow him or her to do so to avoid unnecessary conflict or undue distress.

Bathing

Problems with bathing can have several causes. A person with dementia may be resistant to the idea of requiring assistance with bathing because of embarrassment or a lack of privacy. Some people with dementia may be afraid of the water or of falling, or they may not even recognize what the water is for. Also, they may feel that the room is too cold or the process of bathing is too uncomfortable to deal with.

To make bathing a more pleasant and safe experience for the person with dementia, be sure the room has enough lighting and try playing relaxing music in the background. Be sure the room is warm enough, and test the temperature of the water before letting the person in it. If the person is afraid of the water, pour some over his or her hands first. To prevent falls, install grab bars in the tub and place nonslip tape on the tub's bottom surface. If standing in the shower is a problem, buy a bath bench so the person can sit. Removing glass enclosures on a bathtub can allow you easier access to the person when assistance is needed. Never leave the person unattended in the bath or shower.

Many people with dementia find hair washing in the shower to be distressing because of the water poured over the head and face. Installing a hand-held shower attachment may be helpful. Alternatively, try washing the person's hair in the kitchen sink.

If possible let the person bathe him- or herself, but be sure to instruct the person on each task and guide him or her though each step of the process. Also, set out each item (for example, soap, towel, etc.) in the order it should be used. Providing soap on a rope may allow the person to wash without worrying about dropping the soap.

Try to establish a regular bathing routine. You can allow the person with dementia to choose the manner and time of bathing, but make the choices simple. You are less likely to meet resistance if you establish a bathing routine that is consistent with what the person did before he or she had dementia. If the person puts up a lot of resistance, remember that bathing each day is not a necessity. Sponge baths can be given on the days the person does not bathe.

Creutzfeldt-Jakob Disease

Creutzfeldt-Jakob disease (CJD) is a rare, fatal brain disorder that causes a rapidly progressing dementia. The disease, which affects approximately one in a million people worldwide, has received much attention due to the discovery in England of a handful of people who developed a disorder similar to CJD, most likely by eating beef from cattle that was infected with bovine spongiform encephalopathy (mad cow disease). The disorder was named new variant CJD (vCJD). To date, no cases of vCJD have been acquired in the United States.

According to a recent study, having parents or siblings with any form of dementia more than doubles the risk of CJD. Exposure to brain or nervous system tissue, for example, during a medical procedure, also raises the risk.

CJD is caused by prions, unusual infectious agents that contain no genetic material and consist entirely of a protein that can make copies of itself. Because early symptoms include memory loss and mood changes, CJD is sometimes mistaken for AD, but CJD usually progresses much more rapidly. It mainly afflicts people 50 years of age and older. The majority of patients die within 18 months, some within two to three months after the first signs of the disease appear. Although CJD is transmissible in humans, there is no evidence of an increased risk among family members and physicians who care for CJD patients. No treatments exist for the disease.

Amnestic Syndrome (Amnesia)

People with amnestic syndrome (amnesia) demonstrate severe memory loss but are otherwise of normal intelligence. The exotic nature of the disorder—memories become hidden owing to a head injury, stroke, or encephalitis—has long fascinated scientists and the public.

The first direct evidence that structures in the medial temporal lobe (where the hippocampus is located) play an important role in memory was provided by research on a patient with amnesia. Damage to the temporal lobes due to an accident, severe alcoholism, prolonged low blood pressure, or viral inflammation of the brain cause amnesia. Brain damage from such injuries usually results in anterograde amnesia, an inability to remember anything occurring after the injury. Retrograde amnesia, a loss of memory from a time prior to the accident—such as during childhood—is uncommon.

NEW RESEARCH

Many People With Dementia Continue To Drive

About a quarter of people with moderate to severe dementia continue to drive, even though cognitive impairment is a risk factor for car accidents.

Hawaiian researchers reviewed the medical records of 297 people age 65 and older to look for any indication that their physician had made a diagnosis of cognitive impairment. They also tested the participants' cognitive functioning and asked them if they were currently driving.

Most participants (60%) said they were current drivers. Driving rates declined from 73% in those with good cognitive performance to 38% in participants with intermediate cognitive functioning to 23% of those with poor cognitive performance. Only 5% of people with intermediate cognitive performance had been diagnosed with cognitive impairment by their primary care physician, and only 11% of those with poor cognitive function were recognized as having cognitive problems by their doctor.

"Physician intervention is a key factor in curbing unsafe driving," the authors write. But, if doctors are often unaware of cognitive problems in their patients, as this study suggests, they are unlikely to ask a patient with cognitive impairment to stop driving. However, the authors note that people may still be able to drive safely in the early stages of memory loss.

JOURNAL OF THE AMERICAN GERIATRICS SOCIETY
Volume 50, page 1265
July 2002

Alzheimer Disease

Alzheimer disease—a progressive disorder of the brain that is characterized by deterioration of mental faculties due to the loss of nerve cells and the connections between them—is often accompanied by changes in behavior and personality. The course of the disease is relentless, although the rates of its progress and mental decline vary from person to person. A recent study found that only half of patients with AD survive more than three years after the initial diagnosis. Earlier studies reported survival times of five to nine years. But some individuals can live for 20 years or more after diagnosis.

Degenerative changes in Alzheimer disease. In AD, nerve cells stop functioning, lose connections with each other, and ultimately die. Death of many neurons in key parts of the brain causes those areas to atrophy (shrink) and results in substantial abnormalities of memory, thinking, and behavior.

Early in the disease, destruction of neurons is particularly widespread in parts of the brain controlling memory, especially the hippocampus. This explains why memory impairment is often the first sign of AD. As nerve cells in the hippocampus break down, short-term memory fails and the ability to do familiar tasks begins to decline as well.

The other area of the brain where a great deal of damage occurs is the cerebral cortex, particularly the areas responsible for language, reasoning, perception, and judgment (the temporal, frontal, and parietal lobes). Thus, unwarranted emotional outbursts (referred to as catastrophic reactions), disturbing behaviors (such as wandering), and episodes of extreme agitation appear and become more frequent as the disease progresses.

As additional areas of the brain are affected, the person with AD becomes bedridden, incontinent, totally helpless, and unresponsive to the outside world.

Plaques and tangles. Amyloid plaques and neurofibrillary tangles are the pathological hallmarks of AD. Although discovered only at autopsy, they are required to make a definitive diagnosis of AD. It remains unclear whether these abnormal brain deposits are the cause or a by-product of AD, but researchers have come to understand better how plaques and tangles are formed. This improved knowledge has spawned new attempts to block the underlying process that may lead to their buildup. The success of these strategies may ultimately form the basis of prevention or treatment if these plaques and tangles are, in fact, the cause of AD.

Amyloid plaques develop in areas of the brain that are related

NEW RESEARCH

AD Incidence Decreases In the Very Old

While previous research has shown that the incidence (the number of new cases per year) of Alzheimer disease (AD) approximately doubles every five years after age 65, a new study reveals that once people enter their 90s, the number of new AD cases begins to drop off.

Study participants included 3,308 Utah residents, age 65 and older, who were evaluated for dementia and had their APOE genotype determined. [People with the APOE ε4 allele tend to develop AD at an earlier age; see page 22.]

Although the risk of developing AD increased sharply with age up to around age 90, it began to decline at age 93 in men and age 97 in women. In addition, people with two copies of the APOE ε4 allele tended to develop AD about 10 years sooner than those without APOE ε4, but they did not have higher lifetime rates of AD.

Those who live into their 90s may possess certain genes or other factors that protect them against AD, the authors suggest. Alternatively, many risk factors for AD are also risk factors for coronary heart disease; people who avoid coronary heart disease may be able to live longer without developing AD. Because the incidence of AD does not appear to increase exponentially through life, current projections for the numbers of people who will eventually develop AD may need to be adjusted.

NEUROLOGY
Volume 58, page 209
January 2002

Reality Orientation Therapy

Reality orientation therapy is a behavioral technique designed to orient people with dementia to reality. When using reality orientation, caregivers repeatedly help the person relearn such information as the time of day, the date, and his or her location.

How Is It Performed?

Reality orientation therapy can be carried out either in a group setting at set times or continuously on an individual basis. In group therapy (typically performed at residential care facilities), patients meet regularly in a classroom for 30 to 60 minutes. During the class, a therapist presents and reinforces basic information (name, location, date, names of objects and colors) for the patients with more severe dementia, and discusses sports, television programs, and current events with patients functioning at a higher level. Participants may also engage in word games such as fill-in-the-blank exercises or simple crossword puzzles. The therapist may introduce more information as patients learn more.

Peter Rabins, M.D., (coauthor of this White Paper) prefers to encourage caregivers and anyone else who comes in contact with the patient to engage in continuous reality orientation. In this approach, mistakes are gently corrected and current information is presented throughout the day to help ground the person in his or her surroundings.

A reality orientation board is a central feature of both the classroom and continuous methods. The board can be a bulletin board, blackboard, dry erase board, or any other surface that allows for regular changes in information. Typically, the board includes the day of the week, the date, the weather, the season, the name and time of the person's next meal, the person's location (such as town and state), and the next holiday. At home, the caregiver should place the board where the patient can see it often.

Caregivers should also keep visible a large clock, a calendar, a daily-activities schedule, and possibly a local, state, and world map. If the person is in the early stages of dementia, encourage him or her to wear a watch that displays the date. Also, make available current newspapers and magazines, large-print books, Scrabble sets, crossword puzzle books, or other items that remind the person of current events or stimulate them mentally. If needed, place signs on doors and place arrows around the house to direct the person to certain rooms (the bathroom, kitchen, etc.).

Dr. Rabins advises using statements in everyday conversation that orient the person to the present. For example, say things like, "It is 5:30 in the evening, and we are going to eat dinner." You should also bring up information such as the date and day of the week as well as the names of people and objects frequently encountered. Give positive reinforcement, such as a compliment or smile, when the person makes a statement or engages in behavior that shows an increased awareness.

Be sensitive to the person's capacity to retain information and do not try to push the person beyond his or her ability. Also, remember that the person's abilities can change over time and even from day to day.

Evidence

Reality orientation therapy is supported by a modest amount of research. A meta-analysis of six randomized, controlled trials in people with dementia published in 2000 found that classroom reality orientation produced modest improvements in cognitive function in a group of 125 patients and improved behavior in a group of 48 patients. While the benefits were still present one month after participants stopped attending the classes in one study, it is unclear how long the benefits will last. The authors suggest that adding continuous reality orientation to classroom sessions might produce more lasting effects.

Precautions

One criticism of reality orientation therapy is that when it is applied in a mechanical fashion it does not address the particular needs of an individual person with dementia and may even lead to problems with self-esteem and mood. Indeed, a small percentage of patients become emotionally disturbed or frustrated when attempts are made to bring them into the present. Therapy should be discontinued in such individuals. Also, the persistent repetition of basic information and the frequent correction of the same mistakes may become frustrating for both the patient and the caregiver.

to memory; they are a mixture of abnormal proteins and nerve cell fragments. Their main component is beta-amyloid, a protein that breaks off from the larger amyloid precursor protein. Beta-amyloid is formed when the amyloid precursor protein that is embedded in the cell membrane is broken down for disposal. Enzymes called secretases split the protein in two and form the beta-amyloid fragment.

Researchers recently identified beta-secretase as one of the cleaving enzymes. It cuts amyloid precursor protein in a place that causes beta-amyloid to become insoluble and deposit in the brain. Investigators suspect that blocking beta-secretase activity may prevent production of undesirable forms of beta-amyloid, and experiments are currently under way to test this hypothesis. Still a mystery, however, is what happens to the beta-amyloid segment once it separates from amyloid precursor protein, and how it might cause AD.

Neurofibrillary tangles are the other pathological characteristic of AD. Composed mostly of the protein tau, these twisted, hairlike threads are what remain after the collapse of a neuron's internal support structure, known as microtubules. In healthy neurons, microtubules act like train tracks to carry nutrients from one destination to another. Tau normally serves as the supporting "railroad ties," but in AD the protein becomes hopelessly twisted and disrupts the function of the microtubules. This defect clogs communication within nerve cells and eventually leads to their death.

Researchers are not sure why tau goes awry, but new findings suggest that an enzyme called Pin1 may play an important role in keeping tau intact. When Pin1 binds to an altered tau in test-tube experiments, the protein starts to function as it should and microtubule assembly is restored. Furthermore, researchers found substantially lower levels of Pin1 in the brains of AD patients than in healthy subjects. The significance of these findings remains uncertain, but the presence of an enzyme such as Pin1 may help maintain or restore the proper function of tau—and prevent the formation of tangles. This possibility raises the hope that therapies might be developed to keep tau functioning and prevent AD.

Neurotransmitters. Another characteristic of AD is a reduction in the levels of certain neurotransmitters that are necessary for healthy brain function. The cholinergic neurons in the brain produce acetylcholine, a neurotransmitter crucial to memory and learning. These neurons are plentiful in the hippocampus and the cerebral cortex—two regions of the brain most ravaged by AD. (As is true for plaques and tangles, it is not known whether neuronal loss in these parts of the brain is a cause or an effect of AD.) As the disease progresses, acetylcholine levels drop dramatically and dementia becomes more pronounced. Levels of serotonin, norepinephrine, somatostatin, and GABA—neurotransmitters involved in many brain functions—are diminished in almost half of patients with AD. Such imbalances may lead to insomnia, depression, aggression, and mood or personality changes.

NEW RESEARCH

High Homocysteine Precedes AD

People with high blood levels of homocysteine—an amino acid that is a risk factor for coronary heart disease and stroke—may be at increased risk for developing dementia, new research shows.

Investigators analyzed the blood homocysteine levels of 1,092 people (average age 76) who were free from dementia and tested them for dementia an average of eight years later.

By the end of the study, 111 people were diagnosed with dementia, 83 of them with Alzheimer disease (AD). People with the highest homocysteine levels at the beginning of the study were about two times more likely to be diagnosed with dementia, including AD, at follow-up than people with the lowest levels. The association between homocysteine and dementia appeared unrelated to age, gender, APOE genotype, blood levels of B vitamins, and other health conditions (including stroke) that may contribute to dementia.

High blood homocysteine levels may increase the risk of dementia by damaging blood vessels and neurons in the brain. Vitamin supplementation with folate (also known as folic acid), either alone or in combination with vitamins B_6 and B_{12}, can lower homocysteine levels. However, further research is needed to determine whether such supplementation will lower the risk of dementia.

THE NEW ENGLAND JOURNAL OF MEDICINE
Volume 346, page 476
February 14, 2002

Causes of Alzheimer disease. Despite tremendous advances in the understanding of AD, scientists have yet to pinpoint a true cause of the disorder. Some patients may have a single underlying cause, but in others, a whole host of factors appear to interact in some way to bring on the disease. Old age is the strongest risk factor for AD; others are Down syndrome, a family history of dementia, and the presence of a specific form (ε4) of the gene that makes a protein called apolipoprotein E (see below).

Women are at higher risk for AD than men, and cardiovascular disorders such as high blood pressure, high blood cholesterol, and heart attack are also possible risk factors. A Finnish study published in 2001 found that people with high blood pressure or high blood cholesterol were more than twice as likely to develop AD as those with lower measurements. Another potential risk factor is head injury. Other conditions that have been considered possible triggers of AD, but for which no good evidence supports a causal relationship, are immune system malfunctions, endocrine (hormonal) disorders, slow-acting viruses or bacteria, vitamin deficiencies, exposure to electromagnetic fields, and accumulation of metals such as zinc, copper, aluminum, and iron in the body.

Heredity plays a significant role in AD. A handful of AD patients (fewer than 2%) have the disease as a result of genetic factors. In these families, AD is carried as a dominant trait (which means that half of the offspring will inherit the disorder) on one of three separate chromosomes—1, 14, and 21. However, in other families, genetic predisposition is found both in AD patients and in their relatives who exhibit no AD symptoms. Therefore, environmental risk factors probably combine with a person's genetic makeup either to increase the chances that he or she will develop AD or to cause the disease to begin earlier in life. In one study of identical twins, who share exactly the same genetic material, the age of onset of AD varied by as much as 15 years. By studying people from different ethnic, racial, and social groups, scientists may discover the full range of additional risk factors. These findings, in turn, could provide new insights into what triggers the disease.

Apolipoprotein E. A number of studies have focused on a protein called apolipoprotein E (APOE), which appears to play a role in the formation of amyloid plaques. APOE is one of the lipoproteins that carry cholesterol and other fats in the blood. The gene that directs the production of APOE is located on chromosome 19. It exists in three different versions, known as alleles—APOE ε2, APOE ε3, and APOE ε4. Every person carries two APOE genes, one

Assessing Pain in People with Dementia

Chronic pain is physical discomfort that lasts for an extended period of time and may or may not be caused by a disease. It is a common problem for older people because they are prone to chronic conditions such as arthritis and back problems. Studies have found that 25% to 50% of independent older adults have chronic pain, and 45% to 80% of nursing home residents have serious pain that is not treated adequately.

Chronic pain is a significant problem that can lead to sleep disturbances, depression, anxiety, and decreased mobility and socialization. Fortunately, once recognized, pain can be treated. But people with dementia often cannot express or understand physical problems such as pain. So the caregiver often has the responsibility of recognizing the presence of pain in someone with dementia.

Recognizing pain in someone with dementia requires a special approach. Older people, even those without dementia, often deny that they are in pain. However, they may be more honest if directly asked whether they are aching, hurting, or experiencing discomfort. For people with dementia who cannot respond to these kinds of questions, caregivers need to look for nonverbal clues that the person may be in pain.

The American Geriatrics Society has compiled a list of nonverbal clues, which are listed below. If you notice any of these actions or expressions in a person with dementia, that person may be experiencing pain and you should notify his or her doctor.

Facial Expressions

- Frowning slightly
- Having a sad, frightened, or distorted expression
- Grimacing, wrinkling the forehead, or closing or tightly shutting the eyes
- Blinking rapidly

Verbal or Vocal Expressions

- Moaning, groaning, or sighing
- Chanting, grunting, or calling out
- Breathing noisily
- Asking for help
- Becoming verbally abusive

Body Movements

- Having rigid or tense posture
- Fidgeting
- Pacing or rocking back and forth
- Restricting or changing movement, gait, or mobility

Behavioral Signs

- Refusing food or showing changes in appetite
- Changing sleep patterns
- Suddenly breaking with common routines or beginning to wander

Mental Status Signs

- Crying
- Easily becoming confused, irritable, or distressed

How To Assess Pain

Doctors can assess pain in people with mild to moderate dementia by asking them questions. Often, a doctor will ask the person to rate the pain on a scale from 1 (no pain) to 10 (most severe pain ever experienced). Doctors may also use pictures of faces or a "pain thermometer" to help patients express their level of pain.

If the patient can no longer express himself or herself, the caregiver will need to describe in detail how the patient demonstrates pain and what activities might be triggering it.

Descriptions of the type of pain the patient seems to be experiencing (such as "burning," "aching," or "stabbing") can be useful as well. The doctor will also want to know if any medications or techniques seem to relieve the pain and what prescription and over-the-counter medications the patient is currently taking or has taken in the past (including the dosages).

The doctor will try to determine the cause of the pain, which often originates in muscles, bones, or the nervous system. To do this, the doctor may need to evaluate the patient's physical function (for example, walking ability and range of motion in the joints), perform laboratory tests, and take x-rays.

Treating Chronic Pain

Pain in older adults can and should be treated. Medication is the most common treatment for chronic pain. Acetaminophen (Tylenol), taken periodically throughout the day, is frequently an effective treatment for the types of pain typically experienced by older people.

Nonsteroidal anti-inflammatory drugs (NSAIDs) are also effective but can cause more side effects in older adults. NSAIDs include aspirin, ibuprofen (Advil and other brands), or a cyclooxygenase (COX)-2 inhibitor such as celecoxib (Celebrex), rofecoxib (Vioxx), or valdecoxib (Bextra).

Severe pain can be treated with opioid drugs such as hydrocodone/ acetaminophen (Lorcet, Vicodin) or oxycodone/ acetaminophen (Percocet, Roxicet). Careful monitoring by a doctor can help ensure that these drugs are used safely.

Therapies such as relaxation techniques or massage can also help alleviate chronic pain and are often combined with medication. Pain caused by movement can be reduced by taking medication before the movement or by altering the activity. Pain can also be caused by other problems such as infection or constipation, and treating these conditions can help decrease the pain.

inherited from each parent. A person can therefore have any one of six combinations of these alleles: either a mixed set (for example, ε2/ε4) or a matched pair (for example, ε4/ε4).

Different alleles appear to confer different risks for the development of AD. People who inherit the relatively rare APOE ε2 appear to be at lower risk for AD than others, and if they do get the disease, the age of onset is usually later. APOE ε3 is the most common variety (half the general population is ε3/ε3); researchers believe this allele plays a neutral role in AD. APOE ε4, however, is linked with an increased risk or earlier onset of AD. Individuals with at least one copy of APOE ε4 have a 29% risk of developing AD, compared with a 9% risk in those with no APOE ε4. A person with two copies of APOE ε4 (approximately 3% of the white population) has a 50% chance of developing AD by age 80.

How APOE ε4 increases a person's susceptibility to AD is not yet known. For some reason, APOE ε4 appears to speed up the AD process and lower the age of onset of the disease. The average age when AD symptoms arise is 84 in those with no copies of APOE ε4, 75 in those with one copy, and 68 in those with two copies. Increased risk, however, does not guarantee illness, and the presence or absence of APOE ε4 in a blood sample cannot predict who will get AD. A person can have APOE ε4 and never get the disease. For example, a woman in the Nun Study who died at age 107 had one copy of the APOE ε4 allele but was highly functional when she died.

Lipoprotein(a). A protein known as lipoprotein(a) may play a role in encouraging APOE to bind to and enter neurons. In a 2000 study of 284 patients with AD, elevated levels of lipoprotein(a) increased the risk of late-onset AD among carriers of APOE ε4. In people over age 80, those with the APOE ε4 allele and high levels of lipoprotein(a) had a six times greater risk of AD than those with lower levels. Conversely, high levels of lipoprotein(a) reduced the risk of AD by 60% in noncarriers of APOE ε4 who were over age 80.

Other genes. Studies show that abnormal genes on three different chromosomes—the amyloid precursor protein gene on chromosome 21, the presenilin-1 (PS-1) gene on chromosome 14, and the presenilin-2 (PS-2) gene on chromosome 1—may be directly linked to AD. However, these alterations are uncommon. A defective amyloid precursor protein gene, for instance, has been found in only 25 families worldwide. Passed down from either parent, these genetic abnormalities account for fewer than 10% of early-onset (before age 60) cases of inherited AD. People with an altered amyloid precursor protein gene usually develop AD between 40 and 65 years of age. Individuals who carry a PS-1 mutation may show signs of AD as early as age 30, while people with PS-2 alterations get the disease anywhere from age 40 to 90. Though these three mutations affect only a small number of families, a person carrying one of them will inevitably develop AD.

Beta-amyloid. Other areas of research center on how the beta-amyloid protein affects neurons. In one laboratory study, neurons from the hippocampal area of the brain died when beta-amyloid was added to a cell culture, suggesting that the protein is poisonous to neurons. The authors of another recent study reported that beta-amyloid breaks into fragments and releases free radicals (unstable oxygen molecules) that attack cell membranes. It may be that APOE proteins are involved in the removal of beta-amyloid fragments and that specific forms of the protein are less efficient in doing so.

Aluminum. Much publicity followed the discovery of a possible link between aluminum and AD, when researchers observed larger than expected amounts of the metal in the brains of some people who died of AD. Worried that aluminum might somehow promote the disease, many people began to throw away cans, cookware, cosmetics, antacids, antiperspirants, and other items containing the metal. However, studies of people who were exposed to large quantities of aluminum revealed no increased incidence of dementia. Most likely, the deposition of aluminum in brain tissue is a result—not a cause—of the factors that underlie the dementia. (Incidentally, more aluminum leaches into soft drinks from glass bottles than from aluminum cans, which are coated with a thin layer of plastic.)

Head injury. Scientists are divided over the role of head injury in the development of Alzheimer disease (AD). While some studies have shown that a head injury makes a person more likely to develop AD later in life, other reports have demonstrated no such association. Further research has shown that head injuries do not increase the incidence of AD, but may cause people who are already susceptible to the disease to develop it earlier.

Diagnosis of Alzheimer disease. Although only an autopsy can definitively prove the presence of AD, the clinical diagnosis is usually accurate. The current approach for establishing the cause of memory loss involves both eliminating some potential causes and finding confirmatory support for others. Once other conditions—such as depression, Huntington disease, or hypothyroidism—have been ruled out as causes of dementia, the diagnosis of AD is made on the accumulation of data from the patient's history, mental status exams, and interviews with the patient, family members, and

NEW RESEARCH

Pre- and Poststroke Dementia Increases Mortality

People who have dementia before a stroke (prestroke dementia) and those who develop dementia after a stroke (stroke-related dementia) are at increased risk for dying, new research indicates.

Spanish investigators interviewed the relatives of 324 stroke victims to determine which patients displayed signs of dementia in the five years before their stroke. All available patients were tested three months after their stroke to determine who had dementia symptoms at that time.

About 15% of the patients had dementia before their stroke. After an average follow-up of 16 months, 20% of patients with prestroke dementia were alive compared with 73% of those without prestroke dementia. Nearly 20% of the patients who had survived to three months had dementia that was brought on by the stroke. After an average follow-up of 22 months, 58% of those with stroke-related dementia were alive compared with 95% of those without stroke-related dementia.

"Dementia seems to be one of the most important determinants of mortality in stroke patients," the authors write. One possible explanation may be that patients with dementia are less likely to adhere to their treatment plans after a stroke. Alternatively, doctors may be less likely to prescribe anticoagulant drugs like warfarin (Coumadin) to people with dementia.

STROKE
Volume 33, page 1993
August 2002

Providing Long-Distance Care

People with dementia often have few or no family members living nearby to help them with day-to-day care. In such situations, a family member may need to provide assistance from afar by coordinating local services and delegating tasks to neighbors, family, and friends who live closer to the person with dementia.

Some six million people in the United States have taken on the role of long-distance caregiver. And although this role is inevitably demanding, caregivers can make their jobs less stressful with proper planning and by using a number of services.

Making a Visit

One of the first steps you should take as a long-distance caregiver is to visit the person with dementia to evaluate the situation and determine the person's needs. Preferably, this visit should last a few days. During this time, look for signs of mental or physical decline, problems with bladder or bowel control, malnutrition, depression, and poor mobility. Ask yourself whether the person has poor hygiene or judgment. Does he or she eat nutritious meals and pay bills on time? Does the person wander or end up in unsafe situations?

While visiting, be sure to meet with your relative's doctors, lawyers, and any other professionals he or she sees (or should be seeing) regularly. Discuss the situation with them, and ask them to help in whatever ways they can. Also, visit with the person's friends and neighbors as well as with any relatives who live nearby. Ask for their observations about the person's health, behavior, and safety.

Spend time with your relative. Talk about his or her needs and opinions, and enjoy one another's company. After the visit, call the person on a regular basis and try to ascertain how well he or she is doing, particularly in regard to physical health and cognitive function.

Coordinating Care

The next step is to develop a care plan. During your visit, you likely identified the areas in which the person needs assistance. Now, you need to find out what services are available to address these issues. Here, a geriatric care manager or social worker can be helpful. (To find a geriatric care manager, contact the National Association of Professional Geriatric Care Managers; see the inset box on the opposite page.) These professionals should be able to assist you in finding services in your relative's area and in coordinating care. You can also contact organizations that provide community services. Ask about the details of their services, including the application procedure, the cost, and the length of the waiting list.

Furthermore, ask other relatives and friends who live nearby to stop in and visit the person as often as they can. Find out if they are willing to help with specific tasks, such as grocery shopping or checking to see if the bills are paid. Talk with your relative's neighbors and ask them to look in on the person periodically. Volunteers from local religious or neighborhood organizations may be able to check on the person as well. Tell anyone who visits the person to call you if they notice any problems (for example, the person looks malnourished or disheveled).

Once you have developed a care plan, discuss it with the person's doctors to see if they have any suggestions or input. Also, have a family meeting to discuss the plan. A social worker may be helpful as a mediator. During the meeting, you can delegate responsibilities to different family members. You may need to have periodic meetings or conference calls if the situation changes. Be sure to include the person with dementia in the decision-making process.

It may help to keep a logbook detailing all aspects of the person's care. In this book, write down the names, phone numbers, and addresses of all relatives, friends, neighbors, doctors, and anyone else involved in caring for the person with dementia. Keep contact information on all the organizations involved in providing services to the person. In addition, after every visit, write notes that detail such information as your relative's medical conditions and prescribed medicines.

The log also should contain important financial data, such as the person's bank account, credit card, and tax information. You should keep copies of your relative's will and any advance directives, as well as his or her Social Security number and health insurance information. You also should know the location of important personal documents, such as

friends over a period of several weeks. Diagnoses based on such clinical features are accurate about 90% of the time. Criteria for the diagnosis of AD from the *Diagnostic and Statistical Manual of Mental Disorders* require the presence of memory impairment and at least one other cognitive deficit (such as difficulty communicating) that is severe enough to affect social or job functioning, and that the de-

Organizations That Provide Services

Many organizations can assist you in coordinating care or directing you to local services. In addition to contacting the Administration on Aging, the Alzheimer's Association, and the Alzheimer's Disease Education and Referral Center (see page 46 for contact information), you may also want to get in touch with the following organizations:

American Association of Homes and Services for the Aging (AAHSA)
2519 Connecticut Avenue, NW
Washington, DC 20008-1520
☎ 202-783-2242
www.aahsa.org
AAHSA lists information on providers of assisted-living, home, and community-based services. The organization can help coordinate care through such services as adult day care, transportation assistance, and home health care.

National Council on Aging Benefits Checkup
www.benefitscheckup.org
By filling out an on-line financial information questionnaire, you can find out the federal and state assistance programs for which your relative might qualify.

National Association for Home Care
228 Seventh Street, SE
Washington, D.C., 20003
☎ 202-547-7424
www.nahc.org
The NAHC provides guides and directories that can help you choose and locate home care and hospice agencies in your relative's area. Follow the link for "Agency Locator" at the top of the Web page.

National Association of Professional Geriatric Care Managers
1604 N. Country Club Road
Tucson, AZ 85716-3102
☎ 520-881-8008
www.caremanager.org
Through this association, you can search for geriatric care managers in your relative's area.

Eldercare Locator
☎ 800-677-1116
www.eldercare.gov
Through the toll-free number or the Web site, you can obtain contact information on local agencies that can assist you in coordinating care or refer you to local services. More information is available through the toll-free number than from the Web site.

National Adult Day Services Association (NADSA)
8201 Greensboro Drive, Suite 300
McLean, VA 22102
☎ 866-890-7357 (toll free)
www.nadsa.org
NADSA provides a directory of adult day services and a guide to choosing an adult day center.

a birth certificate. Furthermore, keep travel information handy (such as driving directions, bus schedules, etc.) in case of an emergency.

Moving

Eventually the time may come when the person with dementia is unable to live alone. At this point, you have three main options: move the person to your home, move in with the person, or move the person into an assisted living or residential care facility. You will need to evaluate each option and discuss the situation with your relative's doctor, social worker or geriatric care manager, and other family members. It is possible that a move could be delayed by increasing the amount of services provided or by modifying the person's home.

Here are some things to consider when making your decision: Are there more services, such as respite care, near your home or the care receiver's home? Whose home is better designed and equipped for a person with dementia? Will the move significantly affect other family members, your job, or your financial situation? How rooted is the person in his or her current living environment? Does the person depend on family or friends in the area? Will the move agitate or confuse the person? If neither the person's home nor your home appears to be a reasonable option, investigate residential care or assisted living.

cline is gradual. Laboratory and imaging studies can provide information needed to diagnose many non-AD dementias.

Laboratory tests. Two laboratory tests called the ADmark Assays are available to aid in the diagnosis of AD. One of these assays measures beta-amyloid and tau protein in the cerebrospinal fluid (requiring a spinal tap). Its use is currently discouraged because it is about as accurate as a careful clinical assessment, which needs to be carried out anyway.

The other assay is for the APOE genotype; it bases the *probability* that a person's dementia is due to AD on whether APOE ε4 alleles are present (since some individuals with this allele will never develop AD). This test is not part of routine evaluation of people with dementia.

Some people without dementia request an assay for the APOE genotype, but this is discouraged for several reasons. Most importantly, the presence of an ε4 allele only indicates that the person is at increased risk for developing AD, not that the person will develop AD. Furthermore, according to a panel of experts assembled by the National Institutes of Health, testing for the APOE ε4 gene should not be performed because there is presently no cure for AD and no recommended treatment to lower the risk of developing it. In addition, knowledge of the gene's presence could produce unnecessary anxiety in the individual and lead to discrimination by employers or health insurance companies.

The reaction to atropine eye drops was widely reported as a useful screening test, but it is ineffective in identifying early AD.

Imaging studies. Computed tomography (CT) and MRI scans are used to examine brain structure or function and rule out other possible causes of mental impairment. The use of PET and SPECT is not recommended at this time.

A CT scan uses an x-ray method that makes hundreds of images while rotating 360° around the area that is being studied. A computer processes these images to produce two-dimensional cross-sectional images of the area—like slices from a loaf of bread. This technique can eliminate some causes of dementia other than AD—such as stroke, brain tumor, brain abscess, or hydrocephalus (fluid in the brain). However, specific structures like the hippocampus cannot be visualized. A CT scan can identify enlargement of the lower portions of the lateral ventricles—chambers in the brain that contain and circulate cerebrospinal fluid. Enlargement of these portions of the lateral ventricles, which are adjacent to the hippocampus, indirectly suggests a decrease in the volume of the hippocampus. In clinical studies, this technique has detected 75% to 95% of patients with AD. However, the likelihood of hippocampal atrophy increases in older patients—even in healthy people—and reduces the specificity of the test.

MRI can also detect atrophy and ventricular enlargement. Like CT, this technique forms two-dimensional, cross-sectional images of

NEW RESEARCH

Brain Imaging May Predict AD

A type of functional magnetic resonance imaging (MRI) in which the firing of brain cells can be observed and measured may help diagnose and possibly predict the development of mild cognitive impairment (MCI) and Alzheimer disease (AD), a new study shows.

Researchers studied 5 people with MCI, 10 with AD, and 9 with intact cognition, all in their 60s and 70s. While mentally at rest, the participants underwent an MRI to determine the "functional synchrony" in the firing of brain cells in the hippocampus. The researchers suspected that the synchrony, or balance, of the cells' firing would be high for people with intact cognition but low in those with impaired cognitive function.

People with AD had the lowest levels of functional synchrony. Synchrony levels in patients with MCI were intermediate between those of AD patients and those of people with intact cognition. Also, the participants' scores on the Mini-Mental State Examination correlated well with their levels of functional synchrony.

These findings suggest that imaging studies that determine functional synchrony in the hippocampus—the first brain area typically affected in AD—may help detect patients in the earliest stages of dementia, when interventions may be most useful.

RADIOLOGY
Volume 225, page 253
October 2002

Medications To Treat Alzheimer Disease 2003

Generic Name	Brand Name	Average Daily Dosage*	Wholesale Cost†	How They Work	Comments
galantamine	Reminyl	16 to 24 mg	8 mg: $216	Block acetylcholinesterase, an enzyme that destroys the neurotransmitter acetylcholine. This action elevates the level of acetylcholine in the brain, thereby increasing messages between nerve cells.	Produce slight improvements in memory and reasoning ability, and mental decline is less pronounced. Side effects include nausea, vomiting, diarrhea, loss of appetite, dizziness, fatigue, and possible liver damage. Rivastigmine and galantamine are taken twice a day and are available in liquid form for people who cannot swallow tablets. Donepezil is taken once a day.
rivastigmine	Exelon	6 to 12 mg	3 mg: $224		
donepezil	Aricept	5 to 10 mg	10 mg: $473		

* These dosages represent an average range for the treatment of AD. The precise effective dosage varies from patient to patient and depends on many factors. Do not make any changes in your medication without consulting your doctor.
† Average wholesale prices to pharmacists for 100 tablets or capsules of the dosage listed. Costs to consumers are higher.
Source: *Red Book, 2002* (Medical Economics Data, publishers).

the brain. But MRI uses a powerful magnet rather than x-rays to capture the images. Because it is based on the amount of water in a given tissue, MRI provides a more refined visualization of the brain and, therefore, better resolution.

A promising development in imaging is functional MRI, which not only looks at the structure of the brain, but also at the metabolic processes taking place within it at the time of the scan. For example, functional MRI can detect changes in brain activity that occur as different areas of the brain are stimulated—through memory tests or mathematical tasks, for example. Such images, which show the structure and the metabolic function of the brain, were formerly possible only with a combination of either CT or MRI and another technique—usually PET or SPECT scanning. Functional MRI might become an effective diagnostic tool for AD. Detecting functional abnormalities—which may precede atrophy—can allow earlier diagnosis, and early treatment might prevent or slow the progression of AD.

Progression of Alzheimer disease. Alzheimer disease advances slowly through three symptomatic stages, ranging from mild forgetfulness to severe dementia.

Symptoms of the first stage include impaired memory of recent events, faulty judgment, and poor insight. People may forget important appointments, recent family events, and highly publicized news items. Other symptoms include losing or misplacing possessions, repetition of questions or statements, and minor or occasional disorientation.

As the disease progresses into the second stage, memory problems grow worse and basic self-care skills begin to decline. Patients have trouble expressing themselves verbally or in writing, and may be unable to perform everyday activities such as dressing, bathing, using a knife or fork, or brushing their teeth. They may also suffer from delusions or hallucinations.

In the third stage, almost all capacity for reasoning is lost. Patients end up completely dependent on others for their care. The disorder eventually becomes so debilitating that patients cannot walk or feed themselves, and patients become susceptible to other diseases. Lung and urinary tract infections are common. Pneumonia is the most frequent cause of death.

Treatment of Alzheimer disease. As of yet, no treatment can prevent or halt the mental deterioration associated with AD. The search for effective drug therapy has focused on preventing the destruction of neurons, with the ultimate goal of preserving cognitive function for as long as possible. One avenue researchers have explored is based on the theory that memory deficits in AD are due in part to a deficiency of the neurotransmitter acetylcholine. Scientists have sought ways to boost the amount of acetylcholine in the brain by administering substances containing it, by stimulating the brain to manufacture it in increased quantities, or by preventing the breakdown of the limited quantities of acetylcholine that the brain is able to make. Lecithin and choline, two substances that appear naturally in many foods, are used by the body to produce acetylcholine. Supplements of lecithin and choline, available in health food stores, have been given to AD patients in the hope of improving their mental function, but results have been disappointing.

Cholinesterase inhibitors. Drugs known as cholinesterase inhibitors were the first to be approved by the U.S. Food and Drug Administration (FDA) for the treatment of AD. These medications work by slowing the breakdown of acetylcholine. While they may ease some symptoms associated with AD, they do not halt its progression. According to guidelines published by the American Academy of Neurology in 2001, these drugs are consistently better than placebo, but the average benefit is modest, and the disease continues to progress despite treatments.

Tacrine (Cognex)—the first cholinesterase inhibitor to receive FDA approval—works in only about 20% to 40% of patients with AD. Common side effects are nausea, vomiting, and liver damage.

Tacrine is rarely used, now that a second generation of cholinesterase inhibitors has been developed.

Second-generation cholinesterase inhibitors are similar to tacrine, but produce fewer or less severe side effects. The first one approved by the FDA was donepezil (Aricept). Clinical trials have shown significant improvement in cognitive and overall function in patients receiving donepezil (as compared with those receiving a placebo), with fewer adverse effects than with tacrine. In one 24-week study, at least 80% of the donepezil patients suffered no cognitive decline, compared with 57% of patients taking a placebo. Improvement was greater with higher dosages of the drug: 54% of the patients taking 10 mg of donepezil improved slightly in one cognitive test, compared with 38% of those taking 5 mg and 27% taking the placebo. In a more recent study, patients taking 10 mg of donepezil for one year had half the rate of disease progression of those who received a placebo. The most common side effects of donepezil are nausea, vomiting, and diarrhea.

The second of these drugs to be approved was rivastigmine (Exelon). In four placebo-controlled clinical trials, involving a total of 3,900 people, patients taking rivastigmine had significantly better scores on standard tests of cognitive function than those taking a placebo. One of these trials included 725 patients with AD and found that 24% of the patients in the rivastigmine group showed significant improvements in cognitive function over a 26-week period, compared with 16% of those taking a placebo. The most common adverse effects were nausea, vomiting, loss of appetite, and weight loss.

The newest drug to be approved is galantamine (Reminyl). Its approval was based on data from four placebo-controlled clinical trials involving more than 2,650 patients. Patients taking galantamine scored better on measures of cognitive performance and patient function than those taking a placebo. The most common adverse effects were nausea, vomiting, loss of appetite, diarrhea, and weight loss.

Vitamin E and selegiline. The American Academy of Neurology has concluded that good evidence exists for the use of vitamin E in an attempt to slow the progression of AD. Selegiline (Eldepryl), a medication used to treat Parkinson disease, has more side effects, and there is no advantage to using selegiline if vitamin E is already being used. Although vitamin E is generally safe, large doses have been associated with bleeding in some patients who are deficient in vitamin K.

NEW RESEARCH

AD Drug Effective for Vascular Dementia

In a recent study, researchers report that a medication approved to treat Alzheimer disease (AD)—galantamine (Reminyl)—is also effective for patients with vascular dementia or a combination of AD and cerebrovascular disease (disease of the arteries in or leading to the brain).

Finnish investigators randomized 592 patients who had either vascular dementia or AD with cerebrovascular disease to receive galantamine or a placebo daily.

Six months later, significantly more patients taking galantamine than those taking placebo improved or remained stable on measures of cognitive function (64% vs. 51%) and overall function (74% vs. 59%). Also, patients taking galantamine remained stable in their ability to perform activities of daily living, while patients taking the placebo declined. Further, the galantamine group was more likely to experience improvements in behavioral symptoms than the placebo group. Side effects of nausea and vomiting were more common with galantamine than with the placebo.

The authors conclude that galantamine appears to be as useful for vascular dementia and AD with cerebrovascular disease as it is for the treatment of AD alone. Galantamine "provides a treatment option to a broad range of patients for whom little pharmacological help has been available," they write.

THE LANCET
Volume 359, page 1283
April 13, 2002

Exercise for People with Dementia

While some people see the world of exercise as inhabited only by the young, the fit, and the healthy, research continues to show the benefits of moderate exercise for older persons, those who are not so fit, and those with certain health conditions, including dementia.

Of course, exercise takes on a different dimension for someone with dementia. Memory loss, agitation, confusion, and other symptoms make it difficult, and sometimes unsafe, for such patients to initiate and follow an exercise program on their own. Also, overburdened caregivers may have trouble finding the time and energy to coordinate and supervise such a program. Further, the caregiver may have difficulty deciding what type of exercise is important or appropriate for a person with dementia.

Fortunately, people with conditions like Alzheimer disease do not have to engage in strenuous, time consuming, or highly structured activities to reap the health benefits of moderate exercise. Simple activities like walking, which can be worked into everyday routines, can be of tremendous benefit to both the patient and the caregiver.

Why Exercise?

Physical activity has numerous health benefits, regardless of a person's cognitive status. Engaging in regular exercise helps maintain overall well-being, prevents disease, and decreases the risk of death from cardiovascular diseases, such as heart attack and stroke. It can also increase a person's strength and energy, improve circulation and joint flexibility, and help control blood pressure.

But exercise may also have benefits specific to people with dementia. Caregivers often report that people with dementia display fewer problem behaviors with regular exercise: Patients are calmer and less likely to wander, swear, pace, or display other signs of agitation. They also are better able to maintain their motor skills, balance, and flexibility. These benefits may help them continue to perform personal care activities like bathing and dressing for longer than they otherwise would. Exercise also may promote regular bowel movements in addition to improving mood and sleep. Furthermore, physical activity may make the patient more likely to engage in social interaction and improve his or her ability to communicate. All of these benefits are helpful to the caregiver as well.

While physical activity can improve quality of life for people with dementia, there is no convincing evidence that exercise can prevent memory loss or improve thinking in people with dementia. However, one small study from Italy found improved cognition in men with mild to moderate Alzheimer disease who exercised on a stationary bicycle for 20 minutes a day three times a week.

What to Do

Because of the person's cognitive impairment, the caregiver will usually have to choose the type of exercise and supervise the patient. But what form of exercise should you pick? Walking is one of the first activities to consider. It is a simple yet beneficial exercise that is appropriate for people of any age and does not require any special equipment except loose-fitting clothes and comfortable shoes. At first, go on short strolls with the person and then slowly increase the distance you and the patient walk each day as you both build up endurance. Try to avoid steep inclines and hills. If there are no safe places to walk in your area or the weather is poor, try walking in a local shopping mall. These walks can also be a time when you and the patient bond without the need for verbal communication.

Experimental therapies. For reasons that are not entirely clear, a recent study found that patients with AD who participated in a clinical trial were less likely to be placed in a nursing home over a 3½-year period. Of the patients in clinical trials, 17% entered nursing homes, compared with 37% of eligible nonparticipants and 32% of ineligible patients. This delay could have a number of explanations. For example, it may be due to a direct benefit from the drug being studied, or from improved coping skills that caregivers gained from additional contact with medical personnel during the study. It is also possible that people who elect to participate in clinical trials are different from those who do not. In any case, enrollment in a clinical trial may be beneficial—and may be even more worthwhile

As an alternative to walking, you can choose an activity that the person enjoyed before the illness. If he or she was a dancer, encourage the person to dance or at least engage in some sort of movement to music. If the person liked tennis, provide a racket and allow the person to hit a ball around the backyard or against a wall in a park. Similarly, if golf was a favorite sport, the person may still be good at hitting the ball even though he or she can no longer follow the rules of the game.

Other exercises that older people often enjoy include walking on a treadmill or riding a stationary bike. Weight lifting or using commercially available resistance bands is also an option. If the person has difficulty with balance, exercising can be done while seated in a chair.

Exercising along with the patient allows you to incorporate physical activity into your day as well and is also an effective way to relieve the stress of caregiving. Furthermore, the patient may benefit from being able to follow your lead as you exercise. Be sure to give the person simple, one-step instructions and to demonstrate the activity, if necessary.

Although it is not necessary to exercise every day, try to establish a consistent exercise routine. Attempt to have the activity done at the same time and in the same manner and sequence every time to lessen the chances of having the person become upset or agitated. But be flexible: If the person is resistant to exercising at that time, wait until later and try it again. Try to make exercise fun, and avoid pushing the person to do anything that makes him or her uncomfortable. Remember to have the person warm up before and cool down after exercising by doing stretches and slow walking.

You may want to contact a local senior citizen's center to find out if they offer or know of any group exercise programs that are appropriate for people with mild to moderate dementia. Participation in such a group may make exercising easier because patients can imitate the movements of others; in addition, people with dementia may enjoy interacting with the other people in the group. While the patients may not remember exactly what they have done at each session, they often recall having enjoyed the experience.

Some Cautions

Generally, people with mild to moderate dementia are able to tolerate a moderate exercise program such as walking if they are already able to do things like get around the house and climb stairs on their own without difficulty. However, consult the patient's doctor if you plan to initiate an intense exercise program or if the person has other health conditions like high blood pressure or heart disease. If the person has arthritis or an injury that causes pain, weakness, or stiffness, an occupational or physical therapist may be able to tailor an activity to the patient's needs.

Another important point is not to overdo it. Begin slowly, particularly if the person has not gotten much physical activity recently; then gradually build up the amount of exercise. Should an activity cause discomfort, pain, or swelling, switch to a less intense or different activity. If the person experiences dizziness, muscle strain, shortness of breath, or chronic pain, stop the exercise and consult the person's doctor. Also, you should periodically check for bruises and blisters on the patient's feet if you are walking for exercise.

Over time, the person's disease will progress, and his or her capacity for exercise will likely decrease. Keep this in mind and tone down the intensity of activity when the person can no longer tolerate it as well. If the person persistently refuses to exercise, make sure that depression is not a factor. Persistent refusal is also a sign that the person can no longer exercise.

for patients with AD than for those with other medical conditions, since there is no cure for AD.

A main focus of research on AD continues to be an effort to delay its onset. The following are currently being tested for their usefulness as preventive or therapeutic agents. They are still regarded as highly experimental and are by no means established as effective—but they do offer hope for the future.

Anti-inflammatory drugs. Among the more promising preventive therapies are nonsteroidal anti-inflammatory drugs (NSAIDs)—the class of drugs commonly used to treat arthritis. It is unclear in which way these drugs might be effective.

Evidence first suggesting that NSAIDs may prevent or treat AD came from the observation that patients with rheumatoid arthritis have a low prevalence of AD—as much as 6 to 12 times lower than expected. Researchers initially hypothesized that NSAIDs, taken by these patients for their arthritis, may have provided some protection against the inflammatory component of AD, and preliminary investigations ensued.

But a recent study from Australia contradicted this hypothesis. Researchers found that patients with AD who took NSAIDs scored better on neuropsychological tests than patients with AD who did not take NSAIDs, but both groups had similar amounts of inflammatory plaques and tangles in their brain at postmortem analysis. These researchers concluded that the effects of NSAIDs on the delivery of blood to the brain, rather than their anti-inflammatory effects, may protect against AD.

Other studies have also demonstrated that the risk of developing AD is substantially reduced in patients who have arthritis or a history of using NSAIDs for other reasons. In one study, the risk of developing AD was reduced by half in those who regularly took NSAIDs—mostly ibuprofen (Advil and other brands)—compared with those who did not take these drugs. (Regular use of acetaminophen [Tylenol], which is not a NSAID, did not decrease the risk of AD.)

Nonetheless, NSAIDs are not recommended at this time for the prevention of AD. Long-term treatment with these drugs can be hazardous, particularly in the elderly, and side effects like gastrointestinal disturbances (for example, bleeding and ulcers) can be severe. Further, careful studies are needed before such a recommendation can be made.

Estrogen. Initial evidence suggested that estrogen replacement therapy in postmenopausal women may protect against AD. The most recent placebo-controlled trials, however, indicate that estrogen has no protective effect once the disease has started.

The first reports on the subject found a 35% lower risk of AD in women who had ever used estrogen than in those who had not. Another study reported that women taking estrogen had a 54% lower risk of developing AD than nonusers. Furthermore, results from preliminary trials in Japan and the United States suggested that estrogen supplements improved cognitive function in patients who already suffer from AD.

However, a recent 12-week study conducted in Taiwan showed that estrogen did not improve cognitive function in 50 women with AD who were randomized to receive either estrogen or a placebo. A better designed study, which lasted one year and included 120 women with AD, also found that estrogen replacement had no effect on cognitive function.

The conflict between the earlier and most recent investigations is intriguing. It is possible that drugs that might prevent or delay the onset of AD are of no benefit after the disease has started. This difference is clearer with estrogen, but preliminary evidence suggests that it might be true for NSAIDs as well. However, the evidence suggesting a protective effect for both estrogen and NSAIDs was obtained by reviewing medical records (a research method considered scientifically less rigorous), while patients in the treatment studies were randomized to treatments. Women who choose to take estrogen replacement tend to be from a higher socioeconomic status, are better educated, and have more access to health care, and these factors may have contributed to a lower rate of AD in the nonrandomized studies. Also, estrogen may have an effect on cognition only in the first weeks of treatment and not over the long term.

Only prospective trials, which are now under way, will determine whether estrogen or NSAIDs protect against AD. The decision to initiate estrogen replacement therapy should be considered by every woman on an individual basis after a thorough discussion with her physician. Estrogen may turn out to prevent or delay AD in combination with other treatments, but for now it should be used only for reduction of menopausal symptoms (such as hot flashes and vaginal dryness) and protection against bone loss.

Ginkgo biloba. Ginkgo biloba has been hypothesized to have antioxidant and anti-inflammatory effects within the brain. However, the supplement appears to be ineffective for people with AD. A recent study published in the *Journal of the American Medical Association* shows that the supplement does not improve memory or other cognitive functions in older people who are free of memory impairment, either (see the reprint on page 48). It is possible that it may benefit some patients with unspecified dementia (not AD), but the American Academy of Neurology states that the evidence for ginkgo biloba is weak.

Because ginkgo biloba is considered a food supplement, it is not regulated by the FDA. People who are considering the use of ginkgo biloba should be aware that taking it with aspirin may lead to an increased risk of bleeding.

Statins. Several observational studies suggest that people who take statin drugs to reduce cholesterol may have a lower risk of AD, but these studies did not examine the use of statins in people who

NEW RESEARCH

Antioxidants May Protect Against AD

Results from two recent studies indicate that some antioxidant vitamins from food, but not from supplements, may help prevent Alzheimer disease (AD).

In the first study, researchers analyzed the dietary habits of 5,395 people without dementia (age 55 and older) and followed them for about six years. A high dietary intake of either vitamin C or E decreased the risk of AD by 18%. When people who took supplements were excluded from the analysis, the results remained the same, indicating that the supplements taken had no effect.

In the second study, 815 Chicago residents without dementia (age 65 and older) completed a questionnaire about their dietary habits and were followed for an average of four years. Compared with people who consumed the least dietary vitamin E, those who consumed the most had a 70% lower risk of developing AD. This finding was true only for people who had no APOE ε4 alleles. Intake of vitamin E from supplements, however, had no effect on AD risk.

Antioxidant vitamins may help prevent AD by neutralizing free radicals, which can cause oxidative damage to the brain in specific groups of individuals. Good dietary sources of vitamin C are citrus fruits, broccoli, and sprouts. Sources of vitamin E include grains, egg yolks, milk, and nuts.

JOURNAL OF THE AMERICAN MEDICAL ASSOCIATION
Volume 287, pages 3223 and 3230
June 26, 2002

Alzheimer Disease and Wandering

Nearly 60% of people with Alzheimer disease (AD) will wander away from their homes or caregivers at least once. Two factors help explain why wandering is so common in patients with AD. First, because these individuals are often physically healthy, they are capable of venturing off on their own. Second, they are likely to forget where they are going and be unable to orient themselves. For example, a person with AD may walk outside to get the newspaper, but when he or she turns back to the house it may no longer look familiar. Then, the person may start walking in search of home and become lost. But wandering is not always synonymous with being lost, and it can even be helpful when done within a safe environment (for example, a fenced backyard). Walking helps people with AD become acquainted with their surroundings, reduces anxiety and agitation, and provides exercise.

People with AD may be prompted to wander for a variety of reasons, including being hot, cold, hungry, in pain, bored, or restless. They may also be trying to return to a place from their past, such as a former home or job. A recent study found that people are most likely to wander when they are agitated or angry, when they are in an unfamiliar situation, or when their caregiver is distracted. The study also found that AD patients are more likely to wander away from a grown child (who may leave them alone due to other responsibilities) than from a spouse.

How to Prevent Wandering

Wandering is most likely among patients who are cared for at home, since nursing homes and other care facilities usually have security measures to keep residents safe. Taking the following precautions around the house may prevent wandering:

- Make sure the patient gets enough exercise. Unused energy may prompt wandering, especially during the night. Taking the person for a walk during the day may use up that energy and promote better sleep. In addition, exercise can reduce the anxiety and agitation that lead to wandering.
- If the person tends to wander away from the house, install locks on doors that lead outside and place the locks out of the normal line of vision, either very high or very low. If you don't want to use locks, install an alarm that sounds when the door is opened.
- Avoid leaving the person alone. When you need to leave the house, use respite care (see the feature on pages 40–41) or ask a friend or neighbor to help.
- Remove visual cues that make the person think of going outside—for example, jackets or boots near the back door.
- Hide the car keys. While most people with AD wander on foot, some

already had AD.

Other experimental therapies. Numerous other compounds are currently being tested for their effectiveness against AD. These include the N-methyl-D-aspartate (NMDA) blocker memantine, vitamin C, steroids such as prednisone, colchicine (commonly used to treat gout), nicotine, and drugs designed to interfere with the formation of amyloid plaques and neurofibrillary tangles. There is even a surgical procedure being tested in which a shunt is implanted in the brain to allow the spinal fluid that bathes the brain to drain more freely (see the sidebar on page 38).

The once-promising Alzheimer vaccine is no longer being tested because it triggered brain inflammation in some people. Alternative forms of the vaccine have been identified, but it will take several years to know if they are effective.

Alternative measures. Some of the alternative treatments promoted for memory enhancement include choline, a building block of acetylcholine, which has not proven to be effective; dimethylaminoethanol (DMAE), a nutrient found in seafood; ergoloid mes-

have driven hundreds of miles away from home. Nearby trains and buses are also potential hazards.

- Avoid giving the person sedative medication to prevent wandering. Drugs that are strong enough to accomplish this goal can also cause drowsiness, increased confusion, and incontinence.
- If someone with AD insists on leaving, don't confront or restrain the person. Instead, accompany them on a walk and try to divert their attention—for example, with the offer of a cup of tea back at the house.
- Always dress the person in brightly colored or distinctive clothing that will make it easier to spot him or her. Also, keep track of what the person is wearing each day, and have a recent photo handy in case you need to show it to the police and other searchers.
- Enroll the person in the Alzheimer's Association's Safe Return program. For a $40 registration fee, you will receive materials that make it easier to find a lost person. These include an identification bracelet, name tags to sew into clothing, and access to a 24-hour toll-free number to report that someone is missing. For more information about this program, call 800-272-3900 or visit www.alz.org.

Finding a Lost Wanderer
Someone with AD can wander off even if you have taken all of the above precautions. Here are a few suggestions on what to do when you discover someone is missing:

- Check the entire house, including the basement, before looking outdoors.
- See if any luggage, car keys, or credit cards are missing. These items may provide clues as to where the person has gone.
- Alert friends and neighbors that the person has wandered away, and ask them to notify you if they see the person.
- Call the police. Tell them what the person is wearing, what medical conditions he or she has, and any places the person might have gone.
- If you are leaving to search, make sure someone stays at the house in case the person returns.

Reuniting with a Lost Wanderer
People with AD who become lost are often upset and frightened. When you (or any other searcher) sees the person, approach casually, making sure he or she sees you coming. Tell the person where you both are and why. Do not scold. Instead, calmly say that you have been worried and that you are looking forward to returning home together. If the person does not want to return home immediately, spend some time walking together.

After you have returned home, try to remember that wandering is a part of the disease, and neither you nor the patient is to blame. If one of your security precautions has failed, reassess it and make any necessary changes.

ylates (Gerimal, Hydergine), which are used to treat some mood, behavior, or other problems associated with AD or vascular dementia; piracetam (Nootropil), which may improve the metabolism of acetylcholine; and vasopressin, a hormone produced by the hypothalamus. In addition, a study published in *Neurology* in 2001 found that testosterone injections improved some aspects of memory in older, healthy men.

Since no controlled studies have yet demonstrated that any of these substances improves memory, they cannot be recommended for use in the treatment of AD or any form of memory impairment. One potentially promising agent is huperzine A (hupA), which appears to work in a similar fashion to cholinesterase inhibitors. The results from a Chinese trial comparing hupA to a placebo are encouraging, but further studies are needed to prove effectiveness and safety, especially because it may cause many undesirable side effects.

Standard care for Alzheimer disease. The amount of care necessary for a patient with AD changes over the course of the disorder.

Cholinesterase inhibitors, possibly in conjunction with vitamin E, are recommended for use in the last two stages of AD. Other treatments can be instituted with the appearance of specific symptoms or associated disorders, such as depression or agitation.

According to the American Academy of Neurology, antipsychotic medications can be useful for the treatment of agitation and psychosis in dementia. Newer antipsychotic agents, such as risperidone (Risperdal), olanzapine (Zyprexa), and quetiapine (Seroquel), seem to be better tolerated than traditional antipsychotic agents such as haloperidol (Haldol).

The options for the treatment of depression are medication, psychotherapy, other therapeutic measures such as electroconvulsive therapy, or any combination of these. Treatment for depression is usually highly effective. The first antidepressant medication tried is successful at relieving depression in up to 70% of patients; psychotherapy alone works in about half of patients; and up to 70% of patients improve with electroconvulsive therapy. Examples of the most commonly used medications include sertraline (Zoloft), paroxetine (Paxil), citalopram (Celexa), bupropion (Wellbutrin), and venlafaxine (Effexor). The effectiveness of these drugs and their side effects vary from one individual to another. Some antidepressant drugs can themselves cause side effects that impair memory; therefore, a patient's response to treatment must be carefully monitored. It can take as long as six to eight weeks before depression improves with medication or psychotherapy. Electroconvulsive therapy can work within a couple of weeks.

Coping with caregiving. The daily challenges and frustrations of caring for an individual with AD can leave family members feeling physically exhausted and emotionally drained. Because they are often faced with overwhelming day-to-day responsibilities, most family caregivers tend to neglect their own physical and mental health. Caregivers must pay attention to their own well-being, however—for the ultimate benefit of both themselves and the person with AD.

Caregivers are advised to accept the fact that feelings of love for a relative may be tempered with anger, anxiety, frustration, or embarrassment. These reactions are perfectly natural, and should not be a source of guilt for the caregiver. Equally important are looking after your own health, joining a caregiver support group, scheduling regular respites, asking for help, setting realistic goals, and considering professional counseling if necessary. For more information on respite care, see the feature on pages 40–41.

Choosing a nursing home. As AD progresses, the patient's in-

NEW RESEARCH

Cerebrospinal Fluid Shunt for AD Treatment

Decreased circulation of cerebrospinal fluid (CSF) between the brain's ventricles and the spinal cord, which can lead to the buildup of beta-amyloid and tau in the brain, is a possible contributing factor in Alzheimer disease (AD). Now researchers are finding that improved CSF circulation with the use of a shunt appears to safely slow cognitive deterioration.

In the study, researchers randomly assigned 29 people with AD to receive either a shunt (called Cognishunt) or no treatment. The shunt drains CSF fluid into the abdominal cavity.

One year later, there was a slight decline in cognitive function in patients who received the shunt but a marked decline in those who received no treatment. Further, patients with the shunt had lower beta-amyloid and tau CSF levels at the end of the study than they did at the beginning. Adverse events that may have been related to the device included new-onset seizures, shunt infection, injury to the small intestine, and severe headache. All of these side effects resolved with treatment.

Although this study was not double-blinded and too few people were studied to draw definitive conclusions about the effectiveness and safety of Cognishunt, the results indicate that the device might help clear toxic proteins from the brain that contribute to AD. A larger, controlled trial is now in progress.

NEUROLOGY
Volume 59, page 1139
October 22, 2002

creasing dependency and need for supervision may make it more difficult for the family to provide all necessary care. Because such care often requires the skills of professionally trained people, nursing home placement may be in the best interest of the person with AD.

This decision to place the person with dementia in a nursing home can be hard for the family to accept and may be accompanied by feelings of guilt, sadness, and anger. In addition, the bad publicity some nursing homes have received for giving inadequate and sometimes dangerous care can add to the anxiety. You should keep in mind that many nursing homes do provide excellent care; with some research, you should be able to find a suitable facility.

Before deciding on a nursing home, you may want to explore other residential care programs, such as assisted-living facilities, which provide a combination of housing, personalized assistance, and medical care. Whether such facilities—which vary in size, cost, services, location, and quality—are appropriate for a person with AD depends on the level of care needed.

If a nursing home proves the best option after discussions with the doctor and other members of your family, the first step toward finding a good one is to consult as many people as possible. Helpful information may come from the patient's physician, from friends and acquaintances who have resided in or have a family member in a home, and from the nursing home ombudsperson (who is responsible for investigating complaints). Also, the local chapter of the Alzheimer's Association (see page 46) may have a list of recommended homes or personal references. Remember, also, to visit any candidate nursing home several times before making a final decision. Some factors to consider during those visits are outlined below.

Licensing and regulations. Check to make sure that the nursing home meets basic safety requirements. The home and the administrator should have current licenses from the state, and the home should meet state fire regulations, which include sprinkler systems and fire doors.

Care and services. It is important that the staff be familiar with common issues arising from AD. Therefore, you should ask if the staff is continually trained on AD care issues, what kinds of programs are offered to the residents, how individual care plans are developed, and how different levels of function are supported. Give examples of your patient's behaviors or challenges to find out how difficult situations might be handled. And be sure the

NEW RESEARCH

AD Medications Delay Nursing Home Placement

Cholinesterase inhibitor medications can reduce the rate at which patients with Alzheimer disease (AD) are placed in a nursing home, a new study shows.

Investigators at a research center in Pittsburgh compared 135 AD patients who took cholinesterase inhibitors with 135 AD patients who chose not to take a cholinesterase inhibitor. Treated and untreated patients were matched by age, symptom duration, education, and cognitive performance. They were followed for up to three years.

While patients taking a cholinesterase inhibitor initially experienced less cognitive and functional decline, both the treated and untreated groups eventually became severely impaired at about the same time. Also, medication did not improve survival. However, while 40% of untreated patients were placed in a nursing home over three years, only 6% of treated patients required nursing home placement.

Because taking a cholinesterase inhibitor significantly delayed or prevented nursing home placement, these medications may help patients in ways that were not evident from the measures of cognition and function used in the study, the authors conclude. However, the greatest cognitive and functional benefits of cholinesterase inhibitors are evident early in the course of treatment.

JOURNAL OF NEUROLOGY, NEUROSURGERY, AND PSYCHIATRY
Volume 72, page 310
March 2002

Respite Care

Most people with early or middle-stage Alzheimer disease (AD) can be cared for at home, but such care can be physically and emotionally draining for the caregiver. Respite care, which offers caregivers a temporary break from their duties, can be an invaluable resource. In fact, caregivers who use respite care are able to keep their AD patient at home longer than those who do not use this service. In addition, such caregivers often are healthier and feel happier about their role.

Types of Respite Care

Often, a good way to take a break from caregiving is to have someone you know stay with the AD patient. For those unwilling or unable to rely on family, friends, or neighbors for help, several professional services exist. A few are free, but most involve fees and are not covered by Medicare. The most common types of respite care are in-home care and adult day care.

- **In-home care** includes a range of programs that involve someone coming to your home to provide companion services, personal care, or household help. In-home care providers can be hired privately, through an agency, or through a government program.
- **Adult day care** offers structured recreational programs in a group setting. These programs are usually held in a community center or facility. The services offered may include transportation to and from the program, lunch, exercise, crafts, discussion, and music. Adult day care may be offered from one to five days a week, and a few programs offer evening and weekend hours. Programs may focus just on people with dementia, or they may include people with other illnesses. Some programs may only accept people with dementia who are otherwise physically healthy. You may have more difficulty finding a program that accepts a dementia patient who has difficulty walking or is incontinent.

How to Find Respite Care

A good place to start is your local office on aging, which is usually listed in the government section of the telephone directory. (Note: The actual name of the agency varies from area to area.) Also, the Alzheimer's Association (see page 46 for contact information) and the organizations listed below can refer you to groups and services in your area:

Eldercare Locator
927 15th Street NW, 6th Floor
Washington, DC 20005
☎ 800-677-1116
www.eldercare.gov

National Council on the Aging
409 3rd Street SW, Suite 200
Washington, DC 20024
☎ 202-479-1200
www.ncoa.org

American Association of Retired Persons
601 E Street NW
Washington, DC 20049
☎ 800-424-3410
www.aarp.org

facility provides for the special needs of each patient. Other questions may include:

- Does the facility have its own physician? How are other medical, dental, and vision needs met?
- Can the home accommodate any improvements or declines in a resident's condition? Under what circumstances can a home discharge the person, and how much notice is given?
- What is the policy regarding life-sustaining measures? Although a painful subject to deal with at the time of the patient's admission, it is generally important to record in the resident's chart the wishes of the family and patient regarding terminal care.

Staff. Talk with the staff members who work directly with residents to see if they are competent, friendly, and content in their jobs. Observe how residents are treated and whether they get help when they ask for it. Also, meet with the administrator and direc-

Family Caregiver Alliance
690 Market Street, Suite 600
San Francisco, CA 94104
☎ 415-434-3388
www.caregiver.org

What to Look For

Most referral services do not know the quality of the programs they recommend. So when looking for respite care, you need to do your own research and ask questions. Most respite care providers are reputable and kind, but it is important to be alert to any problems.

Here are a few things to ask a potential in-home care provider:

- Have you had special training and experience in working with people with dementia?
- Have you been certified by the state (if applicable)?
- Do you have references?
- What times are you available?
- Who will substitute if you cannot come to work?
- How can I reach your supervisor if I have a concern?
- Can I see how you interact with the person with dementia before I make a decision?

The following are some questions to ask a potential adult day care service:

- Is the staff continually trained in dementia care?
- What would you do in various situations (for example, if the person with dementia tried to wander off)?
- How are meals prepared?
- What kind of fire emergency plan is in place?
- What kind of activities do you provide?

Adjusting to Respite Care

People with AD accept change slowly, so it may take a month or more for them to adjust to day care or an in-home care provider. Most people respond best if they first have a brief meeting at home with the in-home care provider or someone from the day care center. The primary caregiver should also remain with them for the first few visits to help reassure the patient that everything is fine. Remember that AD patients almost always say they are not interested in respite care, even if they clearly enjoy it. Continue to cheerfully take them to day care or welcome the in-home care provider.

It may be helpful to make respite care seem as attractive as possible. For example, describe an in-home care provider as a friend who has come to visit, or refer to adult day care as "your group" or "the club." Some people with mild dementia like to think they are "volunteering" at the day care center, and most staffs will support this idea.

Frequently, patients will make unfavorable claims about their care, such as "they didn't give me lunch" or "she hit me." The person with dementia may not remember what actually occurred, so ask the respite care provider. If the claims are unfounded, be patient and let the person adjust to the new setting.

Finally, make sure that respite care actually gives you a break. Resist the urge to stay in the house when the in-home care provider is present. You probably will feel better if you leave for a short time, even if you just visit a neighbor or go for a walk. Feelings of guilt about leaving your loved one are common, but remember that getting some rest will help you be a better caregiver.

tors of nursing and social services. They will be able to tell you such things as the number of people each aide must take care of, and how the facility is staffed on weekends and evenings.

Costs. Because nursing home care is expensive, it is important that all costs be clearly outlined and understood. Before making a decision, address how costs will be met and whether paying for them will create a financial burden for family members. Since the laws regarding payment for nursing home care can be complex and vary among the states, be sure to contact a reliable source for accurate information. The Alzheimer's Association, insurance companies, attorneys who specialize in financial planning, Medicare representatives, and some staff members of in-home care programs may be well-informed on payment options. Questions include:

- Does the home accept the patient's funding sources (for example, Medicare)?
- Will the resident receive a refund of advance payments if he

or she leaves the facility?

- How does the home protect cash and assets that are entrusted to it? How are withdrawals noted in order to keep track of the account?
- What charges are extra (for example, television, telephone, laundry, personal care supplies, special nursing procedures)?

Cleanliness and safety. Be sure the nursing home is clean and safe (especially the kitchen and bathroom). Note unpleasant odors, such as mold, garbage, or urine. Persistent odors upon return visits may indicate poor patient care or poor housekeeping. Make sure that the bathrooms have handrails and nonskid floors, the furniture is sturdy, the doors to the outside are secure, and the facility protects the safety of people who wander.

Comfort. Spend time observing everyday life and how people are treated in a variety of facilities. Ask residents and visitors about their opinions of the facility and its staff. See if the residents look happy, comfortable, relaxed, and involved in activities. Ask yourself:

- Is the facility relatively quiet, well lit, and pleasant to be in?
- Is there a well-planned indoor or outdoor wandering path?
- Are there familiar elements in the environment, such as home-like lighting and furnishings, a center of activity, a separate dining room, and areas of personalization in the resident's room?
- Does the facility avoid disorienting sensory stimuli, such as overhead speaker systems, loud alarms, and blaring televisions?

Visiting. Be sure the home is close enough so that family members can visit regularly. Also, confirm that the home has long and convenient visiting hours and that the resident can have privacy with visitors.

Meals and activities. Make sure the food is wholesome, appealing, adequate, and suitable for older people. Find out what services and activities are included in the fee. You should ask if participation in activities is required, and what is done if a resident does not like the food or the activities. Finally, make sure there are creative and effectively planned social activities in addition to supervised daily exercise. ■

GLOSSARY

acetylcholine—A neurotransmitter crucial to memory and learning.

ADmark Assays—Two clinical tests for Alzheimer disease. One measures beta-amyloid and tau protein in the spinal fluid; the other tests for the apolipoprotein E ε4 genotype.

age-associated memory impairment—Normal forgetfulness that increases with age.

Alzheimer disease (AD)—A progressive disorder of the brain that is characterized by deterioration of mental faculties due to the loss of nerve cells and the connections between them. Also called Alzheimer's disease.

amnestic syndrome—Severe memory loss despite maintenance of normal intelligence.

amyloid plaques—Dense deposits of beta-amyloid, pieces of damaged nerve cells, and other proteins. Found in the brains of virtually all people with Alzheimer disease.

amyloid precursor protein—A protein that is split in two by enzymes to produce beta-amyloid.

aphasia—A partial or complete inability to use or understand language.

apolipoprotein E (APOE)—A gene on chromosome 19. The ε4 version of this gene is associated with an increased risk of Alzheimer disease.

beta-amyloid—A sticky, starch-like protein that is the main component of amyloid plaques.

bovine spongiform encephalopathy (BSE)—An infectious disease of cows with manifestations similar to Creutzfeldt-Jakob disease in humans. More commonly known as mad cow disease.

carotid endarterectomy—Surgical removal of a blockage of the carotid artery, the main artery leading from the aorta to the brain.

cerebellum—A fist-sized structure, located at the base of the brain beneath the cerebral cortex, that coordinates movement and balance.

cerebral cortex—The convoluted outer layer of gray matter that constitutes the "thinking" portion of the brain.

choline—A substance used by the body to produce acetylcholine. Present in food.

cholinesterase inhibitors—Medications that slow the breakdown of acetylcholine. Used in the treatment of Alzheimer disease.

colchicine—An anti-inflammatory drug commonly used to treat gout. Currently being tested as a treatment for Alzheimer disease.

complete blood cell count—Measures cellular elements of blood: red blood cells, white blood cells, and platelets. Helps rule out anemia, infections, and vitamin B_{12} deficiency as causes of dementia or factors that can exacerbate dementia.

computed tomography (CT)—An imaging technique that uses x-rays to create a two-dimensional image of the brain or other parts of the body.

Creutzfeldt-Jakob disease (CJD)—A rare, fatal brain disorder that causes a rapid, progressive dementia. Sometimes mistaken for Alzheimer disease.

Cushing disease—A disorder resulting from the overproduction of hormones by the adrenal gland. Also called Cushing's disease.

dementia—A significant intellectual decline or impairment that persists over time in several areas of thinking.

dementia with Lewy bodies—A type of dementia characterized by episodes of confusion, falls, and repetitive hallucinations, as well as signs of parkinsonism early in the disease.

frontotemporal dementia—A spectrum of disorders associated with impaired initiation of plans and goal setting, personality changes, language difficulties, and unawareness of any loss of mental function.

gray matter—The area of the brain, gray in appearance, that contains cell bodies (as opposed to white matter, which contains the nerve fibers that extend from the cell bodies).

hippocampus—A small, S-shaped structure in the brain that appears to play a major role in the process of forging memories.

Huntington disease—A rare, hereditary disorder of the central nervous system characterized by uncontrollable movements and dementia. Also called Huntington's disease.

incontinence—An inability to control urination or defecation.

lecithin—A substance used by the body to produce acetylcholine. Occurs naturally in food.

Lewy bodies—Abnormal structures that are found in cells throughout the brain in people with dementia with Lewy bodies.

long-term memory—Holds information that was learned as recently as a few minutes ago and as long ago as early childhood.

magnetic resonance imaging (MRI)—An imaging technique that uses a powerful magnet, rather than x-rays, to create a two-dimensional image of various areas of the body, including the brain.

microtubules—An internal transport system in nerve cells. Collapsed microtubules form neurofibrillary tangles.

mild cognitive impairment (MCI)—Forgetfulness that is more than normal for one's age but is not associated with certain cognitive problems common in dementia, such as disorientation or confusion. Severity falls between age-associated memory impairment and early dementia.

Mini-Mental State Examination—A test of mental status used to check for any basic cognitive impairment.

neurofibrillary tangles—Found in the brains of virtually all people with Alzheimer disease. Composed mainly of the protein tau. Appear as twisted, hairlike threads and remain after the collapse of the microtubules in the nerve cell.

neuron—Nerve cell.

neurotransmitter—A specialized chemical that relays messages between nerve cells.

nonsteroidal anti-inflammatory drugs (NSAIDs)—A class of drugs, commonly used to treat arthritis, which may be effective in the treatment and prevention of Alzheimer disease.

normal pressure hydrocephalus—A condition characterized by excess fluid in the brain that can result in dementia.

palilalia—Compulsive repetition of a word or phrase with increasing rapidity.

Parkinson disease—A progressive neurological disease characterized by tremors, stooped posture, slow movement, poor balance, and shuffling gait. Also called Parkinson's disease.

parkinsonism—The symptoms of Parkinson disease: tremors; rigid, stooped posture; slowness; and shuffling gait.

Pick disease—A type of frontotemporal dementia characterized by impaired initiation of plans and goal setting, personality changes, unawareness of any loss of mental function, and language difficulties. Also called Pick's disease.

piracetam—An alternative treatment to enhance memory that may improve the metabolism of acetylcholine.

prednisone—A steroid drug with powerful anti-inflammatory effects. Currently being tested as a treatment for Alzheimer disease.

presenilin-1 (PS-1)—A gene on chromosome 14. May be linked to Alzheimer disease.

presenilin-2 (PS-2)—A gene on chromosome 1. May be linked to Alzheimer disease.

prions—Unusual infectious agents that cause Creutzfeldt-Jakob disease.

selegiline—A medication used to treat Parkinson disease that is currently begin tested as a therapy for Alzheimer disease. It has antioxidant effects similar to vitamin E but is associated with more side effects.

short-term memory—Also known as working memory. Sometimes equated with consciousness.

Short Test of Mental Status—A test of mental status given to check for any basic cognitive impairment.

subdural hematoma—A collection of blood between the skull and the brain that can lead to memory problems and loss of consciousness.

vascular dementia—A disorder, often resulting from a series of tiny strokes in the brain, that can lead to dementia.

vasopressin—A hormone produced by the hypothalamus and used as an alternative treatment to enhance memory.

HEALTH INFORMATION ORGANIZATIONS AND SUPPORT GROUPS

Administration on Aging
330 Independence Ave. SW
Washington, DC 20201
☎ 202-619-7501
www.aoa.dhhs.gov

Advocacy agency that works to plan, coordinate, and develop programs for older Americans, such as providing good nutrition, transportation, and senior centers. Local chapters are listed in the government section of the phone book.

Alzheimer's Association
919 N. Michigan Ave., Ste. 1100
Chicago, IL 60611-1676
☎ 800-272-3900
312-335-8700
www.alz.org

Provides general information about Alzheimer disease and issues relevant to caregivers. Local chapters have support group resources and information on caregiving.

Alzheimer's Disease Education and Referral (ADEAR) Center
P.O. Box 8250
Silver Spring, MD 20907-8250
☎ 800-438-4380
www.alzheimers.org

Provides information on Alzheimer disease, including the latest research, new treatments, and referrals, for both health professionals and the general public.

American Stroke Association
7272 Greenville Ave.
Dallas, TX 75231
☎ 888-4-STROKE
800-553-6321 ("Warmline")
www.strokeassociation.org

A division of the American Heart Association; provides referrals to community stroke groups, and information and peer counseling to survivors and caregivers. Call the "Warmline" to subscribe to their magazine, *Stroke Connection.*

American Psychiatric Association
1400 K Street NW
Washington, DC 20005
☎ 888-357-7924
www.psych.org

Medical specialty society that provides clinical patient information about mental illnesses, medication, and psychiatric treatment. Information and brochures are available by contacting the organization's Division of Public Affairs.

National Institute of Mental Health
6001 Executive Blvd.
Rm. 8184, MSC 9663
Bethesda, MD 20892-9663
☎ 800-421-4211
301-443-4513
www.nimh.nih.gov

Dedicated to reducing the personal and economic costs of mental illness. Supports ongoing research on behavior and the brain, provides brochures, and sponsors related programs.

National Institute of Neurological Disorders and Stroke
P.O. Box 5801
Bethesda, MD 20824
☎ 800-352-9424
www.ninds.nih.gov

Leading supporter of neurological research in the United States. Provides list of clinical resource centers and voluntary health agencies.

National Mental Health Association
1021 Prince Street
Alexandria, VA 22314-2971
☎ 800-969-NMHA
703-684-7722
www.nmha.org

National organization dedicated to advocacy and education in all aspects of mental health. Provides books and videos, has branches in communities throughout the country, and offers referrals to local mental health providers.

LEADING HOSPITALS FOR NEUROLOGY AND NEUROSURGERY

U.S. News & World Report and the National Opinion Research Center, a social-science research group at the University of Chicago, recently conducted their 13th annual nationwide survey of 1,484 physicians in 17 medical specialties. The doctors nominated up to five hospitals they consider best from among 6,045 U.S. hospitals. This is the current list of the best neurology hospitals, as determined by the doctors' recommendations from 2000, 2001, and 2002; federal data on death rates; and factual data regarding quality indicators, such as the ratio of registered nurses to patients and the use of advanced technology. Since the results reflect the doctors' opinions, however, they are, to some degree, subjective. Any institution listed is considered a leading center, and the rankings do not imply that other hospitals cannot or do not deliver excellent care.

1. **Mayo Clinic**
   Rochester, Minnesota
   www.mayoclinic.org
   ☎ 507-284-2511

2. **Massachusetts General Hospital**
   Boston, Massachusetts
   www.mgh.harvard.edu
   ☎ 617-726-2000

3. **Johns Hopkins Hospital**
   Baltimore, Maryland
   www.hopkinsmedicine.org
   ☎ 410-955-5000/800-507-9952

4. **New York Presbyterian Hospital**
   New York, New York
   www.nyp.org
   ☎ 212-305-2500

5. **Cleveland Clinic**
   Cleveland, Ohio
   www.clevelandclinic.org
   ☎ 216-444-2200/800-223-2273

6. **UCSF Medical Center**
   San Francisco, California
   www.ucsfhealth.org
   ☎ 415-476-1000/888-689-UCSF

7. **Barnes-Jewish Hospital**
   St. Louis, Missouri
   www.barnesjewish.org
   ☎ 314-747-3000

8. **UCLA Medical Center**
   Los Angeles, California
   www.healthcare.ucla.edu
   ☎ 310-825-9111/800-825-2631

9. **University of Pennsylvania Medical Center**
   Philadelphia, Pennsylvania
   www.pennheath.com/upmc
   ☎ 215-662-4000/800-789-PENN

10. **Methodist Hospital**
    Houston, Texas
    www.methodisthealth.com
    ☎ 713-790-3333

GINKGO BILOBA

Americans spend upwards of $240 million each year on ginkgo biloba, the herbal supplement that—according to some marketing campaigns—can improve memory, concentration, and other aspects of cognition in healthy adults and those with cognitive impairment. However, the following clinical study, reprinted from the *Journal of the American Medical Association,* shows that the supplement does not improve memory or other cognitive functions in older people who are free from memory impairment.

In the research, Paul R. Solomon, Ph.D., and colleagues randomly assigned 230 people (age 60 and older) who did not have dementia to receive either ginkgo (the specific product used was Ginkoba) or a placebo. Ginkgo was taken according to the manufacturer's instructions: 40 mg three times daily with meals. Placebos were taken at the same intervals. The investigators evaluated 14 different measures of cognition.

After six weeks, no differences were found between the two groups on measures of memory, learning, attention, concentration, or naming and verbal fluency. The participants who received ginkgo did not rate their memory as being more improved than people who took the placebo, and spouses, family members, and friends noticed no differences in people who took ginkgo or the placebo.

"When taken following the manufacturer's instructions, [ginkgo] provides no measurable benefit in cognitive function to elderly adults with intact cognitive function," the study's authors write. However, the authors do note that a longer study period or higher doses of ginkgo could produce different outcomes.

While the study results provide clear evidence that ginkgo is not useful for improving memory in healthy adults, the research did not address whether the supplement benefits people with dementia. Some previous research has indicated that the supplement may cause small cognitive improvements in patients with dementia, but Dr. Solomon and his colleagues question whether these improvements (which tend to be much smaller than those achieved with cholinesterase inhibitors) have any significance.

Side effects of ginkgo were not addressed in this trial but can include bleeding, headache, and mild stomach discomfort.

Ginkgo for Memory Enhancement
A Randomized Controlled Trial

Paul R. Solomon, PhD
Felicity Adams, BA
Amanda Silver, BA
Jill Zimmer, BA
Richard DeVeaux, PhD

Context Several over-the-counter treatments are marketed as having the ability to improve memory, attention, and related cognitive functions in as little as 4 weeks. These claims, however, are generally not supported by well-controlled clinical studies.

Objective To evaluate whether ginkgo, an over-the-counter agent marketed as enhancing memory, improves memory in elderly adults as measured by objective neuropsychological tests and subjective ratings.

Design Six-week randomized, double-blind, placebo-controlled, parallel-group trial.

Setting and Participants Community-dwelling volunteer men (n=98) and women (n=132) older than 60 years with Mini-Mental State Examination scores greater than 26 and in generally good health were recruited by a US academic center via newspaper advertisements and enrolled over a 26-month period from July 1996 to September 1998.

Intervention Participants were randomly assigned to receive ginkgo, 40 mg 3 times per day (n=115), or matching placebo (n=115).

Main Outcome Measures Standardized neuropsychological tests of verbal and nonverbal learning and memory, attention and concentration, naming and expressive language, participant self-report on a memory questionnaire, and caregiver clinical global impression of change as completed by a companion.

Results Two hundred three participants (88%) completed the protocol. Analysis of the modified intent-to-treat population (all 219 participants returning for evaluation) indicated that there were no significant differences between treatment groups on any outcome measure. Analysis of the fully evaluable population (the 203 who complied with treatment and returned for evaluation) also indicated no significant differences for any outcome measure.

Conclusions The results of this 6-week study indicate that ginkgo did not facilitate performance on standard neuropsychological tests of learning, memory, attention, and concentration or naming and verbal fluency in elderly adults without cognitive impairment. The ginkgo group also did not differ from the control group in terms of self-reported memory function or global rating by spouses, friends, and relatives. These data suggest that when taken following the manufacturer's instructions, ginkgo provides no measurable benefit in memory or related cognitive function to adults with healthy cognitive function.

JAMA. 2002;288:835-840 www.jama.com

SOME OVER-THE-COUNTER TREATments are marketed as having the ability to improve memory, attention, and related cognitive functions. These claims are generally not supported by well-controlled clinical studies. Ginkoba claims to "enhance mental focus and improve memory and concentration."[1] Several published studies reported beneficial effects of ginkgo on cognition. These studies, however, either report cognitive improvement in only 1 of many memory tests administered[2,3] or report cognitive enhancement in cognitively impaired clinical populations such as patients with cerebrovascular or Alzheimer disease.[4,5] In contrast, advertising claims imply that the compound is broadly beneficial to those both with and without clinically significant cognitive impairments. Specific advertising claims cite more than 50 clinical trials that demonstrate benefit centered around concentration and memory. These studies were conducted for periods ranging from 14 days to 2 months. The manufacturer claims benefit with "at least 4 weeks of uninterrupted use."[6]

The purpose of the present study was to evaluate ginkgo in healthy elderly volunteers in a randomized, double-blind, placebo-controlled trial using standardized tests of memory, learning, attention and concentration, and expressive language as well as subjective ratings by participants and family.

METHODS
Participants

Following approval by the Williams College institutional review board, participants were recruited from newspaper advertisements that solicited individuals who would participate in a study designed to improve memory. An initial telephone interview was conducted to determine if the participant was likely to meet entry criteria for the study. Those who passed the screen provided informed consent and a medical history including current medications, neurologic or psychiatric

Author Affiliations: Department of Psychology (Dr Solomon and Ms Zimmer), Program in Neuroscience (Dr Solomon and Mss Adams, Silver, and Zimmer), Department of Mathematics and Statistics (Dr DeVeaux), Williams College, Williamstown, Mass; and The Memory Clinic, Southwestern Vermont Medical Center, Bennington (Dr Solomon).

Corresponding Author and Reprints: Paul R. Solomon, PhD, Bronfman Science Center, Williams College, 33 Hoxsey St, Williamstown, MA 01267 (e-mail: psolomon@williams.edu).

Figure 1. Study Flow Diagram

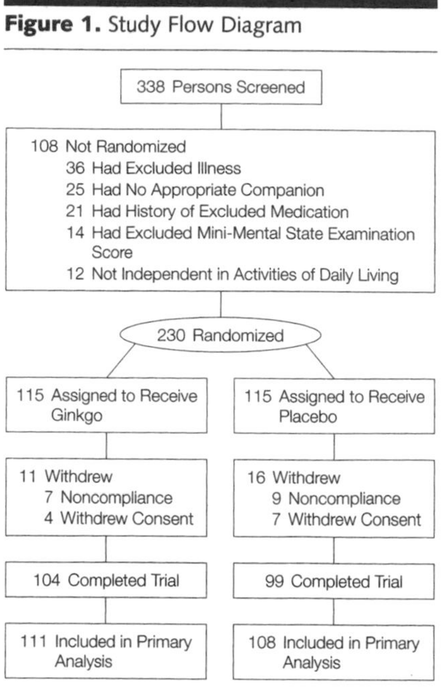

illness, and incidence of head trauma, stroke, mental illness, mental retardation, or life-threatening illness over the last 5 years. Participants were included in the study if they were community dwelling, older than 60 years, and could provide informed consent. They also needed to have a companion who had contact with them on a regular basis (>4 times per week for ≥1 hour) and was willing to complete a questionnaire. The baseline Mini-Mental State Examination[7] score was required to be greater than 26. All participants reported to be independent in instrumental activities of daily living including shopping, transportation, and managing finances. Participants were excluded if they had a history of psychiatric or neurologic disorder or had a life-threatening illness in the last 5 years. They were also excluded if they had taken antidepressant or other psychoactive medications in the past 60 days. A total of 338 community-dwelling participants were screened over a 26-month period from July 1996 to September 1998, and 230 participants (98 men and 132 women) aged 60 to 82 years were randomized in the study.

Study Design

A 6-week double-blind placebo-controlled study was conducted at a single site. FIGURE 1 summarizes the study participation. Participants were randomly assigned to 1 of 2 conditions: ginkgo (Ginkoba, Boehringer Ingelheim Pharmaceuticals)[1] or placebo control (1:1 ratio). Random assignment of participants to each condition was determined by 1 of the investigators (P.R.S.) using a table of random numbers.[8] Medication was placed in sealed envelopes by a research assistant and provided to the participants by 1 of 3 other investigators (F.A., A.S., J.Z.). Dosages for ginkgo were determined by following the manufacturer's label instructions: 1 tablet (40 mg) 3 times a day, with meals. The placebo group took lactose gelatin capsules of similar appearance and on the same schedule as the ginkgo group. At the beginning of the double-blind period, participants were provided with sealed and dated envelopes, each containing medication for 1 day.

One day prior to taking ginkgo or placebo and again at the end of the 6-week double-blind period (while still taking ginkgo and within 3 days of the end of the study), participants underwent neuropsychological evaluation including tests of learning, memory, attention and concentration, and expressive language. They also completed a questionnaire regarding subjective impressions of their memory. Additionally, at the end of the 6 weeks of treatment, the companion was asked to complete a global questionnaire designed to provide an overall impression of change in memory for the participant. Evaluators (F.A., A.S., J.Z.) were blinded to which randomized treatment the participants received.

Participants were contacted by telephone twice (at the end of weeks 2 and 4) during the 6-week period to evaluate compliance. They were excluded from the study if they missed 6 doses in any 2-week period or did not take 3 consecutive doses. At this time, they were asked to stop taking study medication. As an additional measure of compliance, participants were asked to return all dated envelopes at the end of the study.

Outcome Measures

Outcome measures consisted of the following standardized tests of learning, memory, attention and concentration, expressive language, and mental status. Tests of learning and memory included the California Verbal Learning Test (CVLT),[9] in which the participant is asked to learn a 16-item shopping list over 5 trials and then to later recall and subsequently recognize the information; the Logical Memory subscale of the Wechsler Memory Scale–Revised (WMS-R),[10] in which the participant is asked to recall paragraphs both immediately after hearing them and then after a 30-minute delay; and the Visual Reproduction subscale, in which the participant is asked to draw designs both immediately after seeing them and after a 30-minute delay.

Tests of attention and concentration included the Digit Symbol subscale of the Wechsler Adult Intelligence Scale–Revised (WAIS-R),[11] in which the participant must rapidly copy symbols that are paired with numbers; the Stroop Test,[12] which requires the participant not to be distracted by extraneous aspects of stimuli; the Digit Span (WMS-R), which requires the participant to repeat increasingly longer strings of numbers immediately after hearing them; and Mental Control (WMS-R), in which the participant must recite strings of numbers and letters.

Tests of expressive language included the Controlled Category Fluency test,[12] which requires the participant to name members of a particular category (animals) over a 1-minute period; and the Boston Naming Test,[13] which requires the participant to name pictures of items.

Additionally, the Memory Questionnaire[14] as well as a global evaluation completed by a spouse, relative, or friend with whom the patient had regular contact (at least 4 interactions per week) was completed. The Memory Questionnaire consisted of 27 questions that asked the participant to rate how often certain memory lapses occurred. The participant answered on a 4-point scale with descriptors used as anchors: 1 indicating very often, 2 indicating sometimes, 3 indicating rarely, and 4 indicating not at all. The global evaluation was based on the Caregiver Global Impression of Change rating scale.[15] Informants were asked to indicate the option that best described the change in memory over the preceding 6 weeks. The options included: (1) very much improved, (2) much improved, (3) minimally improved, (4) no change, (5) minimally worse, (6) much worse, or (7) very much worse.

All outcome measures, with the exception of the global evaluation, were administered at both the beginning and end of the study. The global evaluation was administered only at the end of the study. Participants who withdrew from the study, or who were dropped because of noncompliance, were asked to return at the end of the study for evaluation. Adverse events were not specifically monitored in this study. Patients who experienced an adverse event were instructed to discontinue study medication and to contact their primary care physician.

Statistical Methods

Analysis for efficacy was performed on 2 participant samples: the modified intent-to-treat primary analysis and the fully evaluable population. The modified intent-to-treat population included all participants who were randomized to treatment, underwent baseline analysis, received at least 1 dose of study drug, and returned for posttreatment evaluation. The fully evaluable population was defined as participants who completed 6 weeks of double-blind treatment and who complied with the standards for taking medication.

Differences in group means for all neuropsychological tests were assessed using both individual *t* tests and repeated-measures analysis of variance in which treatment condition served as the predictor and the cognitive tests served as the repeated measures. The test by condition-interaction term was then tested for statistical significance. Demographic variables were analyzed using the individual *t* tests. Categorical variables were analyzed using the χ^2 test. Results were considered statistically significant if differences reached the .05 level. Nonparametric analyses were used to assess the changes from baseline to week 6 for the Caregiver Global Impression of Change. We sought to detect differences of .05 SD with a power of 90% ($\alpha = .05$), requiring a sample size of 172 participants.[16] JMP version 5.0 (SAS Institute Inc, Cary, NC) statistical software was used for all analyses.

RESULTS

A total of 230 participants were enrolled in the study over a 26-month period, with 203 participants (88%) completing the study (Figure 1). The percentage of participants who completed the study did not differ significantly by treatment group. Of the 27 participants who did not complete the study, 16 (7 ginkgo and 9 placebo) did not comply with the medication dosage regimen and 11 (4 ginkgo and 7 placebo) withdrew consent. All participants were requested to return at the end of week 6 for evaluation.

Modified Intent-to-Treat Analysis

A total of 219 participants (111 ginkgo and 108 placebo) returned at the end of the 6-week period for reevaluation. This included the 203 participants who completed the protocol as well as 13 of 16 participants (6 ginkgo and 7 placebo) who were noncompliant and 3 of the 11 participants (2 ginkgo and 1 placebo) who withdrew consent. The remaining 11 participants (4 ginkgo and 7 placebo) did not return for evaluation and were excluded from the analysis. There were no significant differences between the ginkgo and placebo groups for any of the outcome measures. Neither demographic characteristics nor Mini-Mental State Examination scores varied as a function of treatment condition at baseline (TABLE 1).

There were no significant differences between the ginkgo and placebo groups on any of the objective neuropsychological tests. In general, participants performed better during their second evaluation than during their first, but there were no significant test-by-treatment condition interactions as tested by a repeated-measures analysis of variance ($F_{14,172}=0.099$, overall $P=.31$). Superior performance in all groups at the second testing session was likely due to a practice effect.

Table 1. Demographic Characteristics at Baseline of Participants Who Returned for Week 6 Evaluation (Modified Intent-to-Treat Analysis)

	Mean (SD)		
Characteristic	Ginkgo (n = 111)	Placebo (n = 108)	P Value
Age, y	68.7 (4.7)	69.9 (5.4)	.73
Men, No. (%)	46 (41)	45 (42)	.81
Education, y	14.4 (4.5)	14.0 (3.9)	.85
Mini-Mental State Examination score	28.7 (1.4)	28.8 (1.5)	.53

When tested by individual *t* tests, measures of attention and concentration, including the Digit Symbol subscale of the WAIS-R, the Stroop Test, and the Mental Control and Digit Span (forward and backward) subscales of the WMS-R, showed no significant differences between the ginkgo and placebo groups (TABLE 2 and FIGURE 2). Similarly, tests of verbal and nonverbal learning and memory, including the Logical Memory (I and II) and Visual Reproduction (I and II) subscales of the WMS-R, and the CVLT (initial acquisition, short and long delay, and recognition), also showed no significant differences between the ginkgo and placebo groups. There were no differences in tests of naming (Boston Naming Test) or verbal fluency (Controlled Category Fluency) between the ginkgo and placebo groups. Finally, self-report on the Memory Questionnaire was scored on a scale of 27 to 108 with higher scores indicating more difficulties. There was no difference in the mean reported scores for participants in the ginkgo and placebo groups ($P=.26$).

At the end of the second testing session, participants were asked if they thought they had been taking ginkgo or placebo. Self-report in the ginkgo group indicated that 79 participants (71%) thought they were takingT ginkgo, and self-report in the placebo group indicated that 81 participants (75%) thought they were taking ginkgo ($P=.49$). Informant response to the global rating indicated no difference between the ginkgo and placebo groups ($P=.76$). TABLE 3 shows the distribution of responses.

Figure 2 shows the 95% confidence intervals (CIs) for differences (treatment group minus control) for performance on each test in the modified intent-to-treat analysis. Each interval contains a zero, indicating that none of the differences are statistically significant. Moreover, 7 of the point estimates are positive (favoring ginkgo) and 7 are negative (favoring placebo).

Evaluable Participant Analysis

A total of 203 participants completed the protocol (fully evaluable population). There were no significant differences between the ginkgo and placebo groups for any outcome measure (Table 2).

COMMENT

The results of this 6-week study indicate that ginkgo, marketed over-the-counter as a memory enhancer, did not enhance performance on standard neuropsychological tests of learning, memory, naming and verbal fluency, or attention and concentration. Moreover, there were no differences between ginkgo participants and placebo controls on subjective self-report of memory function or on global rating by spouses, friends, and relatives. These data suggest that when taken following the manufacturer's instructions, this compound provides no measurable benefit in cognitive function to elderly adults with intact cognitive function.

In total, 14 different measures of cognition were evaluated in the present study. Seven of the measures were better in the placebo group, and 7 of the measures were better in the ginkgo group. None of the differences between the means of the 2 groups were statistically significant. The 95% CIs were calculated for each mean difference. Even if one assumes that the true difference between treatments is the up-

Table 2. Neuropsychological Test Results for Ginkgo vs Placebo*

		Modified Intent-to-Treat Analysis						Evaluable Participant Analysis	
		Mean Score at Baseline (SD)		Mean Score at Week 6 (SD)					
Test	Possible Range of Scores (Normative Scores [SD])†	Ginkgo	Placebo	Ginkgo	Placebo	Mean Difference Scores (95% CI of Difference)	*P* Value	Mean Difference Scores (95% CI of Difference)	*P* Value
Digit Symbol (WAIS-R)	0-90‡	46.7 (12.2)	47.8 (10.1)	47.1 (12.4)	47.6 (10.8)	0.65 (−1.45 to 2.76)	.54	0.60 (−1.59 to 2.80)	.59
Mental Control (WMS-R)	0-6 (5 [1])§	5.6 (0.7)	5.5 (0.6)	5.5 (0.6)	5.6 (0.6)	−0.16 (−0.40 to 0.07)	.16	−0.15 (−0.39 to 0.09)	.22
Digit Span (WMS-R)	0-24 (13 [3])§	16.3 (3.6)	15.7 (3.8)	17.2 (3.5)	17.1 (3.1)	−0.44 (−1.29 to 0.41)	.31	−0.43 (−1.31 to 0.45)	.33
Stroop Test (color/word)	0-112‡	58.7 (3.6)	61.1 (11.1)	63.8 (13.6)	63.1 (10.0)	1.51 (−1.12 to 4.14)	.24	0.88 (−1.41 to 3.17)	.33
Logical Memory I (WMS-R)	0-50 (21 [6])§	20.5 (5.1)	23.6 (4.7)	20.6 (5.2)	24.3 (5.5)	−0.53 (−1.71 to 0.65)	.38	−0.42 (−1.66 to 0.81)	.49
Logical Memory II (WMS-R)	0-50 (16 [7])§	16.2 (6.3)	20.3 (7.2)	17.1 (7.9)	22.3 (8.6)	−1.02 (−2.25 to 0.20)	.10	−0.99 (−2.26 to 0.28)	.12
Visual Reproduction I (WMS-R)	0-41 (28 [6])§	31.7 (5.8)	32.4 (5.3)	33.9 (4.6)	35.5 (3.8)	−0.96 (−2.27 to 0.35)	.15	−1.05 (−2.39 to 0.30)	.12
Visual Reproduction II (WMS-R)	0-41 (19 [10])§	21.5 (9.4)	27.5 (8.2)	31.0 (7.9)	31.8 (6.3)	0.19 (−1.52 to 1.90)	.83	0.26 (−1.52 to 2.05)	.77
CVLT (Trials 1-5)	0-80 (45 [9.3])	43.4 (11.5)	43.0 (11.7)	44.2 (11.7)	44.3 (11.8)	−0.58 (−1.90 to 0.74)	.39	−0.36 (−1.73 to 1.01)	.61
CVLT (Short Delay Recall)	0-16 (9 [2.5])	8.9 (2.8)	9.1 (2.9)	10.2 (3.3)	10.2 (3.1)	0.18 (−0.39 to 0.75)	.54	0.28 (−0.31 to 0.86)	.35
CVLT (Long Delay Recall)	0-16 (10 [2.8])	8.6 (3.0)	8.7 (3.1)	9.8 (3.9)	9.8 (3.6)	0.07 (−0.60 to 0.74)	.84	0.15 (−0.56 to 0.86)	.67
CVLT (Recognition Memory)	0-16 (14 [1.7])	13.4 (1.8)	13.4 (1.8)	14.2 (1.6)	14.2 (1.9)	0.03 (−0.40 to 0.47)	.88	−0.07 (−0.52 to 0.38)	.76
Controlled Category Fluency	0-? (17 [4.7])	18.5 (3.9)	19.3 (3.9)	19.4 (4.2)	20.4 (3.8)	−0.16 (−1.10 to 0.79)	.74	−0.14 (−1.13 to 0.86)	.79
Boston Naming Test	0-30‡	25.8 (2.4)	25.3 (2.7)	26.3 (2.5)	26.3 (2.3)	0.46 (−0.07 to 0.99)	.09	0.51 (−0.04 to 1.06)	.06
Memory Questionnaire	27-108‡	81.3 (12.4)	76.8 (12.0)	79.8 (14.7)	76.3 (12.5)	1.00 (−0.75 to 2.76)	.26	1.36 (−0.44 to 3.15)	.13

*CI indicates confidence interval; WAIS-R, Wechsler Adult Intelligence Scale–Revised; WMS-R, Wechsler Memory Scale–Revised; and CVLT, California Verbal Learning Test. Mean difference scores were difference of ginkgo (week 6 minus baseline) and placebo (week 6 minus baseline).
†Normative data are taken from Spreen and Strauss[12] and to the extent available based on age- and education-matched samples. Controlled Category Fluency has no end score due to participants providing as many names of animals as possible.
‡Appropriate age- and education-matched samples are not available for these tests.
§Normative data for the WMS are for an older sample than those used in the present study (range, 71-81 years; midpoint, 76).

per limit of the 95% CI, it would still be difficult to argue that meaningful benefit was derived from taking ginkgo. For example, the Logical Memory portion of the WMS-R measures the participants' ability to recall 2 paragraphs that they initially heard 30 minutes earlier. There are 25 possible discrete items in each paragraph that the participant could recall. The upper limit of the 95% CI for the mean difference between ginkgo and placebo was 0.20 items (ie, participants in the ginkgo group remembered less than 1 item more than participants in the placebo group). Similarly, on the CVLT, participants learn a 16-item shopping list over 5 trials. A perfect score is 80. The upper limit of the 95% CI for the mean difference between ginkgo and placebo was 1.01 items. It would be difficult to argue that either of these differences are of any clinical significance, even if they are real. The results of the Caregiver Global Impression of Change rating scale further support the failure of ginkgo to provide clinically significant improvement in memory. In general, caregivers did not rate changes in memory over the 6-week trial any differently in participants randomized to ginkgo vs placebo participants. Sixty-six percent of those randomized to placebo and 70% to ginkgo were judged by caregivers as showing no change over 6 weeks. Thirty-three percent of placebo and 28% of ginkgo participants were judged as minimally improved, and 3 participants were judged to be much improved; 2 were in the ginkgo group and 1 was in the placebo group (Table 3).

Ginkgo has been evaluated in several double-blind studies that have reported beneficial effects, but these effects were not broad or consistent. Wesnes et al[3] conducted a 3-month double-blind, randomized, placebo-controlled study in 54 patients. Patients were evaluated at weeks 4, 8, and 12. Patients receiving Tanakan (ginkgo extract) performed better on only 2 of 8 tests of memory ($P = .03$) and attention and concentration ($P = .05$) and in each case at only 1 evaluation point. There was not a consistent effect for any outcome measure. Additionally, neither physicians nor patients could distinguish between placebo and compound on an overall scale. Rai et al[2] compared 12 ginkgo-treated with 15 placebo-treated participants who were classified as having mild to moderate memory impairment in a double-blind study and reported significant differences in favor of the gingko group only on the Kendrick Digit Copying task, but not on tests of learning or memory. Rigney et al[17] evaluated 31 participants and 4 doses of ginkgo in a crossover design. They only reported improvement with 1 dose of ginkgo (120 mg), in only the oldest group of participants (50-59 years), and only in 1 of the multiple tests of memory administered. Other studies that have reported positive effects in favor of ginkgo have also either studied small numbers of participants in uncontrolled studies,[18,19] have found benefit in one of many cognitive tasks administered,[20] or have found changes in objective tests relative to controls but not in physician ratings in clinical populations.[4,5] Despite the manufacturer's claims of improved memory in healthy adults, we were unable to identify any well-controlled studies that document this claim.

Recently, ginkgo was reported to be beneficial in a sample of patients with dementia.[4] Mildly to severely demented patients characterized as having either Alzheimer disease or multi-infarct dementia were given either ginkgo (120 mg/d) or placebo for 52 weeks in a randomized double-blind study. The intent-to-treat analysis on 202 patients indicated a 0.1-point decline on the Alzheimer Disease Assessment Scale–Cognitive portion (ADAS-Cog) in the ginkgo group compared with a 1.48-point decline in the placebo group. No subjective differences were reported by either family members or physicians. While provocative, these differences on the ADAS-Cog are significantly smaller than those reported for approved cholinesterase inhibitors in treating patients with Alzheimer disease.[15] Moreover, the failure to find any differences in either physician or family rating raises the issue of whether the small difference on the ADAS-Cog is clinically significant.

Figure 2. Differences (Treatment Group Minus Control) for Performance on Each Test

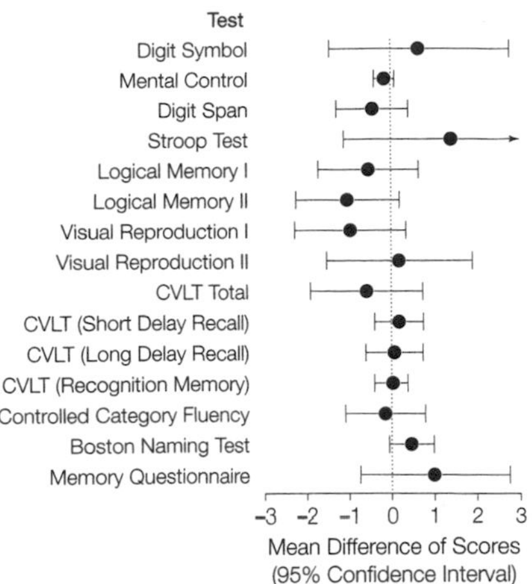

CVLT indicates California Verbal Learning Test. Data are based on the modified intent-to-treat analysis with 111 participants in the ginkgo group and 108 participants in the placebo group.

Table 3. Companion Response on the Caregiver Global Impression of Change Rating Scale*

Response	No. of Responses (%) Ginkgo (n = 110)	Placebo (n = 106)
1 – Very much improved	0 (0)	0 (0)
2 – Much improved	2 (2)	1 (1)
3 – Minimally improved	31 (28)	35 (33)
4 – No change	77 (70)	70 (66)
5 – Minimally worse	0 (0)	0 (0)
6 – Much worse	0 (0)	0 (0)
7 – Very much worse	0 (0)	0 (0)

*Two companions of participants in placebo group and 1 companion of participant in ginkgo group were not available at week 6 to complete the evaluation.

Despite the paucity of well-controlled studies, ginkgo continues to be marketed and widely used.[21,22] Sales in the United States reached $240 million in 1997[23] and more than 5 million prescriptions are written each year in Germany primarily for dementia, cerebral decline, and peripheral arterial insufficiency.[18]

Our study has limitations. It is certainly possible that higher doses or longer periods of exposure than used in this study are necessary to detect changes; however, we administered the compound following the manufacturer's instructions. The manufacturer's label indicates that ginkgo should be administered at a dose of 120 mg/d and that doses of greater than 120 mg show no additional benefit.[6] This is also the dose suggested by the German Commission E.[24] The daily dose in the present study was 120 mg/d. The label also states that a noticeable benefit should be apparent after 4 weeks of usage. The present study evaluated cognition after a 6-week interval. Moreover, there was no indication of a statistical trend toward significance for any of the compounds on any of the measures. Nevertheless, it is possible that longer exposures could produce beneficial effects.

We did not monitor adverse effects in the present study. Although ginkgo is generally characterized as a benign compound,[21] it is not without adverse effects. Reported adverse effects include bleeding, mild gastrointestinal upset, and headache.[25] None of the participants in the present study discontinued treatment due to adverse effects and none spontaneously reported any adverse effects. This finding is generally consistent with studies that did systematically monitor adverse effects.[4]

The issue of quality control has also been raised as a potential source of variance in studies using over-the-counter compounds.[26] One limitation of the present study is that we did not analyze the content of the ginkgo used in this study. However, the manufacturer claims that ginkgo "is processed under strict guidelines . . . ensured through extensive quality control."[6]

We recognize the possibility that ceiling effects may have contributed to the nonsignificant findings in the present study. However, we selected tests that are normalized for the age group that we studied and, as such, have an appropriate range of scores. For example, in the Logical Memory WMS-R scale (Logical Memory I), the potential range of scores is 0 to 50. The ginkgo participants in the present study scored a mean of 20.49 (SD, 5.08) and the placebo participants scored a mean of 23.61 (SD, 4.65). Each of these is well below the maximum score of 50. In addition, none of the participants obtained a maximum score on this scale or any of the other scales used in this study.

We also recognize that the method of blinding in this study could have resulted in unblinding for some participants. However, the finding that participants taking ginkgo as well as those taking placebo reported in equal proportions taking the active compound ginkgo (71% vs 75%) mitigates this concern.

In summary, this study does not support the manufacturer's claims of the benefits of gingko on learning and memory. Treatment over a 6-week period following the manufacturer's dosing suggestions did not produce objective benefit on any of 14 standard neuropsychological tests, nor were any benefits detected in self-report by the participants or observation by a family member or friend.

Author Contributions: *Study concept and design:* Solomon, Silver.
Acquisition of data: Solomon, Adams, Silver, Zimmer.
Analysis and interpretation of data: Solomon, DeVeaux.
Drafting of the manuscript: Solomon.
Critical revision of the manuscript for important intellectual content: Solomon, Adams, Silver, Zimmer, DeVeaux.
Statistical expertise: Solomon, DeVeaux.
Obtained funding: Solomon.
Administrative, technical, or material support: Adams, Silver, Zimmer.
Study supervision: Solomon.

Funding/Support: This work was supported by grants from the National Institute on Aging (AGO-5134-08S2), the Howard Hughes Medical Foundation, and the Essel Foundation.

REFERENCES

1. Ginkoba [package insert]. Ridgefield, Conn: Pharmatron Division of Boehringer Ingelheim Pharmaceuticals; 1997.
2. Rai GS, Shovlin C, Wesnes KA. A double-blind placebo controlled study of *Ginkgo biloba* extract (Tanakan) in elderly patients with mild to moderate memory impairment. *Curr Med Res Opin*. 1991;12:350-355.
3. Wesnes IL, Simmons D, Rook M, et al. A double-blind placebo-controlled trial of Tanaken in the treatment of idiopathic cognitive impairment in the elderly. *Hum Psychopharmacol*. 1987;2:159.
4. LeBars PL, Katz MM, Berman N, et al. A placebo-controlled, double-blind, randomized trial of an extract of *Ginkgo biloba* for dementia. *JAMA*. 1997;278:1327-1332.
5. Taillandier J, Ammar A, Rabourdin JP, et al. Treatment of cerebral aging disorders with *Ginkgo biloba* extract. *Presse Med*. 1986;15:1583-1587.
6. Ginkoba Product Information. Available at: http://www.ginkoba.com. Accessed January 23, 2002.
7. Folstein MF, Folstein SE, McHugh PR. Mini-mental state: a practical method for grading the cognitive state of patients for the clinician. *J Psychiatr Res*. 1975;12:189-198.
8. Games PA, Klare GR. *Elementary Statistics for the Behavioral Sciences*. New York, NY: McGraw-Hill Inc; 1967.
9. Delis DC, Kramer JH, Kaplan E, and Ober BA. *California Verbal Learning Test, Adult Version*. New York, NY: Psychological Corp; 1987.
10. Wechsler DA. *The Wechsler Memory Scale–Revised*. New York, NY: Psychological Corp; 1987.
11. Wechsler DA. *The Wechsler Adult Intelligence Scale–Revised*. New York, NY: Psychological Corp; 1981.
12. Spreen O, Strauss E. *A Compendium of Neuropsychological Tests*. New York, NY: Oxford University Press; 1998.
13. Kaplan EF, Goodglass H, Weintraub S. *The Boston Naming Test*. Philadelphia, Pa: Lea & Fibiger; 1983.
14. Baddeley A. *Your Memory: A User's Guide*. New York, NY: MacMillan Publication Co, Inc; 1982.
15. Knapp MJ, Knopman DS, Solomon PR, et al, for the Tacrine Study Group. A 30-week randomized controlled trial of high-dose tacrine in patients with Alzheimer disease. *JAMA*. 1994;271:985-991.
16. Shua-Haim JR, Comsti E, Gross JS. Aging-associated cognitive decline. *Clin Geriatr Med*. 1997;5:50-60.
17. Rigney S, Kimber S, Hindmarch I. The effect of acute doses of standardized *Ginkgo biloba* extract on memory and psychomotor performance in volunteers. *Psychother Res*. 1999;13:408-415.
18. Allain H, Raoul P, Lieury A, et al. Effect of two doses of *Ginkgo biloba* extract (Egb 761) on the dual-coding test in elderly subjects. *Clin Ther*. 1993;15:549-558.
19. Hindmarch I. Activity of *Ginkgo biloba* on short-term memory. *Presse Med*. 1988;15:1592-1594.
20. Warot D, Lacomblez L, Danjou E, et al. Comparaison des effets de'extraits de *Ginkgo biloba* sur les performances psychomotices et la memoire chez le sujet sain. *Therapie*. 1991;46:33-36.
21. Barrett B, Kiefer D, Rabago D. Assessing the risks and benefits of herbal medicine: an overview of scientific evidence. *Altern Ther Health Med*. 1999;5:40-49.
22. Winocur MZ. *Ginkgo biloba* for dementia: a reasonable alternative. *Psychiatr Pharm*. 1999;39:308-309.
23. Canedy D. Real medicine or medicine show? growth of herbal sales raises issues about value. *New York Times*. July 23, 1998:C1.
24. Blumenthal M, Busse WR, Goldberg A, et al, eds. *The Complete German Commission E Monographs: Therapeutic Guide to Herbal Medicines*. Austin, Tex: American Botanical Council; 1998:136-138.
25. Cupp MJ. Herbal remedies: adverse effects and drug interactions. *Am Fam Physician*. 1999;59:1239-1244.
26. O'Hara M, Kiefer D, Farrell K, et al. A review of 12 commonly used medicinal herbs. *Arch Fam Med*. 1998;7:523-536.

NOTES

NOTES

NOTES

NOTES

NOTES

NOTES

NOTES

NOTES

NOTES

NOTES

NOTES

ISBN 0-929661-37-0
ISSN 1542-1708
Seventh Printing
Printed in the United States of America

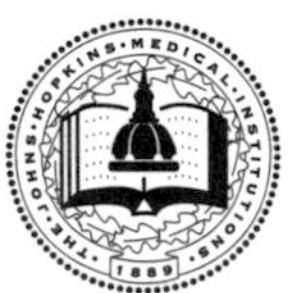

The Johns Hopkins White Papers are published yearly by Medletter Associates, Inc.

Rodney Friedman	Publisher
Devon Schuyler	Executive Editor
Catherine Richter	Senior Editor
Paul Candon	Senior Writer
Kimberly Flynn	Writer/Researcher
Liz Curry	Editorial Associate
Abigail Williams	Intern
Leslie Maltese-McGill	Copy Editor
Bonnie Slotnick	Copy Editor
Scott Hunt	Design Production Manager
Robert Duckwall	Medical Illustrator
Tom Damrauer, M.L.S.	Chief of Information Services
Barbara Maxwell O'Neill	Associate Publisher
Helen Mullen	Circulation Director
Tim O'Brien	Circulation Director
Jerry Loo	Product Manager
Darren Leiser	Promotions Coordinator
Joan Mullally	Head of Business Development

NUTRITION AND WEIGHT CONTROL FOR LONGEVITY

Lora Brown Wilder, Sc.D., M.S., R.D.,

Lawrence J. Cheskin, M.D.,

and

Simeon Margolis, M.D., Ph.D.

2 0 0 3

NUTRITION AND WEIGHT CONTROL FOR LONGEVITY

A healthy diet provides the energy, vitamins, and minerals that the body needs to function properly. In addition, a healthy diet can help to maintain a proper weight. There has been an alarming increase in obesity in the United States. The U.S. Surgeon General and numerous health organizations have initiated a widespread effort to promote awareness among citizens and to alert health professionals to the significant health consequences of this burgeoning epidemic. In this year's White Paper, we discuss how eating well and controlling weight may help prevent disease and prolong life.

■ ■ ■

Highlights:

■ ■ ■

THE AUTHORS

Lora Brown Wilder, Sc.D., M.S., R.D., a registered dietitian, received her M.S. in nutrition from the University of Maryland and her Sc.D. in public health from Johns Hopkins University. She is currently an assistant professor at the Johns Hopkins School of Medicine and is also affiliated with the United States Department of Agriculture and the University of Maryland's Department of Nutrition and Food Science. Dr. Wilder has served on various advisory committees related to nutrition, including committees at the American Heart Association and the National Institutes of Health, and helped set up the first Johns Hopkins Preventive Cardiology Program. In her research, Dr. Wilder has studied the effects of coffee on fatty acids and investigated behavioral strategies to reduce coronary risk factors. Her current research is in the area of dietary assessment methodology. She contributed to *Nutritional Management: The Johns Hopkins Handbook* and has been published in *Circulation*, *American Journal of Medicine*, and *Journal of the American Medical Association.*

▪ ▪ ▪

Lawrence J. Cheskin, M.D., graduated from Dartmouth Medical School and completed a fellowship in gastroenterology at Yale-New Haven Hospital. Currently, he is an associate professor of international health and human nutrition at the Johns Hopkins Bloomberg School of Public Health and an associate professor of medicine at the Johns Hopkins School of Medicine. Dr. Cheskin is also the director of the Johns Hopkins Weight Management Center. In his research, Dr. Cheskin has studied the effects of medications on body weight, the gastrointestinal effects of olestra, how cigarette smoking relates to dieting and body weight, and the effectiveness of lifestyle changes in weight loss and weight maintenance. He is also the author of three books: *Losing Weight for Good*, *New Hope for People with Weight Problems*, and *Better Homes and Gardens' 3 Steps to Weight Loss.* Dr. Cheskin has appeared on television news programs and delivered lectures to both professional and lay audiences on the topics of weight loss and weight management.

▪ ▪ ▪

Simeon Margolis, M.D., Ph.D., received his B.A., M.D., and Ph.D. from the Johns Hopkins University School of Medicine and performed his internship and residency at Johns Hopkins Hospital. He is currently a professor of medicine and biological chemistry at the Johns Hopkins University School of Medicine and medical editor of *The Johns Hopkins Medical Letter, Health After 50.* He has served on various committees for the Department of Health, Education and Welfare, including the National Diabetes Advisory Board and the Arteriosclerosis Specialized Centers of Research Review Committees. In addition, he has been a member of the Endocrinology and Metabolism Panel of the United States Food and Drug Administration.

CONTENTS

NUTRITION AND WEIGHT CONTROL FOR LONGEVITY

Eating right will help you maintain a healthy weight and may protect you against a variety of chronic diseases, including coronary heart disease (CHD), cancer, diabetes, and osteoporosis. Most people recognize the importance of a healthy diet, and yet they do not always follow one: Two-thirds of Americans eat more than the recommended amount of total and saturated fat, according to a U.S. Department of Agriculture (USDA) survey. Moreover, the National Cancer Institute found that only 23% of the population meets the minimum recommendation of five servings of fruits and vegetables a day.

People cite a multitude of obstacles to practicing good nutrition: time constraints, the ready availability of packaged and processed foods; the perception that they will have to give up their favorite foods; and confusion over conflicting information on nutrition and weight loss. And many people harbor the misguided belief that dietary changes made late in life are of little consequence. In fact, changing dietary habits and losing weight in middle or even old age can significantly influence health. This White Paper addresses these concerns, and counters them with simple, effective strategies for achieving good nutrition and, in particular, keeping your weight under control.

Nutrition

This section of the White Paper gives an overview of nutrition principles and specific recommendations—based on research studies—for the intake of various nutrients.

THE BASICS OF NUTRITION

Food provides not only the energy we need to function but also the nutrients required to build all tissues (such as bone, muscle, fat, and blood) and to produce substances used for the chemical processes that take place in our bodies millions of times a day. There are two broad categories of nutrients: macronutrients (carbohydrates, protein, and fats), which supply energy and are needed in large amounts to maintain and repair body structures, and micronutrients, the vitamins and minerals required in small amounts to help regulate chemical processes. Fiber, technically not a nutrient, is also part of a healthy diet.

Calories (technically called kilocalories) are the measure of the amount of energy in a food. One calorie represents the amount of heat needed to raise the temperature of one liter of water by 1° Celsius. Carbohydrates and protein contain four calories per gram; fat contains nine calories per gram; alcohol contains seven calories per gram.

Carbohydrates are starches and sugars obtained from plants. Sugars are known as simple carbohydrates and starches as complex carbohydrates. All carbohydrates are broken down in the intestine and converted in the liver into glucose, a sugar that is carried through the bloodstream to the cells, where it is used for energy. Some glucose is converted into glycogen, which is stored in limited amounts in the liver and muscles for future use. Carbohydrates are converted into fat when intake exceeds immediate needs and glycogen storage capabilities.

Proteins are nitrogen-containing substances that make up muscles, bones, cartilage, skin, antibodies, some hormones, and all enzymes. The proteins in foods are broken down in the intestine into amino acids, the building blocks for body proteins. The body can manufacture 13 of the 22 amino acids present in proteins; these 13 are called nonessential amino acids because they need not be obtained from the diet. The other nine are known as essential amino acids because they must be supplied by food.

Vitamins are organic substances (meaning that they contain carbon) needed to regulate metabolic functions within cells. Vitamins do not supply energy, but one of their functions is to aid in the conversion of macronutrients into energy. Fat-soluble vitamins (A, D, K, and E) are stored in the body for long periods, whereas water-soluble vitamins (the B vitamins and vitamin C) can only be stored for a short time (although vitamin B_{12} is stored for longer periods). See the chart on pages 14–15 for the functions of the individual vitamins.

Minerals are inorganic substances that serve many functions, including helping to maintain water content and acid–base balance (pH) in the body. Macrominerals (calcium, phosphorus, chloride, sodium, magnesium, potassium, and sulfur) are present in the body in large amounts. Microminerals, though no less important, are present in smaller amounts. The most important minerals and their functions are listed in the chart on pages 18–19.

Fiber is present in fruits, vegetables, grains, and legumes. Supplying no nutrients or calories, fiber is not digestible; but it is valuable in helping speed foods through the digestive system and possibly binding toxins and diluting their concentration in the intestine.

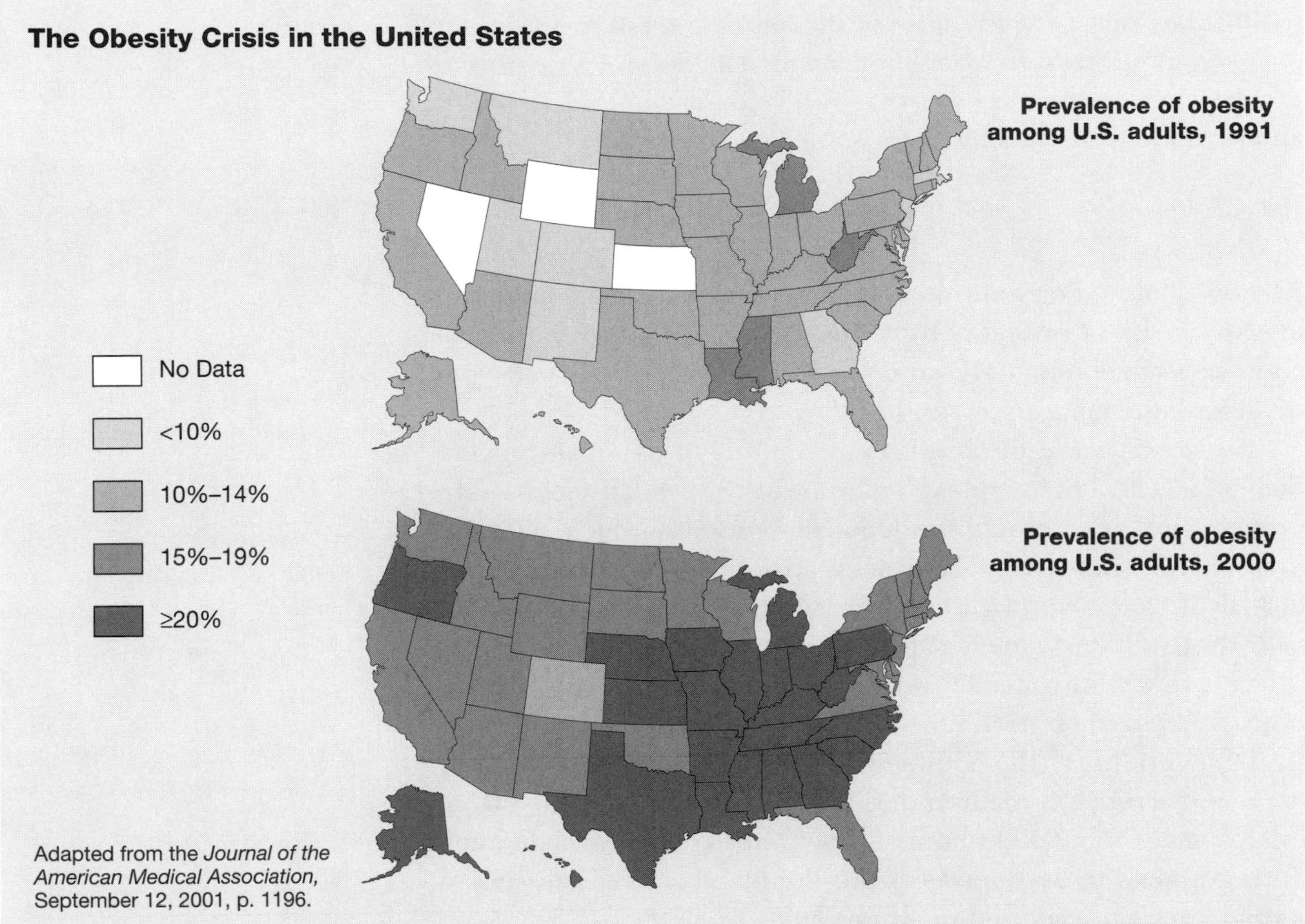

Adapted from the *Journal of the American Medical Association*, September 12, 2001, p. 1196.

One of the greatest health threats facing adults in the United States today is the skyrocketing increase in overweight and obesity. Recent research shows that about two thirds of Americans are either overweight or obese. Since 1980, obesity has doubled among adults in the United States. Overweight and obesity are linked with an increased risk of life-threatening conditions, such as type 2 diabetes, stroke, and coronary heart disease. In addition, obesity can lead to mental anguish due to poor body image, social isolation, and social discrimination. Current research indicates that approximately 300,000 deaths a year in the United States may be attributed to obesity.

Some types of fiber also help to control blood sugar and blood cholesterol levels. See page 53 for information on fiber and weight control.

Water is an essential nutrient because it is involved in all body processes. Since an individual's water needs vary with diet, physical activity, environmental temperature, and other factors, it is difficult to pin down an exact water requirement.

Cholesterol is a waxy, fat-like substance that is produced mainly in the liver, but can also be made by all cells in the body except red blood cells. The liver can produce all the cholesterol the body needs, but cholesterol is also found in all animal products that you eat, such as meats, poultry, fish, eggs, butter, cheese and milk (plant foods have none). For transport in the blood, cholesterol associates with certain proteins to form lipoproteins. Cholesterol is present in the membranes of all cells, acts as insulation around nerve fibers, and serves as a building block for some hormones.

FAT

By now, almost everyone is aware that reducing dietary fat can lessen the risk of several chronic diseases. While a high fat intake contributes to obesity, CHD, and some forms of cancer, not all types of fat have the same effects on health.

Triglycerides are the most abundant fats in foods and in the body's fat cells. Triglycerides contain three types of fatty acids— saturated, monounsaturated, and polyunsaturated—which differ in their chemical structures. Fatty acids are made up of chains of carbon, hydrogen, and oxygen that vary in length and in the number of hydrogen atoms attached to the carbon atoms. The degree to which a fatty acid is loaded with hydrogen determines its "saturation" and impact on health.

Triglycerides are the body's main source of stored energy. They are manufactured in the liver and fat cells as well as obtained from food. It takes about eight hours for all of the triglycerides ingested during a meal to be removed from the blood where, like cholesterol, they are transported on lipoproteins.

Triglycerides consist of any combination of fatty acids. As a result, no food contains just one type of fatty acid. Instead, the fat in a particular food is classified as saturated or unsaturated based on the type of fatty acid that predominates. For example, olive oil is typically thought of as a monounsaturated fat, but it also contains some polyunsaturated and saturated fat: 75% of the oil is monounsaturated, 14% is saturated, and 9% is polyunsaturated. (The percentages do not add up to 100% because other fat-like substances are also present in the oils.)

Fatty acids serve crucial functions in the body: They are required for the membranes of cells, keep skin and hair healthy, and form triglycerides that provide a layer of insulation under the skin. Since the body cannot manufacture them, certain fatty acids must be obtained from foods and are therefore called essential fatty acids. They are required components of cell membranes and can be converted to important hormone-like substances. In addition, dietary fat is needed to help the intestine absorb the fat-soluble vitamins A, D, and E.

Saturated fatty acids carry all the hydrogen atoms that their carbon chains can hold. Saturated fats are solid at room temperature and are found in abundance in animal products, such as meats, cheese, milk, and butter. Tropical oils—palm, palm kernel, and coconut—are also saturated. Saturated fats raise blood cholesterol levels and possibly contribute to certain forms of cancer.

Monounsaturated fatty acids are missing one pair of hydrogen atoms. As a result, two neighboring carbon atoms form what is known chemically as a double bond. The "mono" in monounsaturated indicates that these fatty acids have just one double bond. Liquid at room temperature, they predominate in foods such as olive oil, canola oil, almonds, and avocados. Cholesterol levels drop when monounsaturated fats replace saturated fats in the diet. Researchers discovered the value of monounsaturated oil in part by studying the Mediterranean diet, which is associated with low rates of CHD, and possibly cancer, despite a relatively high total fat intake. Olive oil is the main source of fat in that diet. The Mediterranean diet is also high in fruit, vegetables and grains, and its relatively low content of animal foods may also account for its heart-healthy effects.

Polyunsaturated fatty acids have two or more ("poly," meaning many) double bonds . Also liquid at room temperature, polyunsaturated fats make up the majority of the fatty acids in safflower, sunflower, and corn oils; fish; and some nuts, such as walnuts. Most of the polyunsaturated fats in vegetable fats are called omega-6 fatty acids because the last of the double bonds is located at the sixth carbon atom in the fatty acid chain.

Fish contains both omega-3 and omega-6 fatty acids. All polyunsaturated fats lower blood cholesterol levels when substituted for saturated fats in the diet. Researchers believe that two specific omega-3 fatty acids, eicosapentaenoic acid (EPA) and docosahexaenoic acid (DHA)—found primarily in seafood—may help reduce blood pressure and prevent cardiac arrhythmias (abnormal heart rhythms). Small amounts of omega-3 fatty acids are also found in vegetable sources such as walnuts and soy, canola, and flaxseed oils. While they appear to have some of the benefits of omega-3 fatty acids in fish, more research is required to determine their benefits.

Dietary Fat and Coronary Heart Disease

A diet high in saturated fats increases CHD risk by raising blood cholesterol levels. Body cells use fat as an energy source and need cholesterol as a component of their membranes. Because fat is not

NEW RESEARCH

Soy Foods and Cardiovascular Disease

Replacing animal foods with soy foods reduces the risk of coronary heart disease (CHD), according to recent findings. This appears to be true whether the soy foods are high or low in isoflavones.

Researchers evaluated 41 moderately overweight adults with elevated cholesterol who for a period of one month followed one of three diets: a control diet rich in dairy foods, a soy food diet low in isoflavones (52 g soy protein and 10 mg isoflavones), and a soy food diet high in isoflavones (50 g soy protein and 73 mg isoflavones). Protein sources were low-fat dairy foods and egg substitutes in the control diet and store-bought soy foods, including soymilk and soy burgers, in the soy diets. All three diets were equally low in saturated fat (<5% of calories) and cholesterol.

Compared with the control diet, both soy diets resulted in similar improvements in systolic blood pressure (in men only) and cholesterol levels. Total cholesterol fell by 7% and LDL cholesterol by 8% on the soy diets. Based on these improvements, the risk of CHD was estimated to be 10% lower on the soy diets than on the control diet.

The findings indicate that a variety of soy foods, when substituted for animal protein and in the context of a low-saturated fat, low-cholesterol diet, confer cardiovascular benefits.

AMERICAN JOURNAL OF CLINICAL NUTRITION
Volume 76, page 365
August 1, 2002

An Overview of Fish: The Benefits and the Risks

Seafood is an excellent source of nutrients, including lean protein, vitamins, and minerals. In addition, certain types of fish provide an abundance of beneficial fats called omega-3 fatty acids. While all types of fish contain varying amounts of omega-3 fatty acids, cold-water fatty fish such as salmon, mackerel, albacore tuna, herring, sardines, and lake trout are the most concentrated dietary sources of omega-3 fatty acids. Though there are concerns about certain contaminants in fish, health professionals report that most people can safely eat fish as part of a healthful diet.

Health Benefits of Fish

A growing body of research shows that omega-3 fatty acids may reduce the risk of coronary heart disease (CHD) and certain inflammatory and autoimmune disorders. The cardiovascular benefits attributed to omega-3 fatty acids include protection against sudden cardiac arrest and irregular heart rhythms as well as making blood platelets less sticky, and thus less likely to form blood clots that can cause heart attacks. Furthermore, omega-3 fatty acids can also help lower triglyceride levels and decrease blood pressure slightly in people with hypertension.

What the Studies Show

To date, most studies on the health benefits of fish consumption have been conducted on men, but results from a recent study indicate that heart disease risk is also lower in women who eat fish regularly. As part of a 16-year follow-up of 84,688 women participating in the Nurses' Health Study, investigators noted that fish consumption was associated with a significantly reduced incidence of major CHD events in women. In another recent study, men with no prior cardiovascular disease who consumed a diet rich in fatty fish had a significantly reduced risk of sudden death from CHD.

Current Recommendation

Although the government has not released dietary recommendations for omega-3 fatty acids, the American Heart Association has acknowledged their importance and recommends that Americans consume fatty fish twice a week to benefit from their cardioprotective effects. As part of a balanced diet, fish provide nutritional benefits for healthy people as well as those with CHD.

Fish Oil Supplements

Until more research is conducted on the benefits and risks of fish oil supplements, the American Heart Association does not recommended them as a substitute for fish or as a dietary supplement. In addition, because the U.S. Food and Drug Administration (FDA) does not regulate dosage levels or ingredients used in supplements, it is difficult to know if a supplement contains the levels of an ingredient listed on its label. In fact, recent tests on fish oil capsules showed that a number of brands had far less omega-3 fatty acids than was claimed on the labels.

Contaminants in Fish

While fish supply heart-healthy fats, some types of fish may also harbor toxins such as polychlorinated biphenyls (PCBs) and mercury.

PCBs. Animal studies have shown that PCBs may have adverse effects on the liver, blood, and skin, as well as on the gastrointestinal, nervous, immune, and reproductive systems. Furthermore, the U.S. Environmental Protection Agency (EPA) has classified PCBs as a probable human carcinogen.

Although PCBs have been banned in the United States since 1979, they are nonetheless widely distributed from past use and are highly persistent since they remain present in the environment for a long period of time. Once released into rivers, lakes, and streams, these toxins are introduced into the food chain where they accumulate. In fact, aquatic organisms can contain between 2,000 and 1 million times greater concentrations of

soluble in the watery environment of the bloodstream, the liver wraps the cholesterol and triglycerides in a layer of proteins to transport the fats through the blood. These packages form the three main types of lipoproteins described below.

Very low density lipoprotein (VLDL) carries triglycerides from the liver to other cells. As the triglycerides are removed from VLDL, they are converted into smaller, cholesterol-rich particles, called low density lipoproteins (LDL). Often referred to as "bad" cholesterol, LDL is first oxidized before it is taken up by cells in the arter-

PCBs than that found in the surrounding water, and species at the top of the food chain have the highest concentrations.

According to recent EPA reports, as of 1998, 37 states had released 679 fish advisories informing the public that high concentrations of PCBs had been identified in local fish. To decrease PCB exposure, the EPA suggests removing the internal organs and skin and trimming the fat from fish before cooking. Visit the EPA's Web site at www.epa.gov/OST for more information about PCBs.

Mercury. Bacteria in fresh and salt water convert mercury into methylmercury, a toxin that accumulates in fish. While most fish contain harmless, trace amounts of methylmercury, some larger fish that feed on algae and other fish can accumulate high levels of methylmercury in their tissues. The EPA and the FDA are responsible for regulating and monitoring the safety of seafood. The FDA has issued an advisory indicating that women who are pregnant or are considering becoming pregnant, women who are nursing, and young children should not eat shark, swordfish, king mackerel, or tilefish. High levels of methylmercury in these fish could cause neurological defects or delay mental development in the unborn fetus. Although tuna is not included on the list, there is some concern that it may also contain harmful levels of methylmercury. Nonetheless, the FDA emphasizes that seafood can be an important part of a balanced diet for pregnant women, who can safely eat other kinds of fish. To avoid the risks of methylmercury toxicity while reaping the nutritional benefits of fish, it is prudent to eat a variety of fish and seafood rather than concentrating on one species. For more information about the risks of methylmercury in seafood, visit the FDA's Food Safety Web site at www.cfsan.fda.gov or call toll-free 888-723-3366.

Tips for Buying and Cooking Fish

It is always important to purchase fish from a reputable commercial source. At the supermarket, check the "sell by" or "use by" date, and don't buy fish if the date has expired. Try to make seafood one of your last purchases when buying from a supermarket, and always keep it cold. Place seafood on ice, in the refrigerator or in the freezer, immediately after buying it.

To avoid cross-contamination, never purchase cooked seafood products that are in direct contact with raw seafood products in the display case of your market. Do not purchase frozen seafood if the package is open, torn, or crushed on the edges. If the fish has a strong, ammonia-like or fishy odor or if the flesh does not spring back when pressed, then it is probably not fresh. With whole fish, the eyes should not be cloudy but should be bright and clear and bulging a little. The scales should cling tightly to the skin and the gills should be bright pink or red and free from slime.

Fish needs to be cooked properly (particularly for people who have a compromised immune system), because bacteria and parasites are sometimes naturally present on seafood. To prevent foodborne illness from improperly cooked fish, the U.S. Food and Drug Administration recommends cooking most seafood to an internal temperature of 145° F (63° C) for 15 seconds. If you do not have a meat thermometer, you can check for the doneness of fish in a number of ways. When you think the fish might be done, follow these steps:

- Slide the point of a sharp knife into the flesh; it should slide in easily without resistance.
- Pull the flesh apart slightly to see if the center is at all translucent. If it is, cook the fish for another three to four minutes.
- When the fish is done, it will be opaque throughout (but still moist looking), and the flesh will separate easily into "flakes."

ial walls, where it initiates a series of changes that result in the formation of atherosclerotic plaques. These plaques can eventually hinder blood flow in arteries throughout the body. The formation of a blood clot on the plaques can halt blood flow altogether: Blockage of an artery supplying the heart causes a heart attack, while a blockage in an artery leading to the brain leads to a stroke.

The third type of lipoprotein is called high density lipoprotein (HDL). As it travels through the bloodstream, HDL helps reduce the buildup of arterial plaque by removing cholesterol from arterial walls and returning it to the liver for disposal. For this reason, HDL cholesterol is often called "good" cholesterol.

Measures to prevent the formation of plaques include reducing blood levels of triglycerides and LDL cholesterol while raising HDL cholesterol. The different types of fatty acids in foods have varying effects on the levels of LDL and HDL cholesterol. Saturated fatty acids increase levels of LDL cholesterol, while diets low in saturated fats reduce LDL levels. Although not everyone responds to the same degree, on average, every 1% reduction in saturated fat calories reduces total blood cholesterol levels by about 2 mg/dL, mostly from a drop in LDL cholesterol. Saturated fats raise LDL levels by reducing LDL's removal from the blood by the liver. Polyunsaturated fats overcome this effect by reducing the amount of saturated fat in the diet.

Blood cholesterol levels are also raised by dietary cholesterol, but not as much as by saturated fat. A few foods—eggs, lobster, and shrimp—are especially high in dietary cholesterol.

Another type of fatty acid, trans fats, is formed when food manufacturers add hydrogen atoms to unsaturated fats to make them more saturated and therefore more solid and shelf-stable. The American Heart Association recommends cutting down on trans fats, which are used in many packaged cookies, crackers, and other baked goods; commercially prepared fried foods; and most margarines. Studies suggest that trans fats are even more harmful to health than saturated fats because trans fats not only raise LDL cholesterol, but also lower HDL cholesterol levels more than saturated fats. Elevated levels of blood triglycerides, which are especially common in people with diabetes, may also increase CHD risk.

Eating fish is associated with a reduced risk of CHD. This benefit may be due to special effects of the omega-3 fatty acids found in fish or may simply reflect the fact that many people who eat fish tend to eat less red meat. Data from a recent study strongly suggest that omega-3 fatty acids may be beneficial for the heart. In a study reported in *The New England Journal of Medicine,* blood samples from 94 men who had a heart attack were analyzed and compared with those of 184 men of similar age and smoking status who did not have a heart attack. When blood levels of omega-3 fatty acids were higher, risk for a first or second heart attack declined in both groups. It should be noted, however, that fish oils in capsule form do not lower blood cholesterol levels, although these supplements can reduce triglycerides in people with very high triglyceride levels.

NEW RECOMMENDATION

Limit Intake of Trans Fatty Acids

The only safe intake of trans fatty acids appears to be zero, according to a recent report issued by the Institute of Medicine. The Institute does not specify an official upper intake limit but advises that "trans fatty acid consumption be as low as possible."

Similar to saturated fats, trans fats raise the risk of cardiovascular disease by increasing levels of total and low density lipoprotein (LDL) cholesterol. According to some research, trans fats also lower levels of protective high density lipoprotein (HDL) cholesterol.

Since small amounts of trans fatty acids are naturally present in dairy products and meat, eliminating all trans fats from the diet is impossible. However, the major sources of trans fats—margarines, baked goods, and fried foods that contain hydrogenated vegetable oils—can be limited.

Although food labels do not yet specify trans fatty acid content of foods, the U.S. Food and Drug Administration is currently considering mandatory labeling.

INSTITUTE OF MEDICINE,
NATIONAL ACADEMY OF SCIENCES
Letter report on dietary reference intakes for trans fatty acids
July 2002

For more about fish, see the feature on pages 6–7.

In addition, consuming foods that contain plant stanols and sterols is another way to lower LDL cholesterol. Plant stanols and sterols are added to certain margarines and salad dressings. When used properly, these products, such as the butter substitutes Benecol and Take Control, can help lower total blood cholesterol. The ingredients responsible for the benefit are plant components called sterols, which are chemically similar to cholesterol. When they are ingested, the body mistakes them for cholesterol and tries to absorb them without success. As a result, the absorption of cholesterol is partially blocked. The amount of saturated, unsaturated, and trans fat found in each product is comparable to regular tub margarine; neither contains cholesterol. One and a half tablespoons of Benecol daily or one to two tablespoons of Take Control can lower total cholesterol by up to 10%. The effect is cumulative when the spreads are used with other cholesterol-lowering measures. Sterol products should be used in place of—rather than in addition to—butter or traditional margarine. Consuming more than the recommended amount will not lower cholesterol more than 10%. A week's supply costs about $5.

Dietary Fat and Weight

Fat is a concentrated source of calories—it has nine calories per gram, compared with four calories per gram in protein and carbohydrates. Small amounts of fatty foods, therefore, pack a lot of calories. Reducing fat intake, however, does not guarantee weight loss. Weight is ultimately determined by the total number of calories consumed—whether from fat, carbohydrates, or protein—and the total number expended by metabolism, daily activity, and exercise. Overeating even low-fat foods can result in weight gain.

A low-fat diet combined with regular exercise will help people maintain an appropriate weight, or lose weight if necessary. Weight loss is the most effective way to lower elevated triglyceride levels. It also helps to raise HDL cholesterol levels: In one study, a 5-lb. weight gain lowered HDL levels by 4% in men and by 2% in women; losing weight counteracts this effect. Weight loss is also the first line of treatment for type 2 diabetes. In addition, a weight loss of as little as 5 to 10 lbs. may lower blood pressure enough to make antihypertensive drugs unnecessary. The many factors that affect weight control—and healthy strategies for losing weight—are discussed in detail in the section beginning on page 42.

NEW RESEARCH

Oats Aid in Blood Pressure Treatment

Research has shown that adding oats to the diet can help reduce elevated blood cholesterol levels. Now, two recent reports suggest that oats may also help lower blood pressure and reduce the need for blood pressure medication.

In the first study, researchers randomized 88 adults (age 33 to 67) who were receiving treatment for hypertension to consume a breakfast cereal containing either whole grain oats or refined grain wheat each day. After four weeks, 73% of the oats group was able to stop or reduce the dose of their medication by half compared with 42% of the wheat group. After four weeks, blood pressure decreased by 6/3 mm Hg in the oats group but dropped by only 2/1 mm Hg in the wheat group. However, blood pressure began to rise again when cereal consumption was discontinued after 12 weeks.

In the second study, investigators randomized 18 patients (age 27 to 59) who had untreated hypertension to an oat-cereal group or a low-fiber cereal group. After six weeks, the oats group experienced an 8/6 mm Hg reduction in blood pressure while those in the low-fiber group had almost no blood pressure reduction.

Because oats appear to lower blood pressure in addition to their proven ability to lower elevated cholesterol levels, the authors of the first study suggest that oats may help reduce the overall risk of cardiovascular disease.

THE JOURNAL OF FAMILY PRACTICE
Volume 51, pages 353 and 369
April 2002

Dietary Fat and Cancer

As with CHD, the hypothesis that a high-fat diet promotes the development of certain cancers first came from observational studies of different populations. In cultures where fat consumption is low, such as Japan and China, rates of breast, colon, ovarian, and prostate cancer are also low. In countries where people eat high-fat diets—the United States and Finland, for example—the incidence of these cancers is high. Furthermore, as people emigrate from a country where a low-fat diet is the norm to one where a high-fat diet predominates, and they adopt the dietary habits of their new homeland, their rates of these cancers increase. Thus, some researchers believe that the fat content of the diet, rather than differences in the genetic makeup of people from different countries, is responsible for the increased cancer risk.

Animal studies supported the link between dietary fat and cancer, but human studies have produced conflicting results. While some studies have shown that total fat intake is directly related to cancer risk, others have suggested that a high calorie intake, a diet rich in red meat, or a high intake of saturated fats may be the causative factor. Still other research shows that even if total fat intake is not involved in the development of cancer, it can accelerate progression of the disease.

Research into the role of dietary fat in breast cancer is a good example of the conflicting data on fat and cancer risk. Several studies have linked fat intake to breast cancer development, while others have found no connection. One possible explanation is that dietary fat itself does not raise breast cancer risk, but does so indirectly by promoting weight gain. Several studies have shown that weight gain in adulthood is associated with an increased risk of developing breast cancer. Alternatively, the fat content of the diet in childhood or early adulthood may determine cancer risk, so changes made in mid- to late life may not appreciably decrease risk.

One difficulty with connecting a high-fat diet to cancer is that no measurable factor in the body can be used to determine the increased risk, as with blood cholesterol levels and CHD, for example. It may be that cancer risk is not reduced until fat intake is very low. Because of the relatively high fat content of typical Western diets, modest reductions in fat intake by participants in U.S. studies may be too small to affect cancer risk.

The type of fat in the diet may also be significant. For example, in Mediterranean countries where monounsaturated fats (in the form of olive oil) make up a large part of the diet, women have a

Safe Grilling To Reduce Cancer Risk

Broiling and outdoor grilling are easy, low-fat ways to prepare food. However, studies suggest a potential link between cancer and well-done or charred meat, chicken and fish. To minimize cancer risk while grilling, the American Institute for Cancer Research advises simple measures, such as selecting lean cuts of meat, trimming fat, marinating, precooking, and minimizing fire flare-ups and smoke.

Grilled Foods and Cancer
Studies suggest that grilling and broiling red meat, poultry, and fish at high temperatures can produce harmful substances known as heterocyclic amines (HCAs). These compounds have been shown to cause tumors in animals and may possibly increase the risk of breast, colon, stomach, and prostate cancer in humans. Because they do not contain muscle protein, fruits and vegetables do not produce carcinogens when grilled. Other carcinogens, called polycyclic aromatic hydrocarbons, form when the fat from animal foods drips onto hot coals or stones during grilling. The resulting smoke from flare-ups can then transfer these cancer-causing compounds to food.

Tips for Healthy Grilling
Despite the link between grilled foods and cancer, there is no need to banish grilled foods from your diet as long as you follow a few simple suggestions:

Select lean meats and trim fat. To prevent flare-ups from fat dripping onto flames, coals, or hot rocks, choose lean meats and trim any visible fat before grilling. The leanest cuts of meat are from the loin, flank, and round. Stay away from fatty meats such as sausages and ribs. Before grilling poultry, remove the skin to reduce fat.

Marinate first. Not only does marinating enhance flavor and tenderness, it may also be the most effective way to prevent carcinogens from forming during grilling. Marinating for even just a short time may reduce HCAs by as much as 92% to 99%. Researchers believe the marinade itself may serve as a protective barrier or that antioxidant substances present in the marinade, such as vitamins C and E, may block the development of carcinogens. To be effective, just ½ cup of marinade is required for each pound of meat. Use only very tiny amounts of oil and sweetener in a marinade to minimize the potential for smoke during grilling; smoke can transfer carcinogens to food.

Precook food and grill for a short time at medium to low temperatures. Lower cooking temperatures and shorter cooking times decrease the formation of cancerous compounds. To reduce grilling time, precook meat, fish, and poultry in the oven or microwave. Then, briefly grill to add flavor and to complete cooking. Use small portions of food because they grill faster. Skewered kabobs, for example, require the least cooking time.

Minimize drips. In addition to choosing leaner cuts of meat and poultry to reduce the amount of fat that drips off, you can minimize flare-ups in other ways. If you are cooking over charcoal or lava rocks, do not place the meat directly over them; keep a spray bottle of water handy to extinguish flare-ups. Place a drip pan under the grill rack to catch any drips, or wrap food with aluminum foil punctured with air holes. Handle meat with tongs or a spatula instead of piercing with a fork. If you need to cut into the meat to check for doneness, be sure you do it off the grill, on a plate.

Flip frequently. Research shows that turning a hamburger once per minute while cooking at a temperature of 160° reduces the formation of HCAs. Flipping food frequently will accelerate cooking time, which helps prevent the formation of HCAs. Flipping is also effective in killing bacteria.

Remove charred parts before eating. After grilling, remove the charred part of food. The American Institute for Cancer Research advises against eating charred foods because of the high concentration of potential carcinogens.

For more information about safe grilling, visit the American Institute for Cancer Research Web site at www.aicr.org

lower risk of breast cancer than women in the United States, even though their average total fat intake is about 42% of calories, compared with 35% in the United States.

Recommendations for Fat Intake

1. Above all, keep saturated fat intake to 10% of calories or less. People with CHD, diabetes, or elevated LDL cholesterol levels should get less than 7% of their calories from saturated fat. Meats, poultry skin, and whole-milk dairy products contain the most saturated fat. Limit intake of red meat (beef, pork, and lamb) to two or three servings per week, choose lean cuts, and eat small portions (about 3 oz.). Each week have several meatless meals, such as vegetarian chili or pasta with marinara sauce. Choose low-fat dairy products such as fat-free milk, low-fat yogurt, and reduced-fat cheeses.

2. With few exceptions, limit total fat intake to less than 35% of calories. Most people should not reduce fat intake to less than 20% of calories. For those whose fat intakes have exceeded the recommended amount, fat calories should be replaced with ones from carbohydrates, but not all carbohydrates are equally acceptable. Emphasize whole grains, vegetables, fruits, and legumes (beans and peas) over products that contain a lot of refined carbohydrates, such as sugar and white flour. The American Heart Association (AHA) recommends a diet that includes less-saturated fats and oils. In general, consuming leafy greens and replacing red meat with fish are good ways to improve fat and oil intake. To reduce your use of cooking oils, take advantage of cooking methods that naturally reduce fat: Bake, broil, grill, roast, poach, microwave, or steam foods instead of frying or sautéing them. If you do sauté, use nonstick pans or a vegetable oil spray. Use vegetable oils and butter only in moderation; small amounts of water, wine, or broth can be added instead to prevent foods from sticking. Also, cut down on margarine and salad dressing and, if you use mayonnaise, look for one based on canola oil.

3. Get half your total fat intake from monounsaturated fats. Monounsaturated fats are particularly plentiful in olive oil, canola oil, almonds, walnuts, and avocados. Because these sources are also concentrated sources of total fat, they must be eaten in moderation to maintain a diet containing no more than 35% of calories from fat.

4. Get less than 300 mg of dietary cholesterol per day, and less than 200 mg if you have elevated LDL levels. Although saturated fat raises blood cholesterol levels more than cholesterol from foods, experts still recommend limiting dietary cholesterol.

5. Eat fatty fish twice a week. The omega-3 fatty acids in fatty fish appear to have some protective effect, and fish are a good source of protein and are low in saturated fat. Salmon, sardines, and tuna are all good choices.

6. Be wary of products containing trans fats. Studies show that trans fats have adverse effects on cholesterol levels and may increase the risk of CHD. Fried fast foods, packaged products, such as baked goods, and margarine are major sources of trans fats.

7. Remember that these recommendations need not be followed for each meal or even on a daily basis. It is more important to even out fat intake over the course of a week. If you eat a high-fat lunch, for example, you can compensate by eating a low-fat dinner or a little less fat than usual over the next several meals.

FIBER

For many years, fiber (the indigestible component of plant foods) was thought to be useful only for adding bulk to the diet to prevent constipation. But the shift in the diets of Western societies from ones based on whole grains, vegetables, fruits, and legumes to diets based on meats, refined grains, and processed foods has been associated with an increase in the incidence of CHD and type 2 diabetes; several studies point to a lack of dietary fiber as a primary cause. Some debate has ensued over whether fiber itself has a protective effect or is simply a marker for a healthy diet. But in recent studies, fiber has emerged as an independent factor for the prevention of disease.

Both types of fiber—soluble (sometimes called viscous) fiber, which dissolves in water and forms a gel-like substance, and insoluble fiber, which does not dissolve in water—are important for disease prevention. Most plant foods contain some of each type, but often one or the other predominates. Soluble fiber is found in legumes, barley, oats, and most fruits, while wheat and other whole grains and some vegetables contain insoluble fiber.

The two types of fiber exert different effects in the intestine. Soluble fiber binds bile acids and removes them in the stools. By absorbing many times its weight in water, insoluble fiber increases stool bulk and helps wastes pass more easily and rapidly through the digestive tract.

Fiber and Heart Disease

The connection between fiber and heart disease has focused on the effect of soluble fiber on blood cholesterol levels. In the liver, cholesterol is used to make bile acids. Soluble fiber binds with bile acids in the intestines and removes them in the stool. The liver responds by converting more cholesterol into bile acids. The resulting fall in cholesterol in liver cells leads them to take up more LDL from the blood.

Studies suggest that an increase of 5 to 10 g per day in soluble fiber intake—two to four extra servings of fruits and vegetables—

NEW RESEARCH

Whole Grains and Type 2 Diabetes

Eating a diet rich in whole grains may protect against type 2 diabetes, according to a recent study. Investigators examined the relationship between whole grain consumption and type 2 diabetes in 43,000 men (age 40 to 75) who were followed for up to 12 years.

After adjusting for body mass index (BMI), consuming three daily servings of whole grains was associated with a 30% lower risk of type 2 diabetes than eating only a half serving per day.

Because obesity is a risk factor for type 2 diabetes, nonobese men (those with a BMI of less than 30) particularly benefited from eating whole grains. Nonobese men who consumed three servings of whole grains per day had a 50% lower risk of type 2 diabetes than nonobese participants who ate only a half serving each day. Whole grains foods included brown rice, whole grain breads, popcorn, wheat germ, and bran. The intake of refined grains offered no protection against type 2 diabetes.

The findings suggest that long-term consumption of three daily servings of whole grains may reduce the risk of type 2 diabetes, especially among nonobese men. The authors speculate that the high content of cereal fiber and magnesium in whole grains may underlie their protective effect.

AMERICAN JOURNAL OF CLINICAL NUTRITION
Volume 76, page 535
September 1, 2002

Vitamins: Sources, Actions, and Benefits

This chart describes and provides sources for the 13 vitamins. In addition, it enumerates the adult Recommended Daily Allowances established by the National Academy of Sciences. For some vitamins, not enough is known to recommend a specific amount; in these cases, the Academy has recommended a range called the Estimated Safe and Adequate Daily Dietary Intake.

Vitamin/Food Sources	What It Does/Potential Benefits	Recommended Intake
Vitamin A. Liver, eggs, fortified milk, fish, and fruits and vegetables that contain beta-carotene, such as carrots, sweet potatoes, cantaloupe, leafy greens, tomatoes, apricots, winter squash, red bell peppers, broccoli, and mangoes.	Essential for night vision; helps form and maintain healthy skin and mucous membranes. Beta-carotene is converted in the body to vitamin A; beta-carotene (and other carotenoids) from foods may protect against some cancers and increase resistance to infection in children.	*700 mcg for women; 900 mcg for men.* Vitamin A may be toxic in high doses (over 3,000 mcg), so supplements are not recommended. Beta-carotene supplements may increase lung cancer risk in smokers. In contrast to vitamin A, beta-carotene in food is never toxic.
Vitamin C. (ascorbic acid). Citrus fruits and juices, strawberries, peppers, broccoli, potatoes, kale, cauliflower, cantaloupe.	Promotes healthy gums and teeth; aids in iron absorption; maintains normal connective tissue; helps in wound healing. As an antioxidant, it combats adverse effects of free radicals. May reduce the risk of certain cancers.	*75 mg for women; 90 mg for men.* For supplementation, smokers should add 35 mg a day. Tissue levels are not increased further when supplements exceed 250 mg.
Vitamin D. Milk, fish oil, fortified margarine; also produced by the body in response to sunlight.	Promotes strong bones and teeth by aiding absorption of calcium. Helps maintain blood levels of calcium and phosphorus. May reduce the risk of osteoporosis.	*200 IU for adults age 19 to 50; 400 IU for adults age 51 to 70; 600 IU for adults age 70+.* The limited amount of vitamin D in food often makes it necessary to take a supplement.
Vitamin E. Nuts, vegetable oils, margarine, wheat germ, leafy greens, seeds, almonds, olives, whole grains.	As an antioxidant, it combats adverse effects of free radicals. Consult your doctor before using vitamin E supplements if you are taking aspirin or warfarin.	*15 mg.*
Vitamin K. Cauliflower, broccoli, leafy greens, cabbage, milk, soybeans and eggs. Bacteria in the intestine produces most of the vitamin K needed each day.	Essential for normal blood clotting.	*90 mcg for women; 120 mcg for men.* No supplementation necessary or recommended.
Thiamin (B_1). Whole grains, dried beans, lean meats, liver, wheat germ, nuts, brewer's yeast.	Required for the conversion of carbohydrates into energy; necessary for normal function of the brain, nerves, and heart.	*1.1 mg for women; 1.2 mg for men.* No supplementation necessary or recommended.

Vitamin/Food Sources	What It Does/Potential Benefits	Recommended Intake
Riboflavin (B_2). Dairy products, liver, meat, chicken, fish, leafy greens, beans, nuts, eggs.	Helps cells convert carbohydrates into energy; essential for growth, production of red blood cells, and health of skin and eyes.	*1.1 mg for women; 1.3 mg for men.* No supplementation necessary or recommended.
Niacin (B_3). Nuts, grains, meat, fish, chicken, liver, dairy products.	Aids in release of energy from foods; helps maintain healthy skin, nerves, and digestive system. Large doses may be prescribed by a doctor to lower LDL cholesterol and triglyceride levels and raise HDL cholesterol levels.	*14 mg for women; 16 mg for men.* When used in large doses to lower cholesterol, may cause flushing, nausea, gout, liver damage, and increased blood glucose levels. Do not exceed 35 mg/day unless prescribed by a doctor.
Vitamin B_6 (pyridoxine). Whole grains, bananas, meat, beans, nuts, wheat germ, chicken, fish, liver.	Important in chemical reactions of proteins and amino acids; helps maintain brain function and form red blood cells. May boost immunity in the elderly. May lower homocysteine levels, high levels of which may increase risk of CHD.	*1.5 mg for women age 51+; 1.7 mg for men age 51+.* Megadoses can cause numbness and other neurological disorders.
Folate (B_9). (Also called folic acid or folacin). Leafy greens, wheat germ, liver, beans, whole and fortified grains, broccoli, citrus fruit.	Important in the synthesis of DNA, in normal growth, and in protein metabolism. Adequate intake reduces risk of certain birth defects. May protect against CHD by lowering homocysteine levels.	*400 mcg.* Can be derived from both fortified foods and supplements. Doses should not exceed 1,000 mcg/day.
Vitamin B_{12} (cobalamin). Liver, beef, pork, poultry, eggs, dairy products, seafood, fortified cereals.	Necessary for production of red blood cells; maintains normal functioning of nervous system.	*2.4 mcg.* Strict vegetarians may need supplements. Despite claims, no benefits from megadoses.
Pantothenic acid. Whole grains, dried beans, eggs, milk, liver.	Vital for metabolism of food and production of essential body chemicals.	*5 mg.* No supplementation necessary or recommended.
Biotin. Eggs, milk, liver, brewer's yeast, mushrooms, bananas, grains.	Important in metabolism of protein, carbohydrates, and fats.	*30 mcg.* No supplementation necessary or recommended.

reduces cholesterol levels by about 5%. Other studies have shown that fiber intake directly affects the risk of fatal and nonfatal heart attacks. Data from the Nurses' Health Study indicate that a diet rich in fiber, such as that found in breakfast cereals, promotes a healthy heart. Among 69,000 women (age 37 to 64), participants who ate the most fiber (an average of 23 g per day) had a 23% lower risk of heart attacks and deaths from CHD than women who ate the least (11.5 g per day). Fiber from breakfast cereal was more protective than fiber from fruits and vegetables.

Other research indicates that soluble fiber is more strongly associated with a reduced risk of heart attack and CHD death than insoluble fiber. However, the effect of soluble fiber on blood cholesterol levels does not fully account for the protective effect of dietary fiber. This finding opens the possibility that fiber may work in additional ways—by affecting the body's use of glucose and insulin, for example, or by reducing triglyceride levels. It is also possible that insoluble fiber contributes to these actions.

Fiber and Diabetes

People with type 2 diabetes, which accounts for 95% of all diabetes, are resistant to the actions of insulin. To compensate, the pancreas must secrete more insulin to allow glucose in the blood to enter cells, where it is used for energy. Diabetes develops if the pancreas cannot keep up with the continual demand for large amounts of insulin. Dietary fiber is thought to help prevent diabetes and make it easier for people with diabetes to maintain good control of blood glucose levels because it slows the absorption of sugars from the intestine and diminishes the rise in blood glucose following the ingestion of carbohydrates.

Fiber and Cancer

Colon cancer is the second most common cancer in the United States, where diets tend to be high in fat and low in fiber. Rates are much lower in countries where inhabitants consume a high-fiber, low-fat diet. The relationship between colon cancer and fiber was questioned by a 1999 study that tracked approximately 88,000 female nurses over a 16-year period. Surprisingly, the women who ate the most fiber—nearly 25 g a day—were just as likely to develop cancer and adenomas of the colon as those who ate the least fiber (about 10 g per day). Because the study had limitations in its design and because its findings contradict those of several previous studies, the results cannot be considered definitive.

While debate continues as to whether a high fiber intake can help prevent breast cancer, some research has shown that dietary fiber may lower blood levels of estrogen, thereby possibly reducing breast cancer risk.

Recommendations for Fiber Intake

1. **Consume 25 to 35 g of fiber if under age 50, and 20 to 30 g of fiber if over age 50.** Most people get less than 15 g of fiber daily.
2. **Eat whole grains for insoluble fiber.** Refined grain products—white bread, white flour, white rice, and pasta—are not good sources of fiber. To get insoluble fiber, you must consume the bran (the outer coating of the grain) that is removed in the milling of white flour. Good sources of insoluble fiber include whole grain cereals, whole-wheat bread, whole-wheat crackers, bulgur, and wheat berries.
3. **Eat oats, barley, legumes, and fruits for soluble fiber.**
4. **Increase fiber intake gradually over several weeks.** A sudden increase of fiber in the diet may cause uncomfortable gas pains.
5. **Drink enough water.** Fiber needs fluid to be effective. The standard advice to drink at least eight 8-oz. glasses of water or other fluids every day is being reevaluated, but you should certainly drink whenever you are thirsty.
6. **Do not go overboard on fiber.** A very high intake can interfere with the absorption of some vitamins and minerals.

FOLIC ACID, VITAMIN B_6, AND VITAMIN B_{12}

Several studies have found that a low dietary intake and low blood levels of folic acid and vitamin B_6 are associated with higher levels of blood homocysteine, an amino acid that may increase the risk of CHD, stroke, and peripheral artery disease. In addition, folic acid is essential during the early months of pregnancy to prevent birth defects, such as spina bifida and cleft palate. A lack of vitamin B_{12} can cause a form of dementia in older people that may be mistaken for Alzheimer disease. Many people over age 50 get too little of these B vitamins in their diets. In addition, a decline in the ability to absorb vitamin B_{12} can leave older people vulnerable to a deficiency.

B Vitamins and Heart Disease

Vitamin B_6, and especially folic acid, may be important for the prevention of cardiovascular disease. They affect blood levels of homocysteine by regulating its formation and conversion to other amino acids. It has been known for 30 years that people with a

NEW RESEARCH

High Fiber Diet Has Few Side Effects

Most experts recommend consuming no more than 35 g of fiber per day to reduce gastrointestinal discomfort. Now a study indicates that many people can consume a high-fiber diet without experiencing this side effect.

The study included data from 1,267 women (average age 54) who participated in a 12-month trial that evaluated the effect of diet on breast cancer recurrence. Participants were randomly assigned to either an intervention group that was encouraged to eat at least 30 g of fiber daily or a control group that was instructed to eat five servings of fruits and vegetables per day but received no specific counseling on fiber intake.

Twenty-eight percent of people in the intervention group consumed more than 35 g of fiber daily, as did 8% of those in the control group. After one year, women who consumed 35 g or more of fiber each day, regardless of which group they were in, experienced no more bloating, diarrhea, and upset stomach than the women who ate less fiber. The women who ate 35 g of fiber or more also reported 60% less constipation and 30% less heartburn.

"It is feasible and perhaps beneficial for at least a sizable proportion of healthy women 18 to 70 years of age to consume higher levels of fiber intake than currently recommended," the authors conclude.

JOURNAL OF THE AMERICAN DIETETIC ASSOCIATION
Volume 102, page 549
April 2002

Minerals: Sources, Actions, and Benefits

As with vitamins, the National Academy of Sciences has established Recommended Daily Allowances or Estimated Safe and Adequate Daily Dietary Intakes for minerals. The chart below describes each mineral and gives the Academy's recommendation for intake.

Mineral/Food Sources	What It Does	Recommended Intake
Calcium. Milk and milk products, canned salmon and sardines eaten with bones, dark green leafy vegetables, shellfish, some fortified cereals.	Major component of bones and teeth; helps prevent or minimize osteoporosis; helps regulate heartbeat, blood clotting, muscle contraction, and nerve conduction. May help prevent hypertension.	*1,000 mg for adults age 19 to 50; 1,200 mg for adults age 51+.*
Chloride. Table salt, fish.	Helps maintain fluid and acid–base balance; component of gastric juice.	*No RDA.*
Chromium. Meat, cheese, whole grains, brewer's yeast.	Important in metabolism of carbohydrates and fats. Deficiency may impair the action of insulin.	*25 mcg for women age 19 to 50; 20 mcg for women age 51+; 35 mcg for men age 19 to 50; 30 mcg for men age 51+.*
Copper. Shellfish, nuts, beans, seeds, organ meats, whole grains, potatoes.	Formation of red blood cells; helps keep bones, nerves, and immune system healthy.	*900 mcg.*
Fluoride. Fluoridated water and foods grown or cooked in it, marine fish (with bones), tea.	Contributes to solid bone and tooth formation. Reduces dental cavities.	*3 mg for women; 4 mg for men.*
Iodine. Primarily from iodized salt, but also seafood, seaweed food products, vegetables grown in iodine-rich areas. Widely dispersed in the food supply.	Necessary for the formation of thyroid hormone and thus for normal cell metabolism; prevents goiter (enlargement of the thyroid).	*150 mcg.*
Iron. Liver, kidneys, red meats, eggs, peas, beans, nuts, dried fruits, green leafy vegetables, enriched grain products, fortified cereals. Cooking in iron pots adds iron, especially to acidic foods.	Essential component of hemoglobin (which carries oxygen in red blood cells) and myoglobin (in muscle); part of several enzymes and proteins in the body. Heme iron, found in animal products, is better absorbed by the body than nonheme iron, found in plants.	*18 mg for women age 19 to 50; 8 mg for women age 51+; 8 mg for men. There may be a danger in iron supplements for people who do not know they have hemachromatosis.*

Mineral/Food Sources	What It Does	Recommended Intake
Magnesium. Wheat bran, whole grains, raw leafy green vegetables, nuts, soybeans, bananas.	Aids in bone growth; aids function of nerves and muscles, including regulation of normal heart rhythm.	*310 mg for women age 19 to 30; 320 mg for women age 31+; 400 mg for men age 19 to 30; 420 mg for men age 31+.*
Manganese. Nuts, whole grains, vegetables, fruits, instant coffee, tea, cocoa powder, beans.	Needed for energy production and reproduction. May also be essential for building bones. Excess may interfere with iron absorption.	*1.8 mg for women; 2.3 mg for men.*
Molybdenum. Peas, beans, cereal grains, organ meats, some dark green vegetables.	Aids in bone growth and strengthening of teeth; important in energy metabolism.	*45 mcg.*
Phosphorus. Meats, poultry, fish, dairy products, eggs, dried peas and beans, soft drinks, nuts; present in almost all foods.	Major component of bones and teeth; present in cell membranes and genetic material. Vital for energy metabolism.	*700 mg.*
Potassium. Most foods, especially oranges and orange juice, bananas, potatoes (with skin),tomatoes, potatoes, greens, dried beans, brussels sprouts, dried fruits, yogurt, meat, poultry, milk.	Vital for muscle contraction, nerve impulses, and function of heart and kidneys. Helps regulate blood pressure and water balance in cells.	*1,600 to 2,000 mg minimum.*
Selenium. Fish, shellfish, red meat, nuts, grains, eggs, chicken, garlic, organ meats; amount in vegetables depends on soil.	Part of enzymes that act as antioxidants to prevent cell damage. Needed for proper immune response.	*55 mcg.* Large doses can be toxic.
Sodium. Table salt, salt added to prepared foods (such as cheese, smoked meats, and fast foods), baking soda.	Helps regulate blood pressure and water balance in the body.	*2,400 mg maximum.*
Zinc. Oysters, crabmeat, liver, eggs, poultry, brewer's yeast, wheat germ, milk, beans.	Important in activity of enzymes for cell division, growth, and repair (wound healing), as well as proper functioning of immune system. Maintains taste and smell acuity.	*8 mg for women; 11 mg for men.*

condition called homocystinuria—an inherited metabolic defect that results in extremely high blood levels of homocysteine—develop premature atherosclerosis and often suffer a heart attack or stroke before age 30. Now, researchers have found that people with far more moderate homocysteine elevations are at increased risk for cardiovascular disease.

Just how excess homocysteine contributes to arterial disease is not known. Some animal studies suggest that homocysteine damages the cells lining blood vessels, and paves the way for the buildup of plaque. Other research suggests that homocysteine increases the formation of blood clots, which can obstruct an artery and cause a heart attack or stroke.

There is no doubt that folic acid and homocysteine levels in the blood are inversely related—that is, when folic acid levels are higher, homocysteine levels are lower. Many studies have clearly shown that folic acid supplements lower homocysteine levels. It is not yet clear whether increasing folic acid intake, alone or in combination with vitamin B_6 can lower the risk of arterial disease, but much of the evidence points in that direction. More research needs to be done to determine for certain whether an adequate intake of folic acid and vitamin B_6 can reduce the risk of arterial disease.

Recommendations for Intake of B Vitamins

1. Get plenty of folic acid every day. The Recommended Dietary Allowance (RDA) for this vitamin is 400 micrograms (mcg). Good sources include enriched breads and cereals, dried peas and beans, oranges, orange juice, green vegetables, and whole grains.

2. Eat foods rich in vitamin B_6. Meeting the RDA of 1.3 mg (for women) to 1.7 mg (for men) is all that is necessary. Good sources of vitamin B_6 include fish, meats, poultry, avocados, and bananas.

3. Maintain an adequate B_{12} intake. The RDA for people over 50 is 2.4 mcg per day. People age 50 and older can meet the RDA mainly by consuming foods fortified with B_{12} or with a supplement containing B_{12}. On the other hand, vegetarians who eat no animal products (B_{12} is found only in meat, poultry, shellfish, fish, eggs, and dairy products) need to take a vitamin B_{12} supplement. Vitamin B_6 and iron enhance vitamin B_{12} absorption. People taking supplements of folic acid should also add 1 mcg of vitamin B_{12} daily.

4. People with elevated levels of homocysteine should consider a multivitamin, which will supply these B vitamins. Most multivitamins contain the amounts recommended above.

CALCIUM AND VITAMIN D

Most people are aware that calcium is essential for the formation and strength of bones, but few people realize that it fulfills other important functions. Calcium in the bloodstream is involved in blood clotting, blood pressure control, enzyme activation, contraction and relaxation of muscles (including the heart), nerve transmission, and membrane permeability (controlling the passage of fluids and other substances in and out of cells).

Calcium can be released from bones, which contain 99% of body calcium, whenever blood levels of calcium are too low. Bones are constantly broken down and rebuilt throughout life. This bone turnover becomes a problem only when calcium use outpaces calcium intake because the body will then sacrifice bone in order to maintain blood calcium levels needed for these other crucial functions. Over time, a dietary calcium deficit can cause osteoporosis, a potentially debilitating bone-thinning disorder that increases susceptibility to fractures.

Vitamin D is needed to maintain the body's calcium stores. In addition, vitamin D strengthens the immune system. Although vitamin D is found naturally in only a few foods, the body can usually produce enough in response to sunlight. However, vitamin D formation is reduced in northern or cloudy climates that receive lesser amounts of sunlight. Without this vitamin, ingested calcium is poorly absorbed from the intestine. The ability to generate vitamin D declines with age, so some older people, particularly those who are homebound, are at risk for vitamin D deficiency.

Calcium and Vitamin D and Other Disorders

Calcium may offer a small reduction of blood pressure in people with high blood pressure, and vitamin D may help people with osteoarthritis. Both calcium and vitamin D appear to have a modest protective effect against colon cancer.

Recommendations for Calcium and Vitamin D Intake

1. If you are between the ages of 19 and 50, try to get 1,000 mg of calcium a day. This level of calcium intake helps to maintain calcium stores in bones.

2. At age 51, increase calcium intake to 1,200 mg per day. This amount of calcium is recommended for both men and women; it will help slow the loss of bone that occurs with age.

3. Try to get as much calcium as possible through your diet. Milk

NEW RESEARCH

Calcium May Improve Cholesterol Profile

In postmenopausal women, taking a calcium supplement appears to increase high density lipoprotein (HDL, or "good") cholesterol and improve the ratio of HDL to low density lipoprotein (LDL, or "bad") cholesterol, a new Australian study shows.

Researchers randomized 223 postmenopausal women (average age 72) to receive either 1,000 mg of calcium citrate (Citracal) or a placebo each day for a year. Women were not receiving any other osteoporosis or cholesterol-lowering therapies.

After one year, HDL cholesterol levels had increased significantly (7%) in the women taking calcium, though there were no significant reductions in LDL cholesterol or triglyceride levels in the calcium group. Calcium supplementation also resulted in a significant (16%) increase in the ratio of HDL/LDL cholesterol.

This study suggests that calcium supplementation in postmenopausal women offers benefits beyond helping to maintain bone health. The beneficial effect on HDL cholesterol may have resulted from changes in fat absorption in the intestines.

THE AMERICAN JOURNAL OF MEDICINE
Volume 112, page 343
April 1, 2002

Getting Enough Calcium

While we require calcium for a number of major biological functions, one of the most important roles of this mineral is to maintain healthy bones. An adequate intake of calcium protects against the development of osteoporosis, which causes bones to become porous, brittle, and susceptible to fractures. According to the National Osteoporosis Foundation, approximately 10 million Americans—80% of them women—suffer from osteoporosis. An additional 18 million have low bone mineral density, which is a risk factor for osteoporosis. While postmenopausal women are at highest risk, men also are susceptible to osteoporosis, particularly when they reach age 65.

Calcium Protects Bones

Health professionals generally recommend milk and other dairy foods as a primary source of calcium to protect bones because these foods offer greater concentrations of this essential mineral. You can also help protect against future bone loss by engaging in regular weight-bearing exercise and by not smoking.

Along with calcium, you also need enough vitamin D to ensure proper calcium absorption. Research indicates that the risk of developing vitamin D deficiency is higher after age 50. Fatty fish such as salmon, mackerel, and sardines are rich in vitamin D. Fortified cereals also supply vitamin D. And while most milk is fortified with vitamin D (one cup of fortified milk provides about one quarter of the estimated daily need for vitamin D in adults), other dairy sources of calcium such as yogurt, cheese, and ice cream are generally not fortified. Vitamin D can also be formed in your body during exposure to sunlight.

The Daily Value for Calcium

The U.S. Food and Drug Administration uses the term daily value (DV) to describe the amount of calcium that the general U.S. population needs each day. The amount of calcium in packaged foods is expressed on the label as a percentage of the DV. For example, if a serving of packaged food has 200 mg of calcium, it is listed on the label as 20% DV, since the DV is 1,000 mg. However, to build peak bone mass and prevent osteoporosis, men and postmenopausal women over age 65 require 1,500 mg of calcium daily as well as an intake of vitamin D ranging from 400 to 800 IU a day. Although calcium and vitamin D can be derived from dietary sources, if you are concerned that you are not getting enough of these nutrients to protect your bones, ask your doctor if you should take a calcium and vitamin D supplement.

Lactose Intolerance

Some people have trouble getting enough calcium because they have a fairly common condition called lactose intolerance, a reduced ability to properly digest the milk sugar lactose. An estimated 30 to 50 million Americans suffer from a wide range of symptoms and discomfort associated with lactose intolerance, including cramps, bloating, gas, diarrhea, and nausea. Consult your doctor or a registered dietitian if you experience these symptoms after eating dairy products.

Lactose intolerance is relatively easy to manage; there are a variety of ways to get calcium even if you have trouble digesting lactose (see the inset box). Because symptoms of lactose intolerance are highly variable in their severity, many people can tolerate small amounts of milk or can drink milk when it is consumed with other foods.

and other dairy products are the most concentrated sources. Use only fat-free or low-fat dairy products, however; not only is their reduced saturated fat content a benefit, but they are also slightly higher in calcium than full-fat dairy products. Eating several high-calcium foods over the course of the day can provide the recommended calcium intake: For example, two 8-oz. glasses of fat-free milk, one 8-oz. glass of calcium-fortified orange juice, and one 8-oz. container of plain fat-free yogurt together supply just over 1,200 mg of calcium. Note that the labels "high in calcium," "rich in calcium," or "excellent source of calcium" mean that a serving contains at least 200 mg of calcium. A product that says "contains calcium," "provides calcium," or "good source of calcium" has 100 to 190 mg per serving. And "calcium-enriched," "calcium-fortified," or "more

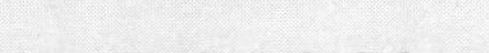

How To Get Calcium

- Select calcium-rich snacks such as pudding, yogurt, and cheese.
- Add milk instead of water to prepare canned soups.
- Try flavored milk (flavored milk has as much calcium as regular milk).
- Eat fortified cereal and drink fortified juice.
- Add nonfat, powdered dry milk to puddings, homemade cookies, breads, and muffins, soups, gravy, and casseroles.
- Drink milk with meals.
- Talk to your doctor about calcium supplements.

How To Get Calcium If You Are Lactose Intolerant

- Consume ample amounts of non-dairy, calcium-rich foods, including calcium-fortified foods.
- Drink soy milk (check the label to see if the milk has been fortified with calcium).
- Drink small amounts of dairy milk (one cup or less) with a meal.
- Drink lactose-reduced milk (it is as nutritious as regular milk).
- Eat yogurt with active or live cultures (yogurt contains less lactose than milk, and the bacteria help to digest the remaining lactose).
- Take lactase enzyme tablets before eating or along with dairy products.
- Add lactase enzyme drops to regular milk.
- Talk to your doctor about calcium supplements.

Nondairy Sources of Calcium

While dairy products are the principal source of dietary calcium, people with lactose intolerance, and those who prefer not to consume dairy foods, can benefit from nondairy dietary sources of calcium. For example, nondairy calcium can be found in some brands of firm tofu (make sure the label says the tofu has been processed with calcium), calcium-fortified juice, dried figs, white beans, canned salmon and sardines with the bones (the bones are soft and edible), as well as soybeans, bok choy, and broccoli. Though spinach contains some calcium, it is also rich in oxalates, which interfere with calcium absorption.

Calcium Supplements

Although food is the best source of calcium, if you are unable to meet your calcium requirement through diet alone, a supplement can help you reach your daily calcium needs. The different types of calcium supplements include calcium carbonate, calcium phosphate, and calcium citrate, each of which contains a different amount of elemental calcium, the amount of calcium in the supplement.

Calcium carbonate and calcium citrate contain the highest percentage of calcium per tablet—40% and 30%, respectively. Studies show that the calcium in citrate-based supplements is more efficiently absorbed than the calcium in carbonate-based ones. Calcium carbonate pills should be taken with meals because calcium absorption from such tablets is improved by the presence of gastric acid. Calcium supplements (as well as dietary calcium) are best absorbed when taken (or consumed) several times a day in amounts of 500 mg or less.

Because calcium supplements are available in a wide range of preparations and strengths, selecting the right one can be complicated. Ask your physician to help you determine which type of calcium supplement is best for you.

calcium" labels mean that the product has 100 mg or more per serving. Sources of calcium that do not have nutrition labels, such as leafy green vegetables or broccoli, contain about 10% of the daily requirement of calcium per serving.

4. Do not hesitate to use supplements to make up for calcium shortfalls. Supplements are warranted for people who are unable to get the recommended amounts of calcium through diet alone. Determine how much calcium you get in your diet, and use supplements to meet the recommended intakes, not to exceed them. Up to 2,500 mg of calcium a day is considered safe for adults. Taking a supplement is not as simple as drinking a glass of milk and knowing that you just got about 300 mg of what is called elemental calcium. (All calcium guidelines refer to elemental calcium.) Elemental calcium must be combined with a weak acid to form a chemical compound in pill, tablet, or liquid supplements. The names of these acids appear in the various suffixes of calcium—for instance, carbonate, citrate, and gluconate.

5. Take calcium supplements with meals. Do not take supplements at bedtime, when the acid content of the stomach is low. Many older people do not produce enough stomach acid between meals to dissolve calcium tablets thoroughly.

6. Expose your skin to sunlight to generate vitamin D production. The recommended intake for vitamin D is 400 IU per day for men and women age 51 to 70, and 600 IU for those over 70. Exposure to sunlight can generate 200 IU in just 10 minutes if the hands and face are exposed. However, sunscreen with a sun protection factor (SPF) of 8 or higher can block the ultraviolet rays needed to produce vitamin D. Therefore, you should spend 10 to 15 minutes outside prior to applying sunscreen. Older people may need slightly longer exposure to compensate for the decreased ability of their skin to synthesize vitamin D in response to sunlight.

7. If you live in a northern climate, consider taking a multivitamin with vitamin D in the winter. Most multivitamins contain 400 IU of vitamin D. People who are homebound or live in a nursing home need vitamin D supplements throughout the year. All people with osteoporosis or low bone mineral density should take 400 to 800 IU of vitamin D—not as a multivitamin but either alone or in combination with a calcium supplement. Consult your physician to see what type of supplement is best for you.

SODIUM AND POTASSIUM

Sodium, found outside cells, and potassium, found mainly inside cells, are minerals that work together to maintain fluid balance in the body. In addition, they are involved in the regulation of muscle contraction and nerve transmission and play an important role in controlling blood pressure.

Although sodium occurs naturally in foods, the average person consumes most dietary sodium from salt and other sodium-containing ingredients (for example, baking soda or monosodium glutamate [MSG]) added to foods in processing, in cooking, or at the table.

Sodium and salt are not the same thing. Chemically, salt is sodium chloride, and only 40% of it is sodium. Keep this in mind when reading the information in this section, since all of the values refer to amounts of sodium, not salt.

NEW RESEARCH

Pre- and Probiotics Promote Health

Prebiotics are indigestible food substances that promote the growth of beneficial bacteria in the digestive tract. Artichokes, asparagus, garlic, and onions contain naturally occurring prebiotics.

According to a recent review, preliminary research suggests that prebiotics may exert anticancer actions and may also enhance the absorption of the minerals calcium, iron, and magnesium.

Probiotics, beneficial bacteria that foster "intestinal balance," are present in active-culture yogurts and fermented milk products. According to the review, probiotics appear to have more robust effects on health than prebiotics.

Although it is far too early to draw conclusions, some evidence suggests that probiotics may help to improve cholesterol levels, fortify immune defenses, guard against cancer, and alleviate inflammatory bowel disease. More compelling evidence indicates that probiotics impede the growth of infection-causing bacteria as well as protect against and ameliorate both viral and antibiotic-induced diarrhea.

The authors conclude that the research on pre- and probiotics is promising; these substances have potentially valuable roles in promoting good health and in countering disease. Additional studies are needed to clearly establish the health benefits and lasting effects of pre- and probiotics.

ANNUAL REVIEWS IN NUTRITION
Volume 22, page 107
January 2002

Sodium, Potassium, and Hypertension

Overall, Americans tend to get too much sodium—about 3,900 mg per day, which is nearly twice the recommended amount—and too little potassium. This imbalance may contribute to high blood pressure. Experts continue to debate whether everyone needs to lower sodium intake to prevent or control high blood pressure. While many experts maintain that everyone should cut back on sodium intake, some hold that sodium reduction is worthwhile only when blood pressure is too high or in those who have a family history of high blood pressure.

Part of the debate results from an incomplete understanding of how sodium increases blood pressure. Researchers know that higher sodium levels promote water retention, which in turn increases blood volume and may ultimately lead to higher blood pressure. Excess sodium is usually excreted in the urine, but 30% to 50% of people with hypertension cannot efficiently get rid of excess sodium. Sodium can also constrict small blood vessels, which causes greater resistance to blood flow. How sodium produces blood vessel constriction remains unknown.

High blood pressure is defined as having a systolic blood pressure (the higher number) of 140 mm Hg or higher and/or a diastolic blood pressure (the lower number) of 90 mm Hg or higher. Studies estimate that if everyone stopped adding salt to their food (which accounts for about a third of the sodium in most people's diets), the number of people who need antihypertensive medication would be cut in half.

The DASH (Dietary Approaches to Stop Hypertension) study provides specific advice for using dietary means to reduce blood pressure. The DASH diet emphasizes fruits, vegetables, and low-fat dairy products to significantly improve blood pressure in people with mildly elevated or normal values. Specifically, the DASH diet consists of 8 to 10 servings of fruits and vegetables plus 2 to 3 servings of low-fat dairy products each day. In addition, the DASH diet promotes plant sources of protein at least once or twice a week. Additional details on the DASH diet can be obtained from the National Heart, Lung, and Blood Institute (www.nhlbi.nih.gov).

The DASH diet provides a well-balanced menu of essential nutrients, particularly potassium, magnesium, and calcium. A large part of the success of the diet may be due to its high potassium content of about 4,400 mg daily (roughly the amount in 11 bananas). Research indicates that potassium lowers blood pressure by relaxing arteries. But the interplay of all essential nutrients, as

NEW RESEARCH

Folate Intake Linked To Lower Stroke Risk

People who consume more folate in their diet appear to have a lower risk of stroke, according to a recent report.

Between 1971 and 1975, researchers asked 9,764 people (age 25 to 74) who did not have cardiovascular disease what they had eaten on the previous day. From this information, the researchers estimated the participants' average baseline folate intake.

During the next 19 years, people who had eaten over 300 micrograms (mcg) of folate per day at baseline had a 13% lower risk of all cardiovascular events (such as a heart attack or stroke) and a 20% lower risk of stroke than those who consumed less than 136 mcg of folate, after adjusting for factors such as diabetes, hypertension, and elevated cholesterol, which contribute to cardiovascular disease.

The researchers speculate that folate may reduce the risk of stroke by decreasing blood levels of homocysteine, a suspected risk factor for cardiovascular disease.

While this study has many limitations, however, because folate is important in other areas of health, it is reasonable that those at risk for stroke should aim to consume 400 mcg of folate per day. Foods rich in folate include dark, leafy green vegetables, legumes, citrus fruits and juices, and whole grain or enriched pastas, breads, and cereals.

STROKE
Volume 33, page 1183
May 2002

well as fiber, is probably just as important as any single vitamin or mineral.

The DASH diet may also help to improve cholesterol levels. In one recent study, the diet reduced total cholesterol an average of 13.7 mg/dL and LDL cholesterol an average of 10.7 mg/dL.

Sodium and Other Disorders

There are several other reasons to reduce sodium in your diet. A high-sodium diet can increase the loss of calcium in the urine, which in turn triggers removal of calcium from bones. A very high intake of sodium (3,000 mg or more per day) can also raise the risk of stomach cancer because sodium irritates the lining of the stomach, especially in people who have had ulcers. Finally, excess sodium contributes to kidney disease as an extension of its effect on hypertension. Chronic high blood pressure damages organs by injuring the blood vessels that supply them, and the kidneys are particularly vulnerable to this effect.

Recommendations for Sodium and Potassium Intake

1. Don't add salt to foods. One teaspoon of salt contains 2,130 mg of sodium. At first, a low-sodium diet may make food taste bland, but within six to eight weeks your palate will adjust, and the amount of salt you once used will make foods taste too salty.

2. If you have hypertension, do not exceed 2,000 mg of sodium daily. Some people who are particularly sodium-sensitive should consume even less.

3. Flavor foods with herbs, spices, and citrus juices. These seasonings can help perk up foods and compensate for the flavor lost from the reduction in salt.

4. Read food labels carefully for sodium content. Packaged and processed foods supply about two thirds of the sodium in the average diet. Minimize your use of high-sodium products, such as luncheon meats, sausages, smoked meats and fish, hot dogs, canned shellfish, canned soups, frozen dinners, condiments (relish, ketchup, soy sauce, and pickles), cheese, and processed snack foods.

5. Remember that sodium comes in many forms, not just salt. Baking soda, monosodium glutamate (MSG), onion salt, garlic salt, and some other flavorings are also sources of sodium.

6. Try salt alternatives. Salt alternatives—such as Cardia and Morton's Lite Salt, which contain about half the sodium of table salt—can be an option for some people. However, people with kidney problems and those taking potassium-sparing diuretics for

How To Select Healthy Foods When Eating Out

The average American eats about four restaurant meals a week. Unfortunately, when we eat out, many of us eat less healthful foods than the food we would have prepared at home. Studies show that most restaurant meals are not only larger in size than home-cooked meals, but they are also higher in calories, saturated fat, and sodium while being lower in fiber and calcium. Fortunately, with a little planning, it is possible to dine out and still eat healthfully by following the advice below:

- Commit yourself in advance to ordering nutritious, healthful meals, and most important of all: adhere to your game plan.
- Eat a piece of fruit, a carrot, or a pretzel before you go out so that you won't be ravenous when you get to the restaurant. Another way to prevent overeating is to drink two glasses of water before your food arrives.
- Avoid fried foods—they are high in fat. Instead of eating fried chicken, request roasted chicken (prepared without the skin or you can remove the skin before eating), and substitute a baked potato for french fries.
- Do not slather butter on baked potatoes, rolls, or corn on the cob. Instead, use butter sparingly or request reduced-fat margarine if the restaurant has it.
- Look for items that say "roasted," "grilled," "steamed," or "poached." These terms (with the exception of "grilled in butter") usually indicate that the foods have been prepared without excess fat.
- Check the menu carefully and identify "light" or "heart-healthy" items. Some restaurants and fast food venues now offer lighter fare for health-conscious customers.
- Select lean cuts of meat such as beef round, loin, sirloin, pork loin chops, turkey, and chicken. Cuts with the name "loin" or "round" are lean. Depending on the cut, steaks can be fatty (prime rib) or lean (sirloin and flank).
- Order dressings and sauces on the side, so you can control the portions. Use them sparingly or not at all. Alternately, request fat-free or low-calorie dressing for salads.
- Instead of a large entrée, choose salads, à la carte items, side dishes, or two appetizers (for example, shrimp cocktail and a salad).
- Order vegetable side dishes and ask that they be served without butter.
- Ask that foods be prepared with olive or canola oil instead of butter, margarine, or shortening.
- Watch portion sizes—typical restaurant servings are often twice the size of a single serving (see pages 60–61 to learn about serving sizes). If the portion is large, eat half of the meal and take the rest home.
- Be cautious at salad bars. Avoid cheeses, croutons, marinated salads, pasta salads, and fruit salads with whipped cream. Instead, choose foods like raw vegetables, fresh greens, fresh fruit, beans, and low-fat dressing.
- Ask for extra plates and spoons or forks to share one rich dessert with everyone at the table. You can still indulge a little and enjoy yourself without overeating. Or simply order lower-fat, lower-calorie alternatives such as fresh fruit, sorbet, gelatin, or angel food cake.
- Get the most nutrition from your calories. For example, order a glass of skim milk instead of soda so you can get the benefit of the calcium and other nutrients in milk.
- See if the managers of your favorite restaurants will offer more vegetarian choices, light dressings, whole grain breads, or greens, such as spinach or kale, which are more nutritious than iceberg lettuce.

hypertension or heart failure should not use these products because they contain more potassium than regular salt. Speak with your doctor first before using these salt alternatives.

7. Look for reduced-sodium packaged foods. Sodium claims made on labels must meet certain standards: Low-sodium foods have 140 mg or less per serving, very-low-sodium means 35 mg or less, and sodium-free has 5 mg or less. Unsalted or no-salt-added foods generally contain only naturally occurring sodium.

8. Get about 2,000 mg of potassium a day. Eat more fruits, vegetables, legumes, and grains. Bananas, kidney beans, lentils, oranges, orange juice, yogurt, cantaloupe, prunes, and potatoes are just a few of the foods that are high in potassium—and low in sodium as well.

ALCOHOL

The role of alcohol in a healthy diet is confusing. While moderate alcohol consumption has some undeniable health benefits, alcohol also adds extra calories, interferes with the action of many medications, and when consumed in excess over a long period of time, can cause some types of heart disease and raise blood pressure. Fatty liver and cirrhosis are major consequences of alcohol abuse. In addition, alcohol is a leading cause of car accidents.

Studies in both men and women have shown that having one to two alcoholic drinks per day is associated with a 30% to 60% reduction in the risk of developing CHD, and also helps protect against ischemic stroke (the type caused by a blood clot in an atherosclerotic carotid or cerebral artery). Just how alcohol prevents CHD and strokes is a subject of much scientific debate, but it is generally accepted that about half of the risk reduction comes from an increase in HDL cholesterol levels. The rest of the protection may be due to alcohol's ability to reduce clot formation in the coronary and cerebral arteries.

For women, however, there is a downside to moderate drinking. Daily consumption of even small amounts of alcohol appears to increase the chances of breast cancer. Studies have shown a 30% to 60% rise in breast cancer risk for women who have one or two alcoholic drinks per day. The risk increases steeply—some studies show it more than doubles—as alcohol consumption rises to three or more drinks per day. Recent alcohol consumption appears to have a greater impact on risk than alcohol consumption early in life.

A report from the Iowa Women's Health Study, involving over

41,000 women, found that the effect of alcohol on breast cancer risk was limited to women taking estrogen replacement therapy (ERT). This result was not confirmed by other studies; however, one study found that in postmenopausal women on ERT, drinking alcohol tripled blood levels of estradiol, a form of estrogen, and estrogen has been shown to promote breast cancer. The researchers who conducted this study speculated that the combination of ERT and alcohol may increase the risk of breast cancer more than either one alone.

Recommendations for Alcohol Consumption

1. If you don't currently drink alcohol, don't start. Experts do not recommend that teetotalers begin drinking alcohol, but instead should take other steps to reduce their risk of CHD.

2. Men who drink should limit themselves to one to two alcoholic drinks per day. This amount of alcohol is enough to reduce CHD risk. However, it may impact the ability to drive and operate other machinery. (A drink is defined as 12 oz. of beer, 5 oz. of wine, or 1½ oz. of 80-proof spirits.)

3. Women who drink, but have no CHD risk factors, should limit alcohol to fewer than seven drinks per week. Having a few drinks per week probably does not increase the odds of getting breast cancer, but it is not known whether this amount of alcohol can prevent CHD.

4. Women who drink and have CHD (or an increased risk for CHD) should have no more than one drink per day. For a woman at risk for CHD, the benefits of moderate alcohol consumption may outweigh the risks. However, keep in mind that there are many ways to reduce CHD risk, but few known ways to reduce the risk of breast cancer.

5. The type of alcoholic drink does not matter. Some studies have emphasized the protective effect of red wine in reducing CHD risk, but most experts agree that wine (red or white), beer, or spirits all have the same effect.

6. Remember that heavy alcohol consumption is a health risk. Heavy drinking (more than two alcoholic drinks per day) can cause a variety of life-threatening diseases, including hypertension, stroke, cardiomyopathy (an enlargement of the heart), and cirrhosis.

7. Certain people should avoid alcohol altogether. They include people with hypertriglyceridemia, pancreatitis, liver disease, porphyria, uncontrolled hypertension, and heart failure. Anyone with a past or current problem with alcohol should not drink. And of course, anyone who is driving should abstain from alcohol.

Nutrition and Disease: Dietary Recommendations

Dietary strategies to help prevent specific diseases are outlined below. Because many of the recommendations overlap, even one or two dietary changes can help protect against several disorders. While there are important dietary recommendations for cancer prevention, the benefits of dietary changes for coronary heart disease (CHD), hypertension (high blood pressure), diabetes, and osteoporosis are based on stronger scientific evidence.

Coronary Heart Disease (CHD) and Stroke

- Limit your intake of saturated fat and trans fatty acids to less than 10% of calories (or less than 7% if you have a high blood cholesterol level). You can accomplish this by restricting your intake of the major sources of saturated fat (fatty meats, full-fat dairy products, and tropical oils) and by restricting your intake of hydrogenated fat (found in commercially prepared baked and fried foods and margarines), the major source of trans fatty acids.
- Center your diet around fish, skinless poultry, and plant-based, unprocessed, whole foods, such as whole grains, fruits, vegetables, legumes (such as beans), and nuts.
- Eat at least two servings of fish per week, particularly fatty fish such as mackerel, salmon, and tuna. Fatty fish provide a type of fat, called omega-3 fatty acids, that is believed to be heart-healthy.
- Include soy foods in your diet—replace foods high in saturated fat and cholesterol with 25 g of soy protein per day. This recommendation is particularly important for those with high levels of total and LDL cholesterol.
- Opt for fat-free and low-fat dairy products. Also choose lean meats in place of higher-fat cuts. The leanest cuts of meat are loin, flank, and round.
- Get at least 15% of total calories from monounsaturated fats such as olive oil. Choose unsaturated fats instead of saturated and trans fats.
- Limit cholesterol to 300 mg per day. If you have high blood cholesterol levels, limit your intake to less than 200 mg per day.
- Get 20-30 g fiber per day (for adults over age 50); include plenty of soluble fiber.
- Consume at least 400 mcg of folate (folic acid) per day from fruits, vegetables, fortified grains, and/or a supplement.
- Limit intake of refined carbohydrates such as white flour and sugar.
- Maintain a desirable weight to prevent metabolic syndrome, a major risk factor for CHD.

Hypertension

- Maintain a desirable weight.
- Limit daily sodium intake to 2,400 mg, the equivalent of about 1¼ teaspoons of table salt (sodium chloride). To achieve a more dramatic reduction in blood pressure, restrict sodium intake to 1,500 mg or less each day, the equivalent of about ⅔ teaspoon of salt.
- Increase intake of fruits and vegetables to get enough potassium. Aim for eight servings per day.
- Consume two to four servings of fat-free or low-fat dairy products each day for adequate calcium and protein.
- Include plenty of whole grains, fish, and poultry.
- Restrict intake of fat, red meat, and sugary foods and drinks.
- Limit consumption of alcohol to no more than one drink per day for women and no more than two drinks per day for men. One alcoholic drink equals one 12-oz. beer, one 5-oz. glass of wine, or one shot (1½ oz.) of 80-proof spirits.

ANTIOXIDANTS

Antioxidants are substances that help to counteract cell damage resulting from the formation of free radicals during normal metabolism. Free radicals are molecules that are highly reactive because they are missing one or more electrons. They seek to combine with other molecules, and can set off a chain reaction that rapidly passes electrons from molecule to molecule. At times, this process can be beneficial: For example, free radicals help the body fight bacteria and viruses. However, the rapid exchange of electrons can also damage cell membranes and DNA. Excess free radical production is now thought to contribute to many diseases, including CHD, cancer, and cataracts.

Type 2 Diabetes
- Maintain a desirable weight.
- Limit saturated fat intake to no more than 7% of total calories.
- Get at least 15% of total fat calories from monounsaturated fat.
- Limit dietary cholesterol to less than 200 mg per day, which requires restriction of all dietary sources of cholesterol, including eggs and shellfish.
- Get at least 25 g of fiber per day; include several servings of whole grains and foods rich in soluble fiber.
- Aim for eight servings per day of a variety of fruits and vegetables. At least one vegetable should be dark green and at least one fruit or vegetable should be orange or red.
- Restrict intake of refined carbohydrates, namely white flour and sugar.
- Choose an overall balanced diet that emphasizes fruits, vegetables, and whole grains.

Osteoporosis
- Consume 1,200 to 1,500 mg of calcium each day. See the feature on pages 22–23 for ways to increase calcium intake.
- Take calcium supplements if the dietary calcium in your diet is low.
- Get an adequate amount of vitamin D (400 to 800 IU per day).
- Limit sodium consumption to 2,400 mg per day.
- Follow a dietary pattern that emphasizes fruits, vegetables, and whole grains.
- Restrict caffeine consumption to less than 300 mg per day. Depending upon brewing methods, the average cup (8 oz.) of coffee contains between 115 and 175 mg caffeine; the average size (12 oz.) soda contains between 30 and 50 mg caffeine, depending upon the brand.

Breast Cancer
- Maintain a desirable weight.
- Limit fat intake, especially saturated fats and trans fatty acids.
- Get at least 25 g of fiber per day. Be sure to include several servings of whole grains.
- Eat at least five servings per day of a variety of fruits and vegetables. At least one vegetable should be dark green and at least one fruit or vegetable should be orange or red.
- Limit alcohol consumption to fewer than seven drinks per week.

Colon Cancer
- Limit your intake of red meat. Choose lean cuts and eat small portions (about 3 oz.).
- Eat several servings of whole grains and at least five servings of a variety of fruits and vegetables each day. Include plenty of spinach, broccoli, tomatoes, oranges, berries, and carrots.
- Consume 1,200 mg of calcium per day by eating calcium-rich foods, such as two to three servings of low fat or fat-free dairy products each day. For additional ways to increase your calcium intake, see pages 22–23.

Prostate Cancer
- Limit intake of fat from animal sources, especially meats and dairy products.
- Limit your intake of red meat. Choose lean cuts and eat small portions (about 3 oz.).
- Eat a diet rich in whole grains and have at least five servings per day of a variety of fruits and vegetables. At least one of the vegetables should be dark green and at least one fruit or vegetable should be orange or red. Include plenty of cruciferous vegetables, such as broccoli, cauliflower, and cabbage.
- Eat several servings of cooked tomato products (such as tomato sauce) per week.

A variety of antioxidants can either neutralize free radicals or repair the damage caused by them. Health problems can arise, however, when the body's production of free radicals overwhelms its natural antioxidant defenses. Foods that contain antioxidants—such as vitamins C and E, the mineral selenium, and a collection of plant pigments known as carotenoids (which includes beta-carotene)—can add to the body's supply of antioxidants. Other substances found in plants, known collectively as phytochemicals (see the section on phytochemicals, page 36), may also act as antioxidants. Each antioxidant has a different mode of action, and many of them appear to work together. For example, vitamin C helps to regenerate vitamin E once it has become oxidized. Therefore, it is important that your diet supplies adequate amounts of all of the antioxidants to achieve this synergy.

Antioxidants and CHD

Numerous studies have shown that people who eat a lot of fruits and vegetables are less likely to develop CHD. Some researchers attribute this benefit to the antioxidants in these foods, especially vitamin C, vitamin E, beta-carotene and other carotenoids. In studies that measured blood levels of these nutrients, high levels were associated with a reduced risk of CHD. However, three large trials have shown that vitamin E supplements provided no benefits in patients with known CHD. A major report recently issued by the Food and Nutrition Board of the National Academy of Sciences—the main authority in the United States for nutritional recommendations—also concluded that vitamin E supplements serve no purpose in helping to reduce CHD. Check with your doctor before taking extra vitamin E if you are taking daily warfarin (Coumadin) or aspirin, because these agents reduce the ability of the blood to clot.

Antioxidants and Cancer

Adequate intakes of beta-carotene and vitamin C have been linked to a reduced risk of cancers of the esophagus, stomach, pancreas, lung, colon, rectum, prostate, breast, ovaries, and cervix. Several studies found that people with low intakes or blood levels of antioxidants have a higher risk of these cancers.

In the studies that showed protective effects, fruits and vegetables—not supplements—were the key sources of these nutrients. In fact, clinical studies with supplements have proven how difficult it is to distinguish between the effect of a food and the effect of one of its many specific components. At best, such studies have produced disappointing results, and a few have even raised the possibility that high doses of a single antioxidant may be harmful. For example, the Physicians' Health Study found that beta-carotene supplements provided no protection against cancer, and two other studies found that beta-carotene supplements increase the incidence of lung cancer in smokers. In none of the three studies did beta-carotene supplements protect against CHD.

Some researchers hypothesize that the large amounts of beta-carotene in the supplements increased lung cancer incidence in these studies because the beta-carotene blocked the absorption of other carotenoids that are protective. This possibility underscores the potential dangers of overloading with one particular nutrient by taking large doses of supplements. Such studies should not stop people from eating foods that supply beta-carotene, which is only one of hundreds of carotenoids in foods. It is virtually impossible to

NEW RESEARCH

Healthy Diet Helps Maintain Mental Functions

Older people who eat a healthy diet are more likely to maintain their cognitive abilities than those who eat less healthful diets, say researchers from Italy.

Investigators interviewed 1,651 men and women (age 65 and older) using a 180-item food questionnaire to rate participants' diets as to the inclusion of various food groups and nutrients. Participants also received a test of cognitive function with an expanded version of the Mini-Mental State Examination.

People who ate a diet low in fat and sugar, moderate in alcohol, and high in fruits, vegetables, and complex carbohydrates were moderately, but significantly, less likely to have cognitive dysfunction than those who ate a less healthy diet. No single component of the diet contributed significantly to the results, suggesting that a combination of factors in a healthy diet contribute to the maintenance of cognitive function.

Because this study could not pinpoint if there are specific dietary components or combinations of components that may be responsible, and because this kind of study (an observational one, not a clinical trial) cannot provide definite proof of a relationship, more research is needed in the area of diet and mental function. Still, this study does add another possible advantage to the long list of reasons to eat a healthy diet.

EUROPEAN JOURNAL OF CLINICAL NUTRITION
Volume 55, page 1053
December 2001

get too much of any particular nutrient from foods alone.

Other carotenoids are still emerging as possibly protective against cancer and other disorders. For example, studies have suggested that tomatoes and tomato-based products are linked to a reduced risk of cancer, particularly prostate cancer. Tomatoes are a leading source of lycopene, the carotenoid that gives tomatoes their red color. The greatest protective effect of tomatoes appears to come from cooked tomato products, such as sauce, since cooking appears to concentrate the lycopene content and increase its absorption. Watermelon is another good source of lycopene.

Selenium is a mineral that has been associated with a reduced risk of developing various cancers. Selenium acts indirectly as an antioxidant; it is an essential component of certain enzymes that inactivate free radicals. Research indicates that people with a high intake of this mineral, and those who live in areas where the selenium content of the soil is high, have a lower risk of lung, colon, and other cancers. Selenium is found in Brazil nuts, fish, wheat germ and other grains, sunflower seeds, turkey, fruits, and vegetables. The amount of selenium in a particular food depends on the amount of the mineral in the soil where the food is grown. Preliminary studies suggest that selenium supplements may help reduce cancer incidence, but further research is necessary.

Antioxidants and Other Disorders

A diet rich in carotenoids, especially lutein and zeaxanthin, has been linked to a reduced risk of developing macular degeneration, an age-related visual disorder that reduces central vision. The retina (the light-sensitive portion of the eye that receives and transmits visual impulses to the brain via the optic nerve) is rich in lutein and zeaxanthin, and studies suggest that these carotenoids protect the macula—the most sensitive portion of the retina—from damaging ultraviolet rays.

In October 2001, researchers from the Age-Related Eye Disease Study (AREDS) reported in the *Archives of Ophthalmology* that taking a combination of antioxidant vitamins and zinc reduced the rate of progression of age-related macular degeneration (AMD) in some people. The AREDS researchers studied 3,640 people, age 55 to 80, who had no AMD, early AMD in one or both eyes, intermediate AMD in one or both eyes, or advanced AMD in one eye. Neither antioxidants nor zinc, alone or in combination, reduced the risk of developing AMD in people without the disease or slowed its progression in those with early AMD. However, people with intermediate

NEW RESEARCH

Tomato Products May Protect Against Prostate Cancer

A recent study has found more evidence that eating tomato products, which contain the antioxidant lycopene, may lower the risk of prostate cancer.

Researchers examined data from 47,365 men in the Health Professionals Follow-Up Study who completed questionnaires about their diet, including their intake of tomato sauce and lycopene (from tomato sauce and other foods such as watermelon and pink grapefruit).

Over a 12-year period, men who ate at least two servings of tomato sauce per week had a 23% lower risk of prostate cancer than men who ate less than one serving per month. Eating two or more servings per week also reduced the risk of metastatic prostate cancer by 35%. Similarly, men with the highest lycopene intake had a 16% lower risk of prostate cancer than men with the lowest lycopene intake.

More studies are needed to firmly establish whether lycopene, alone or in combination with other dietary components, actually reduces prostate cancer risk. In the meantime, it is reasonable for men to consume tomato-based products and other foods with lycopene on a regular basis.

JOURNAL OF THE NATIONAL CANCER INSTITUTE
Volume 94, page 391
March 6, 2002

Impediments to Optimum Nutrition

A nourishing, well-balanced diet can help prevent disabling illnesses like obesity, osteoporosis, heart disease, and type 2 diabetes. Studies show, however, that healthful eating can become more difficult as people grow older. Common obstacles to proper nutrition in older people include declining oral health, diminished absorption of nutrients, swallowing problems, a depressed appetite, and poor digestive health. Fortunately, these obstacles can often be surmounted. In addition to trying the tips below, you may want to ask your physician for a referral to a registered dietitian who can provide personalized advice based on your health needs and food preferences.

Chewing, Tooth, and Mouth Problems

Cavities, dry mouth, gum disease, loss of teeth, and the absence of dentures are common causes of diminished oral health. Declining oral health can alter taste, interfere with eating and the enjoyment of food, and jeopardize nutritional status.

To improve your consumption of food if you have mouth problems or difficulty chewing:

- Choose nutrient-dense foods that are easy to chew and swallow, such as applesauce, casseroles, cottage cheese, custards, fruit smoothies, mashed potatoes, milk shakes, puddings, soups, and yogurt.
- Chop or grind foods to minimize chewing. Try different food consistencies such as liquid, pureed, and soft.
- Moisten foods by adding low-fat sauce or gravy.
- Take small bites of food at a time.

Increased Need for B Vitamins

B vitamins are vital for the breakdown and utilization of carbohydrates, fats, and proteins. In addition, B vitamins help to ensure the proper functioning of the nervous system and the synthesis of red blood cells and genetic material. In addition, B vitamins such as folate, vitamin B_6 and vitamin B_{12}, help to reduce blood levels of homocysteine, a substance linked to heart disease.

Older adults may have greater requirements for certain B vitamins, particularly vitamins B_6 and B_{12}. An insufficient intake of vitamin B_6 may impair immune function in older adults, and the absorption of vitamin B_{12} diminishes with age. Some experts estimate that 10% to 30% of older adults are unable to absorb vitamin B_{12} efficiently from food, due to alterations in the cells lining the digestive tract or diminished secretion of a substance called intrinsic factor that is needed to absorb vitamin B_{12}.

To improve your levels of B vitamins:

- See the chart on pages 14-15 for food sources of B vitamins.
- Consult your physician about possible drug-nutrient interactions that may interfere with healthy levels of B vitamins and other nutrients.
- Consume foods enriched with vitamins, such as breakfast cereals, to boost your intake of folate, vitamin B_6, and vitamin B_{12}. It is important to

AMD or advanced AMD in one eye who took both antioxidants and zinc reduced their risk of progression to more advanced AMD by about 25%; in addition, these individuals lowered their risk of vision loss from AMD by 19%. Because the AREDS supplements contain larger dosages of vitamins and minerals than those present in a normal diet or a typical vitamin tablet, you should check with your primary care physician before starting to take the supplements. This caution applies especially to people receiving treatment for diabetes, heart disease, or cancer. In addition, the AREDS supplements may interfere with over-the-counter or prescription medications or interact with other dietary supplements or herbal preparations.

Vitamin E may help to improve the immune system and memory in older people. One study found that extremely high doses of vitamin E—2,000 IU per day—slowed the progression of Alzheimer disease (although no improvement in symptoms was noted in the patients). These possible effects are promising, but more research is

read the label to find out if the cereal has been enriched with B vitamins. Not all cereals have high levels of B vitamins.
• Consider taking a multivitamin supplement. Experts believe that most older adults can benefit from taking a multivitamin each day to ensure adequate intake of essential nutrients, including B vitamins.

Dysphagia (Difficulty Swallowing)
Every year, more than 10 million Americans, most over the age of 65, see a physician for dysphagia and other problems related to difficulty swallowing. To help minimize the potential for choking from dysphagia:
• Choose soft, east-to-swallow foods.
• Eat small, frequent meals.
• Avoid eating when tired.
• Do not talk or tilt your head back when swallowing.
• Sit upright when eating.

Depressed Appetite
A poor appetite may result from a variety of underlying factors, including illness, depression, and loss of taste or smell. Diminished appetite can also be a side effect of medication. To improve your appetite:
• Share meals with family, friends, and neighbors.
• Increase the flavor and aroma of food by preparing it with herbs and spices or tart ingredients such as lemon or vinegar.
• Have small, frequent meals throughout the day if you tend to feel full quickly.
• Alternate food textures, such as crunchy and soft, and vary taste sensations, such as sweet and sour.
• Avoid caffeine, cigarettes, and very hot or very cold food—all of which may diminish the flavor of food.
• Drink plenty of liquids, particularly if dry mouth—a common side effect of many medications—is depressing your appetite. But be aware that filling up with fluid at the beginning of a meal can decrease the amount of food you eat.

Poor Digestive Health
Digestive ailments, including upset stomach, heartburn, and abdominal discomfort, commonly suppress a healthy appetite and interfere with eating in older adults. To help remedy digestive problems, try the following suggestions:
• Avoid eating near bedtime, because lying down promotes the flow of food back into the esophagus, which can lead to heartburn.
• Avoid alcohol and caffeinated beverages.
• Limit gassy foods such as beans, broccoli, cabbage, brussels sprouts, cauliflower, bran, and carbonated beverages if these are a problem for you.
• Replace raw produce with fruit and vegetable juices and soft canned fruit if you find that raw fruits and vegetables are irritating.
• Eat small, low-fat meals throughout the day.
• Drink beverages between meals, instead of with meals.
• Restrict spicy, fatty, and acidic foods.
• Consult your physician about medical interventions to resolve underlying medical problems.

needed. Make sure to check with your doctor before taking extra vitamin E if you are taking daily warfarin (Coumadin) or aspirin, because all three of these agents reduce the ability of the blood to clot.

Recommendations for Antioxidant Intake

1. Get most of your antioxidants from fruits and vegetables, not supplements. A diet containing five to nine servings of fruits and vegetables per day can easily provide an adequate amount of vitamin C, beta-carotene, other carotenoids, dietary fiber, and phytochemicals, as well as other vitamins and minerals. The beneficial effect of antioxidants may only occur when they are consumed in combination with each other or with other substances, known and not known, in plant foods.

2. Focus on dark green vegetables and orange, red, and yellow fruits and vegetables. Fruits and vegetables of these colors are the most nutritious. They provide substantial amounts of carotenoids and vitamin C, as well as other beneficial nutrients.

3. Be sure to get the RDA for vitamin C: 75 mg for women and 90 mg for men. These amounts are easily obtained through diet. The vitamin chart on pages 14–15 lists some common dietary sources.

4. Don't take selenium supplements. The difference between an adequate and a toxic dose of selenium is quite small. People concerned that they are not getting enough selenium might consider a multivitamin-mineral supplement that contains no more than the RDA for selenium (55 mcg).

PHYTOCHEMICALS

Fruits, vegetables, and other plant foods may protect against disease. From anthocyanins, the red pigment in strawberries and cherries, to allylic sulfides, which are responsible for the pungent flavor of garlic and onions, plant foods contain a plethora of chemical compounds that give them color and flavor and even protect them from insects. These compounds, termed phytochemicals, may be responsible for part of the disease-preventing effect of fruits and vegetables.

Phytochemicals have no traditional nutritive value—that is, they are not vitamins or minerals—but they may have positive effects on the body over the long term. These effects include inhibiting tumor formation, producing an anticoagulant effect, blocking the cancer-promoting effect of certain hormones, and lowering cholesterol levels.

As noted in the antioxidant section (see page 30), studies exploring the effects of supplements (other than possibly vitamin E) have failed to show that a high intake of specific nutrients reduces the risk of disease. These observations leave open the possibility that other substances in plant foods, namely phytochemicals, may be important in disease prevention, either on their own or in combination with the antioxidants.

Phytochemicals are found in a wide variety of plant foods, and indeed many different phytochemicals are often present in a single food—for example, more than 170 have been identified in oranges. The vast number of compounds in fruits, vegetables, grains, and legumes makes it nearly impossible for supplements to substitute for a healthy diet. While the beneficial effects, if any, of phytochemicals have yet to be proven, the following show some promise for disease prevention.

Allylic sulfides. Found in onions and garlic, these substances may enhance immune function, help the body to excrete cancer-causing compounds, and interfere with the development of tumors.

Flavonoids. These compounds function as antioxidants. They may be involved in several actions, including extending the life of vitamin C, inhibiting tumor development, preventing the oxidation of LDL, and controlling inflammation. Various flavonoids are found in a host of fruits and vegetables, as well as in red wine, red and purple grape juice, and green and black tea.

Indoles, isothiocyanates, and sulforaphane. In 1992, researchers at Johns Hopkins found that broccoli, kale, brussels sprouts, and other members of the cabbage family (also known as cruciferous vegetables) contain a potent substance—sulforaphane—that stimulates cells to produce cancer-fighting enzymes. Since then, indoles and isothiocyanates, also present in cruciferous vegetables, have been found to act in a similar manner.

Phenolic acids. Ellagic acid, ferulic acid, and other phenolic acids may prevent damage to DNA. They are found in strawberries, raspberries, tomatoes, citrus fruits, whole grains, and nuts.

Phytoestrogens. These plant substances are converted to estrogen-like compounds by bacteria in the intestine. They are present in many common foods, especially soybeans and soy products such as tofu and soy milk. Lignans and isoflavones are examples of phytoestrogens. Researchers believe that these compounds may help prevent breast cancer by stopping the estrogen produced in the body from entering cells. In addition, the estrogen-like effect produced by these compounds may temper the production of testosterone in men and thus help to thwart prostate cancer. Some reports also suggest that women who eat a lot of soy products have fewer hot flashes associated with menopause.

Soy products may also lower blood cholesterol levels. In a meta-analysis of 38 studies where soy protein replaced animal protein in people's diets, eating an average of 47 g of soy protein per day lowered total cholesterol by about 9%, LDL cholesterol by 13%, and triglycerides by 11%. It is not known whether soy products lower cholesterol levels simply by replacing saturated fats with unsaturated fats (soybeans derive 38% of their calories from fat, mostly unsaturated) or from the isoflavones in soybeans. In one study of 156 men and women on a low-fat, low-cholesterol diet, participants with LDL cholesterol levels averaging 184 mg/dL experienced 9% and 10% reductions in total and LDL cholesterol levels, respectively, while consuming beverages containing 62 mg of isoflavones. Both total and LDL cholesterol levels fell 8% when beverages containing 37 mg of isoflavones were consumed. HDL cholesterol levels and

NEW RESEARCH

Tea Consumption May Protect Against Fatal Heart Attacks

Consumption of black tea—particularly of the antioxidant-containing compounds in tea called flavonoids—is related to a decreased risk of fatal heart attacks, a recent investigation shows.

Dutch researchers obtained dietary, lifestyle, and demographic data from 4,807 people (age 55 and older), who had never suffered a heart attack.

After an average follow-up of almost six years, people who drank more than 12 oz. of black tea each day were 70% less likely to have a heart attack than those who did not drink tea. People who consumed the most flavonoids in their diet, regardless of the source, were 65% less likely to have a fatal heart attack than individuals who consumed the lowest amount of flavonoids.

While some of the association between tea intake and a decreased risk of heart attack could be explained by the fact that tea drinkers tend to be thinner and more educated and smoke less, these factors did not account for all of the decreased risk.

Flavonoids may help reduce the risk of fatal heart attacks by preventing oxidation of low density lipoproteins, inhibiting platelet aggregation, reducing inflammation, and/or improving vascular function, the researchers speculate. Other food sources of flavonoids include fruits and vegetables.

AMERICAN JOURNAL OF CLINICAL NUTRITION
Volume 75, page 880
May 2002

triglycerides were unchanged.

Saponins. These sugar-like compounds have an antibacterial effect. Saponins may strengthen the immune system, prevent microbial and fungal infections, and fight viruses. They are found in potatoes, tomatoes, legumes, oats, soy products, and spinach.

Recommendations for Phytochemical Intake

1. Follow a plant-based diet. Eat five to nine servings of fruits and vegetables and at least six servings of grain products each day, and consume legumes several times a week. Vary the choices to get a wide range of phytochemicals, but focus on dark green vegetables, red and orange fruits and vegetables, and whole grains.

2. Season foods with herbs and spices. Such seasonings also contain phytochemicals. Try using garlic, onions, ginger, basil, oregano, parsley, rosemary, cumin, curry powder, cayenne pepper, red chili pepper, and cinnamon, to name a few.

3. Incorporate soy products. Tofu, soy protein, soy milk, soy flour, soy butter, and meat analogues are all examples. The amounts of soy protein in various soy foods are 8 oz. of soy milk, 4 to 10 g; 4 oz. of tofu, 8 to 13 g; 1 oz. of soy flour, 10 to 13 g; ½ cup of textured soy protein, 11 g; and 3.2 oz. of meat analogue, 18 g. Many soy products taste better than they did several years ago; "veggie" burgers, for example, have become popular, though not all vegetarian burgers are made from tofu (check the label). Tofu and other soy products are mild tasting and pick up the flavor of the foods they are cooked with; try mixing textured soy protein into meat loaf, casserole, or chili recipes. Soy flour can substitute for up to one quarter of the total flour in baking recipes. Tofu can be stir-fried with vegetables or added to soups, and soy butter can be spread on bread in place of peanut butter.

ENHANCED FOODS

As part of an effort to ensure that people eat well, and to help with disease prevention, several areas of food research are devoted to improving the types of foods we eat. These foods include ones that have been enriched or fortified with the addition of healthy components, as well as foods that have been genetically modified to provide certain nutrients. The concept of using food as a way to prevent disease is not new. Beginning in the 1920s, iodine was added to salt to prevent goiters; later, milk was fortified with vitamin D to prevent rickets.

Enriched Food

An enriched food contains nutrients that are added to increase the amount originally present or to replace nutrients lost during processing. An example is white rice that is enriched with B vitamins and iron that were lost during processing.

Fortified Food

Fortified foods are fortified with additional vitamins and/or minerals; they are marketed to promote health and prevent disease. The added nutrients were not present in the original food or were present in lower amounts. Such foods include folic acid-fortified wheat products, calcium-fortified orange juices, and vitamin D-fortified milk.

Functional Food

Although the U.S. Food and Drug Administration(FDA) has made no legal definition of functional foods (see www.cfsan.fda.gov/label.html), many groups use this term to refer to foods with specific health benefits that go beyond traditional nutritional effects. Because there is no uniform definition, the term is applied in different ways. It is sometimes used to refer only to enhanced foods, such as enriched and fortified foods; sometimes the term refers to natural foods with probable benefits. An example is the tomato as a source of lycopene.

Nutraceuticals

Pharmaceutical companies have also started to manufacture functional foods that are intended to have drug-like effects. Broadly known as nutraceuticals, these functional foods rack up billions of dollars in sales. Fruit juice and iced tea with added herbs like ginkgo biloba are examples of nutraceuticals. Experts predict that nutraceuticals could be one of the biggest growth areas in food production. The incredible increase in the number of nutraceuticals on the market in the past few years does not indicate that their health claims have been substantiated. There is little evidence that these products are beneficial, and many of the ingredients used in nutraceuticals have not even been tested in clinical trials.

Genetically Modified Food

Genetic modification of food is another food science initiative, though this technology remains highly controversial. Genetic modification introduces new genes into crops to improve their health benefits or make them hardier. With the world population expect-

NEW RESEARCH

Phytosterols and Cholesterol

Naturally occurring plant compounds called phytosterols can lower cholesterol levels and may reduce the risk of coronary heart disease (CHD), according to a recent review.

Similar in structure to cholesterol, phytosterols are present in all plant foods but are particularly concentrated in vegetable oils, including corn and sunflower oil. The addition of chemically modified phytosterols, called phytosterol esters, to some margarines provide cholesterol-lowering benefits.

While only minute amounts of phytosterols (and phytosterol esters) are absorbed from the digestive tract, these compounds interfere with the absorption of cholesterol from the intestine.

Data from supplement studies indicate that consuming 2 g of phytosterol esters a day safely and effectively reduces levels of LDL cholesterol by about 10%. Furthermore, phytosterol esters complement the cholesterol-lowering effects of statin drugs commonly prescribed for high cholesterol.

According to the review, it is possible that consuming large amounts of phytosterols from supplements and from foods could reduce the risk of CHD. Though more research is needed to evaluate the long-term safety of phytosterol supplements, the data that have accumulated thus far indicate they are quite safe.

ANNUAL REVIEWS IN NUTRITION
Volume 22, page 533
January 2002

ed to double over the next 50 years, a shortage of food is a pressing concern. In addition to honing traditional agricultural techniques to assure a plentiful food supply, research scientists have become increasingly involved in developing genetically engineered food for the same purpose.

Agriculturists have been interbreeding plants of the same or similar species for years to develop crops with improved appearance, durability, or productivity. Genetic modification, however, takes this idea several steps further. It involves identifying and isolating a specific, favorable trait from a plant, animal, bacterium, or virus and then introducing the gene that encodes that trait into another species. For example, crops are currently being modified genetically to resist weed-killing herbicides, repel insects, or contain more nutrients. In addition, genetic modification will most likely influence what we eat and even the medications used to fight disease. Scientists are experimenting with reprogramming plant genes to reduce unhealthy fats, yield biodegradable plastics, and act as antigens, a kind of edible vaccine against infectious organisms. It may be several years, however, before the results of such applications are available to consumers.

Clearly, genetic modification may produce significant agricultural alterations. It may change the makeup of crops and their ability to repel insects and resist toxins. Precisely because of these fundamental changes, genetic modification of food crops has been subject to a lot of controversy, and foods from some such crops are banned from being imported into Europe. Critics argue that we are experimenting with the food supply with a limited understanding of possible far-reaching consequences. The unpredictable consequences of genetic modifications make opponents fear major repercussions to the entire ecosystem. Although genetically altered foods have been tested and are considered safe, long-term studies have not examined their environmental impact. Agriculturists are examining ways to minimize any harmful impact on the environment.

FOOD SAFETY

U.S. consumers have one of the safest supplies of food in the world, but the increasing global exchange of food has recently highlighted the risk of foodborne diseases and suggested the need for an international agreement on standards for food production. In any case, research continues on ways to prevent food contamination.

The National Animal and Disease Center is developing several

RECENT ADVISORY

Sprout Warning

A recent outbreak of food poisoning from alfalfa sprouts has prompted the U.S. Food and Drug Administration (FDA) to renew its 1999 warning against eating raw or lightly cooked sprouts, including alfalfa, clover, and mung bean, which raise the risk of foodborne illness from *E. coli* and Salmonella bacteria.

Children, the elderly, and people with compromised immune systems are at especially high risk and should avoid raw or lightly cooked sprouts. Foodborne illness in these individuals can lead to serious health complications or death.

Common symptoms of foodborne illness in healthy people, which may last for several days, include abdominal discomfort, diarrhea, fever, and nausea.

To prevent food poisoning from sprouts, the government recommends that consumers:

- thoroughly cook all sprouts before consuming;
- request that raw or lightly cooked sprouts not be added to food when dining out;
- avoid eating homegrown, raw or lightly cooked sprouts because a seed may be contaminated with harmful germs, even if the seed is grown in a clean environment; and
- consult a physician if experiencing symptoms of food poisoning.

FOOD AND DRUG ADMINISTRATION
October 2, 2002

Organic Foods

More Americans are turning to organic foods out of a concern for the environment as well as a desire to minimize their exposure to certain chemicals in their food. As a result, the market for organic foods is thriving. Over the past decade, consumer demand for organic foods has increased 20% or more each year in the United States. The Food Marketing Institute estimates that approximately 40% of all U.S. shoppers have purchased at least one organic product. A diverse array of organic goods—from produce to frozen foods—is readily available to consumers, and the popularity of organic foods is expected to continue. But how can consumers be sure that a food labeled organic is really grown organically? And are organic foods better than conventional foods?

What Is Organic?

A national definition of "organic" was recently established by the federal government. This definition encompasses a set of standards that governs the production, labeling, and marketing of organic foods. In order to be called organic, a food must be produced without using bio-engineered foods, herbicides, irradiation, pesticides, synthetic fertilizers, or sewage sludge. Organic livestock must be given 100% organic feed, and antibiotics and growth hormones are prohibited. Only certain substances that are deemed safe and approved by the U.S. Department of Agriculture (USDA) and published in a national list are permitted in the production and handling of organic plants and livestock.

Organic Product Labels

To be sure a food is organic, look on the label for a "USDA Certified Organic" seal. Only products that meet the federal government's criteria for the production, handling, and processing of foods qualify for this seal. While all organic foods carry the basic seal of approval, labels identifying foods as "organic" differ according to the quantity of organic ingredients the food contains:

- **100% organic** means the food contains *only* organically produced raw or processed ingredients, with the exception of water and salt.
- **Organic** indicates that 95% of the ingredients are organically produced and the remaining 5% are from the USDA-approved national list.
- **Made with organic ingredients** denotes that at least 70% of the ingredients in the product are organic. For more information on organic food labels and regulations, visit the USDA's National Organic Program Web site at www.ams.usda.gov/nop.

Is Organic Better?

Currently, there is no scientific evidence that organic foods are safer, better in quality, or more nutritious than conventional foods. In addition, although many consumers perceive organic foods as healthier than conventional foods, a USDA Certified Organic seal does not signify freshness, enhanced taste, or superior quality or nutritional content. Nor does organic guarantee a food is pesticide-free: Up to 5% pesticide residues are permitted in organic foods.

Some reports in the popular media have suggested that certain organic farming methods may make organic foods more likely to harbor harmful microorganisms, particularly *E. coli*. However, current scientific data indicate that both organic and nonorganic foods are equally susceptible to food-borne pathogens, including aflatoxin and *E. coli*. To minimize the risk of foodborne illness, organic foods must be treated with the same proper food handling practices as nonorganic foods.

"Natural" vs. "Organic"

The terms "natural" and "organic" are not synonymous, according to the U.S. Department of Agriculture. In order to be called natural, a food cannot contain artificial ingredients or added colors. A natural product is required to be minimally processed, so that the original raw product is unchanged. When the term natural is used on a label, it must be accompanied by an explanation of the use of the term, such as no artificial ingredients or no added color.

The Politics of Organics

Because organic agriculture helps to protect and recycle natural resources, organically grown foods may have environmental benefits on soil and water resources. However, the unique production expenses required for organic farming lead to higher market costs for organic foods than conventional ones. In addition, some detractors criticize organic farming for its lower crop yields compared with conventional farming. Of key importance is the continuing availability of affordable fruit and vegetables, which are vital for our nutritional needs.

faster and more advanced tests to identify foodborne pathogens, and the USDA and FDA are supporting a "farm-to-table" approach to eliminate and control foodborne toxins at all steps along the chain of food production and consumption. One recent advance uses antibodies that bind to toxins produced by bacteria and fungi (molds) to measure the content of the organisms in foods. Referred to as ELISA (enzyme-linked immunosorbent assay), these highly sensitive tests can identify trace amounts of a toxin and take less time than traditional disease-detection strategies. ELISA test kits to detect bacterial toxins in food are currently in development for use by farmers.

Other strategies to fight foodborne bacteria are evolving from developments in genetic therapy and molecular biology. For example, scientists found that inactivating a gene called DAM can disarm the ability of a strain of salmonella to cause disease. These detection and prevention approaches, combined with proper food preparation and refrigeration techniques, should help to further improve the safety of our food supply.

WEIGHT CONTROL

In addition to adopting good overall nutritional habits, one of the most important ways to preserve good health is to control your weight. By shedding pounds, overweight people can reduce their risk of type 2 diabetes, high blood pressure, and coronary heart disease (CHD). Losing weight may lower low density lipoprotein (LDL) cholesterol, which is often referred to as "bad" cholesterol. Losing weight can also lower triglycerides and even increase high density lipoprotein (HDL) cholesterol, referred to as "good" cholesterol. In addition, weight loss can help to reduce the risk of osteoarthritis and gallstones.

In theory, weight control is a simple matter of balancing energy intake (the calories supplied by food) with energy output (the calories expended by physical activity and metabolism). To lose weight, you need to expend more energy than you take in. In practice, however, the task is clearly not that simple. Obesity—the medical term for excessive amounts of body fat—is a chronic condition, like hypertension or diabetes. While the basic principle of energy balance remains true, several mechanisms—genetic, metabolic, and environmental—control how much you eat and how your body uses and stores energy.

Even if some of the components involved in weight regulation are beyond your control, environmental factors have a significant impact. By manipulating these factors to your advantage, you can successfully lose weight and keep it off.

METABOLISM

A certain amount of calories are needed to supply the energy required for metabolism and everyday activities. When more calories are consumed than are needed, these extra calories are stored primarily as fat—whether the calories come from fat, carbohydrates, or proteins, though dietary fat is converted into body fat most efficiently.

During digestion, enzymes in the small intestine break down carbohydrates into simple sugars like glucose, proteins into amino acids, and triglycerides (dietary fat) into fatty acids and glycerol. Simple sugars and amino acids are rapidly absorbed from the small intestine into the bloodstream. The liver converts other sugars, like fructose and lactose, into glucose, which is used as a source of energy. Amino acids can be used as an energy source but serve mainly as building blocks for body proteins. Fatty acids combine with bile salts to form tiny droplets that promote their entry into cells in the intestinal wall, where they are again formed into triglycerides. The triglycerides are packaged into a type of transport lipoprotein called chylomicrons, which carry the triglycerides to the adipose tissue (fat) for storage of any triglycerides not immediately used to provide energy.

Any excess carbohydrates and protein not immediately used for energy are converted to glycogen and triglycerides in the liver. These triglycerides are transported from the liver on another lipoprotein (very low density lipoprotein) for storage in various parts of the body in individual adipose tissue cells, located just beneath the skin or around the intestines.

To store more fat, the body either creates more fat cells (a process called hyperplasia, which generally occurs only in childhood-onset obesity, during pregnancy, or with rapid weight gain in adults) or enlarges existing fat cells (hypertrophy, the primary way that adults increase their adipose tissue). If faced with a shortage of calories—as when a person diets—the body uses the fat stored in these cells as a source of energy. Unfortunately, once fat cells are formed they can shrink, but they are not eliminated.

FACTORS THAT AFFECT BODY WEIGHT

Controllable factors—such as a high-calorie diet, inappropriate psychological responses to food, and a lack of exercise—play a critical role in the development of obesity. But scientific research has confirmed that more is involved than just a lack of willpower or a sedentary lifestyle.

NEW RESEARCH

Overweight and Obesity on the Rise

Rates of overweight and obesity are higher than ever, according to the Centers for Disease Control and Prevention, which estimates that more than 6 in 10 American adults are overweight.

These disturbing data come from the 1999-2000 National Health and Nutrition Examination Survey, which examined a cross-section of 4,115 American adults age 20 to 74. Height and weight were measured to calculate body mass index (BMI). Overweight was defined as a BMI of 25 or greater, obesity as a BMI of 30 or more, and extreme obesity as a BMI of 40 or higher.

Approximately 65% of adults in 1999-2000 were overweight, compared with 56% in 1988-1994. Obesity rose from 23% in 1988-1994 to 31% in 1999-2000 and extreme obesity climbed from 3% to 5%. While increases were found in all age, gender, and ethnic groups, excessive weight was most prevalent among African-American women: 80% were overweight, half were obese, and 15% were extremely obese.

The findings raise serious concerns about the potential for a surge in obesity-related conditions, including diabetes, heart disease, arthritis, and certain cancers. The authors conclude that immediate action is necessary to thwart the increasingly high prevalence of overweight and obesity.

JOURNAL OF THE AMERICAN MEDICAL ASSOCIATION
Volume 288, page 1723
October 2002

Body Mass Index and Waist Circumference

Body mass index (BMI) and waist circumference measurements are two tools that can be used to determine whether your weight and distribution of body fat might be unhealthy. Current research indicates that a combination of BMI and waist circumference is a better indicator of disease risk associated with overweight and obesity than either of these measurements alone.

Body Mass Index

According to current guidelines from the National Institutes of Health, overweight is defined as a BMI of 25 to 29.9 and obesity as a BMI of 30 and above. (See the inset box to estimate your BMI.) The guidelines recommend that overweight and obese individuals reduce their weight by 10% over a period of six months—the equivalent of losing about one to two pounds per week. However, BMI may not provide an accurate assessment of risk for everyone. For example, BMI may overestimate body fat in extremely muscular individuals. Furthermore, the current guidelines are not age-specific and may be too restrictive for older adults.

BMI by Height and Weight

Without calculating your BMI, you can use this chart to see whether you are at your ideal weight. Find your height in the left-hand column, then read to the right. The middle column shows how much you would weigh if you had a BMI of 25 (overweight); the right-hand column shows your weight with a BMI of 30 (obese).

Height	Body Weight in Pounds BMI = 25	 BMI = 30
4'10"	119 lbs	143 lbs
4'11"	124	148
5'0"	128	153
5'1"	132	158
5'2"	136	164
5'3"	141	169
5'4"	145	174
5'5"	150	180
5'6"	155	186
5'7"	159	191
5'8"	164	197
5'9"	169	203
5'10"	174	207
5'11"	179	215
6'0"	184	221
6'1"	189	227
6'2"	194	233
6'3"	200	240
6'4"	205	246

Waist Circumference

Measuring the circumference of the waist helps to determine fat distribution in the body, specifically abdominal fat, which is an indicator of disease risk. Research shows that the mortality rates and incidence of certain chronic diseases, such as diabetes and high blood pressure, are substantially higher in those with a disproportionate amount of body fat stored in the abdomen.

To measure your waist circumference, wrap a tape measure around your waist at the level of the top of your hip bones; it should feel snug without compressing the skin. Measure after exhaling normally. A normal waist circumference is less than 40 inches in men and less than 35 inches in women. While BMI is a general assessment of body weight and disease risk, waist circumference provides an added and more specific measure of health risk because waist circumference indicates harmful abdominal fat. Even in people of normal weight, an increased waist circumference may be linked to an elevated health risk. And in men and women who are overweight or obese, a high waist circumference increases the already elevated risk of disease. But people with a BMI of 35 or higher have a high risk of disease, regardless of their waist circumference.

Risk Factors That Cannot Be Changed

Although these factors are beyond your control, their impact on weight can be modified by changes in diet and physical activity.

Heredity. Studies show that 80% of children born to two obese parents will themselves become obese, compared with 14% of children born to normal-weight parents. Research on identical twins shows similarly high rates of inheritance. However, studies comparing the weights of adoptees with the weights of their biological and adopted parents indicate that genetic factors are responsible for only about one third of the variance in weight, a figure experts believe is more accurate. Heredity seems to influence the number of fat cells (adipocytes) in the body, how much fat is stored, where it is stored, and the resting metabolic rate. About 80% of obese children become obese adults, though only 20% of obese adults were obese as children.

A number of genes appear to be responsible for the regulation of body weight. A major advance occurred in 1994 when researchers at Rockefeller University discovered that mutations in a gene—termed the obesity (ob) gene—in one strain of mice prevented them from producing leptin, a hormone normally manufactured by adipose tissue cells and released into the bloodstream to inform the brain about the body's level of fat stores. When this communication system works correctly, the hypothalamic area of the brain responds to leptin by reducing appetite and speeding up metabolism to maintain a normal level of body fat. Because mice with the mutated ob gene did not produce leptin, their brains continued to prompt the storage of fat and they became obese. When leptin was injected into these obese mice, they quickly lost weight through a combination of decreased food intake and increased activity.

Mice who had no mutation but had simply been overfed lost some weight with leptin injections, but much less than the leptin-lacking mice. A second strain of obese mice (db) had high leptin levels, but did not respond to leptin because of a mutation in the gene for the leptin receptor in the hypothalamus (the site in the brain that normally receives the leptin message). Unraveling the links between leptin and weight may lead to the development of more effective drugs for weight loss.

Metabolism is the process that extracts and utilizes energy (measured in calories) from food. Even at rest, energy is needed for many functions, such as respiration, heart contractions, and cell repair and growth. The amount of energy used for these basic functions while a person is awake and at rest is known as the resting metabolic rate (RMR), which accounts for about 70% of energy utilization each day (although this percentage is lower in physically active individuals). RMR is affected by weight, age, and the ratio of lean tissue (muscle) to adipose tissue (fat), since muscle is metabolically more active than fat—that is, muscle utilizes more energy even at rest. RMR is also in part genetically determined.

Food intake itself generates energy expenditure because energy is needed to digest food, absorb nutrients, and store excess calories as body fat. This process—called the thermic effect of food or thermogenesis—accounts for 10% to 15% of the body's total daily energy expenditure. Some research suggests that obese people require slightly less energy for thermogenesis, and so more of the calories they eat are stored as body fat rather than used to process food.

Whether or not obese people have an abnormally slow metabolism is a matter of controversy. Because it takes more energy to maintain a greater body mass, a person who weighs 200 lbs. has a higher RMR than one who weighs 150 lbs. In addition, a heavier person expends more calories than a leaner one for any given physical activity. But even when people of the same height, weight, age, sex, and lean body mass are compared, RMR may vary by 20% or more. Consequently, someone who would be predicted to use 1,200 calories through RMR may actually use anywhere from 1,080 to 1,320 calories. This variability could explain why two people who weigh the same may require different amounts of calories to maintain, lose, or gain weight.

Set point theory. According to this theory, each person has a predetermined level of body fat. How the body controls its fat stores is unknown, but the regulatory mechanism, sometimes called the adipostat, is probably located in the hypothalamus. (Other regions of the brain may also play a role.) The adipostat monitors body fat stores, possibly through the actions of leptin on its hypothalamic receptor, and works to maintain the prescribed level of fat, or set point, by adjusting appetite, physical activity, and RMR to conserve or expend energy. Thus, actions perceived to be voluntary, such as eating and physical activity, may be subtly controlled by the set point mechanism.

Factors That Can Be Changed

The following known factors are amenable to individual control.

Dietary intake. Eating more calories than you expend is an important cause of obesity. In fact, regardless of genetic predisposition or any other factors, you cannot gain weight without consuming more calories than you burn. Even small excesses in calorie intake—too small to measure accurately in the most rigorous study—can contribute to obesity over the long term. For example, a person who overeats by just 25 calories a day will consume 9,125 excess calories over the course of a year and so will gain 2½ lbs. (a pound of body fat is equivalent to 3,500 calories). A woman weighing 125 lbs. who starts this pattern at age 20 would weigh 175 lbs. by the time she is 40.

To point to overeating as the cause of obesity is overly simplistic, however. It does not explain why one 125-lb. woman needs 1,800 calories a day to meet her body's energy needs and avoid losing weight, while another 125-lb. woman struggles to avoid gaining weight on 1,200 calories a day.

Numerous other factors contribute to weight gain, including RMR and physical activity. Nevertheless, obese people must be consuming more calories than required by their individual make-ups and activity levels; otherwise they would not store excess body fat. A reduction in calorie intake is essential for weight loss.

Physical activity. Variations in physical activity can have a tremendous impact on total daily energy expenditure. A sedentary person may burn just a few hundred calories above RMR while going about daily activities (working, performing household chores, or walking to the mailbox, for example), whereas an athlete can burn an additional 3,000 calories each day through vigorous exercise. Regular exercise not only burns calories, but it also builds lean muscle mass and raises RMR because muscle requires more energy for maintenance. A low level of activity may be the most important factor responsible for the high and rising rate of obesity in the United States.

Behavioral and psychological issues. Several psychological factors affect weight control. The message to eat often comes from external cues rather than hunger—noon means it's time for lunch, for example. Food and emotions are closely linked; many people use food for comfort or to release tension. Obese people often eat quickly, and eating too fast can lead to taking in more calories than are needed to satisfy hunger. The amount of exercise a person engages in is also shaped by habit and attitudes toward physical activity. Some studies suggest that lean people may expend more energy than obese people in ordinary activities, as well as during formal exercise. For example, lean people may walk around (rather than sit) while on the phone, or may take the stairs rather than an elevator or escalator.

Hormonal (endocrine) abnormalities. An underactive thyroid (hypothyroidism) is often a layperson's explanation for obesity, but even when present, hypothyroidism is rarely a primary cause. Other conditions that may affect weight include polycystic ovary disease; tumors of the pituitary or adrenal glands; an insufficient produc-

NEW RESEARCH

Eating Breakfast Is Associated With Permanent Weight Loss

While skipping breakfast may be a tempting way to cut calories, people who achieve long-term weight loss tend to eat breakfast each day, according to recent findings.

The study involved 2,959 people (average age 46 years, 79% women, 95% white, and 64% married) enrolled in the National Weight Control Registry, which tracks American adults who have maintained a weight loss of at least 30 lbs. for a year or more. Participants completed questionnaires about their weight, diet, and levels of physical activity. The participants had maintained an average weight loss of 71 lbs. for six years.

Almost 80% of the participants reported eating breakfast every day and nearly 90% consumed breakfast four or more days per week. Only 4% reported that they never ate breakfast. Over half of the breakfast eaters said they often or always had hot or cold cereal and/or fruit for breakfast. Compared with breakfast non-eaters, breakfast eaters consumed the same number of calories daily but were slightly more physically active.

Eating breakfast is a behavior common to people who achieve permanent weight loss, conclude the researchers. They speculate that eating breakfast may quell hunger throughout the day and may foster higher levels of physical activity.

OBESITY RESEARCH
Volume 10, page 78
February 2002

The Risks of High-Protein Diets

High-protein diets in various guises have been around since the 1960s, but there has been a recent resurgence in their popularity. Such diets—including *Dr. Atkins' New Diet Revolution, The Zone,* and *Protein Power*—are still promoting the same basic idea that was put forth three decades ago: Eat high-protein, high-fat foods (such as meat and eggs) and restrict carbohydrate-rich foods (such as potatoes, pasta, fruits, and certain vegetables). However, several specific health concerns are associated with a diet that puts such a strong emphasis on the consumption of protein and fat and the restriction of carbohydrates.

Too Much Protein

The amount of protein recommended in high-protein diets exceeds established dietary requirements and may impose health risks. An inordinate intake of protein places extra stress on the liver and kidneys because they have to metabolize and excrete more than the normal amount of waste products. Kidney stones can be caused or aggravated by the high uric acid levels created by high-protein foods. And for those who have diabetes or kidney disease, high-protein diets can speed the progression of kidney disease, even if the diet is followed for a short time (see the sidebar on page 50). Furthermore, some studies suggest that eating too much protein causes excessive calcium loss, which can contribute to osteoporosis.

Too Much Fat

People who lose weight generally assume they are reducing their risk for atherosclerosis; however, a high-protein diet is more likely to harm arteries than help them. Because the protein in high-protein diets is generally derived from animal sources, such as meat, eggs, and cheese, these diets supply large amounts of saturated fat. Saturated fat raises the blood level of low density lipoprotein (LDL), the ("bad") cholesterol, and thus increases the risk for atherosclerosis. Fortunately, most people do not remain on such diets long enough to increase their risk of heart disease.

Low Carbohydrate Intake and Ketosis

The restriction of carbohydrates on a high-protein diet can increase the metabolism of fatty acids and cause ketosis. Ketosis results when excessive amounts of acidic substances known as ketone bodies are released into the bloodstream. Ketosis can be dangerous for people with known or unrecognized heart disease, diabetes, or kidney problems. During pregnancy, ketosis can cause abnormal development of the fetus. It is also worth noting that ketosis can affect the action of certain medications, especially those used to treat high blood pressure.

Nutritional Deficiencies

Inadequate vitamin and mineral intake can result from following a diet that eliminates healthful, carbohydrate-rich foods such as grains, fruits, and vegetables. These foods provide essential vitamins and minerals, as well as fiber, that help to prevent diseases and are necessary for overall health. In fact, one of the basic underlying problems with high-protein diets is their failure to promote a balanced diet and to teach long-term healthful eating habits.

Short-Term Use Is Probably Safe

While there are many limitations and risks with these diets, they may generate weight loss. So, if you are healthy, it is probably safe to stay on a high-protein, low-carbohydrate diet for only a few weeks or months, with proper vitamin and mineral supplements. However, for people with medical conditions such as kidney disease, heart disease, or diabetes, these diets are not a good idea, even in the short term. High-protein, low-carbohydrate diets are best used selectively and under medical supervision.

The Bottom Line: Lose Weight Safely

The hallmarks of a healthy weight-loss diet are flexibility, an emphasis on variety, and an ability to

tion of sex hormones; and insulin-producing tumors of the pancreas. Nevertheless, while they are uncommon, these disorders need to be ruled out by a thorough medical evaluation before determining the best course of action to achieve weight loss.

MEDICAL CONSEQUENCES OF OBESITY

Mortality rates are substantially higher in obese adults, especially in those whose excessive fat is stored in the abdomen rather than in

The Diet Debate

The controversy over high-protein diets leaves many consumers (as well as some health professionals) confused and uncertain about their food choices. Proponents of high-protein diets say that more than 20 years of low-fat recommendations have not lowered the incidence of heart disease in this country, and instead may have contributed to the increase in obesity and type 2 diabetes. On the other side of the debate, defenders of low-fat diets (and those critical of high-protein diets) say that a variety of factors can explain the obesity epidemic.

The low-fat diet perspective. Advocates of low-fat diets state that Americans are eating about 400 more calories a day than they did decades ago. This increase in caloric intake, they contend, has occurred gradually due to the rise in portion sizes as well as declining physical activity levels. Furthermore, when nutritionists sent out the message to reduce fats, many Americans began eating more carbohydrates than were recommended. Also, people assumed that they could eat fat substitutes with abandon. They did not realize that many fat-free foods have just as many calories as their original high-fat versions.

Proponents of low-fat diets cite evidence that diets rich in fruits and vegetables and moderate in protein and fat can help prevent diseases like high blood pressure, prostate cancer, heart disease, and diabetes. They also hold that a low-fat diet helps to control weight because complex carbohydrates have fewer calories than fats.

The high-protein diet perspective. One of the principal beliefs promoted by high-protein diets is that carbohydrates increase the body's production of insulin, which promotes weight gain by speeding up the conversion of food to body fat. Proponents of these diets also maintain that carbohydrates are less filling than other foods, which causes people to consume more calories in an effort to satisfy their hunger.

Advocates of high-protein diets point out that in some people, a low-fat, high-carbohydrate diet can raise triglyceride levels and lower high density lipoprotein (HDL) cholesterol levels—two components of metabolic syndrome, a cluster of conditions that can lead to heart disease and type 2 diabetes.

Once relegated to the realm of quackery, the high-protein diet is now being taken seriously by some researchers who concede that people can lose weight on such diets. A recent study conducted at Duke University Medical Center showed that overweight people who were placed on a very-low-carbohydrate diet program achieved and maintained weight loss during a six-month period. Other studies are also under way to investigate how these diets work.

What to do. For now, as the diet pendulum swings, health experts concede that a low-fat diet may not be the only or best way to lose weight. The question still remains, however, whether high-protein, low-carbohydrate diets are safe and effective on a long-term basis.

accommodate people with diverse needs and food preferences. A safe and effective weight loss program promotes regular exercise and includes all of the recommended daily allowances for vitamins, minerals, and protein. Long-term weight loss can be achieved by a lifelong commitment to portion control (see the feature on portion control on pages 60–61), calorie restriction, and regular exercise. If you need to lose weight, consult your doctor or dietitian to discuss a sensible weight loss plan. Contact the American Dietetic Association at 800-366-1655 or visit their Web site at www.eatright.org for current and accurate nutrition information and to find a qualified nutrition expert.

the hips. In fact, abdominal obesity is particularly dangerous because it leads to resistance to the actions of insulin, the hormone that regulates blood glucose. Insulin resistance results in elevated blood levels of insulin, which is associated with high triglycerides, low HDL cholesterol, high blood pressure, and increased CHD risk, a constellation of conditions called "metabolic syndrome" or "Syndrome X." A person is considered to have metabolic syndrome if he or she has at least three of the following five findings: abdominal obesity, high triglycerides, low HDL cholesterol, high blood pressure, and impaired fasting glucose. Metabolic syndrome and diabetes confer an increased risk of CHD. Abdominal obesity is defined as a waist circumference of 40 inches or more in a man and 35 inches or more in a woman. Excess weight also increases the risk of gallbladder disease and places greater stress on the back, hips, and knees, which may aggravate arthritis. Certain types of cancer also may be more common in overweight people. In addition, obesity is often accompanied by poor self-image, psychological distress, and diminished quality of life. The complications of excessive weight and obesity are a leading cause of preventable deaths, second only to tobacco-related complications.

MEDICAL EVALUATION OF WEIGHT

Anyone who is over age 40 or has health problems should have a thorough medical evaluation prior to beginning a weight loss program. In addition, your physician may refer you to a nutritionist for an assessment of eating habits.

Medical History

The medical history will include the following:

Weight history. Your physician will determine how long you have been overweight, because obesity present since childhood may reflect a genetic predisposition and is often more difficult to treat than adult-onset obesity. Other questions may address dieting history: Have you tried a variety of diets? Is there a pattern of weight loss and gain (called weight cycling or "yo-yo" dieting)?

Medical history. Do you have any symptoms or history of obesity-related disorders (such as CHD, stroke, hypertension, cancer, or diabetes)? Are there any symptoms suggesting an endocrine cause of obesity, such as hypothyroidism?

Family history. Is obesity prevalent in your family? Is there a family history of any obesity-related disorders?

Medications. Drugs that can cause weight gain, increase appetite, or hinder weight loss include corticosteroids, progestins, tricyclic antidepressants, phenothiazines, lithium, sulfonylureas, thiazolidinediones, and insulin.

Depressive symptoms. Depression affects many overweight people, especially those who are severely obese. A thorough evaluation includes questions about mood to determine whether depression needs to be treated along with obesity.

NEW RESEARCH

Low-Carbohydrate Diet Raises Risk Of Kidney Stones and Bone Loss

A recent study examined the effects of a low-carbohydrate, high-protein diet on kidney function and calcium balance over a six-week period.

Researchers evaluated ten healthy people during three consecutive dietary periods: their regular diet (an average of 285 g of carbohydrates per day) for two weeks; a low-carbohydrate (19 g per day) diet for the next two weeks; and a moderate-carbohydrate (33 g per day) "maintenance" diet for the last four weeks.

Levels of urinary citrate—a substance that impedes kidney stone formation—dropped by 41% during the low-carbohydrate phase and remained 24% lower during the maintenance diet. Levels of urinary acid nearly doubled during both the low-carbohydrate phase and the maintenance diet.

Urinary calcium excretion increased by 52% on the low carbohydrate diets. High levels of acid and calcium and reduced amounts of citrate in the urine are associated with an increased risk of kidney stones. The higher urinary output of calcium on the low-carbohydrate diet, unaccompanied by any increase in calcium absorption from the intestine, indicates loss of bone calcium.

While further research is needed to confirm these results, the authors conclude that a low carbohydrate diet raises the risk of kidney stones and bone loss.

AMERICAN JOURNAL OF KIDNEY DISEASES
Volume 40, page 265
August 2002

Physical Examination

Blood pressure, height, weight, and waist circumference are measured. The physician will look for evidence of cardiovascular disease (diseases of the heart and blood vessels), osteoarthritis, and hypothyroidism or other hormonal conditions.

Obesity is often defined as weighing 20% or more above ideal body weight (which varies with height, age, and gender). This definition is somewhat misleading, however, since it is not the amount of excess weight, but the amount of excess adipose tissue—or body fat—that determines the threat to health. It is possible to be overweight without being obese, as in the case of a weight lifter who has built up muscle mass. Moreover, the distribution of body fat is an important predictor of health risk—fat stored in the abdominal area is more harmful than fat stored in the hips, thighs, and buttocks. The degree of obesity is important; a mildly obese person is at less risk for developing obesity-related conditions than someone who is morbidly obese.

In addition to height, age, and gender, a person's ideal weight depends on many factors, including body composition (the proportion of fat and muscle), body shape (where fat is deposited), and general health. The most accurate way to assess the degree of obesity is to measure the amount of body fat. Since this task is not easy to perform, doctors generally rely on surrogate measures, such as body mass index and waist circumference, or use height/weight tables.

The National Heart, Lung, and Blood Institute and the National Institute of Diabetes and Digestive and Kidney Diseases have issued guidelines on the identification, evaluation, and treatment of overweight and obesity. Body mass index and waist circumference were found to be most useful for determining the need for weight loss. The pros and cons of most methods of weight assessment are discussed below.

Height/weight tables. Height/weight tables are the most straightforward way to assess your weight, but there are drawbacks to relying solely on this method. The tables are not based on scientific calculations of ideal weight but instead are derived from height, weight, and mortality data of people seeking life insurance. Moreover, they do not take into account body composition; and, because the tables suggest weight goals that are difficult for most obese people to achieve or maintain, they often lead to frustration for people who are attempting to lose weight.

Body mass index. As the result of the difficulty in directly measuring the amount of body fat and the drawbacks of using

NEW RESEARCH

Being Overweight Raises Cardiovascular Risk

Obesity is a known risk factor for cardiovascular disease. A recent study investigated whether being overweight but not obese also contributes to cardiovascular events.

Researchers examined the relationship between body mass index (BMI) and the development of cardiovascular events (such as heart attacks and strokes) and its associated risk factors in 5,209 white, middle-class adults (age 35 to 75) who were followed for up to 44 years in the Framingham Heart Study. Overweight was defined as a BMI of 25 to 29.9 and obesity as a BMI of 30 or higher.

After differences in age were taken into account, overweight individuals were found to have an elevated risk of hypertension and cardiovascular events, compared with normal-weight participants. Being overweight increased the risk of new onset of hypertension by 46% in men and 75% of women. The risk of cardiovascular disease was 21% higher in overweight men and 20% higher in overweight women compared with 46% in obese men and 64% in obese women.

This long-term population study indicates that being overweight also has an impact on cardiovascular risk, though a smaller one than obesity. Study authors assert that the prevention of weight gain and the treatment of people who are overweight can significantly reduce cardiovascular disease.

ARCHIVES OF INTERNAL MEDICINE
Volume 162, page 1867
September 9, 2002

height/weight tables alone, researchers have turned to a measurement called body mass index (BMI) to define obesity and its severity. BMI is a measurement of your weight as it relates to your height (see the chart in the feature "Body Mass Index and Waist Circumference" on page 44). BMI correlates strongly with the amount of body fat, though it does not measure it directly. Federal guidelines define overweight as a BMI from 25 to 29.9 and obesity as a BMI of 30 or greater. Morbid obesity is a BMI of 40 or greater.

Waist circumference. Fat stored in the abdomen poses a greater health risk than fat stored in the lower body (fortunately, abdominal fat is often the first to go with weight loss.). Typically, men are prone to fat deposition in the abdomen—developing what is commonly called a "pot belly," "beer belly," or "apple shape"—whereas women tend to accumulate fat around the hips, buttocks, and thighs, a distribution called a "pear shape." Some researchers believe that women are naturally programmed to store fat in the lower body for use as an energy reserve during pregnancy and breast feeding. However, women are not immune to accumulating abdominal fat, and weight tends to be stored in a pattern typical to a particular individual (in other words, once a pear, always a pear).

Techniques for measuring body fat. Direct measurement of the amount of body fat is the most accurate way to determine obesity-related health risk. Obesity is defined as fat stores exceeding 25% of total body weight for men or 30% for women. A variety of methods can be used to estimate body fat, including: underwater weighing (hydrodensitometry), dual-energy x-ray absorptiometry (DEXA), and bioelectrical impedance analysis (which involves sending a small current of electricity through the body). These techniques have the advantage of providing a more direct assessment of the proportion of total body weight that is fat. However, none of them is exact, some are expensive and not widely available, and all require trained personnel to administer them. Thus, they are not practical for general use.

Laboratory Tests

Blood will be drawn to measure total and HDL cholesterol, triglycerides, liver function, and blood glucose to screen for some of the complications of obesity. If a thyroid abnormality is suspected, thyroid stimulating hormone (TSH) is often measured.

Bulk Up on Fiber for Weight Control

A diet rich in fiber helps people control their weight. Studies have found that those who consume fiber-rich diets feel less hungry between meals, get fuller more quickly at mealtime, and tend to consume fewer calories throughout the day.

How High-Fiber Foods Help Control Weight

Fiber-rich foods help to promote feelings of fullness and reduce caloric intake in a variety of ways. First, foods high in fiber require more time and effort to chew, so they may reduce the amount of food consumed at a meal. Second, the extra time required to chew high-fiber foods produces more saliva, which, along with the extra water that fiber absorbs, is believed to distend the stomach and create a feeling of fullness. Finally, dietary fiber is thought to block the absorption of some fat and protein in the intestinal tract, thus reducing the calories derived from these nutrients.

The two main types of dietary fiber—soluble and insoluble—contribute to weight control in specific ways:

Soluble fiber (also called viscous fiber) is found in oats, barley, legumes, and dried and fresh fruit. By forming a gel around food particles, this type of fiber slows the passage of food through the stomach and delays hunger signals sent to the brain.

Insoluble fiber is the sponge-like form of dietary fiber (broccoli, potatoes with their skins, apples, beans, whole grain breads and cereals are good sources) that our grandmothers used to refer to as "roughage." This type of fiber supplies bulk by absorbing water in the digestive tract. This bulk in turn contributes to a feeling of fullness, which helps to discourage overeating.

Tips for Adding Fiber to Your Diet

- Be sure to buy whole grain products that say "100% whole wheat" or "100% whole grain."
- Check the Nutrition Facts Panel, and use it to compare products for fiber content.
- Choose brown rice instead of white rice and whole-wheat pasta instead of regular pasta.
- Make your own whole grain breakfast cereal by combining instant oats, toasted wheat germ, and chopped dried fruit.
- Add cooked lentils, barley, or brown rice to burger or meat loaf mixtures.
- Use whole-wheat flour in recipes for cookies, breads, and pancakes: Replace up to half of the white flour with whole-wheat flour.
- In dishes that combine meat and vegetables (such as stir-fries, stews, and salads), double the amount of vegetables called for and use only half the amount of meat.
- Add beans, chick peas, or lentils to tomato sauces and pasta dishes for a delicious meaty texture. One way to increase your intake of high-fiber beans or chick peas is to thin hummus (chick pea dip) or black bean dip with tomato-vegetable juice and some vinegar and use it as a salad dressing.
- Add nutty-tasting ground flaxseeds, which contain both soluble and insoluble fiber, to pancakes, waffles, muffins, and other baked goods. Or sprinkle them over breakfast cereal.

Increasing Your Fiber Intake

To increase both soluble and insoluble fiber intake, consume a variety of fruits and vegetables and a mix of whole grain foods. Experts recommend 3 to 5 servings of vegetables, 2 to 4 servings of fruits, and 6 to 11 servings of whole grains every day to meet the recommended daily intake of 20 to 30 g of fiber for adults over age 50. Consuming the recommended servings of fruits, vegetables, and whole grains each day makes it unnecessary to count grams of fiber or to keep track of how much you are eating of each type of fiber.

If your diet is low in fiber (most Americans consume only about half of the recommended daily intake), increase the amount of fiber you consume, but do so gradually, over a period of several weeks. Do not try to do it all at once because a sudden increase in fiber intake can cause abdominal discomfort. Moderation is especially important for older people whose bowel function may be less than optimal. And most important, if you are not doing so already, make sure to drink plenty of fluid when you increase the fiber in your diet.

LIFESTYLE TREATMENTS FOR WEIGHT LOSS

Successful weight loss requires a three-pronged approach: changing behavior patterns, making dietary adjustments, and increasing physical activity. Culled from medical research, the following guidelines incorporate strategies employed by people who have lost weight and kept it off. Use them to construct a weight loss program on your own or as an adjunct to medical or surgical treatments.

Behavioral Modification

An ability to alter lifelong attitudes toward diet and exercise may ultimately be the key to successful weight management: You must be motivated enough to change habits not for a few weeks or months, but for a lifetime. The importance of this resolve cannot be underestimated.

The desire to lose weight must come from within, rather than from external pressures. A person who wants to shed 20 lbs. to please a spouse is not likely to be as motivated, or as successful, as someone whose goal is to improve health or increase self-esteem. Choosing the right time to start a weight-loss program is also important. People under stress or pressure may not be able to devote the considerable attention and effort required to make lifestyle changes.

If you are motivated and ready to lose weight, the following guidelines will help.

1. Set realistic goals. Remember that weight tables give estimates of ideal weights; you can probably be healthy at weights above "ideal" if you have a nutritious diet and exercise. Instead of attempting to lose a specific number of pounds, make it your goal to adopt healthier eating and exercise habits. If you are obese and feel compelled to set a weight goal, losing 10% to 15% of your current body weight is a realistic objective. The good news is that evidence shows that weight loss of as little as 5% to 10% of body weight can significantly improve risk factors such as blood pressure and blood glucose. The safest rate of weight loss is ½ to 2 lbs. a week.

2. Seek support from family and friends. People who receive social support are more successful in changing their behaviors. Ask family and friends for help, whether this means keeping high-fat foods out of the house or relieving you of some chore so that you have time to exercise. It will be easier to stick to your new eating plan if you are the person responsible for food shopping and preparation, and if everyone in the household eats the same types of foods. (A low-fat diet that includes plenty of fruits, vegetables, and grains will benefit your family's health even if they do not need to lose weight.) You may be more motivated to exercise if you work out with a friend or family member.

3. Make changes gradually. Trying to make many changes quickly can leave you feeling overwhelmed and frustrated. Instead, ease into exercise; do not overdo it. Incorporate low-fat eating in stages. For example, if you typically drink whole milk, switch to reduced-fat (2%) milk, then to low-fat (1%), and then to fat-free milk. With this approach, you will not notice the difference in taste as much. In fact, your taste preferences will actually change—the once-favored high-fat foods will start tasting too rich and greasy after you have eaten low-fat foods for a while. Another tactic is to switch to low-fat foods one meal at a time. For example, concentrate on eating a low-fat breakfast for one week, add lunch the next week, and then dinner the third week.

4. Eat slowly. Many people consume more calories than needed to satisfy their hunger because they eat too quickly. Since it takes about 20 minutes for the brain to recognize that the stomach is full, slowing down helps you feel satisfied on less food. Moreover, eating slowly allows you to better appreciate the flavors and textures of your food.

5. Eat three meals a day, plus snacks. Skipping meals is counterproductive, as is severely reducing food intake, since such strict changes are impossible to maintain and are ultimately unhealthy. People who restrict their eating habits too rigorously often have an "all or nothing" approach: Once they go off their diet, they tend to abandon all efforts and find it difficult to return to healthy eating. In addition, eating the bulk of your calories at one sitting may impair metabolism. You will be more successful in the long run if you allow yourself to eat when you are hungry, eat enough nutritious low-fat food to satisfy that hunger, and spread your calorie intake over the course of the day.

6. Plan for exercise. Choose activities that are convenient and enjoyable for you to do on a regular basis, and then treat exercise like any other appointment—set a time and jot it down in your date book. Many people find it easier to exercise first thing in the morning, before the demands of the day interfere, but others find lunchtime or right after work more convenient. For information on starting an exercise plan, see the feature on page 57.

7. Record your progress. Start a food diary and exercise log to keep track of your accomplishments. Keeping such detailed diaries may seem cumbersome, but they can help you stay motivated, and reviewing the entries can reveal any problem areas. In addition, the information can help facilitate treatment by your nutritionist or doctor.

8. Evaluate your relationship to food. Behavioral and emotional cues frequently trigger an inappropriate desire to eat. The most common cues are habit, stress, boredom, sadness, anxiety, loneliness, and the use of food as a reward. Many people also relate food

NEW RESEARCH

Special Diets and Products Are Not Necessary For Long-Term Weight Control

According to the largest survey ever conducted on long-term weight loss, successful dieters use their own personal strategies—not fad diets, special foods, programs, supplements, or drugs—to lose weight.

Of 4,000 dieters who had achieved a five-year weight loss, 83% followed their own personal diet and exercise plan and only 14% had ever belonged to a commercial weight loss program. More than half reported that they made a consistent effort each day to eat more fruits and vegetables and to cut back on portion sizes, fats, and sweets.

Exercise ranked as a top weight-loss strategy, and dieters who exercised at least three times per week cited it as the key factor in their weight loss. Although walking was the most popular form of exercise, many dieters also lifted weights.

Based on the survey, recommendations include being as active as possible each day; lifting weights; choosing high-fiber, minimally processed carbohydrates; eating lean sources of protein along with carbohydrates, and including small amounts of healthful unsaturated fat from nuts and olive oil.

CONSUMER REPORTS
Volume 67, page 26
June 2002

to love or care and derive comfort from it. Although eating may appear to soothe uncomfortable feelings, its effect is temporary at best and ultimately does not solve any problems. In fact, it may distract you from focusing on the real issues.

9. Recall your accomplishments. Over your lifetime you have probably been successful in tackling many difficult tasks—quitting smoking, learning a new skill, or advancing in the workplace, for example. Reminding yourself of past achievements can help you feel more confident about making the changes that will lead to weight loss.

10. Don't try to be perfect. While losing weight requires significant changes in eating and exercise habits, not every high-calorie food must be banished forever, and you need not exercise vigorously every day. High-calorie foods can be eaten once in a while without hindering weight loss. On days when you have a candy bar, for example, compensate for the extra fat and calories by eliminating a few calories and grams of fat from your diet over the next few days. And "cravings" for high-calorie foods can often be satisfied by small tastes—a piece of chocolate rather than a whole candy bar. It is also acceptable to miss an exercise session. On days when you do not feel like doing formal exercise, take a brisk walk instead. (Remember that calories are also burned during nonexercise activities, such as housework.)

Diet

To determine how many calories you should eat per day, first calculate the number of calories needed to maintain your current weight—roughly 15 calories per pound of body weight in a moderately active person (someone who gets at least 30 minutes of moderate to intense physical activity every day). For example, a moderately active 150-lb. person who consumes 2,250 calories per day will neither gain nor lose weight. A completely sedentary person may require just 12 calories per pound to maintain weight.

A pound of body fat contains 3,500 calories. To lose one to two pounds per week—a gradual and safe rate of weight loss—you must eat 500 to 1,000 fewer calories per day than what is needed to maintain your weight. (The calorie cutback need not be so severe if you also begin to exercise regularly.) Calorie intake should not drop below 1,200 per day in women or 1,500 per day in men (unless the diet is medically supervised and you are taking a vitamin/mineral supplement), since it would be difficult to get all the nutrients you need.

While reducing calorie intake is essential for losing weight,

How To Get Started With An Exercise Plan

Whether it is an early morning walk, a group aerobic class, working out at a health club or doing laps at a pool, a 30-minute workout three or four times a week should provide health benefits. Most people know that exercise is vital for health, but many do not know what types of exercise are safest or how to start an exercise plan. Here are a few tips to help you get started:

- Ask your physician which type of exercise is best for you. This is particularly important if you are over age 50, suffer from a medical condition, or are unsure about your health.
- Engage in activities that involve stretching, aerobic exercise, and strength training. These types of exercise are generally recommended for older adults because they are low-impact and help maintain overall strength, lower blood pressure and strengthen bones.
- Make sure your exercise plan suits your lifestyle. For example, if you are a morning person, select that time to exercise. You may want to consider what you want to achieve from exercise: weight loss, stress reduction, health improvement—these are just a few of the reasons for starting and staying with an exercise plan.
- Avoid boredom with a program that includes exercise that you enjoy and look forward to. Also, it is helpful to alternate diverse activities, such as walking, yoga, tennis, swimming, and weight training.
- Start at a level you can manage and work your way up gradually. If you do too much too quickly, you may get discouraged. In addition, you can damage your muscles and joints.
- If you cannot or do not want to exercise for an extended period, exercise in increments throughout the day. For example, 10 minute blocks of exercise done three times a day provide the same benefits as exercising for 30 minutes. Just make sure to log a total of at least 30 minutes of exercise time. The U.S. Surgeon General and the American College of Sports Medicine agree that at least 30 minutes of moderate activity on most days of the week is a way to reap health benefits. And for people who like to exercise an hour on most days of the week, all the better: A new report by the Institute of Medicine says about 60 minutes of activity a day will help adults maintain a healthy body weight.
- Set realistic goals, particularly if you have never exercised before. That way you will not get discouraged and stop, especially if your aim is weight loss, since it is highly unlikely that you will see dramatic changes right away.
- Ask someone to be your exercise partner if you feel your motivation is waning. Many adults agree that having someone to exercise with helps them keep going.
- Decide if you want to exercise at home or at a health club. Exercising at home offers privacy, avoids commuting time, and is more economical than exercising at a health club. However, if you enjoy being with other people when you exercise, then you should think about joining a health club or enrolling in exercise classes. If you do not want to spend the money on a health club, contact your local YMCA, YWCA, hospital, university, or senior or civic center to find an inexpensive or free program.
- Try to minimize the obstacles to sticking with an exercise program. If you exercise outside your home, be sure that you are comfortable with the exercise facility and that you do not feel out of place. Second, be sure that the exercise facilities are consistent with your goals. And, finally, select one that is conveniently located, near your workplace or home. You will be more inclined to go on a regular basis if it is close by.
- If you are over age 50, and especially if you have a sedentary lifestyle, undergo cardiovascular screening before you start an exercise program. If possible, choose a health club that has a heart-attack emergency plan; ask if the health club has a written emergency plan and automated external defibrillators on hand.
- If you choose to use a personal trainer (either at home or at a gym), seek out a trainer who is properly qualified. A qualified trainer will have a bachelor's degree in exercise science or physical education or will be certified by the American College of Sports Medicine or the National Strength and Conditioning Association.

focusing on calories per se may leave people feeling hungry and frustrated unless the overall composition of the diet is also considered. Replacing dietary fat with complex carbohydrates automatically lowers calorie intake, while allowing a satisfying volume of food. For any given number of calories, you can eat a much larger amount of food on a low-fat diet than on a high-fat diet. The reason for this is simple: Gram for gram, fat contains more than twice as many calories as carbohydrates or protein: nine versus four calories. Fatty foods also contain less water and fiber—substances that help make a food more filling—than foods high in complex carbohydrates. But, all too often, people reduce their intake of fat and instead consume an equal or greater amount of calories in the form of simple and complex carbohydrates.

There are other reasons to reduce the fat content of your diet. Some evidence suggests that a prolonged high-fat diet may trigger an upward adjustment in the body's set point. In addition, fewer calories are burned when dietary fat is converted into body fat than when dietary carbohydrates or protein are converted into fat. Moreover, a low-fat diet can help to lower blood cholesterol levels and may reduce the risk of colon and prostate cancer. And not just the amount, but the type of fat you eat affects your health risks: Saturated fats, found in animal products like meat and cheese, are more harmful than monounsaturated or polyunsaturated fats.

Once you decide on an appropriate calorie intake, you need to determine the amount of total fat you should eat. Most experts now recommend that a diet should derive no more than 35% of its calories from fat (even when substituting monounsaturated for saturated fats). Most people should not reduce fat intake to less than 20% of calories. The AHA does not recommend cutting fat below 15% of total calories for certain groups of people (older adults, for example) owing to concerns over malnutrition and a possible negative effect on blood lipids. The following guidelines will help you adopt a low-fat, high-complex-carbohydrate diet.

1. Eat mostly fruits, vegetables, legumes, and grains. These foods are naturally low in fat and high in fiber. (Fiber provides bulk, which helps to fill you up without adding calories.) The wide variety of these foods provides different textures and flavors, so you will not feel bored or deprived.

2. Do not add fat during cooking. Avoid sautéing foods in butter or oil. Use nonstick pans; coat them lightly with cooking spray if necessary, or try using broth, wine, fruit juice or even water for sautéing. Bake, broil, steam, or roast foods instead of frying them.

3. Choose lean cuts of meat and poultry. Meat and poultry are rich in nutrients and good sources of high-quality protein, but they can also contain a lot of fat. Top round, eye of round, and round are the leanest cuts of beef; tenderloin, top loin, and lean ham are the leanest pork cuts; and light-meat chicken and turkey are leaner than dark meat. Completely trim all external fat from meat before

RECENT RESEARCH

High Fish Intake Is Linked To Low Levels of Leptin

High levels of leptin, a hormone linked with appetite, have been associated with obesity and an increased risk of cardiovascular disease. Low levels of leptin may be linked to diets rich in fish, according to a recent study.

Investigators examined two closely related African tribes in Tanzania who had similar calorie intakes and lifestyles but ate different types of diets. One tribe of 329 people ate a primarily vegetarian diet and the other tribe of 279 people consumed freshwater fish as their major dietary staple. The men and women from both tribes were lean, with an average BMI of about 20.

Leptin levels among the vegetarians were more than twice as high on average than those of the fish eaters, even after adjusting for factors such as age and body fat. Leptin levels among female fish eaters were particularly noteworthy. Although women typically have higher levels of leptin than men, the women fish eaters had substantially lower leptin levels than both female and male vegetarians.

The investigators conclude that one of the benefits of a diet high in fish may be reduced leptin levels. More studies are needed to evaluate different population groups and to determine how eating fish may lower levels of leptin.

CIRCULATION
Volume 106, page 289
July 2002

cooking. Do not eat poultry skin—it contains a lot of fat. But you can leave it on during roasting or baking to help keep the meat moist and tender; just be sure you do not cook the poultry with other ingredients, such as potatoes, that could absorb the fat released from the skin as it cooks. Limit portion sizes to 3 oz.—about the size of the palm of your hand or a deck of cards—and round out the meal with plenty of grains and vegetables.

4. Switch to low-fat or fat-free dairy products. Whole milk and cheeses can contain more fat than meat does. For example, 1 oz. of cheddar has the same amount of fat as a 6-oz. chicken breast or a 3½-oz. sirloin. But do not eliminate dairy products: They are an important source of calcium and protein. Instead, select fat-free milk and fat-free yogurt, along with limited amounts of reduced-fat or part-skim cheeses.

5. Read food labels. The nutrition labels that are required on all packaged foods provide important information about their calorie and fat content, which makes it easy to compare brands. Serving sizes are arbitrary, however, so be sure to compare equal portions.

6. Experiment with reduced-fat, low-fat, and fat-free versions of foods. From fat-free milk to reduced-fat salad dressing and cream cheese, these foods can help you cut fat from your diet. Just because a food is low in fat does not mean you can eat unlimited quantities, however, since it can still provide a lot of calories. For example, some fat-free cakes and cookies contain as many—or more—calories than the regular versions because manufacturers add extra sugar to compensate for flavor lost when fat is removed. To save fat and calories, substitute lower-fat foods in equal amounts for the full-fat versions—for example, eat a cup of low-fat vanilla frozen yogurt (about 3 g fat, 203 calories) instead of a cup of premium ice cream (24 g fat, 356 calories). Resist the urge to have two servings of the frozen yogurt just because it has no fat.

7. Consider the calories in beverages. Although regular soda, fruit juices, and alcoholic beverages are fat free, they contain a significant number of calories. And, with the exception of citrus juices, these beverages are not a good source of vitamins and minerals. Choose calorie-free beverages—water or seltzer, and moderate amounts of coffee and tea—most of the time. Limit your alcohol intake: Try nonalcoholic beer (which has fewer calories than regular beer) or mix wine with seltzer for a lower-calorie wine spritzer. Lessen the calories in fruit juices by mixing them with seltzer, or eat the fruit instead—it has fewer calories than the juice and it satisfies hunger better because of its fiber.

NEW RECOMMENDATION

Fat Substitutes: Use Judiciously

The abundance of available foods that are reduced in fat and/or contain fat substitutes raises concerns about their effectiveness and potential effects on health, according to the American Heart Association (AHA).

While reduced-fat foods and fat substitutes reduce the number of calories consumed from fat and saturated fat, their impact on total caloric intake and body weight in the long term are uncertain. In fact, many low-fat or fat-free foods have equivalent or higher amounts of calories than their full-fat versions. The AHA believes that such strategies as portion control and exercise are likely to have a greater impact on weight than does use of fat-modified products of any kind.

In addition to issues about weight control, one fat substitute, olestra —used in some chips and crackers—inhibits the absorption of fat-soluble nutrients. Vitamins A, D, E, and K are added to offset this effect.

The long-term health effects of fat substitutes are unknown, including their potential interactions with medications and other food ingredients. In summary, the AHA advises, "Within the context of a healthy dietary pattern, fat substitutes, when used judiciously, may provide some flexibility in dietary planning, although additional research is needed to fully determine the longer-term health effects."

CIRCULATION
Volume 105, page 2800
June 2002

Expanded Portion Sizes Contribute to Obesity

Huge servings of food that are well beyond standard portion sizes have become the norm in many American restaurants and fast-food chains. According to the American Dietetic Association, this "portion distortion" has increased the number of Americans who are accustomed to eating super-sized meals. And not surprisingly, the trend toward expanded portion sizes has paralleled the epidemic of obesity in the United States.

The Amount Counts

While fat consumption has dropped in the past 20 years in the United States, serving sizes and total calorie consumption have increased. Large portion sizes became popular in the 1980s, and they have continued to expand. According to recent research, almost all foods and beverages currently sold in the United States are excessive in size and dramatically increased from their original sizes. For example, the average cookie is seven times larger than the government-recommended serving size. And many other foods now exceed standard serving sizes. Hamburgers, french fries, and sodas are two to five times larger than they used to be in the 1970s.

Experts estimate that the dramatic increase in portion sizes could add 15 lbs. a year to the average person. And although the public has been educated about the fat in their diets, they may not realize that consuming other calories due to super-sized portions can lead to weight gain. Unfortunately, many Americans do not understand the importance of eating sensible portions to maintain a healthy weight.

Tips for Controlling Portions

- Learn to recognize the USDA's standard serving sizes and to visualize what they look like.
- Find out how much you are eating when you cook at home by using measuring cups or measuring spoons to determine your typical portions. Or purchase a small scale to weigh food portions, which will help eliminate guesswork.
- Start out with what you have determined are sensible portions for a meal, and do not go back for "seconds."
- Cut back on portions of high-calorie foods, including sweets, spreads, oils, and fast foods.
- Eat meals on a smaller plate.
- Fill your plate with the best proportion of food groups: The American Institute for Cancer Research recommends covering two thirds of your plate with fruits, vegetables, beans, and whole grains, and leaving the remaining one third for meat, fish, poultry, or low-fat dairy products.
- Resign from the "clean plate club."
- Share a portion of food when eating out. Or select small portions, such as a regular burger instead of a quarter-pound burger, or order an appetizer or side dish if the entree is too large.

Determine Daily Portions

The U.S. Department of Agriculture (USDA) devised daily food guidelines (often depicted as the "food guide pyramid") to help people make decisions regarding the amounts of foods to eat. The USDA serving sizes are quite small, and the "portions" you normally eat may be more than one USDA "serving." Exactly how many servings should be in your daily portions depends on your age, gender, body frame size, and level of physical activity. The chart on the next page identifies the size of a serving in the different food groups and provides several easy visual comparisons for a better sense of how big the servings actually are.

8. Watch out for hidden fats. It is easy to overlook the fat and calories contributed by toppings such as margarine, cream sauce, mayonnaise, salad dressings, peanut butter, sour cream, and cheese. Limit the amounts of these items; choose low-fat versions (such as nonfat sour cream or mayonnaise); or find substitutes (for example, tomato sauce instead of cream sauce on pasta).

9. Control portion sizes. Americans tend to eat large portions of food, especially meat, and what many people think of as a serving is usually more than the amount that is listed in nutrition tables and on food labels. For example, a serving of breakfast cereal is about

Food Group	Servings per Day	Serving Size	Visual Clues to Serving Sizes
Grains, breads, pasta, cereals	6 to 11	1 slice bread, ½ cup cooked pasta or rice, ½ cup hot cereal, 1 oz. ready-to-eat cereal	1 slice bread = audiocassette ½ cup pasta, rice, cooked cereal = tennis ball
Fruits	2 to 4	1 piece whole fruit, 1 melon wedge, ½ cup canned fruit or berries, ¼ cup dried fruit, ¾ cup juice, ½ grapefruit, ½ medium banana	1 medium fruit = baseball ¼ cup dried fruit = 1 golf ball or scant handful for average adult
Vegetables	3 to 5	½ cup chopped raw or cooked vegetables, 1 cup raw leafy greens, ¾ cup vegetable juice, ½ cup tomato sauce	1 cup chopped fresh leafy greens = 4 lettuce leaves ½ cup vegetables = ½ baseball or rounded handful for average adult
Dairy products	2 to 3	1 cup milk, 8 oz. yogurt, 1½ oz. natural cheese, 2 oz. processed cheese	1 oz. cheese = 4 dice
Meat, poultry, fish, and alternatives	2 to 3 (5–7 oz.)	2½ to 3 oz. cooked beef, pork, lamb, chicken, turkey, fish, or shellfish, ½ cup cooked beans or tofu*, 1 egg*, 2 Tbsp peanut butter,* ⅓ cup nuts*	3 oz. meat, fish, poultry = deck of playing cards ½ cup cooked beans = ½ baseball or rounded handful for average adult 2 tablespoons of peanut butter = large marshmallow ⅓ cup nuts = level handful for average adult
Fats, sugar, alcohol	Use sparingly	Limit calories from this food group. Choose unsaturated fats, particularly monounsaturated ones. One alcoholic beverage equals one 12 oz. beer, one 5-oz. glass of wine, or one shot (1½ oz.) of spirits.	1 teaspoon or 1 serving of butter or margarine = tip of your thumb

* Counts as approximately 1 oz. of meat.

one cup, but many people fill their bowls with much more than that. To get an accurate picture of the amount of food you normally eat, serve yourself a typical portion, then use a measuring cup, measuring spoons, or a food scale to measure or weigh the food. Next, try serving yourself a smaller portion, eat it slowly, and see if your hunger is satisfied. (Keep in mind that you do not need to feel stuffed to satisfy your hunger.) You can dispense with weighing and measuring food once you become accustomed to estimating smaller portion sizes. Visit the USDA's Center for Nutrition Policy and Promotion Web site at www.cnpp.usda.gov/Pubs/Brochures/index.htm, which provides a useful online brochure, "How Much are you Eating?" For more information about portion sizes, see feature on pages 60–61.

Exercise

Exercise is a valuable element in a weight loss program, but exercise alone results in only modest weight loss, and at a slower rate than calorie restriction. Studies have shown that combining exercise with diet results in greater loss of weight and body fat than dieting alone and is associated with a greater likelihood of maintaining weight loss. And adding exercise to calorie restriction makes the dietary changes easier because they need not be as drastic. It is easy to see why this is so. To lose one pound per week requires a deficit of about 500 calories a day. By adding a half-hour of moderate-to-vigorous exercise per day (enough to burn 250 calories), you reduce the dietary restriction to a more manageable 250 calories per day.

In addition, exercise—especially strength training—helps to maintain muscle mass. Because muscle weighs more than fat, a person who exercises with strength training and cuts calories may lose less weight than one who only cuts calories, but the exerciser will lose more body fat.

The effect of exercise is cumulative. For example, while it takes about nine hours of walking at a normal pace for a 175-lb. person to burn 3,500 calories, the walking does not have to be completed all at once. You can achieve the same calorie deficit if you walk for half an hour each day for 18 days, or 45 minutes for 12 days, or an hour for 9 days. Even if you alternate days or work out only three times a week, you can still burn the same number of calories. You can even break up an exercise session into segments: For example, a 10-minute walk in the morning, 10 minutes at lunch, and 10 minutes in the evening still burn the same number of calories as a single 30-minute walk.

Start an exercise program gradually (for more information on how to start an exercise plan, go to page 57). Pushing too hard at the start may quickly cause frustration and the desire to quit. Trying to do too much, too soon may also lead to muscle strain and soreness, or even injury. Instead, increase your exercise level in the stages described below. And remember that sedentary people over the age of 50 should consult their doctor before starting any vigorous exercise program.

1. Increase your amount of everyday physical activity. The conveniences of modern life have made it easy to become sedentary. Look for ways to counteract the effects of these conveniences: for example, walk rather than drive, or take the stairs rather than an elevator or escalator. When doing errands or shopping, park some distance from your destination and walk the rest of the way. If you take public transportation, get off a few stops early and walk.

Walking up stairs can be a strenuous activity because you lift the full weight of your body with every step. Start slowly—begin by walking down flights of stairs, then start to walk up a flight or two at a time. Gradually increase the number of flights you climb at one time.

2. Add a formal walking program. Walking is appealing because it can be done anywhere, requires no special equipment (other than a supportive pair of shoes), and almost anyone can do it. Set your own pace: You expend approximately the same number of calories during an hour of slow walking as in half an hour of brisk walking. Start by walking for half an hour, three times a week. Once you become comfortable with this level of activity, walk for the same length of time five days a week. Next, gradually increase the duration of your walking to 40 minutes, then 50 minutes, and ultimately 1 hour. As you become more physically fit, you will be able to walk faster and go farther—and thus burn more calories in a given period of time.

3. Vary your activities. If you enjoy walking, make it the foundation of your exercise program. To prevent boredom, and also to work different muscle groups, choose other activities to substitute for walking on some days. Good choices include aerobic dance classes, bicycling, line dancing, or swimming. Swimming is a particularly good activity for older people who may have joint pain from arthritis. The buoyancy of the water lessens the strain on joints. Tennis and golf (provided you walk the course) can also burn calories. The most important rule, however, is to engage in activities that are enjoyable and convenient to do regularly.

4. Start a weight-training program. Working a muscle against resistance increases muscle size and strength. Because muscle takes up about 20% less space than fat, building muscle results in a leaner physique. In addition, having more muscle increases your metabolism, because it requires more energy to maintain muscle than fat tissue. You do not have to become a body builder or lift heavy weights to get the benefits. Working the major muscle groups—chest, arms, legs, and back—with light weights, two to three times a week, is sufficient. If you do not lose weight despite strength training, remember that you want to reduce body fat but not necessarily

NEW RESEARCH

Activity Reduces Levels Of C-Reactive Protein

Recent findings suggest another beneficial effect of exercise: It is associated with lower levels of C-reactive protein (CRP). Elevated blood levels of CRP are a risk factor for coronary heart disease, stroke, and type 2 diabetes.

Researchers evaluated 3,638 healthy American adults (average age 53 years) who participated in the Third National Health and Nutrition Examination Survey (NHANES III). As part of the study, participants gave blood samples for CRP measurements and reported the number of times in the preceding month that they had engaged in physical activity, such as aerobic exercise, yard work, jogging, weight lifting, or walking a mile.

After correcting for other factors, including obesity, which is associated with increased CRP levels, participants who were more physically active were less likely to have high levels of CRP. The more frequent the physical activity, the lower the chance of having an elevated CRP level. People who were active more than 22 times per month were the least likely to have high CRP levels.

The investigators conclude that frequent physical activity is associated with lower levels of CRP. Additional research is needed to determine the duration and intensity of activity that best improve CRP levels.

ARCHIVES OF INTERNAL MEDICINE
Volume 162, page 1286
June 2002

Weight Loss Drugs 2003

Drug Type	Generic Name	Brand Name	Average Daily Dosage*	Wholesale Cost (Generic Cost)†
Noradrenergics	benzphetamine	Didrex	50 mg	50 mg: $89
	diethylpropion	Tenuate	75 mg	25 mg: $51 ($25)
	phendimetrazine	Bontril	105 mg	35 mg: $18 ($20)
		Melfiat	105 mg	105 mg: $80
		Obezine	35 to 105 mg	35 mg: $5
		Phendiet	35 to 105 mg	35 mg: $4
		Prelu-2	105 mg	105 mg: $120
	phentermine	Adipex-P	15 to 37.5 mg	37.5 mg: $170 (30 mg: $90)
		Ionamin	15 to 30 mg	30 mg: $260
		Phentercot	15 to 37.5 mg	30 mg: $12
		Phentride	15 to 37.5 mg	30 mg: $9
		Pro-Fast	15 to 37.5 mg	37.5 mg: $81
Serotonin/ norepinephrine reuptake inhibitor	sibutramine	Meridia	10 to 15 mg	10 mg: $310
Antidepressants	fluoxetine	Prozac	20 mg	20 mg: $311 ($267)
	sertraline	Zoloft	50 mg	25 mg: $252
	bupropion	Wellbutrin	150 to 200 mg	100 mg: $120 ($96)
Miscellaneous off-label uses of approved drugs	topiramate	Topamax	50 to 400 mg	100 mg: $325
	metformin	Glucophage	500 mg	500 mg: $78
Lipase inhibitor	orlistat	Xenical	120 to 360 mg	120 mg: $132

* These dosages represent an average range for the treatment of obesity. The precise effective dosage varies from patient to patient and depends on many factors. Do not make any changes to your medication without consulting your doctor.

† Average wholesale prices to pharmacists for 100 tablets or capsules of the dosage listed. Costs to consumers are higher. If a generic version is available, the cost is listed in parentheses. Source: *Red Book*, 2002 (Medical Economics Data, publishers).

body weight, since muscle is denser and weighs more than fat.

MEDICAL AND SURGICAL TREATMENTS FOR OBESITY

Because the following treatments can be demanding for the patient and carry the risk of adverse side effects, they are appropriate only for people who are severely obese—especially those with, or at high risk for, medical conditions that may be improved with weight loss.

How They Work	Comments
Stimulate the central nervous system and suppress appetite by increasing norepinephrine (noradrenaline) levels in the brain.	Tolerance may develop after a few weeks, slowing the rate of weight loss, but abrupt cessation could cause fatigue and depression. Possible side effects include nervousness, restlessness, difficulty sleeping, irritability, diarrhea, dry mouth, rapid heartbeat, and hypertension. Noradrenergics should be taken with caution by those with mild hypertension and diabetes and not at all by those with arteriosclerosis, moderate to severe hypertension, glaucoma, overactive thyroid, anxiety, a history of drug abuse, or those taking MAO inhibitors. Alcohol should be avoided while taking noradrenergics.
Creates a feeling of fullness by blocking the reabsorption of serotonin and norepinephrine in the brain. May also increase metabolism.	Appears to cause about 5% weight loss over six months. May raise pulse and blood pressure, which should be monitored regularly. Patients with coronary heart disease or uncontrolled hypertension and those who have survived a stroke should not use this drug. Other possible side effects include dry mouth, insomnia, and constipation.
Fluoxetine and sertraline create a feeling of fullness by raising levels of serotonin in the brain. Bupropion raises levels of norepinephrine, serotonin, and dopamine.	Though FDA-approved for depression, these drugs may (as a side effect) cause weight loss. Sometimes prescribed for obese people with depression. Possible side effects include insomnia and fatigue.
An antiseizure medicine that produces weight loss as a side effect. Mechanism unknown.	May cause central nervous system side effects, kidney stones, and acidosis.
Improves insulin sensitivity.	May cause bloating, diarrhea, flatulence, or nausea. Lactic acidosis may occur in patients with heart failure or kidney, liver, or lung disease.
Blocks the action of intestinal and pancreatic lipases (which digest dietary fats). As a result, the undigested dietary fat passes through the intestines and out of the body without being absorbed, carrying with it fat-soluble vitamins that otherwise would have been absorbed in the intestines.	Reduces fat absorption by about 30% and promotes significant weight loss when used with a reduced-calorie diet. May raise blood pressure in some individuals. Other possible side effects include abdominal cramping and diarrhea. Patients must take a daily multivitamin to prevent vitamin deficiency.

Very-Low-Calorie and Low-Calorie Diets

The term very-low-calorie diet (VLCD) is used to describe diets supplying fewer than 800 calories a day. Typically, patients must replace food with a powdered supplement that is combined with a noncaloric liquid (water or diet soda). To prevent deficiencies, the supplement is primarily made of high-quality protein derived from milk, eggs, or soy, along with a small amount of carbohydrates, minimal fat, and added vitamins and minerals. The high protein content of these diets is essential to help preserve muscle mass when calorie intake is so low. Recently, many centers modified their VLCD formulas to contain more calories. Studies have shown that weight loss is about as good on 800 as on 400 to 500 calories a day, and there are probably fewer risks. The term low-calorie diet (LCD) is used to describe diets that supply at least 800 calories per day to slightly below the person's daily caloric expenditure. So for a person needing 2,000 calories per day, a VLCD is 1-799 calories and an LCD is 800-1,999 calories. (Although a program may be referred to as a low-calorie diet, or LCD, we will use VLCD to describe both types, except where the protocols differ.)

Typically lasting 12 to 16 weeks, VLCDs require close medical supervision and are usually administered by weight loss clinics or hospitals. Programs should include regular medical monitoring; behavioral counseling to help you adjust to the diet; and instruction for changing eating patterns once food is reintroduced. Programs may also provide classes and support groups; many place a great emphasis on exercise. Once the VLCD phase is completed, food is slowly reintroduced over 2 to 10 weeks. The cost of participation is around $2,000 to $3,000. Few insurance companies cover this cost. If they do, it is usually covered only if the program is used to help treat a complication of severe obesity.

VLCDs are appropriate for people with a BMI of 35 or higher who have been unable to lose weight with conventional diet and exercise. LCDs are appropriate for individuals with a BMI between 30 and 34.9, especially for those who have coexisting conditions, such as type 2 diabetes, hypertension, high triglycerides, low HDL cholesterol, sleep apnea, or osteoarthritis.

Contraindications to VLCDs include a recent heart attack or stroke, heart rhythm abnormalities (arrhythmias), angina, liver or kidney disease, or type 1 diabetes. However, insulin-treated, obese patients with type 2 diabetes can benefit from VLCDs. For people who can stay on them, VLCDs produce dramatic reductions in weight. On average, participants lose 2.5 to 4 lbs. per week, at a rate that tends to slow as the duration of the VLCD increases to months.

Adding exercise to the program may enhance weight loss. Within three weeks, VLCDs often help lower blood pressure and cholesterol and triglyceride levels. In addition, glycemic control also improves.

Despite the dramatic success possible with VLCDs, they are not a panacea. About 25% of people who start a VLCD cannot adhere to the strict regimen and drop out of the program. Most of those who do complete treatment regain large amounts of weight with-

NEW RESEARCH

Ma-Huang May Cause Heart Attacks, Stroke

Ma-huang, an herbal source of ephedrine that is often used in natural weight-loss products, may cause heart attacks and strokes, even in young people who have no history of cardiovascular disease (CVD).

Investigators collected data from the U.S. Food and Drug Administration (FDA) to determine the number and type of CVD events (heart attacks, strokes, and sudden cardiac deaths) that were associated with Ma-huang use from 1995 to 1997. During this time, the FDA received 926 reports of possible Ma-huang toxicity. These included 37 serious CVD events that occurred shortly after Ma-huang ingestion: 10 heart attacks, 16 strokes, and 11 sudden cardiac deaths. The affected people ranged in age from 20 to 69, and only one had a history of CVD at the time of the event. In all but one of the cases, Ma-huang was taken according to the manufacturer's instructions.

"Persons using or considering using ma huang should be informed of the possibility of associated serious adverse cardiovascular effects," the authors conclude. Although the researchers cannot conclusively say that Ma-huang was the cause of the CVD events in these cases, they suspect that the supplement raises blood pressure by elevating heart rate and cardiac output and constricting blood vessels, which could trigger a heart attack or stroke.

MAYO CLINIC PROCEEDINGS
Volume 77, page 12
January 2002

Dietary Supplements for Weight Loss

The past decade has seen a dramatic increase in the marketing of dietary supplements purported to aid in weight loss. Examples include chitosan, chromium, conjugated linoleic acid, and ephedra (Ma-huang). Despite the enormous popularity of these supplements, there is surprisingly little reliable information about their safety and effectiveness. Consult a physician before taking any kind of dietary supplement.

Effectiveness and Safety

While some weight-loss supplements may have components that could potentially promote weight loss, no well-designed studies in humans have proven the supplements effective. As for the safety of weight-loss supplements, there is limited information available, particularly regarding long-term use. In addition, little is known about the interactions of weight-loss supplements with prescription and other over-the-counter drugs.

Ephedra Under Scrutiny

Ephedra is an herbal stimulant that has been linked to cardiovascular events (such as heart attacks and strokes), neurological damage, and other serious health conditions. In fact, ephedra supplements have been associated with more than 100 cases of serious health problems in over a two-year period. Because of these adverse effects of ephedra, the U.S. Food and Drug Administration (FDA) is currently considering a ban on this dietary supplement.

Dietary Supplements Are Not Tested

While FDA law requires product labels to be accurate, this is difficult to enforce because dietary supplements are exempt from the rigorous testing that is required for drugs and food additives. As a result, the amount of an active ingredient in a supplement often does not conform to the quantity listed on the label. Ingredients may be mislabeled on products or a supplement may contain harmful substances that are not listed on the label.

A dietary supplement, however, can be investigated by the FDA if it appears to pose "a significant or unreasonable health risk" to the public.

Exaggerated and False Claims Are Rampant

Exaggerated and false claims are rampant in the advertisements for weight-loss products. They commonly promise that weight loss will require little sacrifice and will be fast, effortless, and safe. At the same time, the advertisements frequently contradict proven methods of successful weight loss—exercise and cutting calories.

The Federal Trade Commission (FTC) advises consumers to be skeptical of weight-loss products that tout effortless, quick fixes.

There is No Quick Fix

A recent report by the FTC reviewed 300 weight-loss ads that appeared in 2001 in mainstream media (on television, in print, and on the Internet) and found that more than half of the ads included at least one false or unproven claim. According to the FTC report, "The world of weight loss advertising is a virtual fantasy land where pounds "melt away" while "you continue to eat your favorite food" and "amazing pills ... seek and destroy enemy fat."

The Bottom Line

Rapid weight loss is unlikely and can be unsafe when using these products. In addition, the faster weight is lost, the faster it is regained. A maximum 1- to 2-lb. drop per week is recommended for safe, permanent weight loss. The National Institutes of Health, which establishes guidelines on the treatment of overweight and obesity, does not recommend any dietary supplements for weight loss. Exercise, healthy eating, and calorie reduction (500 fewer calories a day for a 1-lb. loss per week) are scientifically proven as safe and effective means of achieving and maintaining a healthy weight.

in a year or two, typically reaching pretreatment weight within five years. In this way, VLCDs are no different from other diets. Most people can stick with dietary restrictions for a limited period of time. VLCDs may be even easier to follow than low-calorie diets that contain real food, because predetermined meals and controlled portion sizes help you to resist temptations.

However, you must learn to overcome the eating and behavioral patterns that contributed to your obesity in the first place—and you ultimately must make daily food choices on your own. As a result, VLCD programs are worthless without detailed attention to long-term maintenance. In one study, patients participated in a VLCD program with intensive behavioral training that included instructions on self-monitoring of eating behavior, guidelines for increasing physical activity, and techniques for counteracting relapse. The behavioral training continued even after the VLCD was finished and the patients returned to eating food. In six months, the patients lost an average of 45 lbs. One year later, they had regained only an average of 5 lbs.

In general, VLCDs are safe when medically supervised. Early side effects of hunger, fatigue, and light-headedness usually subside within two weeks. People who cannot tolerate milk products may react to a dairy-based formula. Later on, dieters may note constipation and intolerance to cold, and the risk of gallstones is increased.

Medications

Whether the treatment of obesity requires medication is a decision that must be made on a case-by-case basis. Drug therapy was never intended to be anything but a last-choice option when no other treatment had worked. And today, the use of medications to help suppress appetite or otherwise alter the body's energy balance remains a controversial area in obesity management. Drugs should be used only in people whose BMI exceeds 30, or exceeds 27 when accompanied by serious medical conditions that could be improved by weight loss. Anorectics—drugs that reduce appetite—do not magically melt away pounds: While they may make it easier to adhere to lifestyle changes, they do not eliminate the need to alter behavior permanently.

For good results, drug therapy must be combined with extensive dietary, exercise, and behavior modifications. Anorectics are not effective for everyone. For example, people whose excessive eating is triggered by habits, stress, or emotions may benefit less from drugs that reduce appetite than those who eat because of hunger. If no weight is lost in the first week or two of use, the drug is unlikely to help and should be discontinued (consult your doctor first). Following are the types of drugs currently in use. The prescription drugs, together with side effects and contraindications, are discussed in the chart on pages 64–65.

Noradrenergics. These drugs increase levels of norepinephrine (noradrenaline) in the brain. Norepinephrine reduces appetite by stimulating the central nervous system. On average, people taking noradrenergics lose about ½ lb. more per week than those taking placebos. A noradrenergic agent called phenylpropanolamine (PPA), present in several medicines including over-the-counter appetite suppressants such as Dexatrim, was recalled by the FDA in November 2000.

Serotonin/norepinephrine reuptake inhibitor. The drug sibutramine (Meridia) enhances both serotonin and norepinephrine levels in the brain. This action promotes feelings of fullness and thus reduces appetite.

Lipase inhibitor. Orlistat (Xenical) blocks the intestinal absorption of about 30% of dietary fat. Side effects—such as cramping, oily anal leakage, and explosive diarrhea—tend to be worse when patients eat greater quantities of fatty foods. These adverse effects discourage the consumption of such foods and contribute to the effectiveness of the drug. Because fat malabsorption associated with orlistat can lead to a loss of fat-soluble vitamins A, D, E and K in the stools, a multivitamin must be taken with this medication.

Antidepressants. Although antidepressants are not approved by the FDA for the treatment of obesity, patients taking the selective serotonin reuptake inhibitors (SSRIs) fluoxetine (Prozac) or sertraline (Zoloft) for depression often experience weight loss. Typically, doctors prescribe these drugs for weight loss if the patient is also depressed. SSRIs increase brain levels of serotonin, which produces feelings of fullness. Thus, some patients taking SSRIs feel less hungry, are less concerned with food, and are better able to control their appetites, though the effect may not last long.

Serotonin releasers. Two drugs, which are no longer on the market, dexfenfluramine (Redux) and fenfluramine (Pondimin), were used to decrease appetite by increasing serotonin levels in the brain. People who took these drugs, however, were at higher risk for heart valve abnormalities and hypertension. The withdrawal of these weight loss drugs from the market in 1997 left many people feeling as if they had been denied the one effective method of weight control.

Dietary Supplements and Herbal Preparations

A wide variety of dietary supplements and herbal preparations have been heavily promoted for weight-loss. A recent critical review of these products found no credible evidence for their safety or effectiveness, with the possible exception of pills containing caffeine and ephedrine. The botanical source of the ephedra in herbal weight-loss preparations is the Chinese herb Ma-huang, and its use has been associated with severe cardiovascular and neurological complications. National Institutes of Health guidelines do not recommend herbal preparations for weight loss. For

NEW RULING

Weight Loss Tax Deduction

Until recently, weight loss expenses were tax-deductible only if losing weight was necessary to treat a disease other than obesity. Now the costs of weight loss for obesity are tax-deductible medical expenses because the Internal Revenue Service (IRS) recognizes that "obesity is medically accepted to be a disease in its own right."

The costs of weight loss programs, behavioral counseling, nutrition counseling, prescription drugs, and surgery are considered deductible medical expenses if a physician diagnoses a taxpayer as being obese.

Taxpayers cannot deduct diet-related foods (since everybody has to buy food), fitness club memberships, cosmetic expenses, or costs already covered by an insurance plan. Any medical expense is deductible only after total medical expenses exceed 7.5% of adjusted gross income. Deductions can be applied retroactively to 1998.

Experts believe that this financial incentive may inspire some obese people to seek and persist with treatment. This new IRS rule raises awareness of obesity as a disease and may prompt additional coverage of obesity treatments by government and insurance programs.

JOURNAL OF THE AMERICAN DIETETIC ASSOCIATION
Volume 102, page 632
May 2002

Surgical Procedures for Weight Loss

Each year, approximately 30,000 Americans undergo bariatric surgery for the treatment of severe obesity. Bariatric surgery is intended for people who either have a body mass index (BMI) of 40 or greater or are 100 pounds overweight and have been unable to lose weight through nonsurgical means. It may also be appropriate for people with a BMI between 35 and 40 who have serious obesity-related complications.

Bariatric surgery does not remove fat tissue by suction or excision; rather it usually involves reducing the size of the stomach. The three commonly used types of bariatric procedures are vertical banded gastroplasty, laparoscopic adjustable gastric banding, and gastric bypass. Most bariatric operations can be performed using laparoscopy, a type of surgery in which surgical instruments are inserted through a small incision in the abdominal wall. Because laparoscopic procedures are less invasive than traditional ones, they are becoming the predominant technique in bariatric surgery. With improved surgical techniques, as well as an increasingly overweight population, bariatric procedures are expected to become more prevalent in the future.

Vertical Banded Gastroplasty

Vertical banded gastroplasty, also called gastric partitioning, is a gastric restriction procedure that divides the stomach into two sections. A stapling instrument is used to section off a golf ball-sized pouch at the top of the stomach, and an inflexible ring (or band) is put in place to encircle the small opening between the pouch and the rest of the stomach.

This procedure allows small amounts of food to pass from the pouch to the remaining portion of the stomach. The likelihood of overeating is reduced because a small quantity of food creates a feeling of fullness.

For the procedure to be effective, patients need to limit their intake of calorie-dense, soft foods, such as ice cream and milk shakes, that readily pass through the pouch.

Side effects of the procedure include stretching or reopening of the stomach pouch, breakdown of the materials used to secure internal structures, and leakage of stomach juices into the abdomen. About 10% to 20% of patients require a follow-up operation, most commonly for an abdominal hernia.

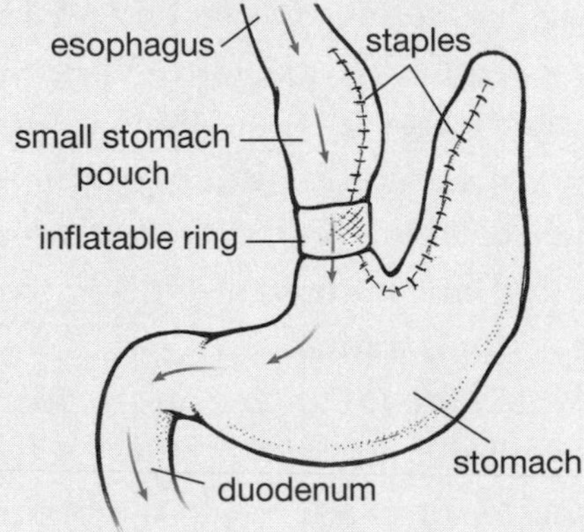

Vertical Banded Gastroplasty

Many patients also experience heartburn and vomiting of solid foods. Vomiting is a special problem because it causes many patients to turn to high-calorie liquids that lead to a significant increase in body weight.

The risk of infection or death from complications of vertical banded gastroplasty is less than 1%. Several studies have shown that vertical banded gastroplasty may result in significant weight loss and improvement in weight-related medical conditions.

Laparoscopic Adjustable Gastric Banding

Approved for use by the U.S. Food and Drug Administration in June 2001, this gastric restriction procedure cuts off a portion of the stomach to reduce gastric volume without sta-

more information, see the feature on dietary supplements on page 67.

Bariatric Surgery

Bariatric surgery is considered for morbidly obese people or for obese people with significant complications of obesity. In either case, the person must have failed to lose weight through other methods. For more information about bariatric surgery, see the feature above.

Liposuction

While the surgical removal of fat may seem like an ideal method of weight reduction, liposuction is, at best, a questionable solution.

pling. Using laparoscopic techniques, an adjustable, hollow, silicone band ("Lap-Band") is wrapped around the upper part of the stomach to create a small pouch. Attached to the band is a flexible tube connected to a miniature access port, which is implanted just beneath the skin of the abdomen. Using this reservoir system, a physician can remove or add saline solution to the band to adjust its fit around the stomach and change the size of the narrow passage that connects the pouch to the lower stomach.

Laparoscopic gastric banding is considered relatively safe and, unlike some other gastric surgeries, is reversible. Clinical trials thus far report significant weight loss, infrequent serious side effects, and a low risk of death. Since this procedure is relatively new, there is little information regarding its long-term safety and efficacy. However, some reported complications related to the band include bleeding, slippage, and obstruction.

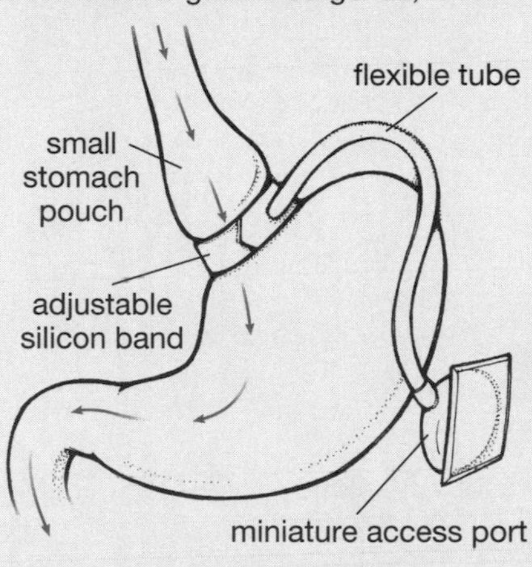

Laparoscopic Adjustable Gastric Banding

Gastric Bypass

Gastric bypass is done in combination with gastric restriction. The volume of the stomach is first reduced by using a stapling tool to create a small upper gastric pouch that is completely separated from the rest of the stomach. The small pouch decreases the quantity of food an individual can comfortably consume. A segment of the small intestine is surgically rerouted to connect directly to the gastric pouch. This procedure allows ingested food to bypass the majority of the stomach as well as part of the small intestine. Since nutrient absorption takes place in the small intestine, the number of calories available to the body is reduced by limiting both the amount of time food spends there and the amount of small intestine exposed to and available to absorb food. The risks associated with gastric bypass are similar to those of vertical banded gastroplasty. However, approximately 30% of bypass patients also develop nutritional deficiencies because many nutrients are normally absorbed in the upper part of the jejunum. Nutritional supplements are recommended, particularly iron, vitamin B_{12}, folate, the fat-soluble vitamins A, D, and E, and possibly calcium. In addition, about one third of bypass patients develop gallstones. Taking bile salts for about six months following surgery can lower this risk, or the gallbladder can be preemptively removed. According to clinical studies, gastric bypass is effective for initiating and sustaining weight loss.

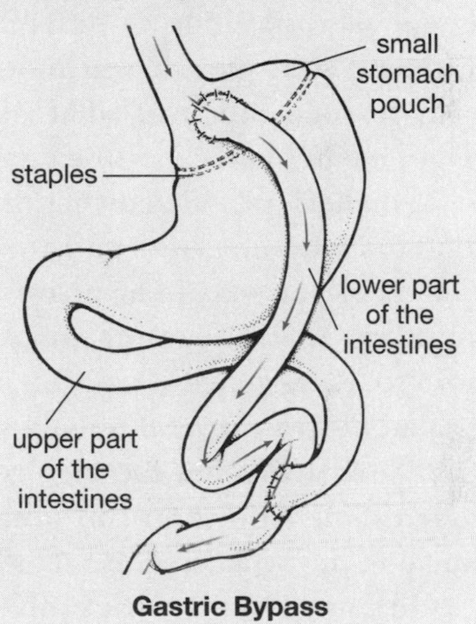

Gastric Bypass

Unlike diet and exercise, fat reduction via liposuction has no proven health benefits. And the procedure cannot help those who are diffusely overweight. Instead, liposuction is appropriate only for people of normal or near-normal weight who have stubborn fat deposits that do not respond to diet and exercise. Candidates should also be in good general health and have skin that is elastic enough to shrink evenly after the surgery—which rules out many people over 50. Finally, liposuction comes with no cosmetic guarantees: While the extracted fat cells will not return, weight can still be gained at other sites in the body.

Common sites of liposuction include the abdomen, hips, buttocks, thighs, legs, upper arms, face, and neck; sometimes several areas are treated at once. Patients must wear a special pressure dressing (such as a girdle or body stocking) over the treated area for several weeks afterwards to help the skin shrink to fit the new contour and to minimize bruising and swelling (which may persist for months). While the overall risk associated with liposuction is low, the more fat that is removed, the greater the risk of complications such as infection or blood clots. Patients interested in liposuction should consult their doctor for an assessment and, possibly, a referral to an experienced plastic surgeon.

MAINTAINING WEIGHT LOSS

Keeping weight off is a bigger challenge than losing the weight in the first place. What distinguishes people who maintain their weight loss from those who lose and then regain weight? The few studies that have examined this question suggest that the answer lies not in genetic predisposition or differences in metabolism, but in the use of coping strategies. If you have lost weight sensibly, you have already learned much of what you need to know about successful weight maintenance. For the most part, all you need to do is continue the behaviors and activities that helped you lose weight. Keep in mind the following strategies.

1. Look for ways to be active every day. Physical activity is just as important in maintaining weight loss as in producing it, maybe more so. Be as active as you can in your day-to-day life, and exercise regularly at least several times a week.

2. Stick with a low-fat, high complex-carbohydrate, portion-controlled diet. While you can occasionally include high-fat foods in your diet, try to keep close tabs on your food choices and portion sizes so you do not slip back into old eating habits.

3. Monitor your eating and exercise habits. Counting calories and fat grams and keeping an exercise log will help you stay on track.

4. Prevent boredom. Experiment with new exercise activities, healthy recipes, and low-calorie foods, such as exotic fruits and vegetables.

5. Do not be alarmed by slight fluctuations in weight. Your weight will vary from day to day depending on your state of hydration—the amount of water in your body. An increase in water weight can be caused by hormonal changes or by eating foods high in sodium.

6. Weigh yourself regularly, but no more than once a day. Once a week may be sufficient. Your goal is not to remain within a pound of your lowest weight, but to maintain your weight within a range.

7. Take lapses in stride. If you have eaten too many cookies or have not exercised in a few days, do not use these lapses as an excuse to give up your efforts. Weight maintenance is a life-long process, not an all-or-nothing contest.

8. Have several problem-solving strategies. Once you have identified your problem areas, think of a variety of solutions. Be flexible. If one solution does not work, try another.

9. Keep your support network strong. Continue to seek help from friends and family.

10. Stay positive. Remind yourself of the great progress you have made. Be proud of your achievement. ■

GLOSSARY

abdominal obesity—Excessive fat in the abdomen indicated by a waist circumference greater than 40 in men and 35 in women.

amino acids—Building blocks of protein. Certain amino acids, also termed essential or "indispensable," must be obtained from the diet because the body does not produce them.

antioxidants—Substances that help the body neutralize free radicals. Beta-carotene, vitamin E, and vitamin C are some examples of the hundreds of naturally occurring antioxidants.

atherosclerosis—An accumulation of deposits of fat and fibrous tissue, called plaques, within the walls of arteries that can narrow the arteries and reduce the flow of blood through them.

bariatric surgery— An operation designed to cause weight loss, often by reducing the size of the stomach. This type of surgery is also called gastric restriction surgery.

bioavailability—A measure of how much and how well a nutrient is absorbed by the body.

body mass index (BMI)—A measurement of weight in relation to height. It is generally considered to be a good indicator of body fat. Calculated by multiplying weight in pounds by 704 and dividing the result by the square of height in inches. Overweight is defined as a BMI between 25 and 29.9 and obesity as a BMI of 30 and over.

calorie—A unit that signifies the quantity of energy in a food. Carbohydrates and protein contain 4 calories per gram; fat contains 9 calories per gram; alcohol contains 7 calories per gram. Technically known as a kilocalorie.

carbohydrates—Foods made up of starches and/or sugars. Sugars are simple carbohydrates while complex carbohydrates are starches that may also contain fiber, vitamins, and minerals. Carbohydrates provide 4 calories per gram.

cardiovascular disease—Disease affecting the heart or arterial vascular system of the body.

carotenoids—A collection of plant pigments that are found in yellow, orange, red, and dark-green fruits and vegetables and may lower the risk of heart disease and certain cancers. Certain carotenoids, particularly beta-carotene, can be converted into vitamin A in the body. Lycopene, lutein, and zeaxanthin are other carotenoids.

cholesterol—A soft, waxy substance present in cells throughout the body. Deposition of blood cholesterol in blood vessels initiates the formation of atherosclerotic plaques. Cholesterol and triglycerides, both fatty substances (or lipids), are transported in the blood in combination with proteins to form three lipoproteins: high density lipoprotein (HDL), low density lipoprotein (LDL), and very low density lipoprotein (VLDL), which carries mainly triglycerides. Because HDL protects against coronary heart disease, it is often called "good" cholesterol. The plaque-forming cholesterol, or LDL, is referred to as "bad" cholesterol. See also dietary cholesterol.

DASH diet—An eating plan that can help control blood pressure and it may also improve cholesterol. Rich in vegetables and fruits, the diet includes low-fat dairy products and is low in saturated fat, total fat, and cholesterol.

diabetes—A disorder characterized by abnormally high levels of glucose (sugar) in the blood.

dietary cholesterol—The cholesterol present in and obtained from animal foods—meats, poultry, fish, shellfish, eggs, and dairy products. Plant foods contain no cholesterol.

dietary supplement—A product (in pill, liquid, or powder form) that is taken in addition to one's regular diet. The supplement can contain a single substance—such as ginkgo biloba, ginseng, or St. John's wort—or a combination of substances.

dysphagia—Difficulty in swallowing food or liquids.

enriched food—A food to which a nutrient or nutrients have been added. Often, the added nutrients were present in the original food but were lost during processing, such as in enriched bread. Sometimes called "fortified food."

enzyme—A protein that accelerates chemical reactions in the body.

essential amino acids— Amino acids that the body cannot synthesize and thus must be consumed in the diet. Lysine is an example. Also known as indispensable amino acids.

essential fatty acids—Fatty acids that are not made by the body and must be obtained from food. Essential fatty acids are necessary for cell structure and are converted into certain hormones that assist in the control of blood pressure, blood clotting, inflammation, and other body functions. Polyunsaturated fatty acids, such as linoleic acid, linolenic acid, and arachidonic acid, are essential fatty acids.

fiber—An indigestible component of fruits, vegetables, grains, and legumes that has numerous health benefits. There are two principal types of fiber: Insoluble fiber does not dissolve in water and helps prevent constipation. Soluble fiber (sometimes called "viscous" fiber) dissolves in water and helps to regulate blood levels of sugar and cholesterol.

fortified food—Food to which a nutrient or nutrients

have been added in order to promote health and prevent disease. The nutrients added to fortified foods are not present in the original food or were present in smaller amounts. Example: vitamin D fortified milk. Sometimes called "enhanced food."

free radicals—Chemical compounds that can damage cells and oxidize low density lipoprotein (LDL) so that it is more likely to be deposited in the walls of arteries.

functional foods—Foods that provide a health benefit beyond the traditional nutrients they contain.

gastric bypass—A type of gastric restriction surgery that reduces the amount of food that can be eaten and absorbed by the body. Gastric bypass involves sealing off a portion of the stomach and bypassing part of the intestine.

genetically modified food— Food that has been genetically altered. A piece of DNA from one plant or animal species is inserted into another species in order to increase food production, decrease the need for pesticides, improve food quality, and/or help prevent diseases in people.

height/weight tables—Tables that display ranges of weights, according to different heights. The information is derived from mortality data of people seeking or obtaining life insurance.

high density lipoprotein (HDL)—A particle in the blood that can protect against coronary heart disease by removing cholesterol from arterial walls. See also cholesterol.

homocysteine—An amino acid that arises from the breakdown of methionine, another amino acid found in animal-derived foods. High blood levels of homocysteine may promote atherosclerosis.

insulin—A hormone that controls the manufacture of glucose by the liver and permits muscle and fat cells to remove glucose from the blood. Also a medication taken by people with diabetes whose pancreas does not make enough insulin.

ketosis—A state in which the blood contains high levels of appetite-suppressing substances called ketones. When carbohydrate consumption is limited and not available for energy, an increased breakdown of fat results in elevated blood levels of ketones. Both poorly controlled diabetes and low-carbohydrate, high-protein diets can lead to ketosis. Side effects of ketosis can include dehydration, dizziness, weakness, headaches, and confusion.

lactose intolerance—A reduced ability to digest the milk sugar lactose that results in abdominal discomfort within 30 minutes to two hours of consuming milk or milk-based foods.

laparoscopic adjustable gastric banding—A minimally invasive, reversible form of gastric restriction surgery that places an adjustable silicone band around the top of the stomach in order to reduce its size and decrease food intake.

leptin—A protein secreted by human fat cells that informs the brain about the body's level of fat stores. Obese people have higher leptin levels than normal-weight individuals.

low density lipoprotein (LDL)—A particle that transports cholesterol in the bloodstream. Its deposition in artery walls initiates plaque formation. A major contributor to coronary heart disease. See also cholesterol.

metabolic syndrome—Also called Syndrome X or insulin resistance syndrome. The presence of at least three of five risk factors (abdominal obesity, elevated triglycerides, low HDL cholesterol, elevated blood pressure, elevated blood sugar) increases the risk of diabetes and coronary heart disease.

metabolism—The chemical process by which the body converts food into energy and various functions. Such activities include food digestion, nutrient absorption, waste elimination, respiration, circulation, and temperature regulation.

minerals—Naturally occurring, inorganic substances required for growth and the maintenance of body functions.

monounsaturated fat—A fat with only one double bond that is capable of absorbing more hydrogen. Monounsaturated fatty acids are widely found in foods; concentrated sources include avocados, almonds, and olive and canola oils. Can lower LDL cholesterol levels when substituted for saturated fat in the diet.

norepinephrine—A stress hormone that promotes satiety (fullness) by stimulating the central nervous system and affecting levels of blood glucose (sugar). Certain weight loss drugs are designed to enhance levels of norepinephrine in the brain. Also called noradrenaline.

obesity—Conventionally defined as a body weight that is 20% or more than what is ideal for a person's height and body type. Obesity is also defined more precisely as a body mass index (BMI) of 30 or higher.

omega-3 fatty acids—Forms of polyunsaturated fat found primarily in fatty fish (such as mackerel, salmon, and tuna), and in small amounts in canola, soybean and walnut oils, walnuts, soybeans, and purslane.

organic food—A product that is grown and produced without the use of petroleum-based fertilizers, sewage sludge-based fertilizers, most conventional pesticides,

GLOSSARY—continued

genetic modification, ionizing radiation, antibiotics, or growth hormones.

osteoporosis—A disorder characterized by fragile, weak bones that result from a loss of bone mass. Increases the risk of bone fracture.

overweight—An excess of body weight that is defined as a body mass index (BMI) of 25 to 29.9.

oxidation—A reaction of any substance with oxygen—an interaction that may generate harmful free radicals, which contribute to the onset of disease. The oxidation of LDL, for example, contributes to its deposition in arterial plaque.

phytochemicals—Compounds from plant foods that may help lower the risk of disease. Flavonoids and soy isoflavones are examples.

plaques—Deposits of fat and fibrous tissue in arteries that can lead to heart disease and stroke.

polyunsaturated fat—A type of fat found in safflower, sunflower, and corn oils. Can help to lower LDL cholesterol when substituted for saturated fat in the diet.

protein—Compounds made up of varying sequences of amino acids. Dietary protein provides four calories per gram.

Recommended Dietary Allowances (RDA)—The average intake of nutrients required to meet the daily nutritional needs of nearly all healthy people.

resting metabolic rate (RMR)—The amount of energy that is spent on basic functions, such as breathing, digestion, heartbeat, and brain activity, while a person is at rest.

saturated fat—A fat found in most animal foods and in tropical oils, such as palm and coconut oils. A major dietary factor in raising blood cholesterol.

serotonin—A chemical in the brain, called a neurotransmitter, that is synthesized from the amino acid tryptophan. Serotonin affects mood and suppresses appetite.

set point theory—A theory that the body maintains a certain weight and body fat level by regulating its own internal controls.

stroke—A sudden reduction in or loss of brain function that occurs when an artery supplying blood to a portion of the brain becomes blocked or ruptures. Nerve cells, or neurons, in the affected area are destroyed by the lack of oxygen and nutrients normally provided by the blood.

thermogenesis—The release of heat energy that occurs when the body breaks down fat and other fuels for energy.

trans fatty acids—Fats formed when food manufacturers add hydrogen atoms to unsaturated fats to make them more saturated and therefore more solid and shelf-stable. Found in margarines, deep-fried fast foods, and store-bought baked goods. Trans fatty acids raise blood cholesterol and lower HDL cholesterol.

triglyceride—A lipid (fat) formed in adipose tissue that serves as the body's major store of energy. Triglycerides released in the liver are carried on lipoproteins, especially very low density lipoprotein. Elevated blood triglyceride levels are associated with an increased risk of coronary heart disease.

vertical banded gastroplasty—A type of bariatric surgery that partitions off a portion of the stomach, leaving room for only about an ounce of food.

vitamins—Organic substances that are required for many metabolic functions including converting food into energy and aiding in the development of bones and tissues. Vitamins themselves do not provide energy. While vitamins are vital to life, they are needed only in minute amounts.

waist circumference—An indicator of abdominal fat. A healthy waist circumference is 40 inches or less for men and 35 inches or less for women. An increased waist circumference confers a health risk.

HEALTH INFORMATION ORGANIZATIONS AND SUPPORT GROUPS

American Council on Exercise
San Diego, CA
www.acefitness.org
☎ 858-279-8227
800-825-3636

American Council on Science and Health (ACSH)
New York, NY
www.acsh.org
☎ 212-362-7044

American Dietetic Association
Chicago, IL
www.eatright.org
☎ 800-366-1655
312-899-0040

American Heart Association
Dallas, TX
www.americanheart.org
☎ 800-242-8721

American Institute for Cancer Research (AICR)
Washington, DC
www.aicr.org
☎ 800-843-8114

American Running Association
Bethesda, MD
www.americanrunning.org
☎ 301-913-9517
800-776-2732

Center for Science in the Public Interest
Washington, DC
www.cspinet.org
☎ 202-332-9110

Food and Nutrition Information Center
Beltsville, MD
www.nal.usda.gov/fnic
☎ 301-504-5719

The Food and Drug Administration
Rockville, MD
www.fda.gov/
☎ 1-888-463-6332

International Food Information Council Foundation (IFIC)
Washington, DC
www.ific.org
☎ 202-296-6540

National Inst. of Diabetes & Digestive & Kidney Disease, Weight-Control Information
Bethesda, MD
www.niddk.nih.gov/health/nutrit/win.htm
☎ 202-828-1025

USDA Meat and Poultry Hotline
Washington, DC
www.fsis.usda.gov/OA/programs/mphotlin.htm
☎ 800-535-4555

LEADING CENTERS FOR WEIGHT CONTROL

The following list of weight control and eating disorder centers was compiled by Dr. Lawrence Cheskin, director of the Johns Hopkins Weight Management Center and coauthor of this White Paper. Listed alphabetically, all of the centers are affiliated with hospitals or universities involved in obesity research.

Duke University Diet and Fitness Program
Durham, NC
www.dukedietcenter.org
☎ 800-235-3853

Johns Hopkins Weight Management Center
Lutherville, MD
www.jhbmc.jhu.edu/weight
☎ 410-847-3744

New York Obesity Research Center St. Luke's-Roosevelt Hospital
New York, NY
cpmcnet.columbia.edu/dept/obesectr/NYORC/
☎ 212-523-4196

Nutrition Research Clinic Baylor College of Medicine
Houston, TX
☎ 713-798-5757

Weight and Eating Disorders Program University of Pennsylvania
Philadelphia, PA
www.uphs.upenn.edu
☎ 215-898-7314

Weight Control Center— New York Hospital
New York, NY
☎ 212-583-1000

Yale Center for Eating and Weight Disorders
New Haven, CT
www.yale.edu/ycewd
☎ 203-432-4610

VITAMINS AND CHRONIC DISEASE

The following report from the *Journal of the American Medical Association* advises all adults to take a daily multivitamin supplement. The recommendation is based on accumulated evidence from more than 100 research studies.

In the article, Kathleen M. Fairfield, M.D., and Robert H. Fletcher, M.D., of Harvard Medical School examine the relationship between vitamins and chronic disease in studies published between 1966 and January 2002. The review focuses on nine major nutrients—folate, vitamins B_6 and B_{12}, provitamin A carotenoids, and vitamins A, C, D, E, and K—because of their close link to disease prevention.

According to the review, although true vitamin deficiencies are rare in developed countries, less-than-optimal intake of certain vitamins is common among American adults. A diminished intake of vitamins may raise the risk of chronic disease, including cardiovascular disease, colon and breast cancer, bone fractures, as well as pregnancies resulting in neural tube defects.

The authors emphasize that while optimal multivitamin doses are beneficial for everyone, high doses of some vitamins, particularly fat-soluble vitamins, are dangerous. A notable example is the toxic effect of excessive amounts of vitamin A. However, taking additional supplements may benefit certain individuals: The elderly are advised to take extra supplements of calcium and vitamins B_{12} and D; and women of childbearing age are advised to consume an additional supplement of 400 micrograms (mcg) of folic acid per day. In addition, most men and nonmenstruating women are advised to select a multivitamin supplement that contains little or no iron.

In an accompanying clinical commentary, the authors note that "most people do not consume an optimal amount of all vitamins by diet alone. Pending strong evidence of effectiveness from randomized trials, it appears prudent for all adults to take vitamin supplements." (However, the authors also point out that because "foods contain thousands of compounds that may be biologically active," supplementation should not be considered a substitute for a good diet.) To meet the supplement recommendation, and to avoid the expense of name-brand vitamins, consumers are advised to purchase inexpensive, generic-brand multivitamins sold at pharmacies or discount shops.

Vitamins for Chronic Disease Prevention in Adults

Scientific Review

Kathleen M. Fairfield, MD, DrPH

Robert H. Fletcher, MD, MSc

Context Although vitamin deficiency is encountered infrequently in developed countries, inadequate intake of several vitamins is associated with chronic disease.

Objective To review the clinically important vitamins with regard to their biological effects, food sources, deficiency syndromes, potential for toxicity, and relationship to chronic disease.

Data Sources and Study Selection We searched MEDLINE for English-language articles about vitamins in relation to chronic diseases and their references published from 1966 through January 11, 2002.

Data Extraction We reviewed articles jointly for the most clinically important information, emphasizing randomized trials where available.

Data Synthesis Our review of 9 vitamins showed that elderly people, vegans, alcohol-dependent individuals, and patients with malabsorption are at higher risk of inadequate intake or absorption of several vitamins. Excessive doses of vitamin A during early pregnancy and fat-soluble vitamins taken anytime may result in adverse outcomes. Inadequate folate status is associated with neural tube defect and some cancers. Folate and vitamins B_6 and B_{12} are required for homocysteine metabolism and are associated with coronary heart disease risk. Vitamin E and lycopene may decrease the risk of prostate cancer. Vitamin D is associated with decreased occurrence of fractures when taken with calcium.

Conclusions Some groups of patients are at higher risk for vitamin deficiency and suboptimal vitamin status. Many physicians may be unaware of common food sources of vitamins or unsure which vitamins they should recommend for their patients. Vitamin excess is possible with supplementation, particularly for fat-soluble vitamins. Inadequate intake of several vitamins has been linked to chronic diseases, including coronary heart disease, cancer, and osteoporosis.

JAMA. 2002;287:3116-3126 www.jama.com

Vitamins are organic compounds that cannot be synthesized by humans and therefore must be ingested to prevent metabolic disorders. Although classic vitamin deficiency syndromes such as scurvy, beriberi, and pellagra are now uncommon in Western societies, specific clinical subgroups remain at risk (TABLE 1). For example, elderly patients are particularly at risk for vitamins B_{12} and D deficiency, alcohol-dependent individuals are at risk for folate, B_6, B_{12}, and thiamin deficiency, and hospitalized patients are at risk for deficiencies of folate and other water-soluble vitamins. Inadequate intake or subtle deficiencies in several vitamins are risk factors for chronic diseases such as cardiovascular disease, cancer, and osteoporosis. In addition, pregnancy or alcohol use may increase vitamin requirements. At least 30% of US residents use vitamin supplements regularly, suggesting that physicians need to be informed about available preparations and prepared to counsel patients in this regard.[1] At a minimum, patients should be queried about their usual diet and use of vitamin supplements.

We searched MEDLINE for English-language articles published from 1966 through January 11, 2002, about vitamins, vitamin deficiencies and toxicity, and specific vitamins in relation to chronic diseases. We paid specific attention to cardiovascular disease, common cancers (lung, colon, breast, and prostate), neural tube defect, and osteoporosis. We reviewed reference lists from retrieved articles for additional pertinent information. The coauthors

Author Affiliations: Division of General Medicine and Primary Care, Beth Israel Deaconess Medical Center, and Channing Laboratory, Department of Medicine, Brigham and Women's Hospital, Harvard Medical School (Dr Fairfield); Department of Ambulatory Care and Prevention, Harvard Medical School/Harvard Pilgrim Health Care, and Department of Epidemiology, Harvard School of Public Health (Dr Fletcher), Boston, Mass.

Corresponding Author and Reprints: Kathleen M. Fairfield, MD, DrPH, Division of General Medicine and Primary Care, Libby 330, Beth Israel Deaconess Medical Center, 330 Longwood Ave, Boston, MA 02215 (e-mail: kfairfie@caregroup.harvard.edu).

Scientific Review and Clinical Applications Section Editor: Wendy Levinson, MD, Contributing Editor.

We encourage authors to submit papers to "Scientific Review and Clinical Applications." Please contact Wendy Levinson, MD, Contributing Editor, *JAMA;* phone: 312-464-5204; fax: 312-464-5824; e-mail: wendy.levinson@utoronto.ca.

reviewed the references jointly and attempted to synthesize the material, placing emphasis on randomized trial data where available. TABLE 2 summarizes the cohort and randomized trial data for the most important vitamin-disease relationships. We reviewed the 9 vitamins that are especially central in the preventive care of adults: folate, vitamins B_6 and B_{12}, vitamin D, vitamin E, the provitamin A carotenoids, vitamin A, vitamin C, and vitamin K. We did not include thiamin (vitamin B_1) or riboflavin (B_2), because of little evidence of their relationship to chronic disease. We include the carotenoid lycopene, although it does not have provitamin A activity and is therefore not a true vitamin. Similarly, vitamin D is not a true vitamin because it can be syn-

Table 1. Clinical Situations in Which Vitamin Deficiency Syndromes Occur

Mechanism	Examples
Poor intake	Food faddism, elderly populations, malabsorption, parenteral nutrition
Abnormal losses	Hemodialysis
Abnormal metabolism	Genetic polymorphisms, alcoholism (mixed with poor intake)
Inadequate synthesis	Vitamin D (northern climates)

Table 2. Summary of Cohort Studies and Randomized Trials of Major Vitamin-Disease Relationships

	Evidence	Summary Points
B Vitamins and CHD	Cohort studies	Low serum folate was associated with increased risk of CHD in a retrospective cohort study.[2] In a large prospective cohort, higher dietary intake of folate and vitamin B_6 was associated with decreased risk of CHD.[3]
	Meta-analysis	Folate lowers plasma homocysteine levels by approximately 25%, and addition of B_{12} lowers it another 7%, but addition of B_6 resulted in no further reduction.[4]
	Additional new clinical trials of B vitamins	Several large clinical trials of folate, B_6, and B_{12} in relation to CHD are under way.[5,6]
Folate and colorectal cancer	Cohort studies	Separate studies of men and women using multivitamins with folate for >10-15 years observed reductions in colon cancer risk.[7,8] Another prospective study found colon cancer risk reductions associated with higher dietary folate in men but not women.[9]
Folate and breast cancer	Cohort studies	Higher folate consumption was associated with decreased breast cancer risk among women consuming alcohol regularly but not among nondrinkers in 3 cohort studies.[10-12]
Folate and neural tube defect	Cohort study	Women consuming a multivitamin with folate during the first 6 weeks of pregnancy were at decreased risk of having a neonate with neural tube defect.[13]
	Randomized trials	Folate supplementation decreased the risk of first[14] and recurrent[15] neural tube defects.
Vitamin E and CHD	Cohort studies	Vitamin E is an antioxidant and affects smooth muscle proliferation and platelet adhesion. Numerous cohort studies showed reduction in CHD risk with higher vitamin E intake.[16,17]
	Randomized trials	Three of 4 randomized controlled trials showed no benefit of vitamin E supplementation on CHD risk.[18-21] In another study, vitamin E reduced the risk of nonfatal myocardial infarctions but not cardiovascular mortality.[22]
Vitamin E and prostate cancer	Cohort studies	Two prospective studies showed decreased prostate cancer risk with increased vitamin E intake, particularly among smokers.[23,24]
	Randomized trial	In the Alpha-Tocopherol Beta-Carotene trial, α-tocopherol supplementation decreased prostate cancer incidence and mortality.[25]
Carotenoids and CHD	Cohort studies	Prospective studies have failed to show an association between carotenoid intake and CHD.[26,27]
	Randomized trials	Beta carotene did not reduce coronary heart disease risk in 5 primary prevention trials.[25,28-31] Two studies suggested increased mortality among smokers supplemented with beta carotene.[18,19]
Carotenoids and lung cancer	Cohort studies	Multiple studies showed inverse associations between beta carotene and lung cancer.[77] Three newer cohort studies have shown inverse associations between alpha carotene (but not beta carotene) and lung cancer.[32-34]
	Randomized trials	Two large randomized placebo-controlled trials found increased lung cancer risk among male smokers receiving beta carotene.[25,28] Three other intervention trials reported no increase in risk but included few smokers.[29,30,35]
Carotenoids and prostate cancer	Cohort studies	Beta carotene was not associated with prostate cancer in several prospective studies.[36] Several prospective studies have found decreased risk of prostate cancer associated with increased lycopene intake.[36-39] Serum studies have been mixed.[23,40,41]
	Randomized trials	One intervention study showed increased prostate cancer incidence and mortality in the group receiving beta carotene[25] and 2 showed no association.[28,30]
Vitamin D and bone mass	Cohort studies, randomized trials	Inadequate vitamin D status is a common problem.[42,43] Vitamin D supplementation decreases bone turnover and increases bone mineral density.[42,44] Supplementation with vitamin D and calcium decreases bone loss and fracture rates in elderly people.[45] It remains unclear whether vitamin D alone decreases fracture rates or whether supplemental calcium is required.

*CHD indicates coronary heart disease.

Table 3. Current Reference Daily Intakes for Vitamins

Vitamin	Daily Value
Vitamin A	1500 μg/L (5000 IU)
Vitamin C	60 mg
Vitamin D	10 μg/L (400 IU)
Vitamin E	20 mg (30 IU)
Vitamin K	80 μg/L
Vitamin B_6	2 mg
Vitamin B_{12}	6 μg/L
Folate	400 μg/L
Thiamin	1.5 mg
Riboflavin	1.7 mg
Niacin	20 mg

thesized by humans, but for the sake of simplicity we use the term *vitamin* to refer to these compounds.

Current recommendations are expressed as daily values, a new dietary reference term that is made up of reference daily intakes (RDIs) for vitamins and minerals, which has replaced US recommended daily allowance, and daily reference values for fats, protein, fiber, sodium, and potassium.[46] TABLE 3 summarizes the RDIs for vitamins.

Folate, Vitamin B_6, and Vitamin B_{12}

Folate and vitamins B_6 and B_{12} are discussed together in relation to coronary heart disease (CHD) because of their joint effects on homocysteine. Elevated plasma total homocysteine level is a major risk factor for coronary disease.[5,47,48] People with the highest homocysteine levels have an approximate 2-fold increase in risk of CHD compared with those with the lowest levels, similar to the increase in risk associated with cigarette smoking or hypercholesterolemia. This effect is independent of other known risk factors.[47]

Folate. Folate (other interchangeable terms include folic acid and folacin) is a water-soluble B vitamin that is necessary in forming coenzymes for purine and pyrimidine synthesis, erythropoiesis, and methionine regeneration.[49] The current RDI for folate is 400 μg. The richest food sources of folate are dark-green leafy vegetables, whole-grain cereals, fortified grain products, and animal products. Since 1996 in the United States, all flour and uncooked cereal grains have been supplemented with 140 μg of folate per 100 g of flour. This practice increases plasma folate levels among nonusers of vitamin supplements from about 4.6 to 10.0 ng/mL in the general population.[50] Higher levels were not chosen because of concern about masking B_{12} deficiency: by treating anemia that might otherwise cause symptoms leading to diagnosis of B_{12} deficiency, neurologic symptoms might progress. We are unaware of reports of folate toxicity. Folate deficiency, generally caused by poor intake or alcoholism, is marked by a macrocytic anemia, and suboptimal folate intake causes fetal neural tube defects. More recently, interest in the scientific community has turned to the role of folate in CHD and cancer.

Vitamin B_6. Vitamin B_6 refers to a group of nitrogen-containing compounds with 3 primary forms: pyridoxine, pyridoxal, and pyridoxamine. They are water soluble and are found in a variety of plant and animal products. The current RDI for vitamin B_6 is 2 mg. The best dietary sources include poultry, fish, meat, legumes, nuts, potatoes, and whole grains.[51] Vitamin B_6 participates in more than 100 enzymatic reactions and is needed for protein metabolism, conversion of tryptophan to niacin, and neurotransmitter formation, among other functions. Deficiency is uncommon, although marginal B_6 status may be related to CHD. True deficiency results in cheilosis, stomatitis, effects on the central nervous system (including depression), and neuropathy. Toxicity is unusual and has been associated with neurotoxicity and photosensitivity with doses higher than 500 mg/d.[49]

Vitamin B_{12}. Vitamin B_{12} (cyanocobalamin) is water soluble and found in animal products only (meat, poultry, fish, eggs, and milk). The current RDI for vitamin B_{12} is 6 μg. It acts as a coenzyme for fat and carbohydrate metabolism, protein synthesis, and hematopoiesis. Deficiency can result from poor intake, including strict veganism, throughout a period of several years or malabsorption from absence of intrinsic factor, from gastric or ileal disease, and among elderly individuals in general.[52] Vitamin B_{12} deficiency results in a macrocytic anemia and neurologic abnormalities: loss of proprioception and vibration sense. There is no determined upper limit for vitamin B_{12} intake because there are no consistent adverse effects of high intake.

B Vitamins and CHD

Many studies have reported increased risk of CHD or ischemic stroke associated with low folate intake or low blood folate levels.[5] Folate, along with vitamins B_6 and B_{12}, is required for the metabolism of homocysteine to methionine. Folate appears to be the critical vitamin in determining plasma homocysteine levels.[53,54] In a meta-analysis,[4] folate lowered plasma homocysteine levels by 25%, and addition of B_{12} lowered homocysteine another 7%, but addition of B_6 did not result in further reductions. A recent report found that folate at 800 μg/d was necessary to minimize homocysteine levels (to 2.7 μmol/L [0.37 mg/L], similar to the effects of folate at 1000 μg/d).[55] Although low serum folate levels have a central role in the pathogenesis of hyperhomocysteinemia, whether folate has direct effects on CHD development remains unclear. Observational studies have consistently shown that elevated homocysteine levels are a risk factor for cardiovascular disease. In a study of elderly patients, mean homocysteine concentrations were significantly higher in participants in the lowest 2 deciles of plasma folate concentration. Serum B_6 and B_{12} levels were also inversely associated with homocysteine levels, but this relationship was weaker than for folate.[56] A smaller study[57] showed similar results.

Low serum folate levels were associated with increased risk of CHD in a retrospective Canadian cohort[2] and a large case-control study.[58] Similarly, higher dietary intakes of folate and vitamin B_6 are associated with decreased risk of CHD.[3] Several large clinical trials of folate, B_6, and B_{12} are under way and will likely clarify the relationships of these vitamins to coronary disease.[5,6] Since the existing evidence is entirely from observational research, it should be viewed with caution until randomized trial results become available.

Most multivitamins provide 400 μg of folate (100% of the current RDI), 3 μg of vitamin B_6 (150% of the RDI), and 9 μg of vitamin B_{12} (150% of the RDI). Until results of trials provide more specific information on vitamin doses required to minimize homocysteine levels, recommending a daily multivitamin for most adults may be the most prudent approach. For patients with premature CHD or a family history of premature CHD, either testing for hyperhomocysteinemia or recommending folate at 800 μg/d is appropriate.

Folate and Cancer

Folate deficiency may contribute to aberrant DNA synthesis and carcinogenesis by decreasing methionine availability and interfering with normal DNA methylation. Recently, interest has grown in the effects of folate supplementation in cancer prevention.[59] Higher dietary folate intake appears to reduce the risk of colon and breast cancer, particularly among moderate consumers of alcohol.

Colorectal Cancer. In the Health Professionals Follow-up Study,[7] men who reported folate ingestion from multivitamins for longer than 10 years had a 25% reduction in colon cancer risk, which increased among moderate alcohol users with low intakes of folate or methionine. The Nurses' Health Study[8] found similar effects for women: those reporting 15 or more years of multivitamin use (with folate) had a 75% reduction in colorectal cancer risk. A recent report from the National Health and Nutrition Examination Survey I (NHANES I)[9] found a statistically significant 60% risk reduction in colon cancer in men and a similar nonsignificant effect in women. Men who used alcohol and consumed diets low in folate and methionine were at highest risk for colon cancer.

A common functional polymorphism in the gene for methylenetetrahydrofolate reductase (*MTHFR*, a major enzyme involved in folate metabolism) is associated with an increased risk of colorectal cancer. Dietary folate and methionine intake modify colorectal cancer risk in people with *MTHFR* polymorphisms.[60-61]

Breast Cancer. Higher folate intake may also reduce breast cancer risk, although possibly only among women who have low folate levels and consume alcohol. Several groups have reported inverse associations between folate consumption and breast cancer risk. It appears that higher intake of folate lowers the excess breast cancer risk associated with alcohol use.[10-12] For example, among Nurses' Health Study participants who used alcohol, multivitamin users had a 25% reduction in breast cancer risk.[10]

Colon and breast cancers are among the most common cancers in Western societies, so folate's potential for helping to prevent these cancers is important. The evidence supporting the protective role of folate for colon and breast cancers is moderately strong but not based on randomized trials. The interaction between alcohol use and folate intake is likely to prove substantial. Subgroups of the population with *MTHFR* polymorphisms may also have higher folate requirements.

Neural Tube Defects. Folate is necessary for embryogenesis, and supplementation reduces the risk of neural tube defects. Multiple observational studies have demonstrated this,[13,62-66] as well as 1 nonrandomized trial[67] and 2 randomized trials.[14,15] Folate supplementation decreases the risk of first occurrence of neural tube defect[14] and recurrent defects in women with a previously affected pregnancy.[15] A recent review suggested that doses well above the current RDI of 400 μg are necessary to maximally reduce the risk of neural tube defects.[68] Because the neural tube closes within 3 weeks of conception (before most women know they are pregnant), supplementing all women who might become pregnant with folate at 800 μg/d is the best way of preventing this birth defect.

Vitamin E

Vitamin E is fat soluble and composed of a family of 8 related compounds, the tocopherols and the tocotrienols. The major chemical forms of vitamin E (based on the location of a methyl group) are the tocopherols α, β, Δ, and γ. α-Tocopherol is the most abundant form in foods and is generally the form used in supplements. However, there is at least some concern[69] that preferential appearance of α-tocopherol in the plasma may displace γ-tocopherol in those taking supplements. Both α- and γ-tocopherol may be associated with prostate cancer reduction.

Vitamin E, like other antioxidants, can scavenge free radicals and may, as a result, prevent oxidative damage to lipid membranes and low-density lipoprotein (LDL). Vitamin E is also needed in immune function, and supplementation enhances cell-mediated immunity in elderly patients.[70] The current RDI for vitamin E is 20 mg (30 IU). Major dietary sources of vitamin E include salad oils, margarine, legumes, and nuts.[71] In people who take supplements (approximately 1 in 3 people), however, the greatest contributor to total intake is supplements. Vitamin E deficiency is rare and is seen primarily in special situations resulting in fat malabsorption, including cystic fibrosis, chronic cholestatic liver disease, abetalipoproteinemia, and short bowel syndrome. Clinical manifestations of vitamin E deficiency include muscle weakness, ataxia, and hemolysis. In adults, 200 to 800 mg/d is generally tolerated without adverse effects, with the exception of gastrointestinal upset. With doses of 800 to 1200 mg/d, antiplatelet effects and bleeding may occur. Doses higher than 1200 mg/d may result in headache, fatigue, nausea, diarrhea, cramping, weakness, blurred vision, and gonadal dysfunction.[49]

Coronary Heart Disease. Vitamin E is postulated to prevent atherosclerotic disease not only by its antioxidant effects, but also by inhibitory effects upon smooth muscle proliferation[72] and platelet adhesion.[73] Observational studies have reported that vitamin E is a protective factor for CHD. The Nurses' Health Study[16] found that women taking vitamin E at more than 67 mg/d (100 IU, or about 20 times the amount in a usual Western diet) had a 44% reduction in major coronary disease. Women who took vitamin E supplements for more than 2 years accounted for the majority of this observed risk reduction. Dietary intake of vitamin E alone, as opposed to supplements, had no impact on the risk of CHD. Similar results were noted in a cohort of men, with protective effects limited to those consuming doses of at least 67 mg/d (100 IU).[17]

Unfortunately, clinical trials have not found that vitamin E supplementation, even in high doses and high-risk patients, protects against CHD. Three of 4 large clinical trials[18-21] examining the effect of vitamin E supplementation in patients with higher risk or preexisting CHD, with varying dose and duration, failed to show a benefit. In the Cambridge Heart Antioxidant Study (CHAOS),[22] α-tocopherol at 267 to 533 mg/d (400-800 IU) reduced the 1-year rate of nonfatal myocardial infarctions among patients with known CHD by 80% but caused no reduction in cardiovascular mortality. The use of vitamin E saved $578 for each patient throughout a 3-year period, largely because of a reduction in hospital admissions for myocardial infarction.[74] In the Alpha-Tocopherol Beta-Carotene (ATBC) trial,[18] the largest such trial completed, no association was observed between vitamin E at 50 mg/d (75 IU) and CHD mortality or angina.[19] Two recent large randomized trials in high-risk patients showed no difference between vitamin E and placebo on cardiovascular events.[20,21] The larger trial used 267 mg (400 IU) of vitamin E and included follow-up for an average of 4.5 years.[20] One recent trial of vitamin E at 533 mg/d (800 IU) in dialysis patients showed reduced risk of cardiovascular events, including myocardial infarction.[75]

Overall, there is strong evidence that vitamin E does not substantially decrease cardiovascular mortality, at least when taken throughout a period of a few years by patients with known coronary artery disease or who are at high risk. However, the observational studies showing a protective effect of vitamin E were all among lower-risk populations, and there are no trial data from similar populations. Vitamin E may still be useful in primary prevention when taken throughout long periods. In addition, some subgroups, including patients receiving dialysis, may benefit from supplementation.

Prostate Cancer. Although the relationship between vitamin E and the major cancers (breast, lung, prostate, and colon) has been evaluated in many studies, the weight of evidence does not support a strong association, with the exception of prostate cancer. There is evidence that α-tocopherol may decrease prostate cancer risk among smokers. In the ATBC trial, in which the participants were all male smokers, α-tocopherol supplementation decreased prostate cancer incidence and mortality.[25] Two other studies supported an association between vitamin E and decreased prostate cancer risk,[23] particularly among smokers.[24]

Studies of vitamin E in plasma and prostate cancer have been mixed. Two older serum studies of α-tocopherol showed no association,[40,41] but a recent plasma study reported inverse relationships for α- and γ-tocopherol.[76] Although few other studies have examined the relationship between γ-tocopherol and prostate cancer, 2 studies showed no association[23] or a modest reduction in risk.[41]

The state of the evidence suggests a possible reduction in prostate cancer risk with α-tocopherol supplements, which may be limited to smokers. The paucity of evidence, in addition to concerns over which form is more likely to have clinical effects, suggests that making recommendations for supplementation is premature.

Carotenoids

Carotenoids are a class of yellow, orange, and red plant-derived compounds. All of the more than 600 known carotenoids are antioxidants, and approximately 50 are vitamins because they have provitamin A activity. Vitamin A refers to preformed retinol and the carotenoids that are converted to retinol by cleavage of a central bond. There is no known deficiency state for carotenoids themselves and no RDI. Carotenoid toxicity includes carotenodermia (yellowing of the skin) and, rarely, diarrhea or arthralgias. Beta carotene has historically received the most attention of the carotenoids because of its provitamin A activity and prevalence in many foods. Two other carotenoids with provitamin A activity, alpha carotene and beta cryptoxanthin, are prevalent in foods and contribute substantially to vitamin A intake. Other carotenoids without provitamin A activity that are relatively well studied because of their higher concentrations in serum include lycopene, lutein, and zeaxanthin.

It was proposed that beta carotene supplementation might prevent cardiovascular disease and cancer because of its antioxidant effects. After disappointing findings from several studies, other carotenoids are now the subject of more intensive investigation. Although much of the early evidence, particularly for cancer prevention, is derived from observational studies of dietary carotenoid intake, some caution must be used in interpreting the findings. Associations between diet and disease in observational studies may be due to the specific carotenoids, other vitamins or compounds in fruits and vegetables, or substitution for dietary meat and fat. Genetic predisposition, underlying nutritional status, smoking, and tissue-specific effects may be important.

Cancer. Many studies have evaluated the relationships between carotenoid intake and cancer. The best evidence is for lung, colon, breast, and prostate cancers. Interest in carotenoids, specifically beta carotene, initially arose because of their antioxidant effects, but retinol and the provitamin A carotenoids may also decrease cancer risk via other mechanisms such as inducing cellular differentiation.

Lung Cancer. Observational studies strongly supported an inverse relationship between beta carotene intake and lung cancer risk. A 1995 review reported inverse relationships for 13 of 14 case-control studies, all of 5 cohort studies of dietary beta carotene intake, and all of 7 studies on plasma levels.[77] Two large cohort studies[32,33] have also demonstrated inverse associations for alpha carotene. A recent report combined updated observational data from the Nurses' Health Study and the Health Professionals Follow-up Study and found significant risk reductions for lycopene and alpha carotene but nonsignificant risk reductions for beta carotene. This report also noted a 32% reduction in risk of lung cancer for people consuming a diet high in a variety of carotenoids.[34]

Two large randomized placebo-controlled trials, the ATBC study[25] and the Beta Carotene and Retinol Efficacy Trial study,[28] assessed the risk of lung cancer among male smokers or asbestos workers receiving beta carotene supplements. Both showed statistically significant increases in lung cancer risk among men who received the supplements. Additional analyses from the ATBC study showed that much of the increased risk was confined to the heaviest smokers (>20 cigarettes per day) and regular alcohol users.[78] Three other intervention trials reported no increase in risk.[29,30,35] These studies all included small proportions of smokers.

These findings provide strong support that, at least among smokers, beta carotene supplementation increases the risk of lung cancer. Alcohol use may modify this risk. Other carotenoids including alpha carotene or total carotenoid intake from foods may be associated with decreased risk of lung cancer, although this evidence remains weak.

Colorectal Cancer. Five randomized trials have shown no reduction in colorectal cancer risk with beta carotene supplementation.[25,28,29,35,79] However, 2 of these did find that among regular alcohol users, beta carotene supplements decreased colon cancer risk.[79,80] Supplementation among alcohol users may be more effective because their serum beta carotene levels appear to be lower.[81-85]

Overall, beta carotene supplementation does not appear to decrease colorectal cancer risk. Because regular users of alcohol have lower beta carotene levels, they may benefit from beta carotene supplements, although there is no strong evidence to support this.

Prostate Cancer. The relationship between beta carotene and prostate cancer has been examined in observational studies and intervention trials. In the largest cohort study of this relationship,[36] beta carotene intake was not associated with prostate cancer risk, and results from other observational studies have been mixed. Several intervention trials have studied the effects of beta carotene supplementation on prostate cancer risk. In the ATBC study, prostate cancer incidence and mortality were increased in the beta carotene supplementation group.[25] However, the increased risk was limited to alcohol users, while nonusers had a 32% lower risk than the placebo group. In the Physicians' Health Study, beta carotene supplementation was not associated with prostate cancer risk overall.[30] However, in the men in the lowest quartile of serum beta carotene level at baseline, those assigned to beta carotene supplements had a 32% reduction in prostate cancer risk.[85] A third large intervention trial of beta carotene revealed no association with prostate cancer.[28]

More recently, investigators have reported on the relationship between the carotenoid lycopene and prostate cancer. Dietary lycopene comes primarily from tomato products, including tomato paste, juice, and sauce, but watermelon, pink grapefruit, and other fruits and vegetables also contribute to intake. Lycopene is not converted to vitamin A, and its effects may be due to its antioxidant activity.[86] Giovannucci et al[36] reported a reduction in prostate cancer risk among men with high lycopene consumption and those with high intakes of lycopene-rich foods, including tomatoes and tomato products. An earlier study among a smaller cohort of Seventh-Day Adventists[37] showed a reduced risk of prostate cancer associated with tomato intake, and 2 additional cohort studies have reported preliminary findings, with similar findings for tomato products.[38,39] Two of 3 studies of plasma or serum lycopene have provided further support for the hypothesis, reporting associations between higher lycopene levels and reductions in prostate cancer risk.[23,40] A third serum-based study[41] found no association but was limited by low serum lycopene levels. There have been no clinical trials of lycopene supplementation for prostate cancer prevention.

In summary, there is insufficient evidence to draw conclusions regarding the relationship between beta carotene and prostate cancer risk and some evidence of an increase in risk among alcohol users. Therefore, beta carotene supplementation for prostate cancer prevention should not be encouraged. The evidence for a protective effect for lycopene is more encouraging, although still inconclusive. Patients should not be encouraged to take lycopene supplements, since the current epidemiological evidence is based on dietary intake and may not reflect a direct benefit of lycopene itself.[86]

Breast Cancer. Observational studies of carotenoids, mainly beta carotene, and breast cancer have produced mixed results. A comprehensive review of the literature in 1997[87] reported that the majority of studies, all observational, did not show reduced breast cancer risk with increased beta carotene consumption. Since that review, 4 cohort studies have all reported no association between dietary carotenoids and breast cancer.[88-91] A fifth cohort study found that premenopausal women, particularly those with a positive family history, have significant reductions in breast cancer risk with increasing dietary alpha and beta carotene, lutein/zeaxanthin, and total vitamin A intake.[92] Six studies of serum carotenoids that were nested within prospective cohorts have yielded mixed results. Results from 4 smaller studies showed no decrease in breast cancer risk with higher serum carotenoids.[93-96] In contrast, 2 larger serum studies found inverse relationships for beta cryptoxanthin, lycopene, and lutein/zeaxanthin.[97,98]

Although recent results from larger serum studies are encouraging, the epidemiological evidence linking carotenoids to breast cancer remains inconclusive. Women with higher serum carotenoids may have higher intake of other nutrients from fruits and vegetables as well, and the carotenoids themselves may not be the protective agents.

Coronary Heart Disease. The antioxidant properties of the carotenoids have raised hope that they might prevent CHD, since oxidation of LDL, with subsequent uptake by foam cells in the endothelium, is a known contributor to the disease.[99] Also, beta carotene specifically is carried on LDL particles and can quench singlet oxygen.[99] Although case-control studies of the association between beta carotene and CHD have been mixed, findings from prospective studies have generally found no effect.[26,27,100] Similarly, beta carotene did not reduce CHD risk in 5 primary prevention studies.[25,28-31] More concerning, 2 studies suggested increased mortality among smokers taking beta carotene supplements.[18,19]

Given the results from multiple trials, along with findings from observational studies, there is no reason to recommend beta carotene supplementation for CHD prevention. There is no evidence to suggest a benefit among any subgroup of the population, and smokers may be at increased risk.

Vitamin D

Vitamin D (calciferol) is not a true vitamin, since humans are able to synthesize it with adequate sunlight exposure. Via photoconversion, 7-dehydrocholesterol becomes previtamin D_3, which is metabolized in the liver to 25-hydroxyvitamin D_3, the major circulating form of vitamin D. In the kidney, this is converted to 2 metabolites, the more active one being 1,25-dihydroxyvitamin D_3. The other metabolite, 24,25-dihydroxyvitamin D_3 appears to have a physiological role as well but is less well studied.[49] For simplicity, we refer to 1,25-dihydroxyvitamin D_3 as vitamin D. The current RDI for vitamin D is 0.01 mg (400 IU). Vitamin D may also be ingested in the diet in the form of vitamin D_3, a prohormone. Food sources include fortified milk, saltwater fish, and fish-liver oil.

Vitamin D deficiency is associated with rickets in children. In adults, vitamin D deficiency leads to secondary hyperparathyroidism, bone loss, osteopenia, osteoporosis, and increased fracture risk.[44] Excessive supplement ingestion (>0.05 mg [2000 IU]) or ingestion by patients with normal renal function can result in toxicity, including soft-tissue calcification and hypercalcemia. Vitamin D acts as a steroid hormone, with effects on calcium absorption, phosphorous homeostasis, bone turnover, and multiple other tissues.

Inadequate vitamin D levels are more common than previously thought, particularly among housebound and elderly people. In a large international study of postmenopausal women, 4% were vitamin D deficient and another 24% had inadequate vitamin D status, as reflected in elevated serum parathyroid hormone levels.[42] In a study among medical inpatients, 57% were vitamin D deficient and 22% were considered severely deficient.[43] Vitamin D deficiency was correlated with poor intake, winter, and being housebound. Another study showed that 50% of a group of postmenopausal women admitted with hip fractures were vitamin D deficient.[101] Among female adolescents in Finland during the winter, 62% had low vitamin D concentrations, and 13% were vitamin D deficient. Low vitamin D levels were associated with low forearm bone mineral densities.[102]

Vitamin D supplementation decreases bone turnover and increases bone mineral density, with measurable decreases in parathyroid hormone.[42,44] Most studies of vitamin D and fracture risk were done with supplemental calcium as well, making the role of vitamin D alone difficult to assess. Supplementation with vitamin D and calcium decreases bone loss and fracture rates in the elderly.[45] Withdrawal of vitamin D and calcium supplements appears to result in return to former bone turnover rates and no lasting benefits in terms of bone density within 2 years of discontinuation.[103] In one trial of vitamin D supplements only, no benefit on hip and other peripheral fractures was observed.[104] An earlier trial of annual vitamin D injection showed a reduction in fracture rates in the upper extremity and ribs only, a finding confined to the women in the study.[152]

As is the case with several other vitamins, there is evidence that host factors such as genetic polymorphisms strongly influence fracture risk and may determine the host response to vitamin D.[105] The *Bsml* polymorphism of the vitamin D receptor has been characterized, and the *BB* genotype is associated with a 2-fold increase in fracture risk after known risk factors are adjusted.[106] This polymorphism may have an effect on accumulation of bone mass during puberty and explain some ethnic differences in bone mass.[107]

In summary, the effects of vitamin D on bone mass are strongly supported by the literature. Dark-skinned people are at higher risk of deficiency (although at lower risk of fracture overall), as are those with little exposure to sunlight. In addition, new evidence suggests that genetic polymorphisms modify the host response to vitamin D. Given the high prevalence of vitamin D deficiency and its effects on bone mass, vitamin D supplementation at 400 IU daily can benefit a large proportion of the population. The addition of calcium may be required to realize the beneficial effects of vitamin D in preventing fracture risk.

Vitamin C

Vitamin C (ascorbic acid) is water soluble and acts as a cofactor in hydroxylation reactions, which are required for collagen synthesis. It is also a strong antioxidant. The current RDI for vitamin C is 60 mg. Food sources of vitamin C include citrus fruits, strawberries, melons, tomatoes, broccoli, and peppers.[108] Vitamin C also promotes hormone synthesis, wound healing, and iron absorption. Vitamin C deficiency results in scurvy, marked by bruising and easy bleeding. Large doses (up to 2000 mg) of vitamin C are generally well tolerated, although doses above this range may result in nausea and diarrhea.[49] Although one study raised some concern that high doses of vitamin C may precipitate calcium oxalate stones,[109] this was not observed in the only large prospective study of this relationship.[110]

Coronary Heart Disease. Because of vitamin C's antioxidant effects, many studies of CHD prevention include vitamin C supplementation. In general, the evidence is unconvincing. Although several studies[111-114] of dietary intake have suggested a modest benefit of increased dietary vitamin C, others[16,17,26,115] have reported no relationship between vitamin C intake and CHD. A single observational study[116] of vitamin C supplementation did show a reduced risk of coronary disease, although no adjustment was made for vitamin E supplementation. Among patients with known CHD, there have been few studies on the role of vitamin C, with generally null results.[117-119] Of 2 prospective serum vitamin C studies, one[120] showed decreased cardiovascular mortality with increasing concentrations, but another[121] showed no relationship. A randomized trial of antioxidants for secondary prevention of CHD failed to show an association for vitamin C.[119] There is some thought that vitamins C and E together might yield additional benefits for preventing CHD, and some observational evidence supports this hypothesis.[122] Two ongoing randomized trials[123,124] will provide additional evidence to help resolve this question.

Cancer. Diets high in vitamin C have been linked to lower cancer rates at several sites. A detailed review in 1995 suggested moderately strong evidence for an inverse relationship between dietary vitamin C (mainly from high fruit and vegetable intake) and cancers of the oral cavity, esophagus, and stomach.[125] Reports from 2 recent prospective studies[120,121] showed increased total cancer mortality among men (but not women) with lower serum vitamin C levels. Recent studies have also supported inverse associations between dietary vitamin C and oral cancer,[126] gastric cancer,[127] and premenopausal breast cancer,[128] particularly among women with a positive family history.[92] A meta-analysis[129] also found decreased breast cancer risk (20% risk reduction) associated with high dietary vitamin C intake. In contrast, a recent cohort analysis[91] showed no overall relationship with vitamin C intake, and a prospective plasma study[130] showed no associations between prediagnostic vitamin C levels and breast cancer risk.

Overall, it does not appear that vitamin C is strongly associated with cardiovascular disease. The evidence is moderately strong that diets high in vitamin C are associated with decreased risk of cancers of the oral cavity, esophagus, stomach, and breast. However, it remains unclear whether this decrease is because of high intake of fruits and vegetables (which offer a wide range of other nutrients) or whether vitamin C itself is the protective nutrient. In addition, there are no studies suggesting that vitamin C supplementation is associated with decreased cancer risk. If diets high in vitamin C do decrease cancers at multiple sites, a large proportion of the population could benefit.

Vitamin A

Vitamin A refers to a family of fat-soluble compounds called retinoids, which have vitamin A activity. Retinol is the predominant form, and 11-*cis* retinal is the active form important for vision. Approximately 50 of the more than 600 carotenoids can be converted to vitamin A. The current RDI for vitamin A is 1500 μg/L (5000 IU). Preformed vitamin A is found only in animal products, including organ meats, fish, egg yolks, and fortified milk. Retinol-binding protein binds vitamin A and regulates its uptake and metabolism. Vitamin A is critical in vision (particularly night vision), the immune response, and epithelial cell growth and repair, among other functions. Vitamin A deficiency is marked by xerophthalmia, night blindness, and increased disease susceptibility. Vitamin A toxicity results in hepatotoxicity, visual changes, and craniofacial anomalies in fetuses (beginning at doses of only 3 times the daily allowance, or 15000 IU).[49,131] Two studies have also reported doubling of hip fracture rates among women with high retinol intake from food or supplements (>1.5 mg/d in one study[132] and 2.0 mg/d in the other[133]). Interest centers on its functions in cancer prevention and immunity, particularly in children in developing countries.[134]

Because of its effects on the epithelium and on immunity, retinol has been investigated as a chemoprotective agent for several cancers. The relationship between retinol and bladder cancer has been studied in multiple case-control and cohort studies. A review in 1996[135] suggested a modest overall association, but this was mainly attributed to carotenoid intake. A recent meta-analysis[136] concluded that diets high in fruits and vegetables were associated with decreased risk of bladder cancer but found no association with retinol. Many groups have also examined the relationship between retinol intake and breast cancer. A review in 1994[137] concluded that existing evidence supported a modest inverse relationship between vitamin A and breast cancer, although it was unclear whether carotenoids or retinol was the key nutrient. Since that review, 3 prospective cohort studies have been published; 2 showed a modest decrease in risk for retinol or total vitamin A,[88,92] and 1 showed no association.[91]

There is interest in vitamin A analogues as chemopreventive agents for breast cancer. One large study[138] of fenretinide given to breast cancer survivors for an average of 5 years showed no decrease in secondary breast cancers. Serum studies of retinol and cancer are unreliable because serum levels are tightly controlled and do not generally reflect intake.[137] No other cancers have been convincingly associated with retinol intake.

Vitamin A may decrease the risk of bladder and breast cancers, but the evidence is weak. There are few studies examining gene-diet interactions with regard to vitamin A, but variation in retinol-binding protein may prove to be an important area of inquiry.

Vitamin K

Vitamin K is fat soluble and essential for normal clotting, specifically for production of prothrombin and factors VII, IX, and X and proteins C and S. It is also necessary for normal bone metabolism. The current RDI for vitamin K is 80 µg/L. Dietary sources of vitamin K include dark-green vegetables, particularly spinach, but it is also synthesized by intestinal bacteria. Vitamin K deficiency, which results in clotting disorders, occurs when either intake is inadequate or intestinal bacteria, which synthesize vitamin K, are altered. Newborn infants are also at risk because of poor placental transfer of vitamin K, lack of intestinal bacteria, and low content in breast milk. For this reason, they receive intramuscular vitamin K at birth. There is no known toxicity state for vitamin K.[49]

Coagulation. In adults, the most critical role of vitamin K relates to clotting. Patients with poor intake throughout a long period are particularly at risk when taking antibiotics, which deplete intestinal bacteria. Other risk factors for vitamin K deficiency include renal or hepatic disease and malabsorption. Most patients present with poor clotting function or hemorrhage.[139,140] An important clinical application of vitamin K occurs in patients taking warfarin, which works by inhibiting the vitamin K–dependent γ-carboxylation of coagulation factors II, VII, IX, and X. Dietary variation in vitamin K consumption can lead to difficulty with warfarin dosing; anticoagulated patients should be given clear instructions on diet.[141] Patients who are excessively anticoagulated can be treated effectively with either oral or parenteral vitamin K.[142,143]

Fracture Risk. There is also newer interest in the role of vitamin K in bone metabolism.[144] Vitamin K is a cofactor in the γ-carboxylation of glutamyl residues on osteocalcin and other bone proteins,[145] raising the question of whether deficiency may contribute to osteoporosis.[146] Lower bone mineral density[147] and higher fracture rates[148,149] have been reported among patients with lower circulating vitamin K levels. In addition, women with low dietary vitamin K levels were at increased risk of hip fracture in 2 prospective cohorts.[150,151]

Vitamin K is essential for normal clotting. Supplementation may prevent fractures, but the evidence for this is not strong.

COMMENT

Although the clinical syndromes of vitamin deficiencies are unusual in Western societies, suboptimal vitamin status is not. Because suboptimal vitamin status is associated with many chronic diseases, including cardiovascular disease, cancer, and osteoporosis, it is important for physicians to identify patients with poor nutrition or other reasons for increased vitamin needs. The science of vitamin supplementation for chronic disease prevention is not well developed, and much of the evidence comes from observational studies.

Funding/Support: Dr Fairfield is supported by career development award CCDA-00-179-01 from the American Cancer Society.

REFERENCES

1. Balluz LS, Kieszak SM, Philen RM, Mulinare J. Vitamin and mineral supplement use in the United States: results from the third National Health and Nutrition Examination Survey. *Arch Fam Med.* 2000;9:258-262.
2. Morrison HI, Schaubel D, Desmeules M, Wigle DT. Serum folate and risk of fatal coronary heart disease. *JAMA.* 1996;275:1893-1896.
3. Rimm EB, Willett WC, Hu FB, et al. Folate and vitamin B6 from diet and supplements in relation to risk of coronary heart disease among women. *JAMA.* 1998; 279:359-364.
4. Homocysteine Lowering Trialists' Collaboration. Lowering blood homocysteine with folic acid based supplements: meta-analysis of randomised trials. *BMJ.* 1998;316:894-898.
5. Eikelboom JW, Lonn E, Genest J Jr, Hankey G, Yusuf S. Homocyst(e)ine and cardiovascular disease: a critical review of the epidemiologic evidence. *Ann Intern Med.* 1999;131:363-375.
6. Bostom AG, Garber C. Endpoints for homocysteine-lowering trials. *Lancet.* 2000;355:511-512.
7. Giovannucci E, Rimm EB, Ascherio A, Stampfer MJ, Colditz GA, Willett WC. Alcohol, low-methionine–low-folate diets, and risk of colon cancer in men. *J Natl Cancer Inst.* 1995;87:265-273.
8. Giovannucci E, Stampfer MJ, Colditz GA, et al. Multivitamin use, folate, and colon cancer in women in the Nurses' Health Study. *Ann Intern Med.* 1998;129: 517-524.
9. Su LJ, Arab L. Nutritional status of folate and colon cancer risk: evidence from NHANES I epidemiologic follow-up study. *Ann Epidemiol.* 2001;11:65-72.
10. Zhang S, Hunter DJ, Hankinson SE, et al. A prospective study of folate intake and the risk of breast cancer. *JAMA.* 1999;281:1632-1637.
11. Rohan TE, Jain MG, Howe GR, Miller AB. Dietary folate consumption and breast cancer risk. *J Natl Cancer Inst.* 2000;92:266-269.
12. Sellers TA, Kushi LH, Cerhan JR, et al. Dietary folate intake, alcohol, and risk of breast cancer in a prospective study of postmenopausal women. *Epidemiology.* 2001;12:420-428.
13. Milunsky A, Jick H, Jick SS, et al. Multivitamin/folic acid supplementation in early pregnancy reduces the prevalence of neural tube defects. *JAMA.* 1989;262:2847-2852.
14. Czeizel AE, Dudas I. Prevention of the first occurrence of neural-tube defects by periconceptional vitamin supplementation. *N Engl J Med.* 1992;327: 1832-1835.
15. MRC Vitamin Study Research Group. Prevention of neural tube defects: results of the Medical Research Council Vitamin Study. *Lancet.* 1991;338:131-137.
16. Stampfer MJ, Hennekens CH, Manson JE, Colditz GA, Rosner B, Willett WC. Vitamin E consumption and the risk of coronary disease in women. *N Engl J Med.* 1993;328:1444-1449.
17. Rimm EB, Stampfer MJ, Ascherio A, Giovannucci E, Colditz GA, Willett WC. Vitamin E consumption and the risk of coronary heart disease in men. *N Engl J Med.* 1993;328:1450-1456.
18. Rapola JM, Virtamo J, Ripatti S, et al. Randomised trial of alpha-tocopherol and beta-carotene supplements on incidence of major coronary events in men with previous myocardial infarction. *Lancet.* 1997;349:1715-1720.
19. Rapola JM, Virtamo J, Haukka JK, et al. Effect of vitamin E and beta carotene on the incidence of angina pectoris: a randomized, double-blind, controlled trial. *JAMA.* 1996;275:693-698.
20. Yusuf S, Dagenais G, Pogue J, Bosch J, Sleight P, for the Heart Outcomes Prevention Evaluation Study Investigators. Vitamin E supplementation and cardiovascular events in high-risk patients. *N Engl J Med.* 2000;342:154-160.
21. deGaetaro G, for the Collaborative Group of the Primary Prevention Project. Low-dose aspirin and vitamin E in people at cardiovascular risk: a randomised trial in general practice. *Lancet.* 2001;357:89-95.
22. Stephens NG, Parsons A, Schofield PM, Kelly F, Cheeseman K, Mitchinson MJ. Randomised controlled trial of vitamin E in patients with coronary disease: Cambridge Heart Antioxidant Study (CHAOS). *Lancet.* 1996;347:781-786.
23. Gann PH, Ma J, Giovannucci E, et al. Lower prostate cancer risk in men with elevated plasma lycopene levels: results of a prospective analysis. *Cancer Res.* 1999;59:1225-1230.
24. Chan JM, Stampfer MJ, Ma J, Rimm EB, Willett WC, Giovannucci EL. Supplemental vitamin E intake and prostate cancer risk in a large cohort of men in the United States. *Cancer Epidemiol Biomarkers Prev.* 1999;8:893-899.
25. The effect of vitamin E and beta carotene on the incidence of lung cancer and other cancers in male smokers: the Alpha-Tocopherol, Beta Carotene Cancer Prevention Study Group. *N Engl J Med.* 1994;330: 1029-1035.
26. Kushi LH, Folsom AR, Prineas RJ, Mink PJ, Wu Y, Bostick RM. Dietary antioxidant vitamins and death from coronary heart disease in postmenopausal women. *N Engl J Med.* 1996;334:1156-1162.
27. Evans RW, Shaten BJ, Day BW, Kuller LH. Prospective association between lipid soluble antioxidants and coronary heart disease in men: the Multiple Risk Factor Intervention Trial. *Am J Epidemiol.* 1998;147:180-186.
28. Omenn GS, Goodman GE, Thornquist MD, et al. Effects of a combination of beta carotene and vitamin A on lung cancer and cardiovascular disease. *N Engl J Med.* 1996;334:1150-1155.

29. Blot WJ, Li JY, Taylor PR, et al. Nutrition intervention trials in Linxian, China: supplementation with specific vitamin/mineral combinations, cancer incidence, and disease-specific mortality in the general population. *J Natl Cancer Inst.* 1993;85:1483-1492.
30. Hennekens CH, Buring JE, Manson JE, et al. Lack of effect of long-term supplementation with beta carotene on the incidence of malignant neoplasms and cardiovascular disease. *N Engl J Med.* 1996;334:1145-1149.
31. Greenberg ER, Baron JA, Karagas MR, et al. Mortality associated with low plasma concentration of beta carotene and the effect of oral supplementation. *JAMA.* 1996;275:699-703.
32. Speizer FE, Colditz GA, Hunter DJ, Rosner B, Hennekens C. Prospective study of smoking, antioxidant intake, and lung cancer in middle-aged women (USA). *Cancer Causes Control.* 1999;10:475-482.
33. Knekt P, Jarvinen R, Teppo L, Aromaa A, Seppanen R. Role of various carotenoids in lung cancer prevention. *J Natl Cancer Inst.* 1999;91:182-184.
34. Michaud DS, Feskanich D, Rimm EB, et al. Intake of specific carotenoids and risk of lung cancer in 2 prospective US cohorts. *Am J Clin Nutr.* 2000;72:990-997.
35. Lee IM, Cook NR, Manson JE, Buring JE, Hennekens CH. Beta-carotene supplementation and incidence of cancer and cardiovascular disease: the Women's Health Study. *J Natl Cancer Inst.* 1999;91:2102-2106.
36. Giovannucci E, Ascherio A, Rimm EB, Stampfer MJ, Colditz GA, Willett WC. Intake of carotenoids and retinol in relation to risk of prostate cancer. *J Natl Cancer Inst.* 1995;87:1767-1776.
37. Mills PK, Beeson WL, Phillips RL, Fraser GE. Cohort study of diet, lifestyle, and prostate cancer in Adventist men. *Cancer.* 1989;64:598-604.
38. Cerhan J, Chiu B, Putnam S, Parker A, Robbins M, Lynch C. A cohort study of diet and prostate cancer risk [abstract]. *Cancer Epidemiol Biomarkers Prev.* 1998;7:175.
39. Baldwin D, Naco G, Petersen F, Fraser G, Ruckle H. The effect of nutritional and clinical factors upon serum prostate specific antigen and prostate cancer risk in a population of elderly California men [abstract]. Paper presented at: 1997 Annual Meeting of the American Urological Association; April 12-17, 1997; New Orleans, La.
40. Hsing AW, Comstock GW, Abbey H, Polk BF. Serologic precursors of cancer: retinol, carotenoids, and tocopherol and risk of prostate cancer. *J Natl Cancer Inst.* 1990;82:941-946.
41. Nomura AM, Stemmermann GN, Lee J, Craft NE. Serum micronutrients and prostate cancer in Japanese Americans in Hawaii. *Cancer Epidemiol Biomarkers Prev.* 1997;6:487-491.
42. Lips P, Duong T, Oleksik A, et al. A global study of vitamin D status and parathyroid function in postmenopausal women with osteoporosis: baseline data from the multiple outcomes of raloxifene evaluation clinical trial. *J Clin Endocrinol Metab.* 2001;86:1212-1221.
43. Thomas MK, Lloyd-Jones DM, Thadhani RI, et al. Hypovitaminosis D in medical inpatients. *N Engl J Med.* 1998;338:777-783.
44. Lips P. Vitamin D deficiency and secondary hyperparathyroidism in the elderly: consequences for bone loss and fractures and therapeutic implications. *Endocr Rev.* 2001;22:477-501.
45. Dawson-Hughes B, Harris SS, Krall EA, Dallal GE. Effect of calcium and vitamin D supplementation on bone density in men and women 65 years of age or older. *N Engl J Med.* 1997;337:670-676.
46. Facts about dietary supplements [National Institutes of Health Clinical Center Web site]. Available at: http://www.cc.nih.gov/ccc/supplements. Accessibility verified April 22, 2002.
47. Graham IM, Daly LE, Refsum HM, et al. Plasma homocysteine as a risk factor for vascular disease: the European Concerted Action Project. *JAMA.* 1997;277:1775-1781.
48. Welch GN, Loscalzo J. Homocysteine and atherothrombosis. *N Engl J Med.* 1998;338:1042-1050.
49. Ziegler EE. *Present Knowledge in Nutrition.* Washington, DC: International Life Sciences Institute; 1996.
50. Jacques PF, Selhub J, Bostom AG, Wilson PW, Rosenberg IH. The effect of folic acid fortification on plasma folate and total homocysteine concentrations. *N Engl J Med.* 1999;340:1449-1454.
51. Dong MH, McGown EL, Schwenneker BW, Sauberlich HE. Thiamin, riboflavin, and vitamin B6 contents of selected foods as served. *J Am Diet Assoc.* 1980;76:156-160.
52. Green R, Kinsella LJ. Current concepts in the diagnosis of cobalamin deficiency. *Neurology.* 1995;45:1435-1440.
53. Nygard O, Refsum H, Ueland PM, Vollset SE. Major lifestyle determinants of plasma total homocysteine distribution: the Hordaland Homocysteine Study. *Am J Clin Nutr.* 1998;67:263-270.
54. Selhub J, Jacques PF, Rosenberg IH, et al. Serum total homocysteine concentrations in the third National Health and Nutrition Examination Survey (1991-1994): population reference ranges and contribution of vitamin status to high serum concentrations. *Ann Intern Med.* 1999;131:331-339.
55. Wald DS, Bishop L, Wald NJ, et al. Randomized trial of folic acid supplementation and serum homocysteine levels. *Arch Intern Med.* 2001;161:695-700.
56. Selhub J, Jacques PF, Wilson PW, Rush D, Rosenberg IH. Vitamin status and intake as primary determinants of homocysteinemia in an elderly population. *JAMA.* 1993;270:2693-2698.
57. Ubbink JB, Vermaak WJ, van der Merwe A, Becker PJ. Vitamin B-12, vitamin B-6, and folate nutritional status in men with hyperhomocysteinemia. *Am J Clin Nutr.* 1993;57:47-53.
58. Robinson K, Arheart K, Refsum H, et al, for the European COMAC Group. Low circulating folate and vitamin B6 concentrations: risk factors for stroke, peripheral vascular disease, and coronary artery disease. *Circulation.* 1998;97:437-443.
59. Kim YI. Folate and cancer prevention: a new medical application of folate beyond hyperhomocysteinemia and neural tube defects. *Nutr Rev.* 1999;57:314-321.
60. Chen J, Giovannucci E, Kelsey K, et al. A methylenetetrahydrofolate reductase polymorphism and the risk of colorectal cancer. *Cancer Res.* 1996;56:4862-4864.
61. Slattery ML, Potter JD, Samowitz W, Schaffer D, Leppert M. Methylenetetrahydrofolate reductase, diet, and risk of colon cancer. *Cancer Epidemiol Biomarkers Prev.* 1999;8:513-518.
62. Smithells RW, Sheppard S, Schorah CJ. Vitamin deficiencies and neural tube defects. *Arch Dis Child.* 1976;51:944-950.
63. Mulinare J, Cordero JF, Erickson JD, Berry RJ. Periconceptional use of multivitamins and the occurrence of neural tube defects. *JAMA.* 1988;260:3141-3145.
64. Bower C, Stanley FJ. Dietary folate as a risk factor for neural-tube defects: evidence from a case-control study in Western Australia. *Med J Aust.* 1989;150:613-619.
65. Werler MM, Shapiro S, Mitchell AA. Periconceptional folic acid exposure and risk of occurrent neural tube defects. *JAMA.* 1993;269:1257-1261.
66. Shaw GM, Schaffer D, Velie EM, Morland K, Harris JA. Periconceptional vitamin use, dietary folate, and the occurrence of neural tube defects. *Epidemiology.* 1995;6:219-226.
67. Smithells RW, Sheppard S, Schorah CJ, et al. Apparent prevention of neural tube defects by periconceptional vitamin supplementation. *Arch Dis Child.* 1981;56:911-918.
68. Wald NJ, Law MR, Morris JK, Wald DS. Quantifying the effect of folic acid. *Lancet.* 2001;358:2069-2073.
69. Giovannucci E. Gamma-tocopherol: a new player in prostate cancer prevention? *J Natl Cancer Inst.* 2000;92:1966-1967.
70. Meydani SN, Meydani M, Blumberg JB, et al. Vitamin E supplementation and in vivo immune response in healthy elderly subjects: a randomized controlled trial. *JAMA.* 1997;277:1380-1386.
71. McLaughlin PJ, Weihrauch JL. Vitamin E content of foods. *J Am Diet Assoc.* 1979;75:647-665.
72. Boscoboinik D, Szewczyk A, Hensey C, Azzi A. Inhibition of cell proliferation by alpha-tocopherol: role of protein kinase C. *J Biol Chem.* 1991;266:6188-6194.
73. Steiner M. Vitamin E: more than an antioxidant. *Clin Cardiol.* 1993;16:I16-I18.
74. Davey PJ, Schulz M, Gliksman M, Dobson M, Aristides M, Stephens NG. Cost-effectiveness of vitamin E therapy in the treatment of patients with angiographically proven coronary narrowing (CHAOS trial): Cambridge Heart Antioxidant Study. *Am J Cardiol.* 1998;82:414-417.
75. Boaz M, Smetana S, Weinstein T, et al. Secondary prevention with antioxidants of cardiovascular disease in endstage renal disease (SPACE): randomised placebo-controlled trial. *Lancet.* 2000;356:1213-1218.
76. Helzlsouer KJ, Huang HY, Alberg AJ, et al. Association between alpha-tocopherol, gamma-tocopherol, selenium, and subsequent prostate cancer. *J Natl Cancer Inst.* 2000;92:2018-2023.
77. van Poppel G, Goldbohm RA. Epidemiologic evidence for beta-carotene and cancer prevention. *Am J Clin Nutr.* 1995;62:1393S-1402S.
78. Albanes D, Heinonen OP, Taylor PR, et al. Alpha-Tocopherol and beta-carotene supplements and lung cancer incidence in the alpha-tocopherol, beta-carotene cancer prevention study: effects of base-line characteristics and study compliance. *J Natl Cancer Inst.* 1996;88:1560-1570.
79. Cook NR, Lee IM, Manson JE, Buring JE, Hennekens CH. Effects of beta-carotene supplementation on cancer incidence by baseline characteristics in the Physicians' Health Study (United States). *Cancer Causes Control.* 2000;11:617-626.
80. Glynn SA, Albanes D, Pietinen P, et al. Alcohol consumption and risk of colorectal cancer in a cohort of Finnish men. *Cancer Causes Control.* 1996;7:214-223.
81. McLarty JW, Holiday DB, Girard WM, Yanagihara RH, Kummet TD, Greenberg SD. Beta-Carotene, vitamin A, and lung cancer chemoprevention: results of an intermediate endpoint study. *Am J Clin Nutr.* 1995;62:1431S-1438S.
82. Fukao A, Tsubono Y, Kawamura M, et al. The independent association of smoking and drinking with serum beta-carotene levels among males in Miyagi, Japan. *Int J Epidemiol.* 1996;25:300-306.
83. Kitamura Y, Tanaka K, Kiyohara C, et al. Relationship of alcohol use, physical activity and dietary habits with serum carotenoids, retinol and alpha-tocopherol among male Japanese smokers. *Int J Epidemiol.* 1997;26:307-314.
84. Albanes D, Virtamo J, Taylor PR, Rautalahti M, Pietinen P, Heinonen OP. Effects of supplemental beta-carotene, cigarette smoking, and alcohol consumption on serum carotenoids in the Alpha-Tocopherol, Beta-Carotene Cancer Prevention Study. *Am J Clin Nutr.* 1997;66:366-372.
85. Cook NR, Stampfer MJ, Ma J, et al. Beta-carotene supplementation for patients with low baseline levels and decreased risks of total and prostate carcinoma. *Cancer.* 1999;86:1783-1792.
86. Giovannucci E. Tomatoes, tomato-based products, lycopene, and cancer: review of the epidemiologic literature. *J Natl Cancer Inst.* 1999;91:317-331.
87. Clavel-Chapelon F, Niravong M, Joseph RR. Diet and breast cancer: review of the epidemiologic literature. *Cancer Detect Prev.* 1997;21:426-440.
88. Kushi LH, Fee RM, Sellers TA, Zheng W, Folsom AR. Intake of vitamins A, C, and E and postmeno-

pausal breast cancer: the Iowa Women's Health Study. *Am J Epidemiol*. 1996;144:165-174.
89. Verhoeven DT, Assen N, Goldbohm RA, et al. Vitamins C and E, retinol, beta-carotene and dietary fibre in relation to breast cancer risk: a prospective cohort study. *Br J Cancer*. 1997;75:149-155.
90. Jarvinen R, Knekt P, Seppanen R, Teppo L. Diet and breast cancer risk in a cohort of Finnish women. *Cancer Lett*. 1997;114:251-253.
91. Michels KB, Holmberg L, Bergkvist L, Ljung H, Bruce A, Wolk A. Dietary antioxidant vitamins, retinol, and breast cancer incidence in a cohort of Swedish women. *Int J Cancer*. 2001;91:563-567.
92. Zhang S, Hunter DJ, Forman MR, et al. Dietary carotenoids and vitamins A, C, and E and risk of breast cancer. *J Natl Cancer Inst*. 1999;91:547-556.
93. Willett WC, Polk BF, Underwood BA, et al. Relation of serum vitamins A and E and carotenoids to the risk of cancer. *N Engl J Med*. 1984;310:430-434.
94. Wald NJ, Boreham J, Hayward JL, Bulbrook RD. Plasma retinol, beta-carotene and vitamin E levels in relation to the future risk of breast cancer. *Br J Cancer*. 1984;49:321-324.
95. Knekt P, Aromaa A, Maatela J, et al. Serum vitamin A and subsequent risk of cancer: cancer incidence follow-up of the Finnish Mobile Clinic Health Examination Survey. *Am J Epidemiol*. 1990;132:857-870.
96. Comstock GW, Helzlsouer KJ, Bush TL. Prediagnostic serum levels of carotenoids and vitamin E as related to subsequent cancer in Washington County, Maryland. *Am J Clin Nutr*. 1991;53:260S-264S.
97. Dorgan JF, Sowell A, Swanson CA, et al. Relationships of serum carotenoids, retinol, alpha-tocopherol, and selenium with breast cancer risk: results from a prospective study in Columbia, Missouri (United States). *Cancer Causes Control*. 1998;9:89-97.
98. Toniolo P, Van Kappel AL, Akhmedkhanov A, et al. Serum carotenoids and breast cancer. *Am J Epidemiol*. 2001;153:1142-1147.
99. Diaz MN, Frei B, Vita JA, Keaney JF Jr. Antioxidants and atherosclerotic heart disease. *N Engl J Med*. 1997;337:408-416.
100. Sahyoun NR, Jacques PF, Russell RM. Carotenoids, vitamins C and E, and mortality in an elderly population. *Am J Epidemiol*. 1996;144:501-511.
101. LeBoff MS, Kohlmeier L, Hurwitz S, Franklin J, Wright J, Glowacki J. Occult vitamin D deficiency in postmenopausal US women with acute hip fracture. *JAMA*. 1999;281:1505-1511.
102. Outila TA, Karkkainen MU, Lamberg-Allardt CJ. Vitamin D status affects serum parathyroid hormone concentrations during winter in female adolescents: associations with forearm bone mineral density. *Am J Clin Nutr*. 2001;74:206-210.
103. Dawson-Hughes B, Harris SS, Krall EA, Dallal GE. Effect of withdrawal of calcium and vitamin D supplements on bone mass in elderly men and women. *Am J Clin Nutr*. 2000;72:745-750.
104. Lips P, Graafmans WC, Ooms ME, Bezemer PD, Bouter LM. Vitamin D supplementation and fracture incidence in elderly persons: a randomized, placebo-controlled clinical trial. *Ann Intern Med*. 1996;124:400-406.
105. Morrison NA, Qi JC, Tokita A, et al. Prediction of bone density from vitamin D receptor alleles. *Nature*. 1994;367:284-287.
106. Feskanich D, Hunter DJ, Willett WC, et al. Vitamin D receptor genotype and the risk of bone fractures in women. *Epidemiology*. 1998;9:535-539.
107. Nelson DA, Vande Vord PJ, Wooley PH. Polymorphism in the vitamin D receptor gene and bone mass in African-American and white mothers and children: a preliminary report. *Ann Rheum Dis*. 2000;59:626-630.
108. Vanderslice JT, Higgs DJ. Vitamin C content of foods: sample variability. *Am J Clin Nutr*. 1991;54:1323S-1327S.
109. Urivetzky M, Kessaris D, Smith AD. Ascorbic acid overdosing: a risk factor for calcium oxalate nephrolithiasis. *J Urol*. 1992;147:1215-1218.
110. Curhan GC, Willett WC, Rimm EB, Stampfer MJ. A prospective study of the intake of vitamins C and B6, and the risk of kidney stones in men. *J Urol*. 1996;155:1847-1851.
111. Kritchevsky SB, Shimakawa T, Tell GS, et al, for the Atherosclerosis Risk in Communities Study. Dietary antioxidants and carotid artery wall thickness: the ARIC Study. *Circulation*. 1995;92:2142-2150.
112. Knekt P, Reunanen A, Jarvinen R, Seppanen R, Heliovaara M, Aromaa A. Antioxidant vitamin intake and coronary mortality in a longitudinal population study. *Am J Epidemiol*. 1994;139:1180-1189.
113. Nyyssonen K, Parviainen MT, Salonen R, Tuomilehto J, Salonen JT. Vitamin C deficiency and risk of myocardial infarction: prospective population study of men from eastern Finland. *BMJ*. 1997;314:634-638.
114. Joshipura KJ, Hu FB, Manson JE, et al. The effect of fruit and vegetable intake on risk for coronary heart disease. *Ann Intern Med*. 2001;134:1106-1114.
115. Gale CR, Martyn CN, Winter PD, Cooper C. Vitamin C and risk of death from stroke and coronary heart disease in cohort of elderly people. *BMJ*. 1995;310:1563-1566.
116. Enstrom JE, Kanim LE, Klein MA. Vitamin C intake and mortality among a sample of the United States population. *Epidemiology*. 1992;3:194-202.
117. Ramirez J, Flowers NC. Leukocyte ascorbic acid and its relationship to coronary artery disease in man. *Am J Clin Nutr*. 1980;33:2079-2087.
118. Hodis HN, Mack WJ, LaBree L, et al. Serial coronary angiographic evidence that antioxidant vitamin intake reduces progression of coronary artery atherosclerosis. *JAMA*. 1995;273:1849-1854.
119. Tardif JC, Cote G, Lesperance J, et al. Probucol and multivitamins in the prevention of restenosis after coronary angioplasty: Multivitamins and Probucol Study Group. *N Engl J Med*. 1997;337:365-372.
120. Khaw KT, Bingham S, Welch A, et al, for the European Prospective Investigation into Cancer and Nutrition. Relation between plasma ascorbic acid and mortality in men and women in EPIC-Norfolk prospective study: a prospective population study. *Lancet*. 2001;357:657-663.
121. Loria CM, Klag MJ, Caulfield LE, Whelton PK. Vitamin C status and mortality in US adults. *Am J Clin Nutr*. 2000;72:139-145.
122. Losonczy KG, Harris TB, Havlik RJ. Vitamin E and vitamin C supplement use and risk of all-cause and coronary heart disease mortality in older persons: the Established Populations for Epidemiologic Studies of the Elderly. *Am J Clin Nutr*. 1996;64:190-196.
123. Christen WG, Gaziano JM, Hennekens CH. Design of Physicians' Health Study II: a randomized trial of beta-carotene, vitamins E and C, and multivitamins, in prevention of cancer, cardiovascular disease, and eye disease, and review of results of completed trials. *Ann Epidemiol*. 2000;10:125-134.
124. Manson JE, Gaziano JM, Spelsberg A, et al, for the WACS Research Group. A secondary prevention trial of antioxidant vitamins and cardiovascular disease in women: rationale, design, and methods. *Ann Epidemiol*. 1995;5:261-269.
125. Byers T, Guerrero N. Epidemiologic evidence for vitamin C and vitamin E in cancer prevention. *Am J Clin Nutr*. 1995;62:1385S-1392S.
126. Negri E, Franceschi S, Bosetti C, et al. Selected micronutrients and oral and pharyngeal cancer. *Int J Cancer*. 2000;86:122-127.
127. You WC, Zhang L, Gail MH, et al. Gastric dysplasia and gastric cancer: *Helicobacter pylori*, serum vitamin C, and other risk factors. *J Natl Cancer Inst*. 2000;92:1607-1612.
128. Freudenheim JL, Marshall JR, Vena JE, et al. Premenopausal breast cancer risk and intake of vegetables, fruits, and related nutrients. *J Natl Cancer Inst*. 1996;88:340-348.
129. Gandini S, Merzenich H, Robertson C, Boyle P. Meta-analysis of studies on breast cancer risk and diet: the role of fruit and vegetable consumption and the intake of associated micronutrients. *Eur J Cancer*. 2000;36:636-646.
130. Wu K, Helzlsouer KJ, Alberg AJ, Comstock GW, Norkus EP, Hoffman SC. A prospective study of plasma ascorbic acid concentrations and breast cancer (United States). *Cancer Causes Control*. 2000;11:279-283.
131. Rothman KJ, Moore LL, Singer MR, Nguyen US, Mannino S, Milunsky A. Teratogenicity of high vitamin A intake. *N Engl J Med*. 1995;333:1369-1373.
132. Melhus H, Michaelsson K, Kindmark A, et al. Excessive dietary intake of vitamin A is associated with reduced bone mineral density and increased risk for hip fracture. *Ann Intern Med*. 1998;129:770-778.
133. Feskanich D, Singh V, Willett WC, Colditz GA. Vitamin A intake and hip fractures among postmenopausal women. *JAMA*. 2002;287:47-54.
134. Fawzi WW, Chalmers TC, Herrera MG, Mosteller F. Vitamin A supplementation and child mortality: a meta-analysis. *JAMA*. 1993;269:898-903.
135. La Vecchia C, Negri E. Nutrition and bladder cancer. *Cancer Causes Control*. 1996;7:95-100.
136. Steinmaus CM, Nunez S, Smith AH. Diet and bladder cancer: a meta-analysis of six dietary variables. *Am J Epidemiol*. 2000;151:693-702.
137. Willett WC, Hunter DJ. Vitamin A and cancers of the breast, large bowel, and prostate: epidemiologic evidence. *Nutr Rev*. 1994;52:S53-S59.
138. Veronesi U, De Palo G, Marubini E, et al. Randomized trial of fenretinide to prevent second breast malignancy in women with early breast cancer. *J Natl Cancer Inst*. 1999;91:1847-1856.
139. Ansell JE, Kumar R, Deykin D. The spectrum of vitamin K deficiency. *JAMA*. 1977;238:40-42.
140. Alperin JB. Coagulopathy caused by vitamin K deficiency in critically ill, hospitalized patients. *JAMA*. 1987;258:1916-1919.
141. Booth SL, Centurelli MA. Vitamin K: a practical guide to the dietary management of patients on warfarin. *Nutr Rev*. 1999;57:288-296.
142. Weibert RT, Le DT, Kayser SR, Rapaport SI. Correction of excessive anticoagulation with low-dose oral vitamin K1. *Ann Intern Med*. 1997;126:959-962.
143. Crowther MA, Julian J, McCarty D, et al. Treatment of warfarin-associated coagulopathy with oral vitamin K: a randomised controlled trial. *Lancet*. 2000;356:1551-1553.
144. Booth SL. Skeletal functions of vitamin K-dependent proteins: not just for clotting anymore. *Nutr Rev*. 1997;55:282-284.
145. Vermeer C, Jie KS, Knapen MH. Role of vitamin K in bone metabolism. *Annu Rev Nutr*. 1995;15:1-22.
146. Binkley NC, Suttie JW. Vitamin K nutrition and osteoporosis. *J Nutr*. 1995;125:1812-1821.
147. Kanai T, Takagi T, Masuhiro K, Nakamura M, Iwata M, Saji F. Serum vitamin K level and bone mineral density in post-menopausal women. *Int J Gynaecol Obstet*. 1997;56:25-30.
148. Hart JP, Shearer MJ, Klenerman L, et al. Electrochemical detection of depressed circulating levels of vitamin K1 in osteoporosis. *J Clin Endocrinol Metab*. 1985;60:1268-1269.
149. Hodges SJ, Akesson K, Vergnaud P, Obrant K, Delmas PD. Circulating levels of vitamins K1 and K2 decreased in elderly women with hip fracture. *J Bone Miner Res*. 1993;8:1241-1245.
150. Feskanich D, Weber P, Willett WC, Rockett H, Booth SL, Colditz GA. Vitamin K intake and hip fractures in women: a prospective study. *Am J Clin Nutr*. 1999;69:74-79.
151. Booth SL, Tucker KL, Chen H, et al. Dietary vitamin K intakes are associated with hip fracture but not with bone mineral density in elderly men and women. *Am J Clin Nutr*. 2000;71:1201-1208.
152. Heikinheimo RJ, Inkovaara JA, Harju EJ, et al. Annual injection of vitamin D and fractures of aged bones. *Calcif Tissue Int*. 1992;51:105-110.

The information contained in this White Paper is not intended as a substitute for the advice of a physician. Readers who suspect they may have specific medical problems should consult a physician about any suggestions made.

Please address inquiries on bulk subscriptions and permission to reproduce selections from this White Paper to Medletter Associates, Inc., 632 Broadway, 11th Floor, New York, NY 10012. The editors are interested in receiving your comments at the above address but regret that they cannot answer letters of any sort personally.

ISBN 0-929661-82-6
ISSN 1542-1899
Second Printing
Printed in the United States of America

The map on page 3 was adapted with permission from the *Journal of the American Medical Association* Vol. 286, No. 10 (September 12, 2001): 1196.

Fairfield, K. and Fletcher, R. "Vitamins for Chronic Disease Prevention in Adults." Reprinted with permission from the *Journal of the American Medical Association* Vol. 287, No. 23 (June 19, 2002): 3116-3126. Copyright © 2002, American Medical Association.

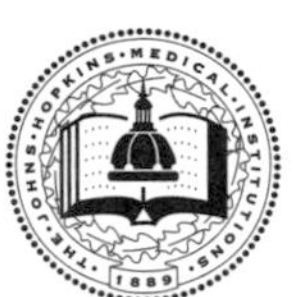

The Johns Hopkins White Papers are published yearly by Medletter Associates, Inc.

PROSTATE DISORDERS

H. Ballentine Carter, M.D.

and

Simeon Margolis, M.D., Ph.D.

2003

PROSTATE DISORDERS

Choosing the best treatment for prostate disorders has long been more art than science. But thanks to new randomized trials, men are finally getting the answers they need. For example, last year a study showed for the first time that radical prostatectomy can reduce the risk of dying from prostate cancer. Research is also revealing what men can do to reduce their risk of benign prostatic hyperplasia (BPH). This year's White Paper reviews the latest knowledge on the causes, diagnosis, and treatment of prostate cancer, BPH, and prostatitis.

▪ ▪ ▪

Highlights:

- The safest way to manage benign prostatic hyperplasia. (page 7)
- Understanding the link between **obesity** and benign prostatic hyperplasia. (page 9)
- The best analysis to date of the safety and effectiveness of **saw palmetto** for benign prostatic hyperplasia. (page 13)
- Are you a good candidate for **transurethral microwave thermotherapy**? (page 20)
- The relationship between low levels of **selenium** and prostate cancer. (page 25)
- How eating **tomato products** may protect against prostate cancer. (page 27)
- Is **PSA screening** overhyped? (page 28)
- The **gene mutation test** that might be able to detect prostate cancer. (page 35)
- For the first time, **surgery** is shown to reduce the risk of dying from prostate cancer. (page 41)
- The tables the professionals use to determine the **best prostate cancer treatment**. (page 42)
- An update on **brachytherapy** and **three-dimensional conformal radiation therapy**. (page 46)
- Are there alternatives to the **herbal supplement PC-SPES**? (page 54)
- The proper way to do **Kegel exercises** to alleviate urinary incontinence. (page 58)
- Why your **choice of surgeon and hospital** is so important. (page 65)

▪ ▪ ▪

www.HopkinsAfter50.com
Visit us for the latest news on prostate disorders and other information that will complement your Johns Hopkins White Paper.

THE AUTHORS

H. Ballentine Carter, M.D., graduated from the Medical University of South Carolina and completed his residency training at New York Hospital-Cornell Medical Center in New York City. Currently, he is a professor of urology and oncology and the Director of Adult Urology at the Johns Hopkins University School of Medicine.

Dr. Carter has written extensively on the diagnosis and staging of prostate cancer. In particular, he has researched prostate specific antigen (PSA) levels: how they change as men age, their variability in men with prostate cancer, and their use in staging, predicting, and managing prostate cancer. At this time, he is working closely with the Baltimore Longitudinal Study of Aging to evaluate the development of prostate disease with age. Dr. Carter has had research articles published in *The Journal of Urology, Urology, Cancer Research,* the *Journal of the American Medical Association,* and the *Journal of the National Cancer Institute.*

▪ ▪ ▪

Simeon Margolis, M.D., Ph.D., received his B.A., M.D., and Ph.D. from the Johns Hopkins University School of Medicine and performed his internship and residency at Johns Hopkins Hospital. He is currently a professor of medicine and biological chemistry at the Johns Hopkins University School of Medicine and medical editor of *The Johns Hopkins Medical Letter, Health After 50.* He has served on various committees for the Department of Health, Education, and Welfare, including the National Diabetes Advisory Board and the Arteriosclerosis Specialized Centers of Research Review Committees. In addition, he has acted as a member of the Endocrinology and Metabolism Panel of the U.S. Food and Drug Administration.

A former weekly columnist for the Baltimore Sun, Dr. Margolis lectures regularly to medical students, physicians, and the general public on a wide variety of topics, such as the prevention of coronary heart disease, the control of cholesterol levels, the treatment of diabetes, and the use of alternative medicine.

CONTENTS

PROSTATE DISORDERS

The prostate is a gland that sits below a man's bladder and in front of his rectum. It is shaped like a crabapple with a narrow core removed. Urine and semen pass through this space via a tube called the urethra.

The prostate has several functions. First, it produces prostatic fluid, which is a component of semen. Second, it serves as a valve to keep urine and semen flowing in the proper direction. Finally, it pumps semen into the urethra during orgasm.

When a man reaches his mid-40s or later, the inner portion of the prostate tends to enlarge and may put pressure on the urethra, a condition called benign prostatic hyperplasia (BPH). BPH affects more than half of men over age 50—about 10 million Americans. Although it can cause a variety of symptoms, BPH is not life-threatening.

Prostate cancer is a much more serious health problem. After skin cancer, it is the second most common cancer in men and is second only to lung cancer as a cause of cancer deaths. The good news is that reliable diagnostic tests and numerous treatment options are available for prostate cancer, and death rates from it are on the decline.

BPH and prostate cancer can have similar symptoms, but have no known relation to each other aside from the fact that they occur in the same organ. Having BPH neither increases nor decreases an individual's risk for prostate cancer: A man may have both conditions at the same time.

A third condition that can affect the prostate is prostatitis, an inflammation of the prostate that may cause pain in the lower back and in the area between the scrotum and rectum. Prostatitis may also cause chills, fever, and a general feeling of being unwell.

STRUCTURE OF THE PROSTATE

The prostate is made up of two kinds of cells: glandular (epithelial) cells and smooth muscle cells. The glandular cells produce part of the fluid portion of semen. The smooth muscles are involuntary muscles (not under the control of the individual), like those of the intestines and blood vessels. They contract to push prostatic fluid into the urethra during ejaculation.

The prostate is arranged in three main regions, or zones. Immediately surrounding the urethra is a thin layer called the transition zone; it is surrounded by the central zone, which is followed by the largest and outermost portion, the peripheral zone. In addition, there are two smaller areas, a tiny periurethral zone, which surrounds the upper urethra, and the fibromuscular zone, a thin layer of smooth muscle that extends along the top and side of the prostate.

Benign Prostatic Hyperplasia (BPH)

BPH is the most common benign (noncancerous) tumor in men. As is true for prostate cancer, BPH occurs more often in Western than in Eastern countries, such as Japan and China, and may be more common among blacks. However, in a recent study of male health professionals, black men were no more likely to have BPH than white men. Not long ago, a study also found a possible genetic link for BPH in men younger than age 65 who have a very enlarged prostate: Their male relatives were four times more likely than other men to need BPH surgery at some point in their lives, and their brothers had a six-fold increase in risk.

Symptoms related to BPH are present in about one in four men by age 55, and in half of men by age 75. However, treatment is necessary only if symptoms become bothersome. By age 80, some 20% to 30% of men experience BPH symptoms severe enough to require treatment. The options for treatment are surgical removal of prostate tissue, heat therapy to vaporize prostate tissue, and medications that either shrink the prostate or relax the prostate muscle tissue that constricts the urethra.

CAUSES OF BPH

In BPH, the enlargement of the glandular tissue and the tightening of smooth muscles may obstruct the urethra. Although the cause of BPH is not understood, normal levels of testosterone (the male sex hormone) and aging are essential for the development of the condition. Experimental evidence from studies in dogs suggests that the female sex hormone estrogen may also play a role in BPH.

The word *hyperplasia* refers to any abnormal accumulation of cells that causes enlargement of a body part or organ. BPH occurs when an increase in the number of prostate cells produces discrete nodules in the prostate. The increase is due to a slowing of the normal rate of death of these cells, rather than to a heightened pro-

Benign Prostatic Hyperplasia (BPH) and Prostate Cancer

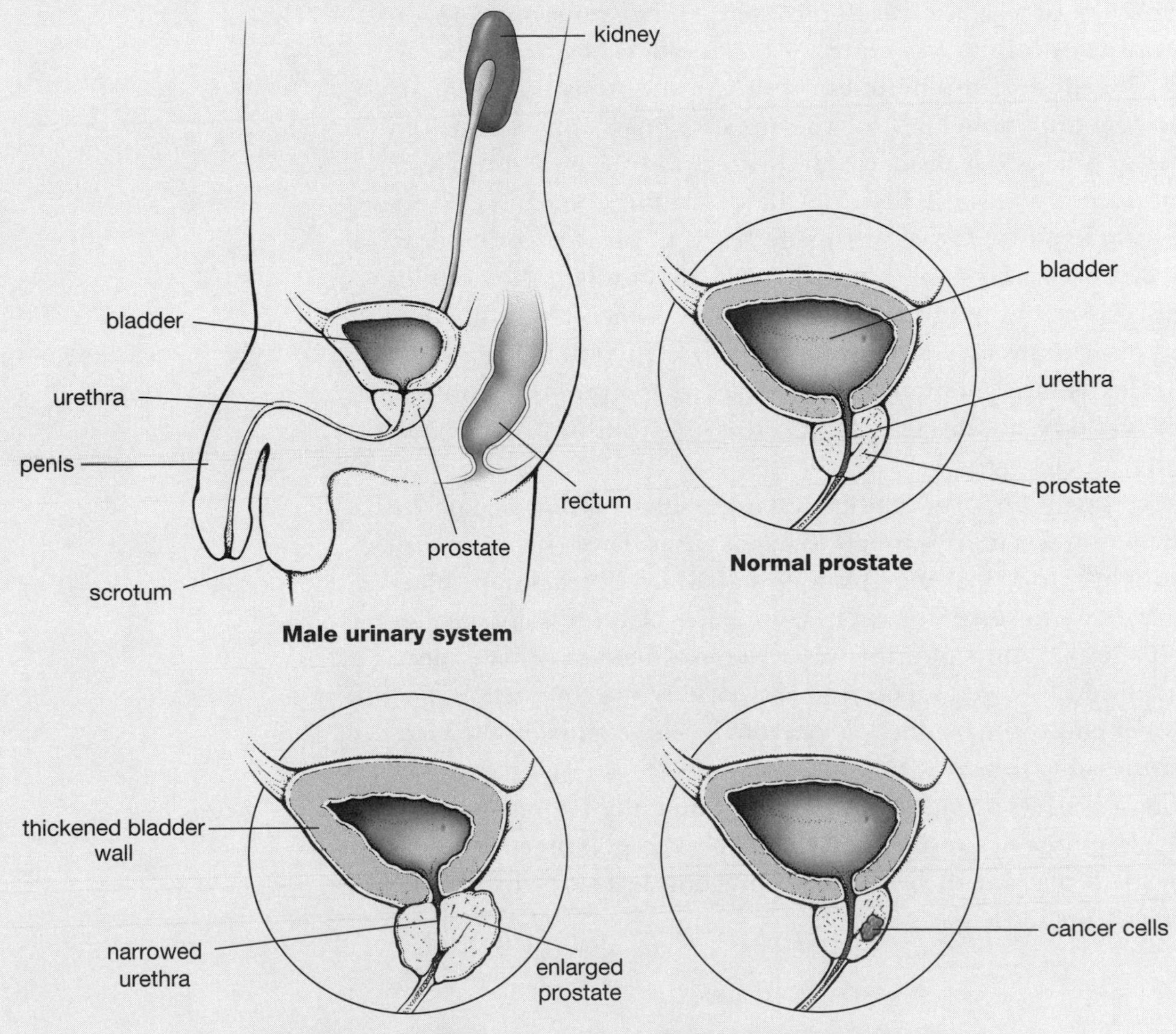

Male urinary system

Normal prostate

Prostate with BPH

Prostate with prostate cancer

The prostate gland is the size and shape of a crabapple and is located at the base of the bladder (in front of the rectum and behind the base of the penis). The gland has several functions: It produces prostatic fluid (a component of semen), acts as a valve to keep urine and semen flowing in the right direction, and releases semen into the urethra during orgasm. The prostate surrounds the urethra and, under normal circumstances, does not interfere with the flow of urine.

In benign prostate hyperplasia (BPH), the inner portion of the prostate gland enlarges. The excess tissue puts pressure on the urethra and may restrict the flow of urine. To compensate, the bladder tries to force urine through the urethra, causing changes in the bladder that result in less effective storage of urine. In about half of men with BPH, these changes lead to urinary symptoms such as slowed or delayed urination, excessive urination at night (nocturia), painful urination, and increased urgency and frequency of urination.

In prostate cancer, a malignant tumor grows within the prostate gland, usually beginning in the peripheral zone, the region next to the rectum. If undetected or untreated, the tumor can grow throughout the prostate and spread to the rest of the body. The tumor can eventually put pressure on the urethra, producing similar symptoms to BPH.

Despite the similarity in their symptoms, BPH and prostate cancer are thought to be unrelated. The presence of one does not affect the risk of developing the other.

duction. The nodules are surrounded by a capsule that contains smooth muscle cells, which can also increase in number.

Whether or not the resulting enlargement puts pressure on the urethra and increases resistance to the flow of urine depends on the location of the nodules. Although the transition zone accounts for only about 5% of the prostate mass, the nodules in men with BPH occur primarily in this region (rarely, it also affects the periurethral zone). Because the transition zone directly envelops the urethra, the excess tissue tends to obstruct urine flow. Contractions of the smooth muscle cells surrounding the nodules can also obstruct the urethra. Consequently, some men with a very enlarged prostate may have no urethral obstruction, while others with mild enlargement may have marked symptoms because a nodule is located where it compresses the urethra, or because smooth muscles tighten.

To compensate for urethral narrowing, the muscular wall of the bladder contracts more strongly to expel urine. These stronger contractions lead to a thickened bladder wall, which decreases the bladder's capacity to store urine. Over time, the bladder holds smaller and smaller amounts of urine, resulting in a need to urinate more frequently. As the urethral obstruction worsens, the contractions can no longer empty the bladder completely. Urine retained in the bladder (residual urine) may then become infected or lead to the formation of bladder stones (calculi). Less often, the kidneys become damaged, either as a result of increased pressure on them from the overworked bladder or because an infection has spread from the bladder to the kidneys.

SYMPTOMS OF BPH

BPH can produce symptoms related to the lower urinary tract. These symptoms include difficulty in starting to urinate, a weak stream, a sudden strong desire to urinate (urgency), an increased frequency of urination, and the sensation that the bladder is not empty after finishing urination. BPH can in fact prevent the bladder from emptying completely (urinary retention), and as the bladder becomes more sensitive to retained urine, a man may become unable to control the bladder (incontinent) because he is unable to respond quickly enough to urinary urgency. A bladder infection or stone can cause burning or pain during urination. Blood in the urine (hematuria) may herald BPH, but most men with BPH do not have this sign.

At times, men with BPH may suddenly become unable to urinate at all, even though their condition is responding to treatment. This problem, called acute urinary retention, requires immediate medical attention at an emergency room. It is easily treated by passing a tube through the penis into the bladder (catheterization). Factors that may trigger acute urinary retention include an extended delay in urination; urinary tract infection; alcohol intake; and the use of certain drugs, such as antidepressants, decongestants, and tranquilizers. Acute urinary retention often occurs quite unexpectedly, and it is impossible to predict whether a man with only modest lower urinary tract symptoms will develop this condition. Although acute urinary retention usually leads to prostate surgery, one study found that one third of men who required catheterization for a bout of acute urinary retention were able to urinate normally after the catheter was removed.

DIAGNOSIS OF BPH

The International Prostate Symptom Score questionnaire, also called the American Urological Association Symptom Index, provides an objective way to assess lower urinary tract symptoms (see page 11 for the questionnaire). This tool helps doctors and patients to decide on treatment. However, it cannot be used for diagnosis, since other diseases can cause lower urinary tract symptoms similar to those of BPH. In addition, as men and women age, the bladder becomes less efficient at storing urine and symptoms of urinary frequency and urgency become more common. Lower urinary tract symptoms may be due to a problem originating in the bladder rather than the prostate.

Therefore, a careful medical history, physical examination, and laboratory tests are required to exclude such conditions as urethral stricture (narrowing of the urethra) and bladder disease (neurological or inflammatory). In fact, some reports indicate that as many as 30% of men who undergo prostate surgery following the usual evaluation show no evidence of urethral obstruction from BPH (meaning their symptoms were due to another cause).

Medical History

A medical history often gives clues to conditions that can mimic BPH, such as urethral stricture, bladder cancer or stones, or abnormal bladder function (problems with holding or emptying urine) due to a neurological disorder (neurogenic bladder). Strictures can result from urethral damage caused by prior trauma, instrumentation (for example, catheter insertion), or an infection, such as gon-

NEW FINDING

Diet May Influence Risk of BPH

The amount and type of food a man eats may affect his risk of benign prostatic hyperplasia (BPH), according to a new study.

More than 33,000 men in the Health Professionals Follow-Up Study completed dietary questionnaires. After eight years, higher intakes of calories, protein, and polyunsaturated fats were associated with an increased risk of BPH. Compared with men in the lowest categories of consumption, BPH risk was 25% higher in men who ate the most calories, 26% higher in men who ate the most protein, and 21% higher in men who ate the most polyunsaturated fats.

The researchers speculate that a high-calorie diet might increase the risk of BPH by leading to abdominal obesity or by causing smooth muscles in the prostate to contract (which can make urinary symptoms worse). A high intake of polyunsaturated fats may raise levels of dihydrotestosterone in the prostate, which causes prostate enlargement. It is not clear why protein may be associated with an increased BPH risk.

Because the associations between diet and BPH risk in the study were not strong, men should consider other health effects—such as the protective effect of polyunsaturated fats on coronary heart disease—before making any changes in their diet.

AMERICAN JOURNAL OF CLINICAL NUTRITION
Volume 75, page 689
April 2002

orrhea. Bladder cancer is suspected when there is a history of blood in the urine. Pain in the penis or bladder area may indicate bladder stones or infection. A neurogenic bladder is suggested when an individual has diabetes or a neurological disease such as multiple sclerosis or Parkinson disease, or describes a recent deterioration in sexual function.

A thorough medical history should also include questions about previous urinary tract infections or prostatitis, and any worsening of urinary symptoms when taking cold or sinus medications. The physician will also ask whether any over-the-counter or prescription medications, supplements, or herbal remedies are being taken, because some of them can worsen or improve symptoms in men with BPH.

Physical Examination

The physical examination may begin with the doctor observing urination to completion to detect any urinary irregularities. The doctor will manually examine the lower abdomen to check for the presence of a mass, which may indicate an enlarged bladder due to retained urine. In addition, a digital rectal exam—to assess the size, shape, and consistency of the prostate—is performed. This important examination, which involves the insertion of a gloved finger into the rectum, is mildly uncomfortable. The detection of hard or firm areas in the prostate raises the suspicion of prostate cancer. If the medical history suggests possible neurological disease, the physical may also include an examination for abnormalities indicating that the urinary symptoms result from a neurogenic bladder.

Laboratory Tests

A urinalysis, which is obtained in all patients with lower urinary tract symptoms, may be the only laboratory test used if symptoms are mild and no other abnormalities are suspected from the medical history and physical examination. A urine culture is added if a urinary infection is suspected. With more severe or chronic symptoms of BPH, blood creatinine or blood urea nitrogen and hemoglobin are measured to rule out kidney damage and anemia.

Measuring blood levels of prostate specific antigen (PSA; see pages 29–32) to screen for prostate cancer is optional unless the digital rectal exam suggests cancer. PSA values alone cannot determine whether symptoms are due to BPH or prostate cancer because both conditions can elevate PSA levels. However, a 2000 study from *The Journal of Urology* found that knowing a man's PSA level is

Managing BPH with Lifestyle Measures

Lifestyle measures can help relieve the symptoms of benign prostatic hyperplasia (BPH) and prevent them from getting worse. For men with mild BPH symptoms, adopting these measures could make it possible to avoid medication or surgery. And for those with more severe symptoms, the measures may improve the effectiveness of drug or surgical treatment. Some of the lifestyle measures you can take to reduce the symptoms of BPH are listed below.

- Try to empty your bladder completely each time you go to the bathroom. This may be easier to accomplish if you urinate while sitting instead of standing.
- Do not delay urination. The bladder empties less efficiently when it is overstretched. In addition, delaying urination can lead to urinary retention in men with BPH.
- Avoid beverages that contain caffeine (for example, coffee, tea, and cola drinks). Caffeine is a diuretic; it increases urine production and leads to more frequent urination.
- Do not consume large amounts of liquids at one time. The bladder in men with BPH stores urine less efficiently and increased urine output causes urinary frequency.
- Avoid drinking any beverages (including water) after 7 P.M. This measure can reduce the number of times you will need to get up to urinate during the night.
- Limit alcohol. Alcohol increases urine production and may weaken bladder muscle tone—both of which can exacerbate BPH symptoms.
- Limit spicy or salty foods. Some men find that spicy food worsens their BPH symptoms, while salty food increases the frequency of urination.
- Avoid over-the-counter antihistamines and decongestants that can contain smooth-muscle stimulants like pseudoephedrine. By stimulating the contraction of muscles in the prostate and bladder neck, these products can obstruct the flow of urine.
- Tell your doctor if you are taking a diuretic, a tricyclic antidepressant, or a medication to treat spasticity. These drugs can worsen the symptoms of BPH, and your doctor may be able to reduce the dose of the drug or switch you to another one.
- Keep active. Retention of urine is common in sedentary men. A study in the November 23, 1998 issue of *Archives of Internal Medicine* found that moderate exercise, such as walking, helps to reduce urinary symptoms.
- Do Kegel exercises. These exercises (see page 58) may prevent urine leakage by strengthening the pelvic floor muscles that help keep the urinary sphincter closed.
- Keep warm. Being cold worsens urinary symptoms by increasing smooth muscle tone in the prostate and bladder neck.

the best way to predict how rapidly his prostate will increase in size over time. In the four-year study of 164 men with newly diagnosed BPH, PSA level was a better predictor of future prostate growth than age or prostate volume.

According to the Clinical Practice Guidelines on BPH from the Agency for Health Care Policy and Research (AHCPR), no further diagnostic tests are needed when the International Prostate Symptom Score is 0 to 7 and no abnormalities are found in the evaluation described above.

Special Diagnostic Tests

Men with moderate to severe symptoms (International Prostate Symptom Score of 8 or higher) may benefit from the following optional tests: uroflowmetry; pressure-flow urodynamic studies; and imaging studies, such as ultrasound or intravenous pyelogram (an x-ray of the urinary tract). In general, imaging studies are reserved for patients with blood in the urine, urinary tract infections, abnormal kidney function, previous surgery on the urinary tract, or a history of urinary tract stones. Cystoscopy should be done only before surgery, not to make decisions on the need for treatment.

Uroflowmetry. This noninvasive test utilizes an electronic recording to measure the speed of urine flow. If the flow rate is slow, obstruction may be present; if the flow rate is high, obstruction is unlikely and there is less chance that therapy for BPH will be effective. Normally, the flow rate is 15 mL per second or greater.

Pressure-flow urodynamic studies. These studies measure bladder pressure during voiding by placing a recording device into the bladder and, often, another into the rectum. The difference between the pressures in the bladder and the rectum indicates the pressure generated by contraction of the bladder muscle. A high pressure with a low flow rate indicates obstruction. However, low pressure with a low flow rate signals an abnormality in the bladder itself, due, for example, to a neurological disorder.

Imaging studies. These tests may be needed to search for structural abnormalities in the kidneys or bladder, to determine the amount of residual urine or the presence of stones in the bladder, or to estimate the size of the prostate. The technique previously used for such studies—x-rays following the intravenous injection of a dye—has largely been supplanted by transabdominal ultrasound.

Filling cystometry. This test involves filling the bladder with fluid, assessing the sensation of urinary urgency felt by the patient, and measuring the pressure within the bladder. According to the AHCPR guidelines, "filling cystometry adds limited information to the evaluation of most men with [lower urinary tract symptoms]." It may be useful, however, in evaluating bladder function in men who cannot urinate or in those with suspected neurological lesions.

Cystoscopy. In this procedure, a cystoscope (a type of telescope) is passed through the urethra into the bladder to provide direct visualization of the urethra and bladder. Cystoscopy is usually performed just before a prostate operation to guide the surgical approach or to look for abnormalities of the urethra or bladder.

WHEN IS BPH TREATMENT NECESSARY?

The course of BPH is not predictable in any individual. Symptoms and objective measurements of urethral obstruction can remain stable for many years and may even improve over time—in as many as one third of men, according to some studies. In one study from the Mayo Clinic, urinary symptoms did not worsen over a 3½-year period in 73% of men with mild BPH.

A progressive decrease in the size and force of the urinary stream and the feeling of incomplete emptying of the bladder are the symptoms most correlated with the eventual need for treatment. Although frequent nighttime urination (nocturia) is one of the most annoying symptoms of BPH, it does not predict the need for future intervention.

If worsening urethral obstruction is left untreated, possible complications are a thickened, irritable bladder with a reduced capacity to store urine, infected residual urine or bladder stones, and a backup of pressure that damages the kidneys.

Decisions regarding treatment are based on the severity of symptoms (as assessed by the International Prostate Symptom Score), the extent of urinary tract damage, and the man's age and overall health. In general, no treatment is needed in those who have only a few symptoms and are not bothered by them. Intervention—usually surgical—is required in the following situations: inadequate bladder emptying resulting in damage to the kidneys; complete inability to urinate after relief of acute urinary retention; incontinence due to overfilling or increased sensitivity of the bladder; bladder stones; infected residual urine; recurrent blood in the urine not responsive to medical therapy; and symptoms that trouble the patient enough to diminish his quality of life.

Treatment decisions are most difficult for men with moderate symptoms. Each individual must determine whether the symptoms bother him enough, or interfere with his life enough, to merit treatment. When selecting a treatment, both patient and doctor must balance the effectiveness of different forms of therapy against their side effects and costs.

NEW RESEARCH

Abdominal Obesity, Insulin Levels May Affect BPH Risk

Obesity is thought to be involved in the development of benign prostatic hyperplasia (BPH). Now a Chinese study shows that abdominal obesity and high blood levels of insulin may be the specific risk factors for BPH.

Researchers collected data on 200 men with BPH and 302 randomly selected healthy men (the control group). They measured the participants' fasting blood levels of insulin and leptin (a hormone produced by fat cells), body mass index (a measure of overall obesity), and waist-to-hip ratio (a measure of abdominal obesity).

Men with the largest waist-to-hip ratios or the highest insulin levels were 2½ times more likely to have BPH than men with the lowest waist-to-hip ratios or insulin levels. The impact of increased blood insulin levels was greatest in those with the lowest waist-to-hip ratios. Body mass index had only a small effect on BPH risk, and leptin levels had no effect.

Abdominal obesity and high blood levels of insulin are associated with lower levels of a protein that binds sex hormones in the blood. As a result, more androgen and estrogen may enter cells of the prostate and increase the risk of BPH.

THE JOURNAL OF UROLOGY
Volume 168, page 599
August 2002

TREATMENT OPTIONS FOR BPH

Currently, the main treatment options for BPH are watchful waiting, medication, surgery, and minimally-invasive therapy. If medications prove ineffective in a man who is not a candidate for surgery (for example, because he is unable to withstand the rigors of surgery) urethral obstruction and incontinence may be managed with intermittent catheterization or with an in-dwelling Foley catheter, which has an inflated balloon at its end to hold it in place in the bladder. A catheter can stay in place indefinitely but is usually changed monthly.

Watchful Waiting

Because the progress and complications of BPH are unpredictable, watchful waiting—meaning that no immediate treatment is attempted—is best for those with minimal symptoms that are not especially bothersome. Physician visits are needed about once a year to review the progress of symptoms, carry out an examination, and perform a few simple laboratory tests.

During watchful waiting, also known as expectant management, men should avoid tranquilizers and over-the-counter cold and sinus remedies that contain decongestants (these drugs can worsen obstructive symptoms). They should also avoid delaying urination and taking in large amounts of fluid or alcohol that can lead to rapid bladder filling. Limiting fluids at night may reduce nocturia. For more information on managing BPH with lifestyle measures, see the feature on page 7.

Phytotherapy

Some people elect to use saw palmetto and other phytotherapeutic agents (plant-derived substances), including African plum, Trinovin, South African star grass, flower pollen extract, soy, stinging nettle, zinc, rye pollen, selenium, purple cone flower, and pumpkin seeds, to manage their BPH symptoms. No solid evidence exists that any of these substances are effective in the management of BPH except for saw palmetto.

A 2002 meta-analysis of saw palmetto that included data from 21 randomized studies and more than 3,000 men with BPH revealed that men taking saw palmetto were more likely to have improved urinary symptoms than men taking a placebo. In addition, saw palmetto users had similar improvements in symptoms to those taking finasteride (Proscar). (For more information on the meta-analysis, see the sidebar on page 13.)

International Prostate Symptom Score Questionnaire

The questionnaire below was developed to help men evaluate the severity of their symptoms from benign prostatic hyperplasia (BPH). This self-administered test can help determine which treatment is needed, if any. Symptoms are classified as mild (1 to 7), moderate (8 to 19), or severe (20 to 35). Generally, no treatment is needed if symptoms are mild; moderate symptoms usually call for some form of treatment; and severe symptoms indicate that surgery is most likely to be effective.

Circle one number on each line.

	Not at all	Less than 1 time in 5	Less than half the time	About half the time	More than half the time	Almost always
1. Over the past month, how often have you had the sensation of not emptying your bladder completely after you finished urinating?	0	1	2	3	4	5
2. Over the past month, how often have you had to urinate again less than two hours after you finished urinating?	0	1	2	3	4	5
3. Over the past month, how often have you found you stopped and started again several times when you urinated?	0	1	2	3	4	5
4. Over the past month, how often have you found it difficult to postpone urination?	0	1	2	3	4	5
5. Over the past month, how often have you had a weak urinary stream?	0	1	2	3	4	5
6. Over the past month, how often have you had to push or strain to begin urination?	0	1	2	3	4	5
	None	**1 time**	**2 times**	**3 times**	**4 times**	**5x or more**
7. Over the past month, how many times did you most typically get up to urinate from the time you went to bed at night until the time you got up in the morning?	0	1	2	3	4	5

Total Score: ___________

Source: American Urological Association.

The adverse effects of saw palmetto are mild and infrequent and include headache, dizziness, nausea, and mild abdominal pain. In the meta-analysis, erectile dysfunction occurred in 1% of men taking saw palmetto and 5% of men taking finasteride.

If saw palmetto is going to work, it usually does so within the first month of treatment. Therefore, you should stop taking it if you experience no improvement in symptoms after a month. If saw palmetto does work for you, continue taking it, but be sure to inform your doctor. The typical dose of saw palmetto is 160 mg taken twice daily. Supplements that contain 85% to 95% free fatty acids and sterols are the most likely to be effective.

Medication

Drug treatment of BPH is a relatively new development; data are still being gathered on the benefits and possible adverse effects of long-term drug therapy. Currently, two types of drugs—5-alpha-reductase inhibitors and alpha-1-adrenergic blockers—are used to treat BPH. Preliminary research suggests that these drugs improve symptoms in 30% to 60% of men taking them, but it is not yet possible to predict who will respond to medical therapy or which drug will work best for an individual patient.

5-alpha-reductase inhibitors. Finasteride (Proscar) blocks the conversion of testosterone to dihydrotestosterone, the major male sex hormone within the cells of the prostate. In some men, finasteride can relieve BPH symptoms, increase urinary flow rate, and actually shrink the size of the prostate, though the drug must be continued indefinitely to prevent recurrence of symptoms. It may take as long as six months, however, to achieve maximum benefits from finasteride. In a study of its safety and effectiveness, two thirds of men taking the drug experienced at least a 20% decrease in prostate size (only about half had achieved this level of reduction by the one-year mark); one third of patients had improved urinary flow; and two thirds felt some relief of symptoms.

Finasteride may be best for men with relatively large prostate glands. An analysis of six studies found that finasteride only improved BPH symptoms in men with an initial prostate volume of over 40 cubic centimeters (cm^3); the drug did not reduce symptoms in men with smaller glands. Since finasteride shrinks the prostate, men with smaller glands are probably less likely to respond to the drug because their urinary symptoms typically result from causes other than physical obstruction (for example, smooth muscle constriction). Another study indicates more specifically that men with greater amounts of glandular tissue will benefit more from finasteride, since this tissue is more responsive to the effects of the drug. Finally, finasteride also reduces the risk of urinary retention and the need for surgery in men with BPH.

Finasteride causes relatively few side effects. Erectile dysfunction (the inability to achieve a full erection) occurs in 3% to 4% of men taking the drug. Finasteride may also decrease the volume of the ejaculate. But adverse effects on sexual function disappear when the drug is stopped.

A study from England found breast enlargement (gynecomastia) in 0.4% of patients taking the drug. About 80% of men who developed gynecomastia had a partial or full remission of their breast enlargement when they stopped taking finasteride. It is possible that gynecomastia might increase the risk of breast cancer. Because it is not clear that breast cancer or even breast enlargement is caused by finasteride, men taking the drug are being carefully monitored until these issues are resolved.

Finasteride can lower PSA levels by about 50% but is not thought to limit the utility of PSA as a screening test for prostate cancer. To get the benefits of finasteride for BPH without compromising the ability to detect early prostate cancer, men should have a PSA test before starting treatment with finasteride; subsequent PSA values can then be adjusted in light of this value. If a man is already on finasteride and no baseline PSA level was obtained, the results of a current PSA test should be multiplied by two to estimate the true PSA level. A fall in PSA of less than 50% after a year of finasteride treatment suggests either that the drug is not being taken as directed or that prostate cancer might be present. Any increase in PSA levels while taking finasteride also raises the possibility of prostate cancer. The fall in PSA levels disappears when finasteride is stopped.

Alpha-1-adrenergic blockers (alpha-blockers). These drugs, originally used to treat high blood pressure, reduce the tension of smooth muscles in blood vessel walls and also relax smooth muscle tissue within the prostate by blocking the effect of nerve impulses signaling the muscles to contract. As a result, daily use of an alpha-blocker may increase urinary flow and relieve symptoms of urinary frequency, urinary urgency, and nocturia. Several alpha-blockers—doxazosin (Cardura), terazosin (Hytrin), and tamsulosin (Flomax)—have been approved by the U.S. Food and Drug Administration (FDA) for the treatment of BPH.

One recent study found that 10 mg of terazosin daily produced a 30% reduction of BPH symptoms in about two thirds of men taking the drug. Lower daily doses of terazosin (2 and 5 mg) produced a smaller improvement. Thus, the authors of this study recommended that physicians gradually increase the dose of terazosin to 10 mg unless troublesome side effects occur. Alpha-blockers can cause such side effects as orthostatic hypotension (dizziness upon standing due to a drop in blood pressure), fatigue, insomnia, and headaches. In this study, orthostatic hypotension was the most frequent side effect.

NEW RESEARCH

Saw Palmetto May Improve Urinary Symptoms in BPH

Saw palmetto, an extract from the dwarf palm tree, may lessen urinary symptoms and improve urine flow in men with benign prostatic hyperplasia (BPH), according to a recent meta-analysis.

Researchers combined data from 21 randomized trials that compared saw palmetto with a placebo or other medications for BPH. The trials included 3,139 men (average age 65) and had follow-up periods ranging from 4 to 48 weeks (average 13 weeks).

Men taking saw palmetto were 76% more likely than men taking a placebo to report that urinary symptoms (such as frequency and urgency) had improved. Saw palmetto and finasteride (Proscar) produced similar improvements in urinary symptoms and peak urine flow. Side effects of saw palmetto were mild and infrequent. Nine percent of men taking saw palmetto withdrew from the trials, compared with 7% of those taking a placebo and 11% of those taking finasteride.

Saw palmetto may be an effective, inexpensive BPH treatment that has fewer side effects than finasteride. However, finasteride may be more effective in certain patients, and the long-term safety of saw palmetto and its ability to prevent the progression of BPH are not known. Also, the amount of saw palmetto contained in supplements varies widely.

COCHRANE DATABASE OF SYSTEMATIC REVIEWS
Issue 3, page CD001423
March 3, 2002

Medications Used in the Treatment of Benign Prostatic Hyperplasia 2003

Drug Type	Generic Name	Brand Name	Average Daily Dosage*	Wholesale Cost (Generic Cost)†
Alpha-1-adrenergic blockers (alpha-blockers)	doxazosin	Cardura	1 to 8 mg	2 mg: $109 ($92)
	terazosin	Hytrin	1 to 10 mg	2 mg: $204 ($161)
	tamsulosin	Flomax	0.4 to 0.8 mg	0.4 mg: $170
5-alpha-reductase inhibitor	finasteride	Proscar	5 mg	5 mg: $266

* These dosages represent an average range for the treatment of benign prostatic hyperplasia. The precise effective dosage varies from patient to patient and depends on many factors. Do not make any changes in your medication without consulting your doctor.
† Average wholesale prices to pharmacists for 100 tablets or capsules of the dosage strength listed. Costs to consumers are higher. If a generic is available, the cost is listed in parentheses. Source: *Red Book, 2002* (Medical Economics Data, publishers).

The authors noted that this problem can be mitigated by taking the daily dose of the drug in the evening. Orthostatic hypotension can also result from taking sildenafil (Viagra) within four hours of taking an alpha-blocker.

In another study of more than 2,000 BPH patients, a maximum of 10 mg of terazosin reduced average International Prostate Symptom Scores from 20 to 12.4 over a one-year period, compared with a drop from 20 to 16.3 in patients taking a placebo.

An advantage of alpha-blockers over finasteride is that they work almost immediately. Another advantage is that they can also treat high blood pressure (hypertension) when it is present in BPH patients. However, whether terazosin is superior to finasteride may depend more on the size of the prostate. When the two drugs were compared in a study published in *The New England Journal of Medicine,* terazosin appeared to produce greater improvement in BPH

How They Work	Special Instructions	Possible Side Effects
Block alpha-1-adrenergic receptors, causing relaxation of muscle tissue in the prostate, bladder neck, and prostate capsule. The result is increased urinary flow and fewer urinary symptoms.	For doxazosin and terazosin, the initial dosage is usually 1 mg to avoid low blood pressure and subsequent lightheadedness or dizziness. Patients requiring higher doses receive them in incremental increases. Take tamsulosin 30 minutes after the same meal every day.	Consult your doctor if you persistently experience headache; unusual tiredness or sleepiness; irritability or restlessness; nausea; abnormal ejaculation or decreased sex drive; diarrhea; back pain; drowsiness or trouble sleeping; chest pain; or runny or stuffy nose. Seek medical attention as soon as possible if you experience lightheadedness or dizziness; a fast, pounding, or irregular heartbeat; chest pain or shortness of breath; lightheadedness or dizziness upon rising from a sitting or lying position; a persistent erection; or swelling in the feet or lower legs.
By blocking the enzyme 5-alpha-reductase, which converts testosterone into dihydrotestosterone (a hormone responsible for prostate growth), the drug causes the prostate to shrink. It is most effective when the prostate is enlarged.	The drug's full effect usually takes about six months to occur. Some men may need to take the drug indefinitely to keep symptoms under control. Women who are or may become pregnant should not handle crushed finasteride tablets because of the potential risk of birth defects in a male fetus.	Side effects are generally uncommon but can include stomach or back pain; erectile dysfunction or decreased sex drive; decreased ejaculate volume; headache; dizziness; or diarrhea. Consult your doctor as soon as possible if you notice breast tenderness and enlargement; skin rash; or swelling of the lips.

symptoms and urinary flow rate than finasteride. But this difference may have been due to the larger number of men in the study with small prostates, who would be more likely to have BPH symptoms from smooth muscle constriction than from physical obstruction by excess glandular tissue.

The alpha-blocker doxazosin was evaluated in three different clinical studies involving 337 men with BPH. Patients took either a placebo or 4 to 12 mg of doxazosin a day. Doxazosin reduced urinary symptoms by 40% more than the placebo and increased peak urinary flow by an average of 2.2 mL per second (compared with 0.9 mL per second in the placebo patients). Despite the previously held belief that doxazosin was effective only for mild or moderate BPH, patients with severe symptoms experienced the greatest improvement. Side effects led to withdrawal from the study by 10% of those on doxazosin and by 4% of those taking a placebo.

In men receiving antihypertensive drugs for the treatment of high blood pressure, the doses may need to be adjusted to account for the blood-pressure-lowering effects of an alpha-blocker. Alpha-blockers may also induce angina (chest pain due to an inadequate supply of oxygen to the heart) in men with coronary heart disease. A doctor will be able to determine which individuals are good candidates for alpha-blockers.

Tamsulosin is a more specific alpha-blocker that primarily targets alpha receptors in the prostate. It has fewer side effects than the other alpha-blockers because it does not lower blood pressure as much. However, some men may benefit from lowering blood pressure and treating lower urinary tract symptoms at the same time.

Combination medical therapy. The National Institutes of Health sponsored a trial called Medical Therapy Of Prostate Symptoms (MTOPS) that is the largest trial ever to compare various types of medical therapy for BPH. The five-year trial involved 3,000 men with BPH symptoms. The men were treated with either finasteride, doxazosin, combination therapy with both drugs, or a placebo.

The results, which were presented at the 2002 meeting of the American Urological Association, revealed that not only is combination therapy safe, it appears to be more effective than monotherapy (either finasteride or doxazosin alone). For example, combination therapy reduced the risk of BPH progression by 67%, compared with 30% to 40% for monotherapy. In addition, combination therapy resulted in greater improvement in urinary symptoms than monotherapy.

As a result of this trial, most men who opt for medical therapy will likely use combination therapy.

Surgery

Surgery for BPH, known as simple prostatectomy, typically involves removing only the inner portion of the prostate, and is performed either transurethrally (through the urethra) or by making an incision in the lower abdomen. Simple prostatectomy for BPH differs from radical prostatectomy for prostate cancer, in which the entire prostate and the seminal vesicles are removed (see pages 40–45).

Surgery offers the fastest, most certain way to improve BPH symptoms. Additionally, less than 10% of patients will require retreatment 5 to 10 years later. But surgery has a greater risk for long-term complications, such as erectile dysfunction, incontinence, and retrograde ejaculation, compared with other treatment options for BPH. (Retrograde ejaculation—ejaculation of semen into the bladder rather than through the penis—is not dangerous, but it may cause infertility and anxiety.) The frequency of these complications varies with the type of surgical procedure.

Surgery is not performed until any urinary tract infection is successfully treated and kidney function is stabilized (if urinary retention has damaged the kidneys). Because blood loss is a common complication during and immediately following most types of BPH surgery, men taking aspirin should stop taking it 7 to 10 days prior to surgery. Aspirin interferes with blood clot formation.

Now that medications are available to treat BPH, fewer patients are opting for surgical procedures. In fact, the rates of transurethral prostatectomy (the most common type of simple prostatectomy; see below) declined by about 50% between 1991 and 1997.

Transurethral prostatectomy (TURP). Transurethral prostatectomy, also called transurethral resection of the prostate (TURP), is considered the gold standard for BPH treatment—the one against which other therapeutic measures are compared. More than 90% of simple prostatectomies for BPH are performed transurethrally by TURP. The procedure is typically performed under general or spinal anesthesia. In carefully selected cases, such as patients with no other medical problems and smaller prostates, TURP may be done as an outpatient procedure.

The procedure involves removal of tissue from the inner portion of the prostate with a long, thin instrument called a resectoscope, which is passed through the urethra into the bladder. A wire loop attached to the end of the resectoscope cuts away prostate tissue and seals blood vessels with an electric current. This can also be accomplished with laser energy (usually a holmium laser) instead of electric current; it is called laser prostatectomy. The loose bits of tissue are collected in the bladder and flushed out of the body through the resectoscope; a sample of this tissue is examined for prostate cancer in the laboratory.

Once the surgery is complete, a catheter is inserted through the urethra into the bladder to prevent blood clot formation; the catheter remains in place for one to three days. After the catheter is removed, most men experience a greater urgency to urinate for 12 to 24 hours. A hospital stay of one to two days is common. Most men experience little or no pain after the procedure, and full recovery can be expected within three weeks.

Improvement in symptoms is noticeable almost immediately after surgery and is greatest in those with the worst symptoms. Marked improvement occurs in about 90% to 95% of men with severe symp-

NEW RESEARCH

BPH Surgery Not More Likely To Cause Sexual Function Problems

Two new studies have found that surgery does not cause more sexual problems than other treatments for benign prostatic hyperplasia (BPH).

The first study looked at 670 Dutch men with BPH before they began treatment and nine months later. Sexual function remained unchanged in 84% of the men, regardless of the type of treatment they received. Men treated with surgery were also less likely than those treated with watchful waiting or medication to experience a worsening in erectile function (5% vs. 11% or 15.5%, respectively).

A British study included 340 men treated for BPH with transurethral prostatectomy (TURP), laser therapy, or watchful waiting. Nearly eight months after treatment, patients in all three groups had reduced ejaculation, but TURP did not cause more ejaculation problems than laser surgery. Both TURP and laser surgery provided similar improvement in erectile function. TURP was better at reducing painful ejaculation than laser surgery or watchful waiting.

The researchers of both studies conclude that surgery may preserve sexual function as well as other BPH treatments and may even be more likely to bring about improvements.

BRITISH JOURNAL OF UROLOGY INTERNATIONAL
Volume 89, page 208
February 2002

BRITISH MEDICAL JOURNAL
Volume 324, page 1059
May 2002

toms and in about 80% of those with moderate symptoms—a rate of improvement that is significantly better than that achieved with medication or watchful waiting. In addition, more than 95% of men who undergo TURP require no further treatment over the next five years.

The most common complications immediately following TURP are bleeding, urinary tract infections, and urinary retention. Longer-term complications include erectile dysfunction, retrograde ejaculation, and incontinence. However, in men with bothersome symptoms, two randomized trials have shown that erectile dysfunction and incontinence occur no more frequently after TURP than with watchful waiting. And in two more recent studies, TURP appeared to cause no more sexual function problems than other treatments for BPH and, in some cases, even brought about improvements (see the sidebar on page 17). (Erectile dysfunction and incontinence can be treated, as discussed on pages 57–66.) Mortality from TURP is very low (0.1%). Laser prostatectomy has been reported to reduce catheterization times and bleeding when compared with standard TURP using electrical current.

Open prostatectomy. An open prostatectomy is the operation of choice when the prostate is so large (more than 80 to 100 g) that TURP cannot be performed safely. There are two types of open prostatectomy for BPH: suprapubic and retropubic. Both require an incision extending from below the navel to the pubic bone. A suprapubic prostatectomy involves opening the bladder and removing the inner portion of the prostate through the bladder. In a retropubic prostatectomy, the bladder is pushed aside and the inner prostate tissue is removed without entering the bladder. Both procedures are performed under general or spinal anesthesia. As in TURP, tissue is checked for prostate cancer.

After a suprapubic prostatectomy, two catheters are placed in the bladder, one through the urethra and another through an opening made in the lower abdominal wall. The catheters remain in place for three to seven days after surgery. Following a retropubic prostatectomy, a catheter is placed in the bladder through the urethra and remains in place for a week. The hospital stay (five to seven days) and the recovery period (four to six weeks) are longer for open prostatectomy than for TURP.

Like TURP, an open prostatectomy is an effective way to relieve symptoms of BPH. But because complications are more common with open prostatectomy than with TURP—and, in some cases, the complications can be life-threatening—open prostatectomy is reserved for otherwise healthy men with the largest prostates. The most common complications immediately after open prostatectomy are excessive bleeding, which may require a transfusion, and wound infection (usually superficial). Because an open prostatectomy is elective surgery, men can donate their own blood in advance, in case they need a transfusion during or after the procedure. More serious complications of an open prostatectomy, though rare, include heart attack, pneumonia, and pulmonary embolism (a blood clot to the lungs). Breathing exercises, leg movements in bed, and early walking can reduce the risk of these complications. Long-term complications, including erectile dysfunction, incontinence, and retrograde ejaculation, are slightly more frequent with open prostatectomy than with TURP.

Transurethral vaporization of the prostate (TVP). Perhaps one of the most promising advances in the surgical treatment of BPH is transurethral vaporization of the prostate (TVP), a modification of TURP. As in TURP, the procedure involves inserting a resectoscope through the urethra. But instead of cutting away tissue with a wire loop, a powerful electrical current—delivered by a grooved roller at the end of the resectoscope—vaporizes prostate tissue with minimal bleeding. A catheter is placed in the urethra after the procedure. Preliminary experience suggests that the procedure can be performed on an outpatient basis, with removal of the catheter in less than 24 hours.

TVP appears to be as effective as TURP. In addition to a reduced risk of bleeding, other advantages of the procedure are its lower cost, fewer complications, and reduced hospital stay compared with TURP. Disadvantages of TVP include less certainty about the long-term outcome of the procedure and the lack of a tissue sample to check for prostate cancer.

Transurethral incision of the prostate (TUIP). First used in the United States in the early 1970s, TUIP also employs an instrument inserted through the urethra. But instead of cutting away prostate tissue, one or two small incisions are made in the prostate with an electrical knife or laser. These incisions alleviate the symptoms of BPH by decreasing the pressure exerted by prostate tissue on the urethra. A sample of tissue is often taken during the procedure to check for prostate cancer. TUIP takes less time to perform than TURP and can be done on an outpatient basis under local anesthesia in most cases.

TUIP is effective only in men with smaller prostates (less than 40 g). The degree of symptom improvement in these men is slightly less than that achieved with TURP, but the duration of symptom re-

NEW RESEARCH

TUMT May Provide Long-Term Symptom Relief for Men With BPH

One type of transurethral microwave thermotherapy (TUMT) appears to relieve symptoms of benign prostatic hyperplasia (BPH) for up to six years after treatment, according to a recent study from Sweden.

Researchers used a TUMT device that is not available in the United States. (The overall TUMT method is the same for all devices, but they use different levels of power and heat.) The researchers treated 371 men with BPH by performing TUMT for either 30 or 60 minutes.

One to six years after treatment, 76% of the participants said they had benefited from the treatment and 22% said their symptoms were completely gone. In addition, 41% of the men who needed a catheter before TUMT were temporarily or permanently catheter-free after the procedure. International Prostate Symptom Scores and quality of life scores improved in both groups, but they improved more with the 60-minute treatment than with the 30-minute treatment.

TUMT gave better symptom relief for patients with moderate—rather than severe—flow obstruction and for those with mainly irritative symptoms of BPH. The researchers also conclude that TUMT is an effective alternative to transurethral prostatectomy (TURP).

SCANDINAVIAN JOURNAL OF UROLOGY AND NEPHROLOGY
Volume 36, page 113
Number 2, 2002

Transurethral Microwave Thermotherapy

Transurethral microwave thermotherapy (TUMT), a minimally invasive treatment for benign prostatic hyperplasia (BPH), is growing in popularity. Three TUMT devices—the Prostatron, Targis, and Thermatrx treatment systems—are currently available as alternatives to transurethral prostatectomy (also known as TURP) for the treatment of BPH. (The company that markets the Prostatron and Targis systems refers to TUMT as cooled thermotherapy.)

In TUMT, microwave energy is sent through a special catheter to heat the prostate and destroy excess tissue while keeping the urethra cool. The procedure is performed on an outpatient basis and does not require general anesthesia. Patients often recover quickly and generally have less severe complications than with TURP. However, TURP still appears to produce more significant and long-lasting benefits.

Who Benefits From TUMT

TUMT is for men with moderate prostate volumes (30 to 100 mL) and moderate to severe symptoms (an International Prostate Symptom Score of 12 or above; see page 11). The procedure is typically reserved for men who do not benefit from or cannot tolerate medication for BPH. TUMT is not effective for men who have prostates that extend into the bladder. In addition, it should not be performed in men with an active urinary tract infection or a history of prostate cancer, bladder cancer, or pelvic trauma; in those who have undergone TURP; or in those who want to father children (because TUMT can affect ejaculation).

Preparation

Your urologist will provide specific instructions on how to prepare for TUMT. You likely will be required to ingest nothing (no food, drink, or medication) for six hours before the procedure. Upon arriving at the urologist's office or hospital outpatient clinic, you might be given an oral pain medication to reduce any discomfort and an antianxiety medication to relax you. Also, you will be asked to urinate just before the treatment.

The TUMT Procedure

First, a local anesthetic may be placed within the urethra. Then, the urologist inserts a specialized catheter through the urethra and positions the catheter in the prostate; a temperature sensor is placed in the rectum. An antenna inside the catheter directs the microwave energy to the prostate. The microwave energy generates enough heat to increase the temperature of the prostate to above 113° F. Cool water circulating through the catheter prevents damage to the urethra from the heat. The system automatically shuts down if the temperature in the rectum or urethra becomes too hot.

During the treatment, you might feel spasms in your bladder, a warming feeling, or an urgent need to pass urine or stool. While the procedure itself lasts only 30 to 60 minutes, the entire visit can take up to three hours.

After the Procedure

Someone will need to drive you home after the procedure. Because you are likely to experience irritation and inflammation in and around your urethra, a catheter is placed in the urethra to drain urine from your bladder. Depending on the specific TUMT procedure, catheterization can last from two days to two weeks. Even after the catheter is removed, you may experience discomfort in your lower abdomen or urinary urgency and frequency. Contact your doctor if you experience severe abdominal pain, a high fever, an inability to urinate, or painful urination after removal of the catheter.

You will probably need to rest at home for several days after TUMT. Also, your urine may have a pinkish hue for the first few days after the procedure. BPH symptoms are likely to improve gradually over the next few weeks or months as the irritative symptoms resolve. The delay in improvement occurs because the body needs time to absorb and discard the prostate tissue destroyed by the heat.

Benefits

In several studies, men have experienced a 40% to 70% reduction in BPH symptoms and a 14% to 60% increase in peak urinary flow rate 12 weeks after TUMT. Quality-of-life scores also improve significantly after TUMT.

lief is similar. Since the incidence of retrograde ejaculation is lower than with TURP, TUIP is an option for men concerned about their fertility.

Minimally-Invasive Therapy

A variety of minimally-invasive procedures have been introduced over the past decade. The goal of these procedures is to alleviate low-

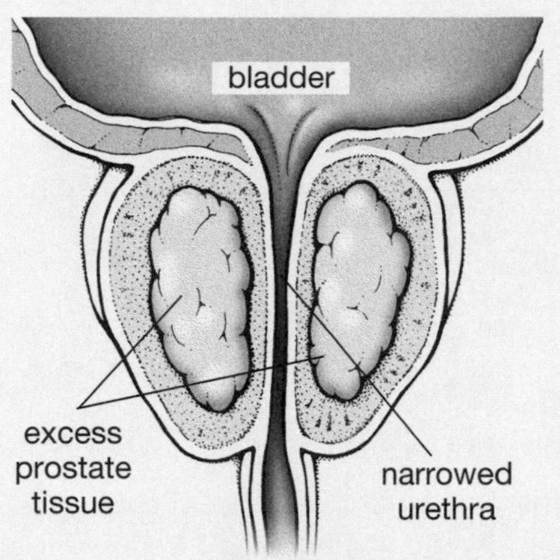

Before TUMT

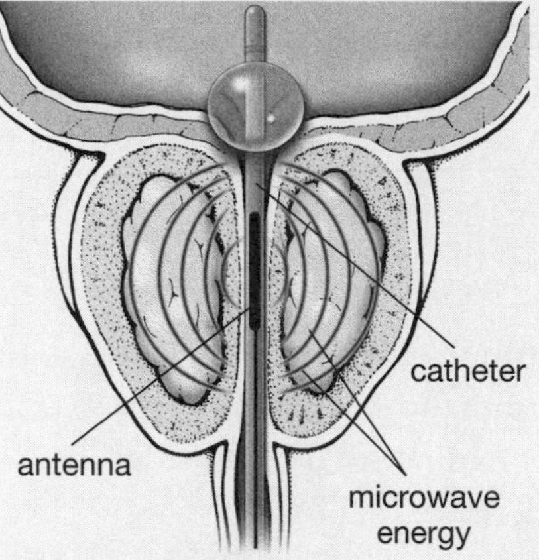

During TUMT

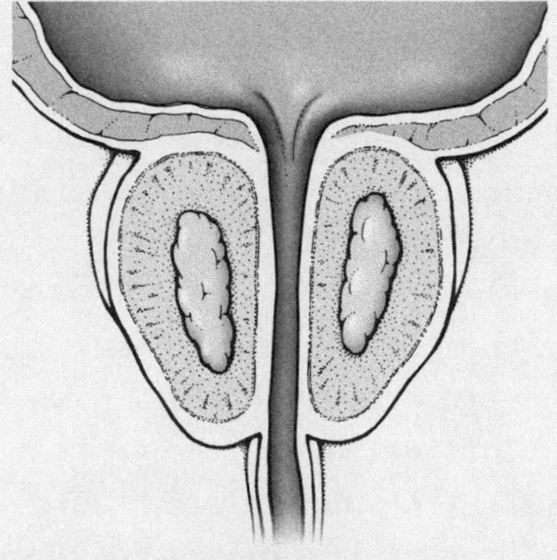

After TUMT

In one report, 80% of TUMT patients experienced a significant improvement in symptoms compared with 33% of men who took the alpha-blocker terazosin (Hytrin). The same report also found that TUMT had a significantly lower failure rate than terazosin. Some experts have suggested that patients may benefit from taking an alpha-blocker during the weeks immediately after TUMT, before the procedure begins to have its full effects.

Other research has found that the improvements with TUMT do not last as long as those with TURP. One study reported that 62% of men were satisfied with the results of TUMT after one year, but only 23% remained satisfied four years later. After four years, two thirds of TUMT patients had sought additional treatment. (If TUMT does not relieve symptoms, men can subsequently undergo a repeat TUMT or consider a different minimally-invasive treatment, medication, or TURP.)

Side Effects

Most investigators have found that the complications of TUMT are usually minor, can be managed easily, and generally pass with time. Overall, about 38% of men experience at least one complication after TUMT. These include acute incontinence in 3% of men, urinary retention (lasting an average of about 18 days) in 11%, and urinary tract infection in 13%. Urinary tract infection is more common with TUMT than with TURP, most likely because men are usually catheterized longer after TUMT. Unlike TURP, TUMT carries a low risk of major complications, such as bleeding.

TUMT is less likely to affect sexual function than TURP. In fact, TUMT may be a good alternative to TURP for sexually active men. About 17% of men experience difficulties with sexual function after TUMT, compared with 36% after TURP. Retrograde ejaculation occurs in 0% to 28% of TUMT patients but in 48% to 90% of TURP patients. Retrograde ejaculation is the ejaculation of semen into the bladder rather than through the penis. It is not dangerous but may cause infertility and anxiety.

The U.S. Food and Drug Administration has received reports of 16 serious heat-related injuries following TUMT, including significant damage to the urethra or penis. These injuries were generally not related to problems with the device itself, but with improper patient selection or failure of the physician to follow the proper procedures. Be sure to choose a urologist who is experienced in the use of TUMT.

er urinary tract symptoms while reducing the morbidity associated with surgery.

Minimally-invasive therapy for BPH uses heat to vaporize tissue in the prostate, a procedure known as thermoablation. It is unclear exactly how thermoablation works—it may improve symptoms by reducing smooth muscle tone within the prostate, or perhaps tissue destruction is the only factor at work.

Minimally-invasive therapy has several disadvantages compared with TURP. First, it takes more time after the procedure for symptoms to improve. Second, the urinary retention rate is as high as 40%. Third, up to 50% of men need further treatments. The advantages of minimally-invasive therapy over TURP are that it is performed as an outpatient procedure, and that there is a reduction in adverse events such as bleeding, incontinence, and retrograde ejaculation.

The most commonly used minimally-invasive therapies at this time are transurethral microwave thermotherapy (TUMT), transurethral needle ablation (TUNA), interstitial laser coagulation (ILC), and water-induced thermotherapy (WIT).

Transurethral microwave thermotherapy (TUMT). In TUMT, a catheter is inserted through the urethra and microwave energy at temperatures above 113° F is delivered to the prostate. At the same time, a cooling system prevents damage to the surrounding tissues, particularly the urethra. TUMT is associated with fewer risks than surgery, and if BPH symptoms return, the procedure can be repeated or the patient can undergo TURP. For more information about TUMT, see the feature on pages 20–21.

Transurethral needle ablation (TUNA) and interstitial laser coagulation (ILC). With TUNA and ILC, a needle is placed through the urethra for delivery of radiofrequency energy (TUNA) or laser energy (ILC) into the prostatic tissue. Larger prostates require several needle punctures.

One advantage of these approaches is that the surgeon can target specific areas of the prostate; other minimally-invasive therapies deliver heat to the entire prostate. However, TUNA and ILC usually require intravenous sedation in addition to topical anesthesia.

In a randomized study that compared TUNA and TURP, International Prostate Symptom Score improvements were comparable and similar to those of TUMT. But in a multicenter study in the United States, TUNA failed in 27% of men who then underwent TURP.

The multicenter experience with ILC demonstrated a 60% improvement in symptom scores with a major complication rate lower than 2%. Catheterization was required for five days on average after the procedure.

Water-induced thermotherapy (WIT). WIT is a newer therapy that relies on conduction of heat to prostate tissue from a water-filled balloon that is inflated inside the prostatic urethra (the portion of the urethra that is located within the prostate). The catheter is insulated to prevent damage to tissues other than the prostate. Treatments can be performed on an outpatient basis using only topical anesthesia.

One study of 125 men treated with WIT found that the improvement in symptom scores was significant, and that treatment results tended to last. It appears that catheterization times (one to five weeks) may be longer for WIT than for other minimally-invasive therapies. Ongoing randomized studies will help determine the value of WIT compared with other minimally-invasive therapies.

Other Treatments

A number of other treatment options for BPH are currently being investigated. These options tend to be less invasive and have fewer complications than simple prostatectomy.

Ultrasound. High-intensity, focused ultrasound (HIFU) also destroys prostate tissue with heat. In this case, ultrasound waves—emitted from an instrument inserted into the rectum—form cavities within the prostate. The destroyed tissue sloughs away and is flushed out of the body in the urine. Because it produces high temperatures, HIFU requires anesthesia.

One benefit of HIFU is its ability to focus the ultrasound precisely and spare surrounding tissues from damage. In a small study of 15 men, the procedure resulted in an average 48% improvement in the International Prostate Symptom Score and a 51% increase in urinary flow rate. However, nearly three quarters of the men had urinary retention that resolved in a few days, and almost half experienced hematospermia (blood in the semen) for up to three months. In another study, 44% of men who underwent HIFU required TURP within four years. In addition, no tissue is available to test for prostate cancer.

Stents. Stents are plastic or metal devices placed in the urethra (via a catheter) to keep it open. This option is used most often in elderly men who have acute urinary retention and whose ill health makes them unable to withstand more aggressive treatments such as prostatectomy. The primary advantages of stents are that they can be placed quickly (in about 15 minutes) under regional anesthesia; men can leave the hospital the same day or the next morning; and little convalescence is required. However, patients may experience bothersome voiding symptoms (urgency, frequency, or painful urination) for days to weeks after the procedure. Another concern with these devices is the need for precise positioning within the urethra. Additionally, little is known about the long-term effects of stents. If necessary, a stent can be removed, in most cases without damaging the urethra.

NEW FINDING

Dietary Calcium May Decrease Prostate-Protective Hormone

A diet high in calcium-rich dairy foods has been hypothesized to increase the risk of prostate cancer, and a new study suggests that decreased levels of a prostate-protective hormone may be the reason.

Researchers examined data from 20,885 men in the Physicians' Health Study who completed biannual questionnaires about their dietary habits and body mass index for 11 years.

Compared with men who consumed 150 mg of calcium or less from dairy foods per day, men who ate more than 600 mg of calcium daily had a 32% higher risk of prostate cancer. This increased risk seemed to be due to the calcium in food, not the fat, since skim milk was the most common dairy product consumed.

Overall, men who consumed more calcium from dairy products had lower blood levels of 1,25-dihydroxyvitamin D3, a hormone that is thought to slow the growth of prostate cancer cells. When blood levels of calcium are low, there is increased formation of the hormone to increase blood calcium levels. When blood levels of calcium are high, production of the hormone decreases.

The researchers are not recommending that men lower their calcium consumption based on these findings. They say that more research is needed.

AMERICAN JOURNAL OF CLINICAL NUTRITION
Volume 74, page 549
October 2001

Prostate Cancer

According to the American Cancer Society, in 2002 an estimated 189,000 new cases of prostate cancer were discovered and 30,200 men died from the disease. Newly diagnosed prostate cancer cases increased after the introduction of the prostate specific antigen (PSA) test, reached a peak in 1992, and then declined. It is not unusual to observe an increase in incidence followed by a fall in incidence after the introduction of an accurate screening test. This sequence occurs because the screening process discovers cases that would have gone undetected. Although deaths from prostate cancer are decreasing, it is not clear that widespread PSA testing is responsible.

Some experts theorize that every man will develop some degree of prostate cancer if he lives long enough. Autopsy studies have shown microscopic evidence of prostate cancer in 15% to 30% of men over the age of 50 and in 60% to 70% of men who reach age 80. A male born today has a 16% chance of being diagnosed with prostate cancer at some time in his life and a 3% chance of dying from the disease.

Experts disagree on how the PSA test should be used and how prostate cancer should be treated once it is diagnosed. Those opposed to widespread PSA screening point to the tremendous costs of testing every man over age 50, plus the uncertain benefits of treatments for prostate cancer.

CAUSES OF PROSTATE CANCER

The underlying cause of prostate cancer is unknown. Like other cancers, however, multiple sequential events over a period of many years are probably necessary to produce a cancerous change in a prostate cell.

The first step in the cancer process is the action of an initiator that produces an alteration (mutation) in the genetic makeup of a cell. But the subsequent action of a cancer promoter, which stimulates growth of the abnormal cell, is necessary for cancer to progress.

Age, race, and family history are important risk factors for prostate cancer. Environmental factors may also play a role. No association has been found between prostate cancer and socioeconomic status, education, occupation, or the presence of benign prostatic hyperplasia (BPH). However, research has raised the possibility that a high fat intake and lack of exposure to sunlight may play a role in the development of prostate cancer. Although several studies found a link between vasectomy and increased prostate cancer risk, an expert panel determined that vasectomy did not cause the increase.

Age

As a man ages, his risk of prostate cancer increases dramatically. This age-related increase is greater for prostate cancer than for any other type of cancer. The average age at the time of diagnosis is between 65 and 70, and the average age of death is between 77 and 80.

Race

In the United States, prostate cancer is significantly more common in blacks, and a recent study found that Jamaica has the highest incidence of prostate cancer in the world. Death rates from prostate cancer have declined primarily in whites and remain twice as high in blacks as in whites.

Family History

Evidence of a genetic component in prostate cancer comes from studies of families with multiple affected members. The risk grows with the number of additional affected relatives and with the discovery of prostate cancer in another family member before the age of 55. Thus, a man who has one brother with prostate cancer is twice as likely to develop the disease as a man with no affected relatives; when two first-degree relatives (brother or father) have prostate cancer, the risk increases fivefold; and a man with three first-degree relatives with prostate cancer has an 11-times greater risk.

A number of genetic alterations are linked with prostate cancer. For example, mutations in the p53 gene, which normally limits cell growth, have been associated with more than 50 types of cancer, including prostate cancer. The first hereditary prostate cancer gene, known as HPC1, was discovered in 1996 by a team of researchers from Johns Hopkins and Sweden. One third of inherited prostate cancers may be attributed to an alteration of HPC1. More recently, the same research team mapped a second prostate cancer gene to the X chromosome, one of the two chromosomes that determine gender. Defects in this gene, termed HPCX, may be responsible for 16% of hereditary prostate cancers. Inherited gene defects that raise the risk of other types of cancer—such as BRCA1 and BRCA2 mutations, which heighten a woman's susceptibility to breast and ovarian cancer—have also been implicated in prostate cancer.

In men who inherit an alteration of HPC1, the risk of developing prostate cancer by age 85 may be as high as 90%. However, this

NEW RESEARCH

Low Selenium Levels Associated With Increased Prostate Cancer Risk

The amount of the mineral selenium in the blood tends to decrease with age, and men with the lowest selenium levels may be at increased risk for prostate cancer, according to a new study.

Researchers examined the medical records of 52 men who were diagnosed with prostate cancer and had their blood selenium levels measured an average of four years before the diagnosis. Ninety-six age-matched men without prostate cancer were used as a control group.

In both groups, the older the men, the more likely they were to have decreased blood selenium levels. Even after adjusting for factors such as body mass index and smoking and alcohol history, men with higher selenium levels were at lower risk for prostate cancer. When the subjects were divided into four groups (quartiles) based on their selenium levels, men in all three of the upper quartiles had a lower risk of prostate cancer than men in the lowest quartile. In addition, men with the lowest blood selenium levels (8 to 11 micrograms per deciliter) had a four to five times greater risk of prostate cancer than men with higher blood selenium levels.

The researchers conclude that studies are needed to test whether selenium supplements can protect against prostate cancer, and if so, how.

THE JOURNAL OF UROLOGY
Volume 166, page 2034
December 2001

figure is based on subjects who had an unusually high incidence of prostate cancer in their family, and other studies may find a smaller risk. Mutations of BRCA1 and BRCA2 are associated with a 16% increased chance of prostate cancer. Not yet established is the risk of prostate cancer from other gene mutations.

Rare gene mutations like HPC1 confer a high risk for developing prostate cancer but probably account for a minority of prostate cancers. It is more likely that most prostate cancers result from the inheritance of genes that function normally but differ between individuals (polymorphic). Interactions between each person's genetic makeup and the environment probably explain the variations in risk of developing prostate cancer among different races and individuals.

Environmental Factors

Much effort has been devoted to a search for environmental factors that might serve as promoters for prostate cancer. The incidence of microscopic prostate cancer is similar among men in the United States and in all the other countries that have been examined. But the mortality rates from prostate cancer differ from one country to another and even within different regions of the United States. These differences suggest that some environmental factor or factors influence the progression of prostate cancer from microscopic tumors to clinically significant ones. Two possible factors are diet and sunlight exposure.

Diet. The majority of studies on the relationship between dietary fat and prostate cancer have found that a higher fat intake is associated with an increased risk of prostate cancer. Fat makes up 30% to 40% of the calories in the American diet, compared with 15% in Japan. These differences in fat intake may help explain the much lower death rate from prostate cancer in Japan, as well as the great variability in mortality rates around the world. Another possibility is that people who eat a high-fat diet are less likely to eat healthful foods such as vegetables.

A high intake of vegetables may lower the risk of prostate cancer. According to a study of 628 men with prostate cancer published in the *Journal of the National Cancer Institute* in 2000, men who ate 28 or more servings of vegetables a week had a 35% lower risk of prostate cancer than those who ate 14 or fewer servings per week.

Cruciferous vegetables, such as cabbage and broccoli, appeared to provide a further protective effect: Men who ate three or more servings of cruciferous vegetables a week (in addition to other vegetables) had a 41% lower risk of prostate cancer than those who ate less than one serving a week. Cruciferous vegetables are rich in substances that induce enzymes to detoxify environmental carcinogens, including the free radicals found in the human diet.

In addition, a 2000 study from Johns Hopkins found that gamma-tocopherol, the type of vitamin E that is most abundant in foods, appears to protect against prostate cancer. The effect was stronger than that offered by alpha-tocopherol, the predominant type of vitamin E in vitamin supplements.

Sunlight exposure. According to one study, sunlight may protect against prostate cancer by promoting the body's production of vitamin D. Vitamin D is synthesized in the skin during exposure to the ultraviolet (UV) radiation in sunlight. When the incidence of prostate cancer mortality was examined in white men in 3,073 counties in the United States, areas with the lowest amounts of UV radiation had the highest mortality rates. Overall, deaths from prostate cancer were highest in the Northeast and lowest in the Southwest.

In addition, a laboratory study found that physiological concentrations of the active form of vitamin D change the makeup of prostate cancer cells so that they are less likely to spread. Further studies are needed to determine whether vitamin D supplements can prevent or treat prostate cancer. Spending at least half an hour in the sunlight each day and drinking fortified milk are the best ways to get vitamin D; megadose supplements can be toxic. For those who take supplements, the recommended dose of vitamin D is 400 to 800 IU daily.

SYMPTOMS OF PROSTATE CANCER

In its early stages, prostate cancer usually causes no symptoms. As the prostate enlarges, a man may experience difficulty in beginning to urinate, nocturia, and urinary urgency and frequency—symptoms indistinguishable from those of BPH, except that they may appear more abruptly when due to cancer. The onset of erectile dysfunction or a decrease in the firmness of erections may follow cancerous invasion of the nerves controlling the erectile process. In some men, the first symptoms of prostate cancer result from its spread to distant sites—for example, severe back pain from cancer that has spread to the vertebrae.

DIAGNOSIS OF PROSTATE CANCER

Abnormalities in either a digital rectal exam or PSA test raise the suspicion of cancer and should be evaluated further. Diagnosing

NEW RESEARCH

Tomato Products May Protect Against Prostate Cancer

A recent study has found more evidence that eating tomato products, which contain the antioxidant lycopene, may lower the risk of prostate cancer.

Researchers examined data from 47,365 men in the Health Professionals Follow-Up Study who completed questionnaires about their diet, including their intake of tomato sauce and lycopene (from tomato sauce and other foods such as pizza, watermelon, and pink grapefruit).

Over a 12-year period, men who ate at least two servings of tomato sauce per week had a 23% lower risk of prostate cancer than men who ate less than one serving per month. Eating two or more servings per week also reduced the risk of metastatic prostate cancer by 35%. Similarly, men with the highest lycopene intake had a 16% lower risk of prostate cancer than men with the lowest lycopene intake.

More studies are needed to firmly establish whether lycopene, alone or in combination with other dietary components, actually reduces prostate cancer risk. In the meantime, it is reasonable for men to consume tomato-based products and other lycopene-containing foods on a regular basis.

JOURNAL OF THE NATIONAL CANCER INSTITUTE
Volume 94, page 391
March 6, 2002

How Valuable Is PSA Screening?

The prostate specific antigen (PSA) test measures levels of PSA in the blood. Originally approved by the U.S. Food and Drug Administration to evaluate the effectiveness of treatment for prostate cancer, the PSA test was subsequently approved as a screening test for the disease. Although prostate cancer mortality has dropped since the PSA test began to be widely used to screen for prostate cancer, some experts have questioned its usefulness.

Problems with the PSA Test

The PSA test has always been recognized as an imperfect tool. For example, the test is associated with false positives (that is, abnormal test results in men who do not have prostate cancer) because other prostate disorders such as benign prostatic hyperplasia (BPH) and prostatitis can also raise PSA levels. These false positive tests lead to unnecessary prostate biopsies as well as anxiety. False negatives can also occur (normal test results in men who have prostate cancer).

Another problem with the PSA test is overdetection—the detection of cancers that might never have been manifest otherwise. Treating such cancers will not extend a man's life and is therefore unnecessary.

Overdetection is of particular concern in older men, because it is estimated that without treatment an early cancer can take an average of 17 years to progress and cause death. Many older men with early PSA-detected cancers will not live long enough for their prostate cancer to cause harm—even if it goes untreated. Instead, they will die from some other cause like heart disease or stroke.

If a screening test effectively reduces cancer deaths, then populations that are more intensively screened should have the greatest reduction in cancer deaths. But population studies have yet to show this relationship between the intensity of PSA testing and mortality—a relationship that would suggest that PSA testing effectively reduces prostate cancer deaths. More studies are needed to definitively determine whether PSA saves lives. Two large randomized trials, one in the United States and another in Europe, are currently under way and should provide some answers when the studies are completed around 2005. In the meantime, the results of recent research have created a lively debate.

In Defense of PSA

Clinical studies show that an elevated PSA is the single best predictor of the presence of prostate cancer. In addition, since the introduction of PSA screening, prostate cancer is being diagnosed at an earlier stage, and there has been a decrease in the number of men diagnosed with advanced prostate cancer.

Studies show that the PSA test detects prostate cancer approximately five to seven years earlier than a digital rectal exam (DRE), which was the only method of detecting prostate cancer before the availability of the PSA test. Because they are found earlier, cancers detected by the PSA test are usually more treatable than those found by DRE.

Research also shows that prostate cancer deaths have decreased by about 1.6% each year since 1991, when the PSA test began to be widely used as a screening tool in the United States. Also, in a Canadian study, men who received PSA screening were 67% less likely to die from prostate cancer than men who were not screened (though the study was not randomized and screened men were

prostate cancer at an early stage can be difficult, however, because the cancer cells tend to spread diffusely through the prostate and into surrounding tissues, rather than forming a solid mass as is the case in most other forms of cancer.

Digital Rectal Examination

The frequent absence of a solid, palpable mass makes it difficult to detect early prostate cancer with a digital rectal exam. Used alone, a digital rectal exam misses 30% to 40% of prostate cancers, and most are detected when it is too late for treatment to be effective. The most reliable way to detect prostate cancer in its early stages is to combine digital rectal exams with measurement of PSA.

followed for a longer period of time than nonscreened men). Further, prostate cancer death rates are not dropping in several European countries that do not promote PSA screening.

Why PSA Is Being Questioned
Although prostate cancer mortality has declined since the introduction of PSA screening, there is conflicting evidence as to whether PSA screening is responsible for the decrease. Some experts maintain that the decrease in mortality is too small and occurred too soon after the introduction of widespread PSA testing to be explained by screening.

Several recent studies have questioned the relationship between PSA testing and reduced mortality from prostate cancer. One was the population-based Canadian study mentioned previously. This study also found that the intensity of PSA testing was not associated with a decrease in prostate cancer mortality in different areas of the country and in different birth cohorts (see the sidebar on page 31). Other population data from England and Wales demonstrate that mortality declines similar to those in the United States are occurring even though PSA testing has not been widespread in these countries.

A third study on PSA testing has created even more uncertainty. In 1993, free PSA screening was offered to men between the ages of 45 and 80 in the Austrian state of Tyrol, but not to men in the rest of Austria. Before the screening program, the rate of prostate cancer mortality in Tyrol was similar to that in the rest of Austria. After the screening program began, prostate cancer mortality decreased significantly in Tyrol compared to the rest of the country. However, it is likely that the mortality decline was due—at least in part—to increases in the rates of radical prostatectomy that occurred in the decade prior to the onset of screening in Tyrol.

Recommendations
Currently, the American Cancer Society and the American Urological Association recommend an annual PSA test and a DRE beginning at age 50 after a discussion of the risks and benefits of screening with a doctor. Men at increased risk for prostate cancer—such as black men, men with a family history of prostate cancer, or veterans exposed to Agent Orange—should begin screening at age 40 or 45. However, the U.S. Preventive Services Task Force, which advises the Centers for Disease Control and Prevention, does not currently recommend PSA screening for prostate cancer.

The Bottom Line
The decision to screen for prostate cancer should be based on a discussion with your doctor about the benefits and limitations of the test. You should also consider whether you are willing to undergo a biopsy and treatment if cancer is detected. When given the option, approximately 70% of men choose to be tested.

When to begin testing and how often to repeat it are also topics of debate. Studies by Dr. H. Ballentine Carter, co-author of this White Paper, found that men in their 40s and 50s who had above-average PSA levels were three to four times more likely to develop prostate cancer over the next 20 to 30 years than men who had lower-than-average PSA levels. Also, testing men at age 40, age 45, and then every other year after age 50 was shown to be a better screening strategy (saved more lives and was less costly) than yearly testing beginning at age 50. As a result, PSA screening may be more useful if it is begun earlier in all men.

Prostate Specific Antigen

The PSA test was first approved by the FDA in 1986 as a way to determine whether prostate cancer had been treated successfully and to monitor for its recurrence. However, PSA tests are now FDA-approved for detection and are widely used to screen for the presence of prostate cancer.

Clinical studies have demonstrated the following important facts about PSA and prostate cancer: 1) An elevated PSA is the single best predictor of the presence of prostate cancer. 2) PSA detects prostate cancer about five to seven years earlier than digital rectal exams. 3) Most cancers detected with PSA testing are curable, whereas most cancers detected with digital rectal exams are no longer curable. 4) Serial PSA testing of a population leads to virtual elimination of advanced prostate cancer.

However, it is not clear whether using the PSA test to screen for prostate cancer actually reduces the death rate from the disease. Consequently, some experts are questioning the value of the test as a screening tool. To learn more about the debate over PSA screening, see the feature on pages 28–29.

PSA, an enzyme produced almost exclusively by the glandular cells of the prostate, is secreted during ejaculation into the prostatic ducts that empty into the urethra. PSA liquefies semen after ejaculation so that sperm are released. Little PSA enters the blood unless some abnormality of the prostate disrupts the normal architecture of the gland and creates an opening for PSA to pass into the bloodstream. Thus, high blood levels of PSA can indicate the presence of cancer. The percentage risks of cancer based on PSA levels are below:

- PSA levels under 4 ng/mL (nanograms per milliliter) are "normal" at age 50 to 70; levels below 2.5 ng/mL are "normal" at age 40 to 50;
- 4 to 10 ng/mL, 20% to 30% risk;
- 10 to 20 ng/mL, 50% to 75% risk; and
- Above 20 ng/mL, 90% risk.

PSA screening for prostate cancer should start at age 50 for white men and at age 40 or 45 for black men and those with a family history of prostate cancer. The earlier start for black men reflects their greater risk of cancer at an earlier age. The most effective screening strategies in terms of when to start testing and how often to test are still being investigated.

A number of factors may affect the results of the PSA test. For example, men should abstain from sex for two days prior to a PSA test. This recommendation is based on the finding that ejaculation on the day or two before a PSA test may increase PSA levels in the blood (although other studies have been equivocal on this point). This temporary increase in PSA may lead some men to undergo an unnecessary biopsy. Digital rectal exams and biopsies of the prostate may also affect PSA levels, though the change caused by a digital rectal exam is not thought to be significant enough to result in a false-positive test result. A biopsy, however, may elevate PSA levels for as long as four weeks.

In the past 10 years, researchers have developed several ways to improve the capability of PSA to detect prostate cancer. These include assessing PSA in relation to prostate size (PSA density); monitoring annual changes in PSA (PSA velocity); measuring the ratio of free to total PSA (percent free PSA); and adjusting PSA for a patient's age (age-specific PSA).

PSA density. Calculated by dividing the PSA value by the volume of the prostate (as determined by transrectal ultrasonography; see pages 33–34), PSA density takes into account the size of a man's prostate when evaluating his PSA level. Thus, doctors can better distinguish between BPH and cancer: The higher the PSA density, the greater the chance of cancer, because elevated PSA is more likely to indicate cancer if prostate enlargement does not explain the increase. PSA density appears most useful for men with PSA levels of 4 to 10 ng/mL. According to several studies, a PSA density exceeding 0.15 indicates a higher risk of cancer.

PSA velocity. This technique monitors annual changes in PSA values, which rise more rapidly in men with prostate cancer than in men without the disease. A 1992 study from Johns Hopkins and the National Institute of Aging found that an increase in PSA levels greater than 0.75 ng/mL per year was an early predictor of prostate cancer in men with PSA levels between 4 and 10 ng/mL. PSA velocity is especially helpful for detecting early cancer in men with only mild PSA elevations and a normal digital rectal exam, but it is useful in predicting the presence of cancer only when changes in PSA are evaluated over 1½ to 2 years or longer.

Percent free PSA. The PSA in the blood is either bound (attached to proteins) or unbound (free). Men with prostate cancer have a higher percentage of bound PSA and a lower percentage of free PSA, compared with men with BPH. Available data suggest that measuring the percentage of free PSA in the blood (to determine the ratio of free to total PSA) improves the distinction between PSA elevations due to cancer and those caused by BPH. In men with PSA levels between 4 and 10 ng/mL, using a percent free PSA cutoff of 24% to determine the necessity for a prostate biopsy (that is, no biopsy if percent free PSA is greater than 24%) would discover more than 90% of prostate cancers and reduce by 20% the number of unnecessary biopsies. Therefore, this approach holds promise for reducing unnecessary biopsies due to false-positive PSA results.

Age-specific PSA. PSA increases with age because the prostate gradually enlarges as men grow older. Some years ago, researchers suggested adjusting PSA levels for the age of the patient. In other words, higher levels would be considered normal in older men and lower levels considered normal in younger men. However, it has not been shown that using lower levels to prompt biopsy in young men increases the likelihood of finding curable cancers, nor

NEW RESEARCH

PSA Screening May Not Reduce Prostate Cancer Death Rate

Screening for prostate cancer with prostate specific antigen (PSA) has increased the number of men diagnosed with prostate cancer but has not necessarily decreased the number of men dying of the disease, according to a new study.

Researchers calculated the change in prostate cancer incidence between 1989 and 1993 and the change in prostate cancer mortality between 1995 and 1999 for all Quebec men age 50 and older. The population was divided into 15 age groups and 15 regional groups.

Prostate cancer incidence increased in all the age and regional groups, but mortality did not fall in all the groups. When mortality did decrease, the size of the decrease did not correspond with the size of the increase in prostate cancer incidence six years earlier.

The lack of correspondence between prostate cancer incidence and mortality was probably due to the PSA test detecting cases of prostate cancer that were not life-threatening, the researchers write. An alternative explanation is that not enough time had elapsed since the onset of widespread testing to see an effect on mortality from the detection and treatment of early disease. Two large randomized trials currently under way may provide answers, perhaps as early as 2005, to the question of whether PSA testing saves lives.

CANADIAN MEDICAL ASSOCIATION JOURNAL
Volume 166, page 586
March 5, 2002

Prostate Biopsy

A prostate biopsy is recommended when prostate cancer is suspected, either because of an elevated prostate specific antigen (PSA) level or an abnormal finding on a digital rectal exam (DRE). The procedure is the only certain way to determine the presence of cancer.

Each year doctors perform prostate biopsies on some 800,000 men. Many men worry that the procedure will be painful, although it usually causes only minor discomfort. Because high levels of anxiety can increase discomfort during a prostate biopsy, men should learn as much as possible about the procedure beforehand to help reduce any anxiety they may have.

Preparation

Your doctor will likely tell you to stop taking any anticoagulant or antiplatelet drugs, like warfarin (Coumadin) or aspirin, 7 to 10 days before the biopsy to prevent bleeding during or after the procedure. Also, doctors typically prescribe antibiotics before the biopsy to help prevent any infections that could occur if bacteria from the rectum enter the prostate or bloodstream during the procedure.

On the day of the biopsy, your intestines must be cleaned with an enema, which can usually be done at home according to your doctor's instructions. The enema clears excess bacteria from the rectum and gives the doctor better access to the prostate during the biopsy.

The Procedure

A prostate biopsy is usually done in a urologist's office and takes about a half hour to perform. Some patients receive a mild sedative just before the procedure.

A transrectal ultrasound-guided biopsy (TRUS) is the most common method used. The procedure is performed while you are lying on your side on a table. Some doctors put an anesthetic lidocaine gel (Xylocaine) into the rectum to help minimize discomfort.

The doctor first performs a DRE to identify any areas of the prostate that warrant special attention during the biopsy. Next, the doctor gently inserts a thin ultrasound probe into the rectum; the probe emits sound waves that are converted into video images, allowing visualization of the prostate gland. Some doctors will inject lidocaine anesthetic into the tissues surrounding the prostate gland, using ultrasound to direct the injection needle. Some, but not all, studies suggest that this practice decreases patient discomfort.

Most prostate cancers cannot be seen on ultrasound, and therefore, ultrasound is used primarily to ensure that the prostate gland is adequately sampled throughout. Areas that appear abnormal on ultrasound are specifically targeted.

Fitted to the ultrasound probe is a spring-loaded device called a biopsy gun that quickly drives small needles through the wall of the rectum and into the prostate. In less than a second, the needles remove samples of tissue about one sixteenth of an inch in diameter. The doctor collects tissue samples in the areas of the prostate that contain abnormalities, as well as in a predetermined, carefully spaced pattern throughout the prostate. While the experts do not agree on the optimal number of samples needed, doctors usually take between 8 and 12.

If the anus is too narrow to comfortably insert the ultrasound probe, heavier sedation may be required and the biopsy is performed in a monitored operating room instead of the urologist's office. In patients who have had their rectum removed because of cancer, a perineal approach is sometimes necessary. In the perineal biopsy technique, the doctor injects the perineum (the region between the scrotum and anus) with a local anesthetic. A needle is then inserted through the perineum and into the prostate to obtain a sample. An ultrasound probe positioned against the perineum is used to guide the needle. The needle is inserted at different angles to obtain a number of tissue samples.

Risks

Biopsies taken using the TRUS method typically cause little discomfort, even without the use of anesthesia or sedatives. Some men find the procedure to be painless, while others report a sensation similar to the snapping of a rubber band against the skin each time a sample of tissue is taken.

Common side effects from prostate biopsies include minor rectal bleeding, blood in the stool or urine (for a few days and sometimes longer) and blood in the semen (giving it a pinkish hue for a few weeks

that using higher levels in older men interferes with the chance of detecting curable cancer. For now, a level of 4 ng/mL is considered the upper limit of normal in men over age 50. The use of PSA levels above 2.5 ng/mL to suggest a higher risk of cancer in younger men may be appropriate since younger men are less likely to have prostate enlargement.

and sometimes longer). Men may experience soreness in the biopsied area for several days after the procedure. Rare but serious complications such as infection (signaled by painful urination, penile discharge, or fever), severe swelling or redness near the biopsied area, prolonged or heavy bleeding, or difficulty urinating require immediate medical attention.

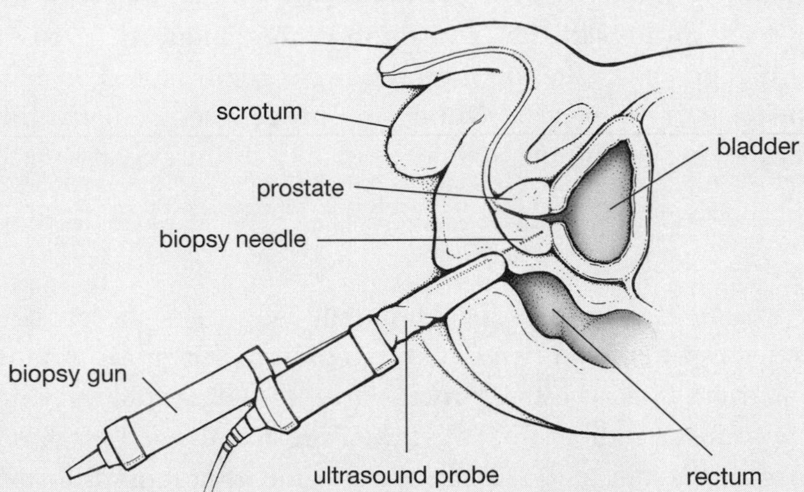

The Biopsy Results

After the biopsy, the tissue samples are sent to a lab where a pathologist examines the cells under a microscope for the presence of cancer. If the pathologist detects cancer, he or she will indicate how aggressive the cancer is by assigning it a Gleason score (see pages 36–37). Results are usually ready in three to five days. In nearly three quarters of prostate biopsies, no prostate cancer is detected. Instead, the elevated PSA levels or abnormal DRE findings that led to the biopsy may be the result of prostatitis, benign prostatic hyperplasia, or some nonmedical condition such as sexual activity within 48 hours of the PSA test.

In some cases, pathologists find prostatic intraepithelial neoplasia (PIN)—cells that many experts consider precancerous with the potential of eventually becoming cancerous. In the past, urologists believed that PIN indicated that cancer was likely to be present but was missed by the biopsy, and they recommended repeating the biopsy. A number of recent studies suggest that this is not the case and that a repeat biopsy is usually not necessary when PIN is discovered. (The finding of PIN alone does not mean that a man should begin treatment for prostate cancer.) If the pathologist finds atypical cells (cells suspicious but not diagnostic of cancer), however, a repeat biopsy is necessary. About 50% of men with atypical cells on an initial biopsy will be found to have cancer on a repeat biopsy.

In some men who test negative for prostate cancer, a repeat biopsy may be recommended if the DRE was highly suggestive of cancer, the PSA level has increased quickly, the percentage of free PSA is low (especially if it is less than 10% to 15%), or the PSA level is persistently high (over 10 ng/mL). In such cases, prostate cancer may actually be present but was missed on the initial biopsy. A small proportion of cancers—10% to 20%—occur in the transition zone (the area of the prostate farthest away from the rectum and therefore more difficult to sample), rather than the peripheral zone (where most cancers arise and where most of the tissue samples are taken during a biopsy). Therefore, a repeat biopsy may concentrate on taking tissue samples from the transition zone to ensure that cancer was not missed in this area.

Limitations

Despite advances in the technology and techniques used in prostate biopsies, they are still an imperfect way to detect cancer. Biopsies miss about 15% of prostate cancers, and they may not reveal the true aggressiveness of a detected cancer. As a result, a biopsy is not the only test that helps guide treatment. Doctors factor in the results of PSA tests, DREs, and sometimes body scans, in addition to the man's symptoms, age, overall health and life expectancy, and personal feelings and opinions about certain treatments when determining a course of therapy. Fortunately, when prostate cancer is detected at an early stage, the man has an excellent chance of being cured.

Transrectal Ultrasonography

If a digital rectal exam, a PSA test, or both are suspicious for cancer, transrectal ultrasonography is used to determine the size of the prostate, direct the needles used for prostate biopsy, and identify areas of possible cancer to ensure that they are sampled. The procedure takes 15 to 20 minutes and is performed on an outpatient basis. Some physicians recommend the use of local analgesics such as lidocaine (Xylocaine) to reduce discomfort during the procedure. With the patient lying on his side, an ultrasound probe (about the size of a finger) that generates the ultrasound waves is gently passed three to four inches into the rectum. Ultrasound images are taken with the probe in several positions as it is gradually withdrawn from the rectum.

Biopsy

When prostate cancer is suspected, needle biopsies of the prostate are carried out to obtain tissue for a microscopic diagnosis. Almost three quarters of all prostate cancers arise in the peripheral zone, which accounts for about 65% to 75% of prostate tissue. Less often, cancer occurs in the central or transition zone. (For more information on prostate biopsy, see the feature on pages 32–33.)

Other Diagnostic Tests

Other routine tests include urinalysis and blood tests for anemia. Elevated levels of acid phosphatase are more common when prostate cancer has spread to other organs, but the acid phosphatase test is rarely used today because it usually provides no more information than that obtained with a PSA test. If surgery is contemplated, general health status—particularly cardiovascular and pulmonary function—is assessed to decide whether the person is a suitable candidate for surgery.

Determining the extent of prostate cancer is important in arriving at a prognosis and choosing the treatment best suited for a given individual. Digital rectal exam results, PSA findings (higher PSA levels are associated with a greater chance of advanced disease), and evaluation of the biopsy specimen give the urologist a good idea of whether the cancer is confined to the prostate or has spread outside the gland (surgery is unlikely to be curative if the cancer has spread). In some cases, patients may be injected with a radioactive material and undergo a bone scan to determine whether the prostate cancer has spread to bones. Some physicians do not order a bone scan when PSA levels are less than 10 ng/mL because the chance of a positive scan is very low (less than 0.5%). However, other physicians prefer to have the scan done even if the risk of spread is low, so that it can act as a baseline for comparison if later studies are needed. Patients with PSA levels of 20 ng/mL and higher should have a bone scan.

A test called ProstaScint is available to detect prostate cancer

NEW RESEARCH

High Levels of Enzyme May Aid In Diagnosis of Prostate Cancer

An enzyme that appears to be elevated in prostate cancer cells may help in the diagnosis of prostate cancer when biopsy results are ambiguous and prostate specific antigen (PSA) levels are between 4 and 10 ng/mL, two studies find.

In the first study, researchers tested 342 tissue samples from patients who had prostate biopsies. Tissue samples with localized prostate cancer cells had significantly higher levels of expression of the gene for the enzyme alpha-methylacyl coenzyme A racemase (AMACR) than tissue samples containing noncancerous cells.

In the second study, researchers measured mRNA for AMACR in tissue samples from 168 men undergoing radical prostatectomy. The level of expression of AMACR mRNA was up to nine times greater in the samples from men with prostate cancer than in the samples from men with benign prostatic hyperplasia.

Researchers from both studies found that high expression levels of AMACR accurately predicted prostate cancer and that low levels predicted an absence of cancer. They say that larger studies are needed to prove the utility of AMACR to aid in the diagnosis of prostate cancer.

JOURNAL OF THE AMERICAN MEDICAL ASSOCIATION
Volume 287, page 1662
April 3, 2002

CANCER RESEARCH
Volume 62, page 2220
April 15, 2002

cells that have spread. ProstaScint uses antibodies that attach to a protein, called prostate specific membrane antigen, on prostate cancer cells. These antibodies mark cancer cells with a radioactive isotope that is then picked up by a special scanner. The potential value of this test is the avoidance of an unnecessary operation by detecting the spread of cancer before surgery is attempted. The scan is also used to detect residual disease after surgery for prostate cancer. However, the value of the ProstaScint scan is limited by false-positive and false-negative results.

When cancer is thought to be confined to the prostate (based on digital rectal exam, PSA, and biopsy results), computed tomography (CT), magnetic resonance imaging (MRI), and ProstaScint scans are not routinely used. However, a CT scan may be done to look for enlarged lymph nodes if spread of cancer is suspected. In some cases, the urologist may recommend a laparoscopic biopsy, in which a surgeon uses an instrument with a light and a camera (laparoscope) to view the lymph nodes near the prostate. A blood test, using an assay based on the reverse transcriptase polymerase chain reaction, or (RT)-PCR, is also being evaluated for its ability to determine whether cancer has spread beyond the prostate. It uses a form of biological amplification to detect the presence of prostate cells in the blood. More research will be needed before this test can be used to guide patient management.

After determining the extent and location of the cancer, doctors use two methods to describe the cancer's clinical stage. These are the Whitmore-Jewett and TNM (tumor, node, metastasis) systems.

The Whitmore-Jewett system uses stages A, B, C, and D to describe the extent of the tumor. Each stage is further subdivided into two categories to indicate severity within a particular stage (for example, stage A1 or A2). In stage A, cancer has been identified from prostate tissue taken during surgery for BPH but is not detectable during a digital rectal exam. Stage B cancer is detectable during a digital rectal exam but is still confined within the prostate. In stage C, the cancer is palpable and has spread beyond the prostate capsule to nearby tissues, such as the seminal vesicles. And in stage D, cancer cells have spread (metastasized) to the lymph nodes or to organs and tissues beyond the pelvis.

The TNM system assigns a T number to a tumor according to its extent (T1 to T4); an N+ if cancer has spread to lymph nodes; and an M+ to indicate the presence of distant metastases. In addition, T1 and T2 are further subdivided by a, b, and c (for example, T1a). In T1, the tumor is not palpable during a digital rectal exam and is not

NEW RESEARCH

Gene Mutation Test Could Help Detect Early Prostate Cancer

A test that detects chemical changes associated with a gene mutation could be used as a screening tool for prostate cancer, a new study suggests.

Glutathione S-transferase, an enzyme that detoxifies drugs, is encoded by the gene GSTP1. Methylation, a metabolic process that inactivates the GSTP1 gene, is the most common genetic event associated with prostate cancer. GSTP1 methylation is more common in men with early-stage prostate cancer than in those with normal prostates or diseases such as benign prostatic hyperplasia (BPH).

Could levels of GSTP1 methylation reveal valuable diagnostic information? To find out, researchers at Johns Hopkins examined prostate biopsy samples from 21 men with high prostate specific antigen (PSA) levels. Elevated levels of methylated GSTP1 correctly predicted the presence of prostate cancer in 10 of 11 patients; low levels correctly predicted the absence of cancer in 10 of 10 patients.

If further studies show that elevated levels of methylated GSTP1 accurately predict the presence of prostate cancer, methylated GSTP1 could be helpful in detecting early prostate cancer that is missed during a prostate biopsy.

JOURNAL OF THE NATIONAL CANCER INSTITUTE
Volume 93, page 1747
November 21, 2001

visible with imaging techniques. T2 cancer is palpable but still confined to the prostate. T3 and T4 describe palpable tumors that have spread locally beyond the prostate into surrounding structures. The most commonly diagnosed stage of cancer today is T1c, indicating that the cancer cannot be felt during a digital rectal exam, but PSA levels are elevated.

WHEN IS PROSTATE CANCER TREATMENT NECESSARY?

The choice of treatment for prostate cancer depends on the clinical stage of the cancer (extent of disease) and the age and general health of the individual. While one third of men over age 50 have minute prostate tumors, only 10% of them develop cancer serious enough to pose a health problem. However, investigators have found in healthy men who have more than a 10-year life expectancy that about 80% of prostate cancers detected by PSA testing are significant tumors that warrant treatment. Still, with increased use of PSA, some men will be diagnosed with small prostate cancers (which cannot be felt during a digital rectal exam but are detected through ultrasound or biopsy) that pose no immediate threat and, indeed, may never need treatment. A recent study has estimated that about 15% of cancers detected with PSA testing fall into this category.

Possible complications may also factor into a man's decision to postpone treatment. If he opts for surgery or radiation, he risks the possibility of bowel, urinary, or sexual problems. If he chooses watchful waiting (no treatment is provided, but the possibility of cancer growth is closely monitored), he may be anxious about the progress of the disease.

Doctors use several methods to help predict the seriousness of the cancer and the need for treatment. One method is the Gleason score (which ranges from 2 to 10). It is based on how malignant (cancerous) the biopsied cancer cells appear to the pathologist. The pathologist assigns a grade of 1 to 5 to the two most prevalent cancer patterns within the biopsy tissue, and adds them together to determine the score. Well-differentiated cells—cells that differ only slightly in appearance from normal prostate cells—have a low grade of malignancy and are given a low Gleason score. The lower the Gleason score, the better: A score of 2 to 4 indicates a greater probability of an insignificant cancer; higher scores suggest a greater likelihood of a significant, life-threatening cancer. Men with "high-grade" disease (defined as a Gleason score of 7 to 10) are considered poor candidates for watchful waiting, since the high score indicates the presence of an aggressive cancer. Less than 10% of men suspected of having prostate cancer, based on a digital rectal exam and PSA, have well-differentiated tumors.

Another method for predicting which prostate cancers require treatment was investigated at Johns Hopkins. In this study, the vast majority of prostate tumors detected by PSA were significant in terms of size and grade. To help predict cancer significance more accurately, the researchers factored in PSA density, the number of positive biopsies, the percentage of the biopsied tissue that contains cancer cells, and cancer grade. According to their research, men are more likely to have insignificant cancer (a very small tumor), and thus be suitable candidates for watchful waiting, if they fulfill the following criteria: a nonpalpable tumor by digital rectal exam; PSA density less than 0.15; signs of cancer in no more than two biopsy samples of prostate tissue; less than 50% of any single biopsy contains cancer cells; and a Gleason score of less than 7. Watchful waiting may be a rational choice for older men whose tumors have the above characteristics.

Age also plays an important part in deciding whether to treat prostate cancer aggressively. Because prostate cancer generally progresses slowly, older men with small tumors can choose watchful waiting more safely than younger men. Men in their 50s and early 60s with prostate cancer are likely to live long enough for their disease to become life-threatening; men in their late 70s and 80s are likely to die of another cause first.

TREATMENT OPTIONS FOR PROSTATE CANCER

The standard management options for prostate cancer include watchful waiting, radical prostatectomy, radiation therapy, and hormone treatment to lower levels of the male hormone testosterone. Radiation therapy can be delivered from an external source (external beam radiation therapy) or by implantation of radioactive seeds (brachytherapy). Cryotherapy (freezing the prostate) is also used to treat prostate cancer.

Radical prostatectomy and radiation therapy can potentially cure prostate cancer in its early stages. Hormone therapy is not curative and is generally used only to slow the progression of the disease once it has spread to other sites. Though various forms of chemotherapy are effective in treating some types of cancer, they have been less successful for prostate cancer. (Men with prostate cancer who wish to discuss specific treatments with those who have already undergone

NEW RESEARCH

Watchful Waiting Can Be Valuable Treatment Option for Some Men

Watchful waiting is a reasonable option for older men who are thought to have early-stage prostate cancer, a new study reports.

Researchers at Johns Hopkins identified 81 men (average age 65) who were believed to have small-volume prostate cancers based on their biopsy findings and prostate specific antigen (PSA) levels. These men decided to delay treatment but were closely monitored with PSA tests and digital rectal examinations every six months and prostate biopsies every year. If the disease appeared to be progressing, the researchers recommended treatment with radical prostatectomy or radiation.

After an average of 23 months, the disease progressed in 25 men (31%). In these men the initial PSA density was higher and the percentage of free PSA was lower than in men whose disease did not progress. After finding out that their disease had progressed, 13 of the 25 men underwent radical prostatectomy, and 12 of the 13 (92%) had small tumors that were still curable.

Since the vast majority of the men who delayed treatment by a few years were still able to benefit from radical prostatectomy, the researchers conclude that watchful waiting—with strict adherence to follow-up—can be a valuable treatment option for some older men with small-volume prostate cancers.

THE JOURNAL OF UROLOGY
Volume 167, page 1231
March 2002

Deciding on Management for Prostate Cancer

Once a biopsy of the prostate confirms the presence of prostate cancer, a man must begin the process of choosing a management option. While the management choices for many cancers are somewhat limited, the options for prostate cancer are quite varied and include watchful waiting, radical prostatectomy, radiation therapy, and hormone therapy.

Because prostate cancer progresses slowly, men can take time to consider the management options. During this time, they should learn as much as they can about the various management options (see pages 37–57), consider their own feelings and expectations, and talk with those close to them about the choices. When considering management options, men and their doctors

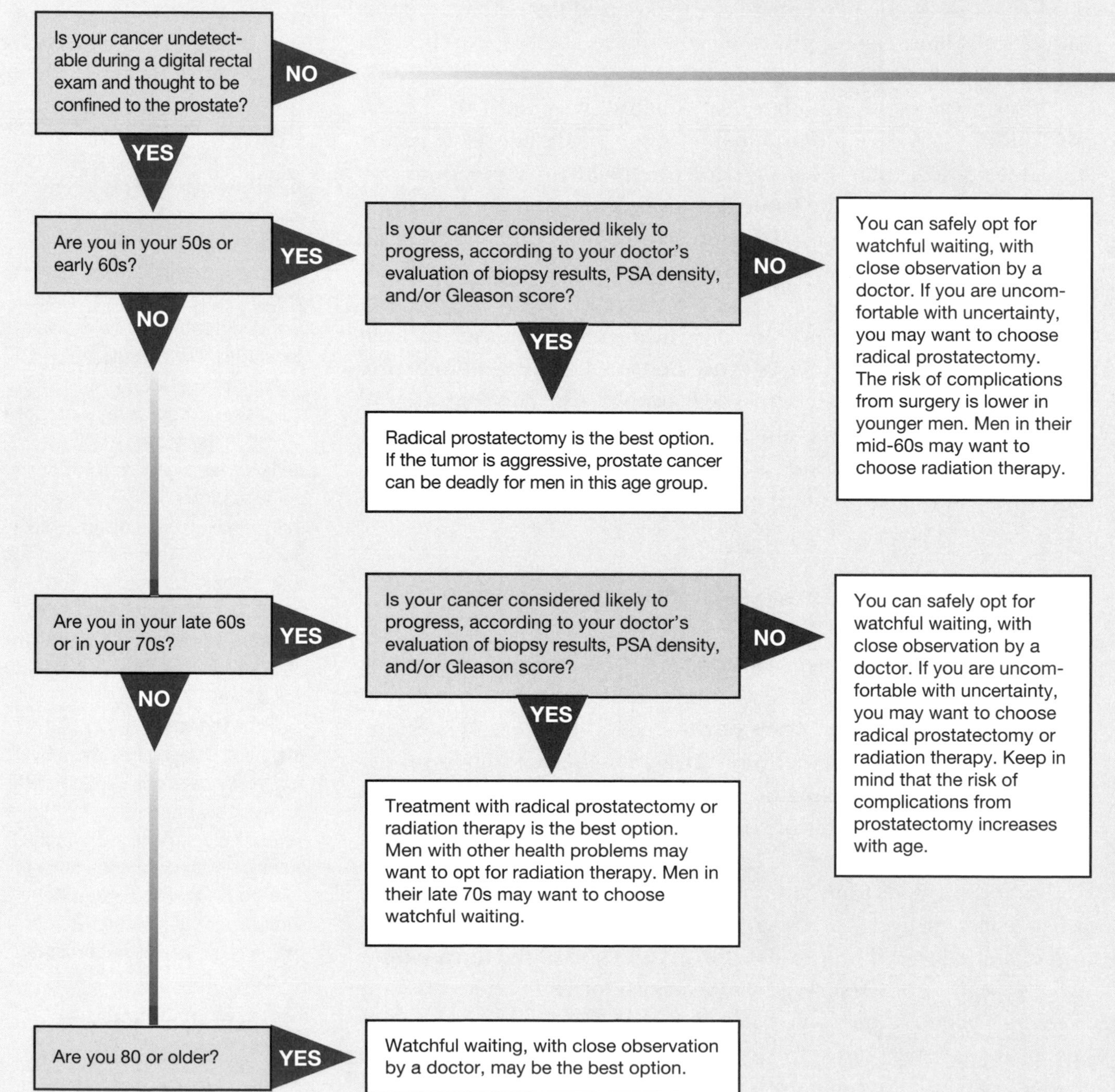

must take into account the stage of the cancer and the Gleason score as well as the man's age, life expectancy, and overall health. Men should also learn about the potential side effects of various therapies and decide which effects they are willing to tolerate. Furthermore, they should consider consulting physicians from different fields (urologists, radiation oncologists, and medical oncologists) to get a broader spectrum of opinions.

The flow chart printed below is meant as a general guideline. It provides men who are otherwise in good health with an idea of what the best course of action might be for their specific circumstances. However, no one guideline can apply to all prostate cancer patients; each case must be considered on an individual basis.

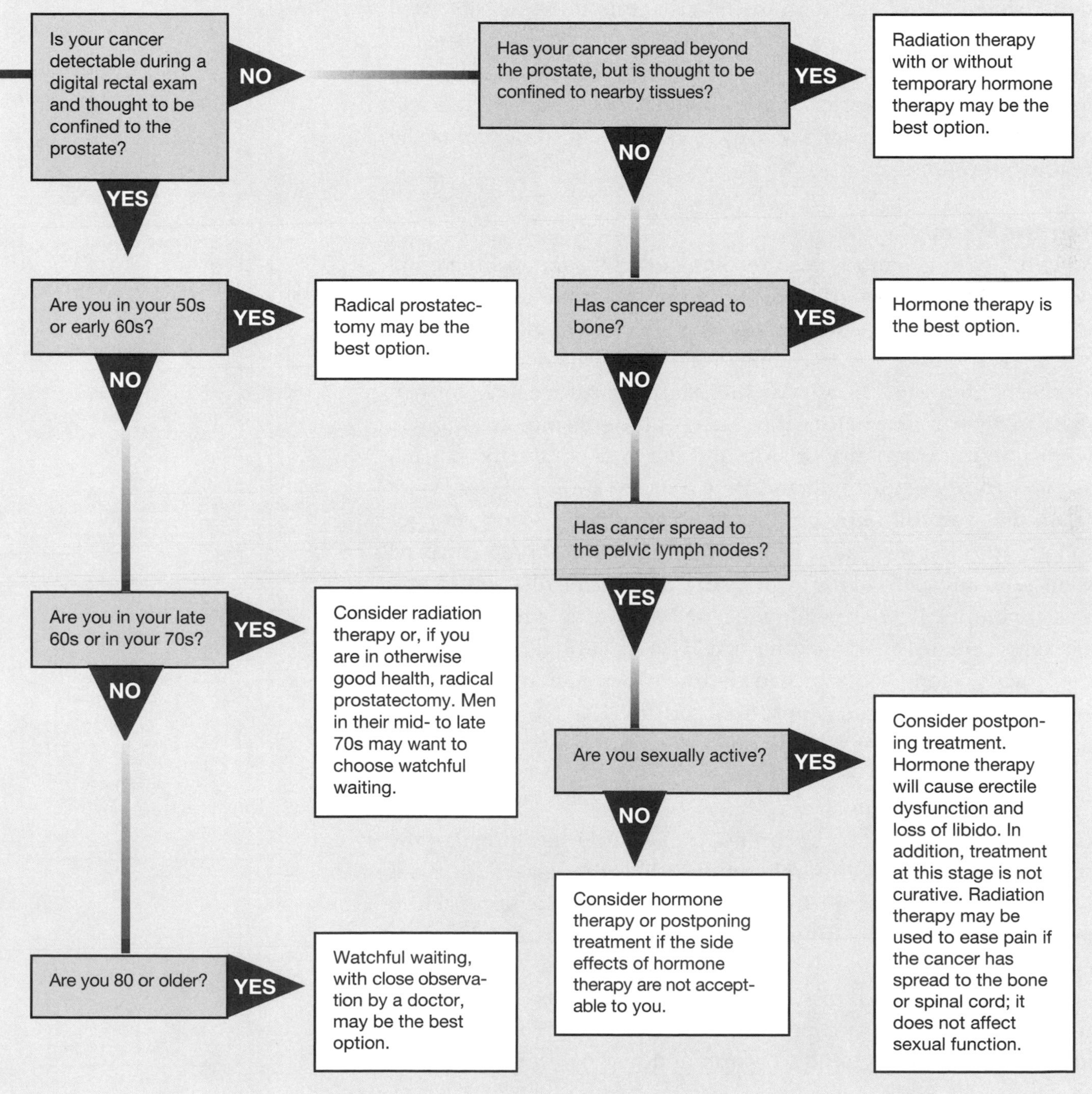

them should contact the support groups listed on page 73.)

Bear in mind that a particular doctor's specialty may influence the treatment he or she recommends. A 2000 study published in the *Journal of the American Medical Association* found a wide variety of beliefs and practices regarding prostate cancer treatment between 504 urologists and 559 radiation oncologists. For patients with cancer limited to the prostate and a life expectancy of 10 years or more, 93% of urologists chose radical prostatectomy as the preferred treatment, while 72% of radiation oncologists responded that external beam radiation therapy and surgery are equally effective. Because both groups of doctors were more likely to recommend the treatment that they themselves deliver, the authors suggested consulting with a member of each specialty to get a balanced picture of the treatment options.

Watchful Waiting

Watchful waiting is most often recommended for men who are unlikely to live long enough to benefit from treatment and for those who have disease that is too far advanced to cure. In addition, some men who are thought to have small-volume cancers may opt for this approach. Men who choose watchful waiting must see a doctor regularly to determine whether the cancer is progressing. Recommendations on the frequency of visits and the tests conducted at each visit vary from doctor to doctor. Dr. Carter, co-author of this White Paper, uses the following guidelines for men age 75 and younger who are in otherwise good health: PSA testing and a digital rectal exam semi-annually, along with yearly transrectal ultrasound and prostate biopsy. Recommendations for PSA testing and digital rectal exams remain the same after age 75, but yearly ultrasound and biopsy are no longer performed routinely. Between appointments, a man of any age should report to his doctor if he has blood in the urine, difficulty voiding, or new onset of pain.

Radical Prostatectomy

Radical prostatectomy is not curative if the cancer has spread to the lymph nodes in the pelvis. Therefore, when the risk of spread is judged to be high, some surgeons use a laparoscopic approach to obtain samples of the lymph nodes before the planned prostatectomy; others sample the lymph nodes at the time of the scheduled prostatectomy and discontinue the operation if the cancer has spread. However, it is uncommon today (because of PSA testing) to find disease that has spread to lymph nodes at the time of surgery.

If enlarged lymph nodes are discovered on a CT scan or MRI in men with prostate cancer, aspiration of cells from the lymph nodes with a fine needle should be performed to determine whether the cancer has metastasized.

Radical prostatectomy was developed at Johns Hopkins at the beginning of the 20th century. The operation was not popular at first because of the high frequency of erectile dysfunction and urinary incontinence. But in the early 1980s, Patrick Walsh, M.D., a urologist at Johns Hopkins, developed a new approach to the operation. He devised a "road map" that allows surgeons to remove the prostate with a lower chance of damaging the structures important for erections and urinary control.

This anatomical, or "nerve-sparing," technique has reduced the risk of severe incontinence to 1% to 3% and the chance of mild incontinence to around 10%. One group of researchers reported successful recovery of erections in 68% of men treated with nerve-sparing surgery. Dr. Walsh has performed radical prostatectomy on more than 2,000 men with early prostate cancer, preserving potency in 90% of men in their 40s, 75% of those in their 50s, and 60% of those in their 60s. Full recovery can take more than a year in some cases. When erectile dysfunction does occur after surgery, it can usually be treated successfully (see pages 60–66).

Nerve-sparing radical retropubic prostatectomy begins with a vertical incision in the abdomen from the pubic area to the navel. (Some surgeons make the incision into the perineum, which is located between the scrotum and the rectum; in this case the procedure is called a perineal prostatectomy.) If appropriate, samples of the pelvic lymph nodes may be removed and tested for signs of cancer. The surgeon then cuts and ties the group of veins that lies atop the prostate and urethra (the dorsal vein complex) in order to minimize bleeding—which can obscure the operative field and increase the risk of complications. Next, the surgeon severs the urethra, taking care to avoid the urethral sphincter muscles in order to preserve urinary continence.

At this point, the "nerve-sparing" aspect of the procedure comes into play: The tiny nerve bundles that sit on either side of the prostate—those required for an erection—are carefully dissected away from the prostate but are otherwise left intact. (If the cancer has spread to these nerves, however, they will be removed.) The surgeon then cuts through the bladder neck (the junction between the bladder and the prostate) to completely separate the prostate and removes some of the surrounding tissues, including the semi-

NEW FINDING

Prostatectomy Reduces Mortality Rate From Prostate Cancer

A new study is the first to show that radical prostatectomy is more effective than watchful waiting for preventing prostate cancer deaths.

Swedish researchers randomly assigned 695 men under the age of 75 with early-stage prostate cancer (found mostly by digital rectal exam) to watchful waiting or radical prostatectomy. During a follow-up of 6.2 years, 9% of the watchful waiting group and 5% of the prostatectomy group had died of prostate cancer, but the overall death rate from any cause was the same in both groups. Distant metastases were 14% more likely in the watchful waiting group than in the prostatectomy group.

The prostatectomy group experienced more erectile dysfunction (80% vs. 45%) and more urinary leakage (49% vs. 21%) than the watchful waiting group. More men in the watchful waiting group had a weak urinary stream.

In an accompanying editorial, Johns Hopkins prostate expert Patrick Walsh, M.D., says these results are encouraging. However, more research is needed to determine whether prostatectomy is as valuable for men in the United States, where 75% of tumors are found through prostate specific antigen (PSA) testing and thus at an earlier stage than in Sweden. Also, longer follow-up is needed to determine the long-term mortality rate.

THE NEW ENGLAND JOURNAL OF MEDICINE
Volume 347, pages 781, 790, and 839
September 12, 2002

Partin Tables

Before deciding on a treatment for prostate cancer, it is useful to know whether the cancer has spread from the prostate to the adjacent tissue, seminal vesicles, or lymph nodes. Although it is not possible to conclusively determine this information before surgery, the Partin tables, printed below, help predict the chance that a cancer is confined to the prostate or has spread. The prediction is based on the patient's prostate specific antigen (PSA) level, biopsy Gleason score, and clinical stage.

To use the Partin tables, you first need to know the stage of your cancer to determine which of the four tables applies to you. After finding the right table, deter-

Clinical Stage T1c
(nonpalpable, PSA elevated)

PSA Range (ng/mL)	Pathological Stage	Gleason Score 2–4	5–6	3+4=7	4+3=7	8–10
0–2.5	Organ confined	95	90	79	71	66
	Extraprostatic extension	5	9	17	25	28
	Seminal vesicle (+)	—	0	2	2	4
	Lymph node (+)	—	—	1	1	1
2.6–4	Organ confined	92	84	68	58	52
	Extraprostatic extension	8	15	27	37	40
	Seminal vesicle (+)	—	1	4	4	6
	Lymph node (+)	—	—	1	1	1
4.1–6	Organ confined	90	80	63	52	46
	Extraprostatic extension	10	19	32	42	45
	Seminal vesicle (+)	—	1	3	3	5
	Lymph node (+)	—	0	2	3	3
6.1–10	Organ confined	87	75	54	43	37
	Extraprostatic extension	13	23	36	47	48
	Seminal vesicle (+)	—	2	8	8	13
	Lymph node (+)	—	0	2	2	3
>10	Organ confined	80	62	37	27	22
	Extraprostatic extension	20	33	43	51	50
	Seminal vesicle (+)	—	4	12	11	17
	Lymph node (+)	—	2	8	10	11

Clinical Stage T2a
(palpable <½ of one lobe)

PSA Range (ng/mL)	Pathological Stage	Gleason Score 2–4	5–6	3+4=7	4+3=7	8–10
0–2.5	Organ confined	91	81	64	53	47
	Extraprostatic extension	9	17	29	40	42
	Seminal vesicle (+)	—	1	5	4	7
	Lymph node (+)	—	0	2	3	3
2.6–4	Organ confined	85	71	50	39	33
	Extraprostatic extension	15	27	41	52	53
	Seminal vesicle (+)	—	2	7	6	10
	Lymph node (+)	—	0	2	2	3
4.1–6	Organ confined	81	66	44	33	28
	Extraprostatic extension	19	32	46	56	58
	Seminal vesicle (+)	—	1	5	5	8
	Lymph node (+)	—	1	4	6	6
6.1–10	Organ confined	76	58	35	25	21
	Extraprostatic extension	24	37	49	58	57
	Seminal vesicle (+)	—	4	13	11	17
	Lymph node (+)	—	1	3	5	5
>10	Organ confined	65	42	20	14	11
	Extraprostatic extension	35	47	49	55	52
	Seminal vesicle (+)	—	6	16	13	19
	Lymph node (+)	—	4	14	18	17

mine into which of the five PSA ranges your PSA level falls. Then, follow this row across to find the column that corresponds to your Gleason score. The four numbers are the percent chance that your cancer is organ confined or has spread to nearby tissues (extraprostatic extension), the seminal vesicles, or the lymph nodes.

For example, a man with a stage T2a tumor, a PSA level of 11 ng/mL, and a Gleason score of 5 will have a 42% chance of having his cancer confined to the prostate, a 47% chance of cancer that has spread to adjacent tissue, a 6% chance of seminal vesicle involvement, and a 4% chance of lymph node involvement.

Clinical Stage T2b
(palpable >½ of one lobe, not on both lobes)

PSA Range (ng/mL)	Pathological Stage	Gleason Score 2–4	5–6	3+4=7	4+3=7	8–10
0–2.5	Organ confined	88	75	54	43	37
	Extraprostatic extension	12	22	35	45	46
	Seminal vesicle (+)	—	2	6	5	9
	Lymph node (+)	—	1	4	6	6
2.6–4	Organ confined	80	63	41	30	25
	Extraprostatic extension	20	34	47	57	57
	Seminal vesicle (+)	—	2	9	7	12
	Lymph node (+)	—	1	3	4	5
4.1–6	Organ confined	75	57	35	25	21
	Extraprostatic extension	25	39	51	60	59
	Seminal vesicle (+)	—	2	7	5	9
	Lymph node (+)	—	2	7	10	10
6.1–10	Organ confined	69	49	26	19	15
	Extraprostatic extension	31	44	52	60	57
	Seminal vesicle (+)	—	5	16	13	19
	Lymph node (+)	—	2	6	8	8
>10	Organ confined	57	33	14	9	7
	Extraprostatic extension	43	52	47	50	46
	Seminal vesicle (+)	—	8	17	13	19
	Lymph node (+)	—	8	22	27	27

Clinical Stage T2c
(palpable on both lobes)

PSA Range (ng/mL)	Pathological Stage	Gleason Score 2–4	5–6	3+4=7	4+3=7	8–10
0–2.5	Organ confined	86	73	51	39	34
	Extraprostatic extension	14	24	36	45	47
	Seminal vesicle (+)	—	1	5	5	8
	Lymph node (+)	—	1	6	9	10
2.6–4	Organ confined	78	61	38	27	23
	Extraprostatic extension	22	36	48	57	57
	Seminal vesicle (+)	—	2	8	6	10
	Lymph node (+)	—	1	5	7	8
4.1–6	Organ confined	73	55	31	21	18
	Extraprostatic extension	27	40	50	57	57
	Seminal vesicle (+)	—	2	6	4	7
	Lymph node (+)	—	3	12	16	16
6.1–10	Organ confined	67	46	24	16	13
	Extraprostatic extension	33	46	52	58	56
	Seminal vesicle (+)	—	5	13	11	16
	Lymph node (+)	—	3	10	13	13
>10	Organ confined	54	30	11	7	6
	Extraprostatic extension	46	51	42	43	41
	Seminal vesicle (+)	—	6	13	10	15
	Lymph node (+)	—	13	33	38	38

Adapted from *Urology*, December 2001, p. 845–846.

nal vesicles and vas deferens (the main duct that carries semen). Finally, the bladder neck is narrowed with stitches and reconnected to the urethra. A Foley catheter (inserted through the urethra to drain urine from the bladder) is left in place for two to three weeks to allow time for the rebuilt urinary tract to heal. Rare complications of radical prostatectomy include narrowing of the urethra (urethral stricture), damage to the rectum, and the surgical and anesthetic risks (including death) that accompany any operation.

Some surgeons are using laparoscopy to perform radical prostatectomy. The laparoscopic procedure takes two to four times as long to perform, and it is unclear how cancer control rates, incontinence, and erectile dysfunction compare with those of the standard approach. This approach is being used at Hopkins in some patients, but it is still considered investigational.

PSA is the most sensitive indicator of disease status after any treatment for prostate cancer. An undetectable PSA level (usually less than 0.2 ng/mL) after radical prostatectomy indicates that all benign and malignant prostate tissue has been removed. A detectable PSA in the postoperative period means that the tumor had spread to other tissues and was not totally excised at the time of surgery. A subsequent rise in PSA levels indicates local recurrence or growth of the cancer in other sites.

For men with localized prostate cancer (stage T1 and T2) before treatment, the chance of recurrent cancer—indicated by detectable PSA levels—10 years after treatment is around 30%. A detectable PSA indicates recurrent disease months to years before the cancer is visible by CT scan or bone scan. The ProstaScint scan has been used to determine the site of residual cancer after surgery in men who have detectable PSA levels and no evidence of disease on other imaging tests (for example, CT scan, bone scan, or MRI). When evidence indicates that residual cancer is limited to the pelvis, radiation therapy is a treatment option for men with detectable PSA levels after radical prostatectomy. A detectable PSA in the first year after surgery indicates a high probability that the disease has spread beyond the pelvis and that radiation will not successfully eradicate the cancer.

In a groundbreaking study, researchers at Johns Hopkins took the first steps toward clarifying what happens to patients with a detectable PSA after surgery. For up to 15 years (average 5 years), they followed nearly 2,000 patients after radical prostatectomy who were all treated by a single surgeon, had localized prostate cancer, and received no hormone therapy unless metastatic disease became apparent by radiographic imaging. Results were promising even in the 304 (15%) men in the study with detectable PSA levels in the years following surgery. Overall, their five-year disease-free (no sign of metastatic cancer) survival rate was 63% following the first detectable PSA, and metastatic cancer was not apparent for an average of eight years. These results should reassure men who experience rising PSA levels following surgery. At the same time, these findings serve as a reminder that continued regular monitoring is essential after surgery.

External Beam Radiation Therapy

External beam radiation therapy is an excellent treatment option for prostate cancer, especially for older men with medical illnesses that make surgery dangerous and for men with more advanced cancer (stage C or T3) that cannot be completely removed surgically.

It is also used as a palliative treatment (meaning a treatment aimed at delaying the progression of disease, relieving pain, and limiting disease complications, rather than curing a disease). For a patient with prostate cancer that has metastasized to the bones, palliative treatment can diminish pain and lessen the likelihood of bone fractures. Palliative treatment can also be used to treat neurological symptoms resulting from compression of the spinal cord if cancer has spread to the spine.

Some men with stage A (T1) or B (T2) cancer select radiation therapy after weighing the pros and cons of radiation vs. surgery. Although no adequate study has directly compared radical prostatectomy with radiation, available evidence suggests that patients choosing either approach have a similar chance of having no evidence of cancer present five years after treatment for stage T1 or T2 disease. Radiation therapists are working to improve external beam radiation therapy by targeting maximal radiation doses to the prostate more precisely, thereby minimizing the damage to surrounding tissues (a technique called three-dimensional conformal radiation therapy; see the feature on pages 46–47).

Complications of radiation therapy mostly involve adverse effects on the urinary tract, which can lead to increased frequency and urgency of urination, and bowel damage, which may cause diarrhea, rectal bleeding, exacerbation of hemorrhoids, and cramps. These symptoms usually disappear days to weeks after completing treatment. Urinary incontinence is rare; it occurs in less than 1% to 2% of patients. Erectile dysfunction occurs in 40% to 60% of men, depending on their age and sexual function before treatment. In some

NEW RESEARCH

Migrating Brachytherapy Seeds Do Not Appear Harmful to Lungs

Radioactive seeds implanted in the prostate during brachytherapy may migrate to the lungs more often than previously thought. However, these migrated seeds do not appear to cause short-term harm, according to a new study.

Researchers reviewed the medical records of 58 patients who underwent brachytherapy and had chest x-rays within 90 days of the procedure. At least one seed had moved to the lungs in 21 (36%) of the patients. (Previous studies had suggested that seeds migrate in 6% to 29% of patients.) Fourteen of these patients agreed to lung-function testing; nine had normal lung function and the other five had a history of smoking or chronic obstructive pulmonary disease prior to brachytherapy.

The type of seeds used did not appear to increase the risk of migration, but the risk increased slightly with the number of seeds implanted. Radioactive seeds are thought to move into the lungs from the heart after entering the circulatory system from blood vessels around the prostate.

The researchers stress that although migrated seeds did not appear to cause any short-term lung problems, long-term follow-up is needed. Doctors should discuss the possibility of seed migration with men considering brachytherapy.

UROLOGY
Volume 59, page 555
April 2002

The Newest Types of Radiation Therapy

Radiation therapy is the second most common treatment for early-stage prostate cancer (radical prostatectomy is the first). The standard way to deliver radiation therapy is to aim beams of radiation at the tumor from outside the body, a technique called external beam radiation therapy (EBRT).

Because radiation to the prostate can harm the nearby rectum, bowel, and bladder, researchers have developed refinements of and alternatives to standard EBRT. Three-dimensional conformal radiation therapy (3DCRT) is the most popular refinement. Brachytherapy, also known as "seed" therapy, is an alternative to standard radiation therapy.

3DCRT

In 3DCRT, the oncologist "conforms" the radiation beams to the precise shape of the tumor. Custom shaping of the beams permits higher doses of radiation to the tumor, while avoiding healthy tissue and nearby organs. This refinement improves the chance of a cure and reduces the risk of complications.

3DCRT requires considerable planning on the part of the radiation oncologist. The first step involves performing dozens of computed tomography (CT) scans. This information is fed into a computer to create a three-dimensional image of the prostate, seminal vesicles, bladder, urethra, and rectum. The radiation oncologist then maps out the precise areas for the radiation to target. Like standard EBRT, the therapy is administered five days a week for about seven or eight weeks. Common side effects may include mild fatigue, increased urinary frequency or urgency, and changes in bowel function like frequency of bowel movements, bowel urgency, and diarrhea.

3DCRT has distinct advantages over standard EBRT. Studies have shown that 3DCRT markedly reduces the acute side effects that occur during traditional radiation treatment. For example, in one study symptoms of bowel and bladder irritation requiring medication were reduced from 57% with conventional EBRT to 36% with 3DCRT.

Because the radiation doses used with 3DCRT are significantly higher than those delivered with conventional EBRT (about 81 Gray instead of 65-70 Gray), 3DCRT may increase the chance of a cure. A 2000 study published in *Urology* detailed the results of a group of men who underwent 3DCRT at Fox Chase Cancer Center. The researchers reviewed the medical records of 471 men treated between 1987 and 1995 for prostate cancer that was confined to the prostate. Most men were treated with 3DCRT; 408 men received radiation alone, and the rest received radiation plus hormone therapy. Among those who received radiation alone, biochemical control (defined as stable prostate specific antigen [PSA] levels) was achieved in 60% of men after five years and 59% of men after eight years.

A further refinement of 3DCRT is intensity-modulated radiation therapy (IMRT), in which the intensity of each beam is raised or lowered to meet the needs of the patient. This additional fine-tuning may provide improvement over standard 3DCRT. In a 2000 study published in *The Journal of Urology*, IMRT reduced the rate of rectal side effects, but not bladder

cases, erectile dysfunction does not develop until several years after radiation therapy.

Current data would suggest that PSA levels greater than 0.5 to 1.0 ng/mL indicate residual cancer after radiation therapy; a rising PSA based on three consecutive readings after the lowest point indicates progression of the disease following radiation therapy. There is growing evidence that this definition of failure used by radiation therapists overestimates disease-free survival. In older men, radiation therapy is a reasonable option because total eradication may not be necessary and control of the cancer may be sufficient.

Brachytherapy

Another method of treating prostate cancer with radiation is to implant radioactive seeds within the prostate (interstitial brachy-

side effects, when compared with standard 3DCRT.

Brachytherapy

In brachytherapy, a computer guides the implantation of 80 to 120 radioactive "seeds" (tiny metal pellets) directly into the tumor in the prostate. The radiation works in the immediate area of the tumor and delivers a highly concentrated, yet confined, dose of radiation over a continuous period—24 hours a day for several months.

During brachytherapy, the patient does not become radioactive and poses no health threat to his family, friends, or coworkers. Most of the radioactivity is absorbed directly into the prostate, and the pellets remain in the body after they lose their radioactive energy. The seeds can migrate to other parts of the body, such as the lungs, but so far this does not appear to cause any problems (see the sidebar on page 45).

Brachytherapy can often be performed on an outpatient basis; it typically takes about an hour to implant the seeds. The procedure is extremely convenient because a man can return to normal activity, including work, within several days. However, recent studies have highlighted a greater risk of irritative urinary and bowel side effects with brachytherapy when compared to EBRT. In addition, long-term effectiveness of brachytherapy in terms of eradicating cancer is not known.

In the absence of randomized trials, your doctor must rely on the results of observational and retrospective studies to compare the results of different types of treatment for prostate cancer.

In a study published by Johns Hopkins experts in *Urology* in 1998, 76 radical prostatectomy patients from Hopkins were matched (by stage, grade, and PSA) as closely as possible to the published results from 122 brachytherapy subjects from the Northwest Institute. All of the men had clinically localized prostate cancer. Seven years after treatment, progression-free survival was 98% in the radical prostatectomy group and 79% in the brachytherapy group.

A retrospective study published in 1998 in the *Journal of the American Medical Association* compared data from men with clinically localized prostate cancer who had undergone one of three types of treatment. The study authors concluded that, five years after treatment, survival was better with radical prostatectomy or EBRT than with brachytherapy alone for men with intermediate or high-risk cancers (cancers with adverse features such as high stage, grade, or PSA). However, there were no statistical differences in outcome among men with low-risk cancers (those with no adverse features) who had radical prostatectomy, EBRT, or brachytherapy.

Brachytherapy is not used alone to treat men with high-risk cancers because it treats only cancer cells inside the prostate, not those that might have extended beyond the prostate. The clinical research committee of the American Brachytherapy Society recommends that brachytherapy be used only in men with early-stage cancer (T1 to T2a) who have a Gleason score between 2 and 6 and a PSA less than 10 ng/mL (that is, low-risk cancers).

Some radiation oncologists are combining brachytherapy with EBRT (both standard and conformal) in an effort to improve survival rates, but this technique is not proven to be more effective than 3DCRT alone. In addition, side effects are greater with combination therapy.

therapy). This approach had not been considered as effective as external beam radiation therapy in controlling prostate cancer; however, improved methods for placement of radioactive seeds have led to a resurgence of interest in the technique.

To learn more about the effectiveness and safety of brachytherapy, see the feature above.

Cryotherapy

Cryotherapy (freezing the prostate) is accomplished by placing probes through the perineum and into the prostate. The advantage of this approach is its minimal invasiveness. However, patients should be aware that no long-term studies are yet available to demonstrate that cryotherapy is as effective for treating prostate cancer as radical prostatectomy or external beam radiation therapy. In addition, its side effects, such as erectile dysfunction, can be substantial.

Like brachytherapy, cryotherapy preserves the section of the urethra that passes through the prostate. Since 10% to 20% of early-stage prostate cancers are located within millimeters of the urethra, these treatments may fail to totally eliminate the cancer. In fact, enthusiasm for cryotherapy as a treatment for early-stage prostate cancer has diminished over the last few years with reports of incomplete cancer eradication.

Hormone Therapy

The discovery that male sex hormones (androgens), and testosterone in particular, are required to maintain the size and function of the prostate led to the development of treatments designed to interfere with these effects of testosterone. Preventing testosterone from acting on prostate cancer cells can temporarily cause the cancer to regress, or at least to grow more slowly. However, because some prostate cancer cells are able to grow without testosterone (called androgen-independent or -insensitive cells), the tumor continues to grow despite the withdrawal of this hormone. Thus, hormone therapy is useful, but not curative.

In general, hormone therapy is reserved for men whose prostate cancer has spread to other tissues (stages D1, D2, N+, or M+) and cannot be completely eradicated by surgery or radiation. The goals of hormone therapy are to prolong life and relieve symptoms, such as bone pain and urinary problems. Most men (90%) with D2 (M+) stage cancer live for more than six months but less than 10 years; about half survive for 3 years or less, and about one quarter live for 5 years. The prognosis for a man choosing hormone therapy depends on the makeup of his prostate cancer—in other words, the ratio of androgen-dependent cells to androgen-independent cells. The greater the number of androgen-dependent cells within the tumor, the more likely the cancer will respond to androgen withdrawal. The return to PSA levels less than 4.0 ng/mL within three to six months of initiating hormone therapy portends a good response to the treatment. A rising PSA while on hormone therapy means that the disease is progressing.

There is no general agreement as to when to begin hormone treatment in men whose cancer has spread. Survival may not be significantly different if hormone treatment is started before or after the detection of metastatic disease on x-rays or scans. All effective forms of hormone therapy produce erectile dysfunction and loss of libido (sex drive)—and none is curative regardless of when treatment begins. Since an earlier start appears not to prolong life, early therapy may not be worth the erectile dysfunction, loss of libido, and other side effects (such as hot flashes or loss of energy) or the costs of hormone therapy.

There are two approaches to testosterone withdrawal, also called testicular androgen blockade or castration. The first is surgical removal of the testicles, which produce about 95% of the body's testosterone (surgical castration). The second is administration of a variety of drugs that interfere with the manufacture or actions of testosterone (medical castration).

The signal to synthesize testosterone originates in an area of the brain called the hypothalamus. At regular intervals, the hypothalamus secretes luteinizing hormone-releasing hormone (LH-RH), which stimulates the pituitary gland to produce luteinizing hormone (LH) and follicle-stimulating hormone (FSH). LH signals Leydig cells in the testicles to secrete testosterone into the bloodstream; FSH stimulates sperm production. When testosterone reaches the prostate, it is converted to dihydrotestosterone (DHT)—a more potent form of testosterone—by the enzyme 5-alpha-reductase. The drugs used for medical castration inhibit this sequence of events at various stages.

The most significant side effects of androgen withdrawal are erectile dysfunction in about 90% of patients and loss of libido. Others include breast enlargement; weight gain; loss of muscle mass; and decreased bone mass (osteoporosis). About two out of three men have hot flashes—like those experienced by women during menopause. These are not harmful and are probably caused by the effects of low androgen levels on the hypothalamus, which regulates body temperature. Hot flashes can often be managed with low doses of oral estrogen (1 mg per day), medroxyprogesterone (Provera), or megestrol acetate (Megace). Androgen withdrawal does not cause the voice to change in pitch, as some people fear.

Surgical castration. Surgical removal of the testicles, known as bilateral orchiectomy, is the easiest and oldest way to interrupt the effect of testosterone on prostate cancer cells. The operation can be performed in about 20 minutes with a spinal block or local anesthetic; the patient can usually go home the same day. Patients on anticoagulant therapy may not be candidates for surgical castration, since they are at risk for uncontrolled bleeding.

Surgical castration involves opening the scrotum with a small incision, removing each testicle individually, and then closing the

NEW RESEARCH

Hormone Therapy May Increase Risk of Coronary Heart Disease

Treating prostate cancer with hormone therapy may cause circulatory and metabolic changes that can increase the risk of coronary heart disease (CHD), according to a recent study.

Twenty-two men (average age 67) with prostate cancer were treated with hormone therapy for three months. Then 14 of the men discontinued therapy, while the other 8 continued therapy for another three months. All patients were tested for CHD risk factors before and after treatment.

At three months, all patients had increases in arterial stiffness, which is thought to contribute to CHD. At six months, the group that continued therapy still had increased arterial stiffness, while the group that discontinued therapy had returned to pretreatment levels. The drop in testosterone levels caused by hormone therapy most likely led to the increased arterial stiffness, as well as to changes such as increased fat mass and increased insulin levels—metabolic changes that lead to premature CHD. Hormone therapy did not increase blood pressure or blood levels of cholesterol or glucose.

The researchers say that more studies are needed on this topic because men with prostate cancer are in an age group that is likely to develop CHD as well.

JOURNAL OF CLINICAL ENDOCRINOLOGY AND METABOLISM
Volume 86, page 4261
September 2001

Medications Used in Hormone Treatment of Prostate Cancer

Drug Type	Generic Name	Brand Name	Average Dosage*	Estimated Cost† (Generic Cost)
Estrogens	estrogen, conjugated	Premarin	3.75 mg daily	1.25 mg: $105
Luteinizing hormone-releasing hormone analogs	goserelin	Zoladex 3.6 Zoladex 10.8	3.6 mg injected monthly 10.8 mg injected every 3 months	3.6 mg: $470 10.8 mg: $1,410
	leuprolide	Eligard Lupron Oaklide	7.5 mg injected monthly 7.5 mg injected monthly 7.5 mg injected monthly	7.5 mg/mL, 1 mL vial: $644 5 mg/mL, 2.8 mL vial: $442 ($385) 5 mg/mL, 2.8 mL vial: $367 ($385)
	leuprolide implant	Viadur	72 mg released annually	$5,684 annually
	triptorelin	Trelstar Depot Trelstar LA	3.75 mg injected monthly 11.25 mg injected every 3 months	3.75 mg: $437 each 11.25 mg: $1,311 each
Antiandrogens	bicalutamide	Casodex	50 mg daily	50 mg: $1,297
	flutamide	Eulexin	750 mg daily	125 mg: $254 ($209)
	nilutamide	Nilandron	300 mg daily	150 mg: $1,007

* These dosages represent an average range for the treatment of prostate cancer. The precise effective dosage varies from patient to patient and depends on many factors. Do not make any changes in your medication without consulting your doctor.

† Average wholesale prices to pharmacists for 100 tablets or capsules (or for each injection or implant, where indicated) of the dosage amount listed. If a generic version is available, the cost is listed in parentheses. Costs to consumers are higher. Source: *Red Book, 2002* (Medical Economics Data, publishers).

scrotum. Neither the operation nor the recovery is painful. In a variation of this procedure, called a subcapsular orchiectomy, just the contents of the testicles are removed. The empty shell of each testicle is left in place to produce a more satisfactory outward appearance. However, some surgeons do not use this technique for fear that some testosterone-producing cells may be left behind.

The effect of orchiectomy is almost immediate. Within 12 hours after the procedure, testosterone levels fall to what is known as the castrate range. Because it is so effective, this level of testosterone reduction is used as the standard for comparison with all other treatments. Orchiectomy costs about $2,000.

Even though it is the most effective and least expensive form of androgen withdrawal, only about one quarter of men choose surgical castration. Obviously, significant psychological issues influence the decision to have this operation, which cannot be reversed. Men who are psychologically troubled by orchiectomy may prefer a medical approach to castration. Medical treatments can be as ef-

How They Work	Comments
Estrogen targets the hypothalamus to block the release of luteinizing hormone-releasing hormone (LH-RH). In the absence of LH-RH, the pituitary gland does not release luteinizing hormone (LH), which is required to stimulate the production of testosterone by the testicles. Estrogen also acts directly on the pituitary.	Estrogen tablets lower testosterone to the castrate range over a two-week period. If estrogen is discontinued, testosterone levels return to normal. Side effects include possible cardiovascular problems (such as heart attack or blood clots), enlargement of the breasts, nausea, vomiting, fluid retention, erectile dysfunction, and loss of libido.
Initially, these drugs stimulate the release of LH by the pituitary gland, prompting a jump in testosterone production. After several weeks, however, they block LH formation by the pituitary, and testosterone levels fall to the castrate range.	These drugs are equivalent to treatment with surgical castration in delaying progression of cancer. LH-RH analogs pose less cardiovascular risk than estrogen. Their side effects include erectile dysfunction, loss of libido, hot flashes, weight gain, loss of energy, and loss of bone and muscle mass. Viadur is an implant that must be replaced annually.
To stimulate prostate cells, testosterone must first bind to specific androgen receptors within the cells. Antiandrogens bind to these androgen receptors, thus preventing androgens (including testosterone) from stimulating the cell.	Since antiandrogens (taken orally) do not block testosterone production, most patients preserve their potency. However, these drugs are not effective alone, and so are used in combination with castration or LH-RH analogs. Side effects are breast enlargement, diarrhea, and possible liver damage. Men taking flutamide should have their liver function checked after the first few months of treatment.

fective as orchiectomy, and the side effects of androgen withdrawal—whether surgical or medical—are similar. Despite these side effects, it is important to remember that androgen withdrawal prolongs life for most men.

Estrogen preparations. A synthetic form of the female hormone estrogen is used to lower testosterone levels to the castrate range by blocking the release of LH from the pituitary gland, thereby shutting down the production of testosterone. Daily doses of estrogen are as effective as surgical castration, though the hormone takes longer to work; testosterone levels fall over a two-week period.

The most significant side effect of estrogen preparations is an increased risk of cardiovascular complications. These include heart attack, inflammation of the veins (phlebitis), blood clots (thrombi) that can break off and travel to the lungs (pulmonary embolism), and swelling of the legs (edema). Because of these risks, patients with a history of heart disease or thrombophlebitis should not use estrogen therapy. In others, these side effects can be minimized by using low doses of the drug. In addition, taking an aspirin every other day helps to lower the risk of a heart attack and thrombophlebitis; edema can be treated with diuretics. Estrogen can also cause nausea and vomiting. And like castration, estrogen can cause breast enlargement and erectile dysfunction. With the advent of LH-RH analogs, estrogens are not widely used. However, there is renewed interest in diethylstilbestrol (DES), a form of estrogen used in the 1960s for advanced prostate cancer.

LH-RH analogs. These are synthetic products with chemical structures almost identical to natural luteinizing hormone-releasing hormone. Initially they behave like LH-RH and stimulate the release of LH from the pituitary gland, causing a "flare," or jump, in testosterone production. But after a short period they block LH release and reduce testosterone secretion from the testicles. The result is testosterone levels similar to those that occur after surgical removal of the testicles. The testosterone flare, which may be severe enough to increase bone pain significantly in men with prostate cancer that has spread to bones, is usually treated with an antiandrogen (see below) until testosterone levels fall to the castrate range about two to three weeks later.

Commonly used LH-RH analogs are leuprolide (Eligard, Lupron, and Oaklide), goserelin (Zoladex), and triptorelin (Trelstar). LH-RH analogs are traditionally given as injections every month or every three months. Another option is an implanted drug delivery system (Viadur) that releases leuprolide continuously for one year. Injectable drugs cost about $4,000 to $5,000 per year.

Side effects of the LH-RH analogs are erectile dysfunction, loss of libido, hot flashes, weight gain, loss of energy, and decreased bone and muscle mass. (Bisphosphonates such as pamidronate [Aredia] are being investigated for use with LH-RH analogs in an effort to prevent bone loss.) In addition, some patients experience irritation at the injection sites. LH-RH analogs are less likely to cause breast enlargement, nausea, vomiting, and thromboembolism than estrogen. In addition, they do not carry the same cardiovascular risk as estrogen. LH-RH analogs are equivalent to estrogen and surgical castration in delaying progression of cancer and prolonging survival.

Antiandrogens. To stimulate prostate cells (both cancerous and noncancerous), androgens must first bind to specific receptors within the cells. Certain drugs, such as flutamide (Eulexin), bicalutamide (Casodex), and nilutamide (Nilandron), bind to these receptors and prevent androgens from stimulating the cells. Since antiandrogens do not block testosterone production—which sets them apart from the other choices for hormone therapy—their use preserves potency in some patients. However, a recent study comparing bicalutamide with castration did not report the proportion of men who maintained the ability to achieve erections sufficient for intercourse. Flutamide is a widely used antiandrogen, though it can cost between $150 and $300 per month. The usual dosage is two 125-mg capsules, three times a day.

However, antiandrogens used alone may not be as effective as castration (testosterone levels can double with flutamide), so researchers are currently evaluating their use with other drugs, such as finasteride (see pages 12–13), to improve their performance. In addition, antiandrogens may cause hot flashes, breast enlargement (in about half to three quarters of men), diarrhea, and, in rare instances, liver damage. (One study found significant liver damage in 3 of every 10,000 users.) To recognize early liver damage, men taking flutamide must have their liver function tested a few months after starting treatment. Signs of liver problems include nausea, vomiting, fatigue, and jaundice. Nilutamide may temporarily slow the ability of the eyes to adapt to darkness. This side effect lasts for about four to six weeks.

A rise in PSA during hormone therapy indicates disease progression. In 40% to 75% of men on antiandrogens who have a rising PSA, withdrawal of the medication results in a decrease in PSA. Why this occurs is not clear—it may be due to a mutation in the cancer cells that results in their being stimulated by antiandrogens.

Total androgen blockade. Since the adrenal glands also produce small amounts of androgens, some doctors use antiandrogens with surgical or medical castration to block the possible effect of adrenal androgens on prostate cells. The combination of an LH-RH analog or surgical castration to halt production of testicular androgens and an antiandrogen to block the effect of adrenal androgens is referred to as total androgen blockade or suppression. Despite promising preliminary findings in the 1980s, numerous studies have failed to demonstrate that total androgen blockade prolongs life more than standard medical or surgical castration. If there is a benefit, it is probably small. A recent analysis of many studies found no difference in survival between men on combined therapy and those who underwent surgical castration or took LH-RH analogs alone. The results of the largest clinical trial to date, which compared total androgen blockade (orchiectomy plus flutamide) to orchiectomy alone, demonstrated no survival advantage with total androgen blockade. Total androgen blockade costs between $7,000 and $9,000 per year.

NEW RESEARCH

Estrogen Therapy Safer for Bones Than LH-RH Analogs

Luteinizing hormone-releasing hormone (LH-RH) analogs can effectively treat prostate cancer, but they can also cause bone loss and osteoporosis. Now a new study shows that estrogen may lower testosterone levels without harming the bones.

Researchers treated 54 men with localized prostate cancer with radiation therapy, orchiectomy, LH-RH analogs, or estrogen in the form of diethylstilbestrol (DES). Fourteen of the men received DES in addition to LH-RH analogs or orchiectomy. A control group of 24 men with benign prostatic hyperplasia (BPH) received no hormone therapy. The researchers then periodically measured the subjects' urinary levels of N-telopeptide, an indicator of bone loss.

After 18 months, the average blood testosterone level was greatly reduced in all groups except the radiation and BPH groups. Men in the BPH, radiation, DES, DES plus LH-RH, and DES plus orchiectomy groups all had similar levels of N-telopeptide in their urine. However, men receiving orchiectomy or LH-RH analogs alone had N-telopeptide levels that were more than twice as high.

The researchers conclude that estrogen therapy in the form of DES, either alone or in combination with LH-RH analogs or orchiectomy, can both treat prostate cancer and protect bones.

THE JOURNAL OF UROLOGY
Volume 167, page 535
February 2002

The Recall of PC-SPES

The recall of PC-SPES last year left many prostate cancer patients with a mixture of emotions: confusion, anger, and despair. It also left them with a host of unanswered questions. How could prescription medications have gotten into a so-called "natural" supplement? Had the supplement's manufacturer intentionally defrauded desperate cancer patients? And what would patients who had experienced good results with the treatment do now that it was no longer available?

We may never know all the details of the PC-SPES recall. But there is still good news for men who found that PC-SPES worked for them when other treatments had failed.

A History of PC-SPES

PC-SPES was a nutritional supplement containing eight herbs that was purported to shrink prostate cancer tumors. It was developed by a pharmacist in the early 1990s and, starting in 1996, was manufactured in China for a California-based company called BotanicLab. The supplement was taken by as many as 10,000 American men, most of them with advanced prostate cancer that no longer responded to hormone therapy such as luteinizing hormone-releasing hormone (LH-RH) analogs or antiandrogens.

The supplement did seem to be effective at reducing prostate specific antigen (PSA) levels. A 2002 review of more than a dozen uncontrolled studies revealed that PSA levels dropped in 80% to 90% of hormone-sensitive patients (those not yet resistant to hormone treatment) and 65% of hormone-insensitive patients (those no longer responding to hormone therapy) taking PC-SPES. Some patients even experienced tumor shrinkage, along with improved pain control and better quality of life.

PC-SPES also produced some side effects: blood clots in the legs and lungs, breast enlargement, nipple tenderness, hot flashes, and loss of libido. The similarity of these side effects to those produced by estrogen therapy suggested that the supplement might have estrogen-like activity. Estrogen is an effective treatment for prostate cancer, but it was largely replaced by LH-RH analogs in the 1970s because it tended to cause blood clots and other cardiovascular side effects.

Then, in early 2001, a man taking PC-SPES started to bleed excessively. Doctors found the anticoagulant warfarin (Coumadin) in his blood, which led to the discovery that PC-SPES contained warfarin. Other supplements from BotanicLab were tested and found to contain ingredients such as alprazolam (Xanax), an anti-anxiety drug. The distributor recalled the supplements, and the National Center for Complementary and Alternative Medicine halted four studies of PC-SPES that it was funding.

Finally, at the annual meeting of the American Association for Cancer Research in April 2002, researchers from California and the Czech Republic revealed more startling news: Much of the PC-SPES produced between 1996 and 1999 contained diethylstilbestrol (DES), a type of estrogen, and indomethacin (Indocin), a powerful anti-inflammatory drug. Batches of the supplement produced after 1999 contained warfarin and smaller amounts of DES and indomethacin. These findings were later published in the *Journal of the National Cancer Institute*.

The researchers hypothesized that the manufacturers in China added

Neoadjuvant hormone therapy. In neoadjuvant hormone therapy, temporary androgen blockade is used prior to—or combined with—surgery or radiation therapy in an attempt to increase the chances of eradicating all cancer. Available evidence suggests that androgen blockade before surgery does not increase the probability of an undetectable PSA level after surgery for men with localized (T1 or T2) or locally advanced (T3) prostate cancer. In addition, the use of hormone therapy before surgery makes it more difficult to perform a nerve-sparing procedure and more difficult to assess the true pathological extent of disease.

Preliminary data suggest that hormone therapy combined with radiation may increase survival for men with high-grade, locally advanced (T3 or T4) disease. Further studies are needed to clarify

DES to the supplement because they knew it would have an effect on prostate cancer; they included warfarin and indomethacin to counteract the increased risk of blood clots associated with DES. It is unclear whether the company in California knew of the tampering.

Renewed Interest in DES

DES was used in the 1960s as a treatment for men with advanced prostate cancer. Interestingly, the results with PC-SPES have prompted renewed interest in DES. Studies show that DES seems to be just as effective against prostate cancer as LH-RH analogs and antiandrogens, without increasing the risk of osteoporosis (see the sidebar on page 53).

Few doctors prescribe DES because it increases the risk of blood clots. But some researchers have suggested that using DES at lower doses than those used in the 1960s might reduce the risk. Another option may be to combine DES with aspirin. Of course, men will still have to deal with the other side effects of estrogen, such as breast enlargement and loss of libido.

If you are one of the thousands of people who responded well to PC-SPES, the good news is that you may be able to get similar or even better results with DES. Taking DES requires a doctor's prescription, which ensures that you will receive a standard dose—usually 1, 3, or 5 mg a day. The study of PC-SPES published in the *Journal of the National Cancer Institute* found that a daily dose of PC-SPES could contain anywhere from 0 to 0.5 mg of DES, depending on the lot number. In addition, DES costs only $30 a month—a far cry from the $250 to $400 a month that men were spending on PC-SPES.

Eli Lilly stopped marketing DES several years ago, but a pharmacist can prepare the medication for you (a process called compounding) if you have a doctor's prescription. The International Academy of Compounding Pharmacists (www.IACPrx.org or 800-927-4227) can direct you to a compounding pharmacist near you.

What You Need To Know About Herbal Supplements

The discovery that a supposedly natural remedy contained several undisclosed prescription drugs is frightening, especially because about 30% to 40% of men with prostate cancer use some type of complementary or alternative medicine. Unfortunately, dietary supplements do not have proven safety and efficacy because the U.S. Food and Drug Administration (FDA) does not regulate them. This means that dangerous supplements such as ephedra are readily available over the counter and that other products may be contaminated with or contain prescription drugs.

The only real protection you have against taking a harmful or ineffective supplement is to avoid all products that have not been approved by the FDA. You can reduce your risk of taking an inaccurately labeled supplement by buying supplements that meet U.S. Pharmacopeia standards (look for the "USP" symbol on the label), but this does not imply that the supplement is safe or effective.

Be sure to tell your doctor if you decide to take any complementary or alternative remedies and if you experience any side effects from them. This is for your own safety, as well as for the safety of others who might take the product.

which patients are most likely to benefit from this approach and the optimal length of time to use androgen blockade.

Intermittent androgen suppression. In this approach, androgen blockade is achieved chemically (using an LH-RH analog alone or in combination with an antiandrogen) until PSA levels fall. Treatment is then discontinued until PSA begins to climb again. The rationale for this approach, though not tested scientifically, is the belief that hormone therapy encourages the growth of androgen-insensitive cancer cells (the cells that ultimately cause the tumor to continue to grow despite hormone therapy). Some doctors believe that cycling therapy on and off may delay the emergence of these deadly cells. In addition, intermittent androgen suppression is associated with fewer side effects since men discontinue therapy for periods of time. More studies are needed to determine if this approach is better, or possibly worse. When animals with prostate cancer were treated with either intermittent or continuous androgen suppression, those treated with continuous therapy survived 50% longer. Intermittent androgen suppression is considered experimental and should be used only in trials adequately designed to compare intermittent and continuous therapy.

PC-SPES. PC-SPES was an over-the-counter product marketed as a natural herbal remedy for prostate cancer in the United States from 1996 to 2002. It was removed from the market after the discovery that the product contained several potentially harmful agents: the synthetic estrogen DES, the potent anti-inflammatory drug indomethacin (Indocin), and the blood thinner warfarin (Coumadin). For more information about the PC-SPES recall, see the feature on pages 54–55.

Other options. Levels of testosterone can be reduced within 24 hours with ketoconazole (Nizoral); this drug is approved by the FDA to treat fungal infections, but it also inhibits the synthesis of adrenal and testicular androgens. Ketoconazole is used selectively when lowering androgens rapidly could be beneficial (for example, to alleviate pain). The drug raises luteinizing hormone levels, which might eventually override its effect on testosterone and limit its utility for long-term treatment. Ketoconazole also can have an adverse effect on the liver.

Finasteride, used to treat BPH, is not effective in the treatment of advanced prostate cancer when used alone. It blocks the conversion of testosterone to DHT and thus lowers DHT levels within prostate cells. Since finasteride and flutamide together preserve sexual function in some men, the combination has been studied as a treatment option for advanced prostate cancer. The rationale is that by lowering DHT levels, finasteride may increase the ability of flutamide to block testosterone actions. However, preliminary evidence suggests that this approach is less effective in lowering PSA levels than androgen withdrawal with surgical castration or LH-RH analogs.

Once hormone therapy is no longer effective, other options are available to relieve cancer pain and help patients maintain their quality of life. Patients must realize that it is always possible to get effective pain relief with large enough doses of the proper medications. A wide range of medications—nonsteroidal anti-inflammatory drugs and corticosteroids, as well as morphine and other narcotics—may be used to stop pain. Mitoxantrone (Novantrone)—a chemotherapeutic agent used to treat a form of leukemia—is approved for reducing pain from metastatic prostate cancer. It is used in combination with the steroid prednisone (Deltasone and other brands). In addition, bone pain can be treated with bisphosphonate drugs such as zoledronic acid (Zometa), radiation aimed at specific sites of bone metastases (spot radiation), or injections of strontium-89 (a radioactive substance that targets bone metastases). Surgery, such as transurethral prostatectomy (also called transurethral resection of the prostate, or TURP), can be performed to treat urinary symptoms due to locally advanced disease (see pages 17–18).

MANAGING SIDE EFFECTS OF TREATMENT

The two side effects of prostate cancer treatment that concern men the most are urinary incontinence and erectile dysfunction. As treatments improve, these complications will become less common. When they do occur, however, it is important to realize that there are effective ways to alleviate them.

Urinary Incontinence

Because surgery or radiation therapy may irritate the urethra or bladder or damage the urinary sphincter muscles that contract to prevent urine from flowing out of the bladder, some degree of incontinence is common immediately after treatment.

For example, sudden involuntary bladder contraction, or urge incontinence, is common for a few days after catheter removal following TURP for treatment of BPH. In the initial period after radical prostatectomy, it is more typical for men to experience stress incontinence, which occurs during moments of physical strain, as when sneezing, coughing, or lifting heavy objects. Recovering bladder control can be a slow process and may take up to six months, but fortunately severe incontinence occurs in less than 1% of men after surgery for BPH and in less than 10% of men after radical prostatectomy or radiation therapy for prostate cancer.

A number of methods can be used to reduce incontinence. These include lifestyle measures, Kegel exercises, collagen injections, and artificial sphincter implantation. In addition, absorbent products, penile clamps, external collection devices, catheters, and medications can help men cope with the problem.

Lifestyle measures. Simple changes in behavior can help. An unhealthy diet and lack of exercise can lead to obesity, which increases pressure on the bladder. Because constipation can also worsen symptoms, it is important to include high-fiber foods, such as

NEW RESEARCH

Choosing Hormone Therapy May Affect Quality of Life

Some men with localized prostate cancer (stage T1 or T2) elect conservative treatment during the first year after diagnosis, choosing no treatment (watchful waiting) or hormone therapy rather than surgery or radiation. The choice of treatment appears to affect quality of life, according to a recent study.

Researchers surveyed 311 sexually potent men who chose either watchful waiting (74%) or hormone therapy (26%). The men answered quality-of-life questionnaires six months and one year later. Before treatment, both groups of men had similar urinary symptoms.

One year after diagnosis, 80% of the hormone therapy patients and 30% of the watchful waiting patients had erectile dysfunction. The hormone therapy patients experienced more breast swelling (20% vs. 4%) and hot flashes (58% vs. 11%) than the watchful waiting patients. Also, hormone therapy patients reported having more physical discomfort and limitations. However, more hormone therapy patients (56%) than watchful waiting patients (45%) reported being pleased with their treatment decision.

The researchers say that doctors should discuss the potential for declines in sexual function and vitality when patients are making treatment decisions.

JOURNAL OF THE NATIONAL CANCER INSTITUTE
Volume 94, page 430
March 20, 2002

Kegel Exercises for Postsurgery Incontinence

Temporary urinary incontinence can be a problem after surgery for benign prostatic hyperplasia or prostate cancer. While there are numerous effective treatments for incontinence (including collagen injections, artificial sphincter implantation, and various medical products), certain physical techniques, used alone or in combination with these treatments, can help a man achieve continence sooner. One of these techniques, called Kegel exercises, helps strengthen and retrain the pubococcygeal, or pelvic floor, muscles that are involved in urinary control.

A gynecologist named Arnold Kegel, M.D., developed these exercises in the 1940s as a way to help women who became incontinent after giving birth. Also known as pubococcygeal exercises or pelvic floor exercises, the technique later proved useful for some men who became incontinent after prostate surgery. Kegel exercises involve the contraction and release of the pelvic floor muscles, which help control the bladder, bowel, and urethra (and, in women, the uterus and vagina, as well). When relaxed, the pelvic floor muscles allow urine to flow through the urethra; when contracted, these muscles help prevent urine flow.

Finding the Muscles

Many people (especially men) find it difficult to locate and isolate the pelvic floor muscles, particularly after prostate surgery, which can weaken these muscles. So, don't be discouraged if you initially have trouble finding or contracting them.

Men can use one of four techniques to find their pelvic floor muscles. First, try to slow or stop the stream of urine while voiding. The muscle you use to do this is the pelvic floor muscle. Second, watch yourself in a mirror and attempt to move your penis without using your hands. If you can do this without moving muscles in your stomach, buttocks, or legs, you are using your pelvic floor muscles. Third, the pelvic floor muscles are used when trying to stop yourself from passing gas. As before, be sure not to clench your buttocks or tense your abdominal muscles. Lastly, if you are not sure that you are contracting the right muscle, you can insert your finger into your anus; you will feel it tense on your finger if you are clenching the pelvic floor muscle.

The Technique

Although there is no standard routine for performing Kegel exercises, a good way to begin is to do 45 repetitions a day. Each repetition involves contracting the pelvic floor muscles for three seconds and releasing them for three seconds. Divide the 45 repetitions into three sets of 15 each. Do each set in a different position: one set while sitting, one set while standing, and the last set while lying down. This is important because you will likely encounter situations in everyday life when you will have to consciously hold in urine in any of the three positions.

To ensure that you are using the right muscles, place your hand on

leafy green vegetables, fruits, whole grains, and beans, in the diet. Caffeine and alcohol consumption should be limited since they increase frequency of urination. If nighttime urination is a problem, liquid consumption should be stopped several hours before bedtime so that sleep is not interrupted.

Kegel exercises. Kegel exercises are performed by squeezing and relaxing the pelvic floor muscles that support the bladder and surround the urethra. By strengthening these muscles (which can be located by stopping or slowing urine flow in midstream), Kegels may help improve bladder control. For more information about Kegel exercises, see the feature above.

Collagen injections. Collagen can be injected around the bladder neck to increase bulk and provide increased resistance to urine flow at times of stress. However, follow-up injections are often needed because collagen is a naturally occurring protein that is broken down within the body.

your stomach while performing a Kegel exercise. Your abdominal muscles should be relaxed, and you should be able to breathe freely. If you feel your abdominal muscles tense you are using the wrong muscles, and this can add pressure to your bladder, which may worsen incontinence.

At first, you may need to do the Kegel exercises in private so you can focus. But after you become accustomed to doing the exercises, you should be able to perform them almost any time without anyone noticing that you are doing them. If initially you cannot complete a set of 15 exercises, break up the set into smaller portions. If you can successfully complete all three sets each day, do not hesitate to do more anytime throughout the day. Kegel exercises are associated with no harmful effects.

In addition, continue doing the Kegel exercises even if you don't notice an improvement in urinary control after a few days. It will probably take about two weeks to see an improvement, and you may need to do the exercises for a few months before gaining the full effect. The exercises appear to have the greatest benefit in the first few months after prostate surgery.

The Evidence

While study results regarding the effectiveness of Kegel exercises have been mixed, a report in the January 8, 2000 issue of *The Lancet* provides some of the strongest evidence for their benefit after prostate surgery. In this Belgian study, 102 men, who experienced incontinence after radical prostatectomy, were randomized either to a treatment group, which performed 90 Kegel exercises a day after catheter removal, or to a control group, which performed no Kegel exercises. After three months, 88% of the Kegel group was continent compared with 56% of the control group. After one year, the treatment group had a 95% continence rate, while 81% of the control group was continent.

Another recent study found a benefit for Kegel exercises after transurethral prostatectomy (TURP) for benign prostatic hyperplasia. In the study, 58 men who underwent TURP were randomized to an experimental group that performed Kegel exercises three times daily or to a control group that did not perform the exercises. The exercise group showed less urinary frequency, dribbling, and incontinence in the first three weeks after surgery, although after four weeks both groups had regained a similar level of urinary function. Still, the exercise group showed greater improvements in quality of life at week four.

Although most men who experience incontinence after prostate surgery eventually regain bladder control on their own, these studies show that Kegel exercises can help men regain continence more quickly. Because there appears to be little risk involved in doing Kegel exercises, the authors of *The Lancet* study recommend that men who undergo prostate surgery begin performing Kegel exercises one day after their catheter is removed.

Artificial sphincter implantation. In this procedure, a doughnut-shaped rubber cuff is implanted around the urethra to keep urine in the bladder. The fluid-filled cuff is connected by a thin tube to a bulb implanted in the scrotum which, in turn, is connected to a reservoir within the abdomen. The fluid in the cuff creates pressure around the urethra to hold urine inside the bladder. When the urge to urinate is felt, squeezing the scrotal bulb transfers fluid from the cuff to the reservoir and deflates the cuff for three minutes so urine can drain through the urethra. Afterward, the cuff automatically refills with fluid and urine flow is again stopped.

Absorbent products. Wearing absorbent pads or undergarments is the most common way to manage incontinence. Typically used directly after surgery, these products can be used for minor to severe incontinence.

Penile clamps. These devices, which compress the penis to prevent urine from leaking, may be an option for managing severe incontinence. Penile clamps are not recommended for use immediately after treatment because they prevent the development of the independent muscle control that is needed to regain urinary continence.

External collection devices. These condom-like devices can be pulled over the penis and held in place with adhesive, Velcro straps, or elastic bands. A tube drains fluid from the device to a bag secured on the leg. Often used with a penile clamp, it should be avoided right after surgery since muscle control will not return if a patient does not use and develop the appropriate muscles on his own.

Catheters. A Foley catheter is a small tube that is inserted through the urethra and allows urine to flow continuously from the bladder into a bag. This option is not recommended for long-term use after the postoperative period because it can cause irritation, infection, and possibly loss of muscle control.

Medications. Certain medications may improve continence either by increasing constriction at the outlet of the bladder into the urethra or by preventing excessive contractions in the bladder itself. In general, however, drugs are not effective for severe cases of incontinence. Medications such as oxybutynin (Ditropan), tolterodine (Detrol), and propantheline (Pro-Banthine) may reduce urge incontinence by decreasing involuntary bladder contractions. Nasal decongestants, like pseudoephedrine, or the antidepressant imipramine (Tofranil) can reduce stress incontinence by increasing smooth muscle tone at the bladder neck. Because pseudoephedrine is a stimulant that can increase heart rate and blood pressure, it should only be used with medical advice. The drug may cause nervousness, restlessness, and insomnia and may have adverse effects in patients with asthma or cardiovascular disease.

Erectile Dysfunction

Men who must undergo radical prostatectomy or radiation therapy for prostate cancer often fear they will be unable to resume sexual activity after treatment. While these procedures may result in erectile dysfunction, they do not affect libido or the ability to achieve orgasm. This is in contrast to hormone therapy, which lowers testosterone levels and decreases libido.

The penis is made up of nerves, smooth muscle, and blood vessels. Within the organ are two cylindrical chambers—the corpus cavernosa, or corporal bodies—that extend from the base to the tip on either side. When a man has an erection, smooth muscle tissue within the penis relaxes, causing these spongy chambers to dilate and fill with blood. The swollen corporal bodies press against and close the veins that normally allow blood to flow away from the penis; as a result, the penis remains engorged with blood. After orgasm, the smooth muscle contracts and blood once again flows out of the penis.

This process is initiated by signals passing through nerve bundles that run toward the penis along either side of the prostate. Radical prostatectomy can cause erectile dysfunction when one or both of these nerve bundles is damaged during surgery. Nerve damage does not affect sensation in the penis, but it does impair the ability to achieve a normal erection. Radiation treatment can also result in erectile dysfunction by damaging these nerves or the arteries that carry blood to the penis.

The first treatment used in erectile dysfunction is either a vacuum pump or an oral drug. If these are ineffective or inappropriate, another option is vasodilators, which must be injected or inserted into the penis. Surgical implantation of a prosthesis is an option for men who do not respond to less-invasive forms of treatment.

Vacuum pumps. A simple, noninvasive treatment for erectile dysfunction is the vacuum pump—an airtight tube that is placed around the penis before intercourse. An attached pump withdraws the air from the tube and creates a partial vacuum that causes the penis to become engorged with blood. A constricting ring is then placed at the base of the penis to prevent blood from flowing out. Erections last about half an hour; leaving the constricting ring on for a longer period may be harmful.

Vacuum pumps are highly effective devices, but many men find them cumbersome to use. In an Israeli study of 85 men with erectile dysfunction after radical prostatectomy, 78 responded to the device but only 7 were still using it a year later.

Oral drugs. Sildenafil (Viagra) is one of the biggest advances in the pharmacological treatment of erectile dysfunction. This drug is the first in a new class of drugs known as phosphodiesterase type 5 inhibitors.

Normally, sexual arousal increases levels of the substance cyclic guanosine monophosphate (cGMP) in the penis. Higher levels of cGMP relax smooth muscles in the penis and allow blood to flow into its two inner chambers. Sildenafil works by blocking the actions of an enzyme called phosphodiesterase type 5, which is found primarily in the penis. This enzyme causes erections to subside by breaking down cGMP. By maintaining increased cGMP levels, sildenafil enhances both relaxation of smooth muscles in the corpus

NEW RESEARCH

Nerve-Sparing Prostatectomy Does Not Increase Cancer Recurrence

Sparing the nerves responsible for urinary and sexual function during a radical prostatectomy does not appear to increase the risk of prostate cancer recurrence, according to a new study.

Researchers looked at the medical records of 734 men who had radical prostatectomies for localized prostate cancer: 240 had nerve-sparing procedures and 494 had standard surgery. The men were evaluated for the presence of positive surgical margins (meaning an increased risk of residual tumor left behind), and their prostate specific antigen (PSA) scores were measured periodically up to nine years after surgery.

The risk of prostate cancer recurrence, determined by a rise in PSA levels, at three years after surgery was 10% for patients who had the nerve-sparing procedure and 17% for patients who had a standard prostatectomy. At five years after surgery, the risk of recurrence was 14% for the nerve-sparing operation and 21% for the standard procedure. There was no difference in the rate of positive surgical margins between the two groups.

The nerve-sparing procedure did not appear to increase the risk of recurrence even in men who had high Gleason scores and high PSA levels before surgery, so the researchers recommend that a nerve-sparing prostatectomy be performed whenever possible.

JOURNAL OF CLINICAL ONCOLOGY
Volume 20, page 1853
April 1, 2002

When Prostate Cancer Returns

With most types of cancer, a person is considered disease-free if the cancer has not returned within five years of treatment. Prostate cancer may be the exception to this rule, since it progresses slowly and may not reappear for 5 to 10 years after treatment. For example, a recent study looked at 2,782 men who had cancer confined to the prostate and underwent radical prostatectomy. Of the cancer recurrences that occurred within the first 10 years of surgery, 20% occurred after the first 5 years. Therefore, all men who have been treated for prostate cancer need continued monitoring of their condition.

Types of Cancer Recurrences
Prostate cancer can recur in one of the following three ways:

- In a **local recurrence**, the cancer reappears in the original area (in the prostate itself or the seminal vesicles if the prostate was not removed, or in the prostate bed or pelvis if the prostate was removed).
- In a **regional recurrence**, the cancer reappears near the original site (usually in the lymph nodes around the prostate).
- In a **metastatic recurrence**, the cancer reappears in another place in the body, most often the bones.

Who Is at Risk and Why
The risk of prostate cancer recurrence varies with the clinical stage and grade of the cancer; a higher stage or grade at the time of treatment is associated with a greater chance of recurrence. Recurrence rates also vary with the type of treatment. Although research shows that radical prostatectomy and radiation therapy produce a "cure" in about 80% of patients, the definition of "cure" used by radiation therapists may inflate the success rate for radiation therapy. In addition, studies with longer follow-ups may reveal increased failure rates for treatments that leave the prostate intact (like radiation therapy), compared with those in which the prostate is removed (radical prostatectomy). Good data are not yet available on recurrence risks after newer procedures like cryotherapy.

There are many reasons why prostate cancer can return after treatment. For example, radiation therapy may not eradicate all the cancer cells despite the fact that the cells are all contained within the prostate. Or, the cancer may have spread undetected outside the prostate before treatment was initiated.

How a Recurrence Is Discovered
A PSA test is one way to detect a recurrence of prostate cancer. After treatment, the PSA level should drop. With radical prostatectomy, the PSA should be undetectable about three to four weeks after surgery if all the cancer has been eradicated. With radiation therapy, the lowest PSA value (referred to as the nadir) may take one to three years to achieve. But most radiation therapists agree that a PSA that is not eventually maintained at a level below 0.5 to 1.0 ng/ml indicates a failure to cure.

A rising PSA after any treatment for prostate cancer indicates cancer progression. If the cancer has spread beyond the prostate, the PSA will rise quickly; if the cancer recurs locally,

cavernosa and engorgement of these chambers with blood. As a result, men with erectile dysfunction can respond naturally to sexual arousal.

The sildenafil tablet becomes effective about an hour after it is ingested, though it may begin to work as soon as 30 minutes after the dose and persist for as long as four hours. Unlike other therapies for erectile dysfunction, however, sildenafil does not produce erections in the absence of sexual stimulation. The drug should be taken only once a day, but men can engage in intercourse more than once while the tablet is effective.

Sildenafil was tested in a total of 21 clinical trials that involved more than 3,000 men of varying ages (the average age was 55). Study participants had experienced mild, moderate, or complete erectile dysfunction for an average of five years; erectile dysfunction resulted from a wide range of conditions including previous pros-

the PSA level may not rise for years.

A single PSA test does not provide enough evidence that prostate cancer has returned. If the PSA is detectable, a second test should be conducted to rule out laboratory error. A PSA that is rising provides more definitive evidence of residual disease than a single measurement. If the PSA is rising, further tests such as a computed tomography (CT) scan or bone scan may be useful to identify the presence of cancer outside of the prostate.

Recurrent prostate cancer can be detected in other ways besides a PSA test. During a digital rectal examination (DRE), a doctor may feel a new hardness or mass in a man whose prostate was not removed. New symptoms such as bone pain, urination problems, blood in the urine, increased fatigue, weight loss, weakness, or loss of appetite should not be viewed as the first signs of disease progression, since a rising PSA would predate these symptoms by years.

Treatment

Treatment for recurrent prostate cancer depends on the suspected location of the recurrence and how the cancer was treated initially. Though the exact details of your cancer will determine the best course of treatment for you, the following are general guidelines on what to do if you have:

A rising PSA but no symptoms and no evidence on a CT scan or bone scan that the cancer has spread. In this case, watchful waiting may be the best option. Studies have shown that starting therapy immediately offers no benefit over delaying therapy until symptoms appear. In addition, the side effects from treatment of a recurrence, such as loss of sexual function, can significantly reduce quality of life. Watchful waiting requires regular examinations, including measurement of PSA and serum creatinine (to assess kidney function) every 6 months and a bone scan every 6 to 12 months.

A local recurrence after radical prostatectomy. Radiation therapy may be used to destroy cancer cells that were left behind in the prostate bed. Radiation therapy is more likely to be beneficial if PSA levels remained undetectable for more than a year after radical prostatectomy, indicating a higher likelihood of cancer in the prostate bed only.

A local recurrence after radiation therapy. If radical prostatectomy is performed, there is an increased risk of injury to surrounding structures (the urinary sphincter, rectum, and erectogenic nerves) because the radiation therapy causes scarring in the prostate and surrounding tissue. This increases the risk of complications such as incontinence and erectile dysfunction. Cryotherapy may be an option, although its benefits are unproven. Hormone therapy may cause the tumor to regress temporarily, but watchful waiting may be a better option.

A regional or metastatic recurrence. Hormone therapy (see pages 48–57)—ridding the body of as much testosterone as possible—is usually the treatment of choice for metastatic prostate cancer. When the cancer has not spread to the bone, many men may prefer to delay hormone therapy to avoid its side effects. Men with cancer that has spread to the bone should begin hormone therapy.

tate surgery, diabetes, high blood pressure, and psychological causes. Overall, sexual intercourse was successful about 70% of the time after taking sildenafil, and the drug was effective in men with erectile dysfunction attributed to a wide variety of underlying causes. Specifically, in men who developed erectile dysfunction after radical prostatectomy, sildenafil improved erections in 43% of patients, compared to 15% of those taking a placebo. It is thought that after radical prostatectomy, sildenafil is effective only in men with at least one intact neurovascular bundle (the nerves that supply the corpus cavernosa).

Several trials are now investigating how well sildenafil works following prostate treatment. One study of 28 men who underwent radical prostatectomy found that sildenafil worked in 80% of men with both nerves intact, but in none who had both nerves cut. More recently, 91 radical prostatectomy patients were stratified according to procedure: 72% of those with both nerve bundles intact responded to sildenafil, while 50% of those with one nerve bundle responded. Interestingly, 15% of men who had non–nerve-sparing surgery achieved erections—most likely because some nerve tissue remained intact.

Less research has been conducted on the effects of sildenafil in men suffering from erectile dysfunction following radiation therapy, but it is thought that sildenafil should be effective if erectile dysfunction has resulted from damage to the arteries and not the nerves. In a preliminary study, sildenafil worked in 77% of 35 men who took it following radiation. And a 1999 study of sildenafil in 62 men undergoing brachytherapy reported an 80% response rate.

Side effects of sildenafil are generally mild and short-lived; the most common are headache, facial flushing, and indigestion. In rare cases, and usually at higher doses, the drug may temporarily interfere with the eye's ability to distinguish between the colors green and blue. However, sildenafil is dangerous in men who use nitrates—a class of drugs (including nitroglycerin) prescribed for angina—since the combination may cause a precipitous drop in blood pressure. A number of deaths have resulted from this drug combination, and deaths have also occurred in men with severe coronary heart disease—even in those who were not taking nitrates. In addition, the drug should be used with caution by men with low blood pressure, those taking multiple drugs to control blood pressure or drugs such as erythromycin (Ery-Tab and other brand) or cimetidine (Tagamet), and those with liver or kidney disease. Sildenafil can also cause low blood pressure and fainting if taken within four hours of taking an alpha-blocker.

The discovery of sildenafil is certainly a breakthrough in the treatment of erectile dysfunction, but it is important to remember that it does not work in all men. For example, since the drug has no effect on libido and works only when a man is sexually aroused, it will not help men with decreased libido caused by hormone therapy for prostate cancer.

Still, sildenafil offers an excellent therapeutic option for many men suffering from erectile dysfunction. The drug, which is available only by prescription (in 25-, 50-, or 100-mg doses), costs about $10 a tablet. Insurance coverage for sildenafil depends on the insurer and the cause of erectile dysfunction.

Vasodilators. Erections can be produced directly by vasodilators, drugs that widen the blood vessels and allow the penis to become engorged with blood. Vasodilators include papaverine, phentolamine, and alprostadil; the most common of these is alprostadil.

Alprostadil can be injected directly into the base of the penis with a needle or inserted into the urethra in pellet form through a delivery system called MUSE. Both approaches have drawbacks, however. Injections can cause pain, scarring, and priapism—a painful, prolonged erection that must be treated medically—and MUSE can cause urethral burning. Low doses should minimize the risk of such side effects.

Since vasodilators cause erections by dilating blood vessels—an event that occurs after a nerve signal travels along the neurovascular bundles to the penis—they may work when sildenafil (Viagra, see pages 61–64) does not (such as when the neurovascular bundles are no longer intact). Moreover, researchers recently theorized that regular injections of vasodilators (regardless of sexual activity) might help bring about the return of normal erections—presumably by re-establishing regular blood flow to the penis.

In a small 12-week study, 67% of radical prostatectomy patients who received alprostadil injections ultimately achieved normal erections, compared with just 20% of those who did not receive injections. In addition, an Israeli study published in 2001 found that injection therapy with a vasodilator was more effective than either vacuum pumps or sildenafil. A study of 270 radical prostatectomy patients assigned to MUSE suggested that it may be successful in stimulating erections in 40% of cases.

Surgery. Several types of surgically implanted devices can provide erections sufficient for sexual intercourse. In one approach, a semi-rigid device—a rod-shaped piece of silicone inserted into the penis—is bent downward into the erect position before intercourse; afterward, it can be folded upward close to the body. A more commonly used device consists of two hydraulic chambers implanted into the penis and connected to a fluid-filled pump placed in the scrotum. An erection is created by pumping fluid into the chambers.

Future treatments. Erectile dysfunction is an expanding field of research, with new treatments on the horizon. One new drug known as apomorphine (Uprima) seeks to target mechanisms in the brain to stimulate an erection. It may be available within the next year or two; although it may not be as effective as sildenafil, it will at least provide another option for men who cannot take sildenafil.

A topical preparation of alprostadil, called Topiglan, shows some promise for men with erectile dysfunction. This preparation is applied to the head of the penis. Further research is necessary, but if

NEW RESEARCH

Busy Surgeons and Hospitals Have Fewer Surgical Complications

Surgeons and hospitals that perform a large number of radical prostatectomies have a lower complication rate, a study finds.

Researchers reviewed the records of 11,522 men who underwent a radical prostatectomy between 1992 and 1996 and grouped the patients' surgeons and hospitals based on how many prostatectomies they performed a year.

Life-threatening complications were significantly less common in patients of high-volume surgeons than in patients of low-volume surgeons (26% vs. 32%). The rate of late urinary complications (those occurring a month to a year after surgery) was 20% in patients treated by high-volume surgeons and 28% in patients of low-volume surgeons.

High-volume hospitals also had fewer life-threatening complications than low-volume hospitals (27% vs. 32%). Late urinary complications were less common in high-volume hospitals than in low-volume hospitals (20% vs. 28%). Neither hospital nor surgeon volume affected rates of mortality or urinary incontinence more than one year after surgery.

The researchers conclude that a patient is less likely to experience life-threatening or late urinary complications if treated at a high-volume hospital by a doctor who performs many radical prostatectomies.

THE NEW ENGLAND JOURNAL OF MEDICINE
Volume 346, page 1138
April 11, 2002

Topiglan works, it could further revolutionize erectile dysfunction treatment: An ointment would ease the mode of delivery while reducing the risk of adverse effects.

Prostatitis

Prostatitis is a common condition in which the prostate becomes infected or inflamed. The disorder usually causes severe pain in the perineum—the area between the rectum and scrotum. Men may also feel pain in their groin, genitals, and lower back. While these symptoms largely define prostatitis, additional problems can include an urgent or frequent need to urinate, which some physicians may mistake for benign prostatic hyperplasia (BPH).

But prostatitis can be a far more disturbing condition. In addition to pain in the pelvic region, a number of men with prostatitis complain of painful ejaculation. Some patients, however, say that ejaculation provides pain relief. In fact, researchers do not fully understand how the disease evolves in all cases, and as a consequence, few effective treatments are available. According to one study, patients with prostatitis report a diminished quality of life that is on par with those who have recently suffered a heart attack.

Part of the problem in treating prostatitis is that the disease comes in several forms. Some patients experience acute flare-ups, with sudden and continuous pain that lasts for several days at a time. More common, however, is chronic prostatitis, which may last for several weeks, only to disappear and then start up again. It usually affects men in their early 40s, and it is one of the leading reasons why patients visit a urologist.

Prostatitis is further differentiated by bacterial and nonbacterial causes. Nearly 95% of patients are thought to develop prostatitis from nonbacterial origins, which have yet to be identified. In addition, some men may have signs of inflammation, such as white blood cells in their semen, but none of the painful symptoms of prostatitis. A related condition, called prostatodynia, causes the same symptoms as prostatitis, but with no laboratory signs of infection or inflammation.

CAUSES OF PROSTATITIS

While the causes of bacterial prostatitis are obvious and easy to detect, researchers have only theories on why men develop the more

Types of Prostatitis

Prostatitis, an infection or inflammation of the prostate, can take several forms. Each produces similar symptoms, but the causes and treatments vary. The acute bacterial form is the easiest to treat but comprises only 1% to 5% of prostatitis cases. The most common form (95% of cases) and the most difficult to treat is chronic nonbacterial prostatitis. A third form called chronic bacterial prostatitis is relatively uncommon; it occurs more frequently in older men and is caused by recurrent or inadequately treated infection. A related condition called prostatodynia is now included in the category of chronic nonbacterial prostatitis/pelvic pain syndrome.

Type:	Acute bacterial prostatitis	Chronic bacterial prostatitis	Chronic nonbacterial prostatitis/ pelvic pain syndrome
Symptoms:	Fever, chills, low back pain, painful urination, urinary urgency and frequency, and urinary retention.	Low back pain, perineal pain (discomfort between the scrotum and rectum), testicular or lower abdominal pain, urinary frequency, and painful urination.	Low back pain, perineal pain, testicular or lower abdominal pain, urinary frequency, and painful urination.
Cause:	Bacteria normally present in the urinary tract or large intestine enter the prostate, usually from the urethra. Prostate biopsy can introduce bacteria from the rectum into the prostate.	Bacteria in the urinary tract.	Unknown. May be due to chlamydia or ureaplasma (microorganisms that can infect the bladder) from the urethra or increased tension in the muscles of the bladder neck (the junction between the bladder and the prostate) and the prostatic urethra (the portion of the urethra that is located within the prostate).
Diagnosis:	Digital rectal exam (DRE) and analysis of urine sample.	DRE, analysis of urine sample before and after prostate massage, and analysis of prostate secretions.	DRE, analysis of urine sample before and after prostate massage, and analysis of prostate secretions.
Findings:	Prostate is tender, swollen, warm, and firm. Bacteria are present in urine.	Prostate is enlarged, boggy (soft), or firm, bacteria in urine after a prostate massage, and white blood cells in prostatic fluid.	No findings on DRE, white blood cells may or may not be present in the prostatic fluid, and no bacteria in the urine sample taken after prostate massage.
Treatment:	Antibiotics for four to six weeks.	Antibiotics for 12 to 16 weeks.	If white blood cells are present in the prostatic fluid, a six-week course of doxycycline (Apo-Doxy, Doryx) may eradicate chlamydia or ureaplasma. If no white blood cells are present, alpha-blockers and anti-inflammatory drugs may relieve symptoms.
Self-care:	Over-the-counter pain relievers, bed rest, increased fluid intake, and stool softeners if constipation is a problem.	Exercise, warm baths, and prostate massage.	Warm baths, ice packs, prostate massage, and avoidance of spicy foods, red wine, and caffeine.
Prognosis:	Responds very well to antibiotics.	Can be difficult to treat. If the condition returns, low-dose antibiotics may be needed indefinitely.	Can be very difficult to treat, but relief of symptoms can be successful.

prevalent, nonbacterial form. Some men find that stress, emotional problems, or even coffee seems to trigger flare-ups. Other possible culprits include zinc deficiency, tight sphincter muscles, insufficient ejaculation, and dehydration. Scientists have attempted to confirm these potential causes, but the evidence is inconclusive.

Some experts suggest that nonbacterial prostatitis is not really a prostate problem at all. Rather, flare-ups could be the result of a pelvic muscle spasm or some other cause that mimics symptoms originating in the prostate. Another theory under investigation is that prostatitis is caused by an autoimmune disorder. In this scenario, the immune system mistakenly attacks healthy prostate tissue and promotes inflammation, not unlike the way rheumatoid arthritis targets the joints. Indeed, researchers recently found that men with chronic prostatitis had increased levels of the same pro-inflammatory molecules that are elevated in the joint tissue of rheumatoid arthritis patients.

DIAGNOSIS OF PROSTATITIS

As part of the initial evaluation, the patient's urine is examined to determine if the disease stems from a bacterial cause. Cultures are taken from normal urine flow (both urethral and bladder specimens), and from urine voided after a prostate massage—a process in which the doctor methodically strokes the prostate until fluid is pushed out into the urethra. A prostate massage is not performed if fever and chills accompany a bout of acute prostatitis. Acute flare-ups may also cause a steep rise in prostate specific antigen (PSA) levels, so PSA testing for prostate cancer should be avoided during these episodes.

A symptom questionnaire recently developed by the National Institutes of Health (NIH) may also help in assessing the disease through answers to questions on three different aspects of prostatitis: pain, urinary symptoms, and quality of life. After scoring the answers, a physician can determine the impact of a patient's symptoms and to what degree treatments are working.

TREATMENT OF PROSTATITIS

Treatment is fairly straightforward for bacterial prostatitis. A patient is given antibiotics for a period of 4 to 16 weeks. Appropriate antibiotics include carbenicillin (Geocillin, Geopen), trimethoprim/sulfamethoxazole (Bactrim, Cotrim), doxycycline (Apo-Doxy, Doryx), and fluoroquinolones like ciprofloxacin (Cipro). Bacterial prostatitis is the most curable form of the disease, although some patients may not respond to treatment, or symptoms may reappear once the antibiotics are stopped.

While antibiotics typically are reserved only for bacterial diseases, many patients with persistent symptoms receive antibiotics and a prostate massage for nonbacterial prostatitis and prostatodynia, followed by high doses of alpha-blocker drugs (used for BPH). Prostatodynia may improve when treated with muscle relaxants and alpha-blockers. Men who experience pain are usually helped by anti-inflammatory medications. A warm bath may also work for some, while ice packs are better for others.

If ejaculation is not painful, sex or masturbation may improve symptoms. A new study from Turkey found that prostatitis patients who ejaculated at least twice a week over a six-month period were likely to experience greater relief of symptoms than those who ejaculated less frequently. Still, many men are frustrated because there is no breakthrough therapy that provides consistent relief from nonbacterial prostatitis. Fortunately, major research efforts are currently under way, such as the NIH-funded Chronic Prostatitis Cohort (CPC) Study. Experts are optimistic that the CPC Study and other research will provide important new insights on improving management of chronic prostatitis. ■

GLOSSARY

5-alpha-reductase inhibitors—A class of drugs used to treat benign prostatic hyperplasia (BPH). They block the conversion of testosterone into dihydrotestosterone, the major male sex hormone within the cells of the prostate.

acid phosphatase—An enzyme found in the prostate gland. Levels in the blood were used in the past to determine the stage of prostate cancer but are no longer used routinely with the advent of PSA testing.

acute urinary retention—A complete inability to urinate that requires immediate medical attention.

age-specific PSA—An adjustment of the PSA value that accounts for the natural, gradual increase in PSA that occurs with age as the prostate enlarges.

alpha-1-adrenergic blockers—A class of drugs used to treat benign prostatic hyperplasia (BPH) that work by relaxing smooth muscle tissue within the prostate. Also called alpha-blockers.

androgen—A sex hormone, such as testosterone, found in higher levels in males than in females.

antiandrogens—Drugs that bind to androgen receptors in cells, preventing androgens from stimulating the cells.

benign prostatic hyperplasia (BPH)—Noncancerous enlargement of the prostate gland due to an increase in the number of prostate cells.

bladder calculi—Calcium stones that may occur in the bladder.

bladder neck—The junction between the bladder and the prostate.

brachytherapy—A treatment for prostate cancer that involves the implantation of radioactive seeds into the prostate.

castration—Elimination of testosterone from the body. See **medical castration** and **surgical castration**.

catheterization—A procedure in which a tube is inserted into the urethra to drain urine from the bladder. Used after prostate surgery and in the case of acute urinary retention.

cryotherapy—The application of extreme cold to treat a disease, such as prostate cancer.

cystoscopy—Passage of a cystoscope (a type of telescope) through the urethra into the bladder to directly view the urethra and bladder.

digital rectal exam (DRE)—An examination in which a doctor inserts a lubricated, gloved finger into the rectum to feel for abnormalities of the prostate and rectum.

dihydrotestosterone (DHT)—The most potent androgen inside prostate cells; formed from testosterone by the enzyme 5-alpha-reductase.

epithelial cells—See **glandular cells**.

expectant management—See **watchful waiting**.

external beam radiation therapy—A therapy for prostate cancer that uses an x-ray machine to aim high-energy radiation at the prostate.

filling cystometry—A test that involves filling the bladder with fluid, assessing the sensation of urinary urgency felt by the patient, and measuring the pressure within the bladder.

Foley catheter—A small tube inserted through the urethra that allows urine to drain from the bladder into a bag. Has a balloon at its tip so that it remains in place when filled with water.

follicle-stimulating hormone (FSH)—A pituitary hormone that stimulates sperm production by the testes.

glandular cells—Cells in the prostate that produce part of the fluid portion of semen. Also called epithelial cells.

Gleason score—A classification system for prostate cancer, based on the microscopic appearance of cancer cells, that is used to predict the seriousness of the cancer and the need for treatment. Scores range from 2 to 10 and are derived by adding the two most prevalent cancer grades, which range from 1 to 5. A lower score indicates that the cancer is less aggressive.

hematuria—Blood in the urine.

hormone therapy—Usually a treatment for prostate cancer that has spread. Slows the progression of cancer by preventing testosterone from acting on cancer cells but does not cure the cancer.

HPC1—The first prostate cancer gene to be discovered.

imaging studies—Tests that produce an image of the body; for example, ultrasound, computed tomography (CT), magnetic resonance imaging (MRI), and x-rays.

incontinence—An inability to control bladder function.

intermittent androgen suppression—A technique in which androgen blockade with medications is discontinued once PSA levels fall and restarted when PSA levels begin to rise again.

Kegel exercises—Exercises to strengthen the pelvic floor muscles. Can help men recover bladder function faster after prostate surgery.

laparoscopy—A technique in which a tiny instrument containing a light and camera is inserted into the body through a small incision. Used for a variety of surgical and diagnostic procedures, including radical prostatectomy.

libido—Sex drive.

luteinizing hormone (LH)—A pituitary hormone that stimulates the release of testosterone from the testicles.

luteinizing hormone-releasing hormone (LH-RH)—A hormone released by the hypothalamus that stimulates the pituitary gland to produce luteinizing hormone (LH) and follicle-stimulating hormone (FSH).

luteinizing hormone-releasing hormone (LH-RH) analogs—Medications with chemical structures almost identical to natural LH-RH. They block the release of luteinizing hormone (LH) from the pituitary gland, thus reducing testosterone secretion from the testicles.

medical castration—The administration of medication to interfere with the manufacture or actions of testosterone.

metastatic prostate cancer—Prostate cancer that has spread from the prostate to other parts of the body.

neoadjuvant hormone therapy—The use of hormone therapy prior to, or combined with, surgery or radiation therapy in an attempt to increase the chances of eradicating all the cancer cells.

neurogenic bladder—A dysfunction of the bladder due to a malfunction of the nerves that control the bladder.

nocturia—Frequent nighttime urination; a symptom of benign prostatic hyperplasia (BPH) and other diseases.

orchiectomy—See **surgical castration**.

penile clamp—A device that compresses the penis to prevent urine from leaking.

percent free PSA—The amount of PSA not attached to blood proteins divided by the total amount of PSA. Men with prostate cancer have a lower percentage of free PSA than men with benign prostatic hyperplasia (BPH).

perineal prostatectomy—A type of radical prostatectomy in which the incision is made into the perineum instead of into the abdomen.

perineum—The area between the scrotum and rectum.

phytotherapy—The use of plant-derived substances to treat a medical condition such as benign prostatic hyperplasia (BPH).

pressure-flow urodynamic studies—Tests that measure bladder pressure during urination by placing a recording device into the bladder and often into the rectum as well.

ProstaScint—A new test for detecting prostate cancer that has spread to other parts of the body.

prostate—A gland the size and shape of a crabapple that surrounds the upper portion of the male urethra. Its main function is to produce part of the fluid that makes up semen.

prostate specific antigen (PSA)—An enzyme produced by the glandular cells of the prostate and secreted into the seminal fluid that is released during ejaculation. High blood levels may indicate the presence of prostate cancer but can also be caused by benign prostatic hyperplasia (BPH) and infection.

prostatic intraepithelial neoplasia (PIN)—A precancerous change within the prostate that is thought to have the potential to develop into cancer.

prostatitis—An inflammation of the prostate that may cause pain in the lower back and in the area between the scrotum and rectum.

prostatodynia—A condition that causes the same symptoms as prostatitis but is not associated with infection or inflammation.

PSA density—The PSA level divided by the volume of the prostate. Allows the doctor to better distinguish between benign prostatic hyperplasia (BPH) and cancer by taking prostate volume into account when assessing the PSA level.

PSA velocity—A measurement of the changes in PSA values over time. PSA velocity is greater in men with prostate cancer than in those without the disease.

radical prostatectomy—A type of surgery for prostate cancer that removes the entire prostate and the seminal vesicles.

residual urine—Urine retained in the bladder after voiding. It can become infected or lead to the formation of bladder stones.

retrograde ejaculation—Ejaculation of semen into the bladder rather than through the penis.

retropubic open prostatectomy—An operation for benign prostatic hyperplasia (BPH) used when the prostate is too large for the surgeon to perform transurethral prostatectomy (TURP). It involves pushing aside the bladder so that the inner prostate tissue can be removed without entering the bladder.

simple prostatectomy—A type of surgery for benign prostatic hyperplasia (BPH) that typically involves removing only the inner portion of the prostate. It is performed either through the urethra (TURP) or by making an incision in the lower abdomen (retropubic or suprapubic prostatectomy).

smooth muscle cells—Muscle cells in the prostate that contract to push prostatic fluid into the urethra during ejaculation.

stent—A plastic or metal device placed in the urethra to keep it open.

suprapubic open prostatectomy—An operation for benign prostatic hyperplasia (BPH) performed when the prostate is too large to allow for TURP. Involves opening the bladder and removing the inner portion of the prostate through the bladder.

GLOSSARY—continued

surgical castration—Surgical removal of either the testicles (bilateral orchiectomy) or the contents of the testicles (subcapsular orchiectomy) that produce testosterone.

thermotherapy—A treatment for benign prostatic hyperplasia (BPH) that involves heating the prostate to more than 110° F. Resulting tissue and nerve damage alleviates symptoms.

TNM system—A system for describing the clinical stage of a cancerous tumor using T numbers that indicate whether the tumor is palpable or not and if palpable, the extent of the tumor (e.g., T1 and T2), as well as N+ for cancer that has spread to the lymph nodes and M+ for cancer that has spread to other parts of the body.

total androgen blockade—A treatment for prostate cancer that interferes with the production and action of both testicular and adrenal androgens by combining an antiandrogen with a luteinizing hormone-releasing hormone analog or surgical castration.

transrectal ultrasonography—A procedure that uses an ultrasound probe inserted into the rectum to develop images of the prostate. Used to guide needle biopsy of the prostate to diagnose prostate cancer.

transurethral incision of the prostate (TUIP)—A treatment for benign prostatic hyperplasia (BPH) in which one or two small incisions are made in the prostate with an electrical knife or laser. Symptoms of BPH are alleviated by decreasing the pressure the prostate exerts on the urethra.

transurethral microwave therapy (TUMT)—A benign prostatic hyperplasia (BPH) treatment that employs microwave energy emitted from a catheter inserted in the urethra to heat and destroy prostate tissue.

transurethral needle ablation (TUNA)—A benign prostatic hyperplasia (BPH) treatment in which prostate tissue is destroyed with heat that is delivered by low-energy radio waves through tiny needles at the tip of a catheter inserted into the prostate through the urethra.

transurethral prostatectomy (TURP)—The "gold standard" treatment for benign prostatic hyperplasia (BPH). A long, thin instrument called a resectoscope is passed through the urethra into the bladder and used to cut away prostate tissue and seal blood vessels with an electric current. Also called transurethral resection of the prostate.

transurethral vaporization of the prostate (TVP)—A procedure for benign prostatic hyperplasia (BPH) that uses a powerful electrical current to vaporize the prostate tissue with minimal bleeding.

urethra—The canal through which urine is transported from the bladder and out of the body. In men, the urethra also carries semen that is released during ejaculation.

urethral stricture—Narrowing of the urethra.

uroflowmetry—A noninvasive test for benign prostatic hyperplasia (BPH) that measures the speed of urine flow.

vasodilator—A drug that allows the penis to become engorged with blood by widening the blood vessels. Used as a treatment for erectile dysfunction. Examples are papaverine, phentolamine, and alprostadil.

watchful waiting—An approach to the management of benign prostatic hyperplasia (BPH) or prostate cancer in which no treatment is immediately attempted, but the patient is carefully monitored. Also known as expectant management.

Whitmore-Jewett system—A system for describing the clinical stage of a cancerous tumor using the letters A, B, C, and D, with D denoting the most advanced stage.

HEALTH INFORMATION ORGANIZATIONS AND SUPPORT GROUPS

American Cancer Society
1599 Clifton Rd., NE
Atlanta, GA 30329
☎ 800-ACS-2345
www.cancer.org

National, community-based organization that answers questions about cancer, provides information on specific cancer topics, and makes referrals to treatment centers or self-help organizations. Free publications on prostate cancer. Sponsors a support group called Man to Man.

American Foundation for Urologic Disease
1128 North Charles St.
Baltimore, MD 21201
☎ 800-242-2383
800-808-7866 (US TOO)
410-468-1800
www.afud.org

Supports research and seeks to educate the public with brochures and education packets on urological diseases. Call for information about US TOO, a support group for prostate cancer survivors and their families.

Cancer Care
275 7th Ave.
New York, NY 10001
☎ 800-813-HOPE
212-712-8080
www.cancercare.org

Provides support for patients and families through financial assistance, educational materials, referrals to local community resources, and one-on-one counseling (at the 800 number).

Cancer Information Service National Cancer Institute
Public Inquiries Office
31 Center Dr., MSC 2580
Building 31, Room 10A03
Bethesda, MD 20892-2580
☎ 800-4CANCER
cis.nci.nih.gov

Nationwide network with 19 regional offices. Provides information about early detection, risk, and prevention of cancer, local services, and details of ongoing clinical trials. Publishes free literature.

The National Kidney and Urologic Diseases Information Clearinghouse
3 Information Way
Bethesda, MD 20892-3580
☎ 800-891-5390
301-654-4415
www.niddk.nih.gov/health/kidney/nkudic.htm

National clearinghouse that provides access to a health information database. Also publishes a newsletter and provides educational material. Write, call, or visit the Web site for information.

Prostate Cancer Education Council
1800 Jackson St.
Golden, Colorado 80401
☎ 303-316-4685
www.pcaw.com

The Council is a group of doctors and health professionals who produce educational materials on prostate cancer and are working on a long-term study on prostate screening.

LEADING HOSPITALS FOR UROLOGY

U.S. News & World Report and the National Opinion Research Center, a social-science research group at the University of Chicago, recently conducted their 13th annual nationwide survey of 1,484 physicians in 17 medical specialties. The doctors nominated up to five hospitals they consider best from among 6,045 U.S. hospitals. This is the current list of the best urology hospitals, as determined by the doctors' recommendations from 2000, 2001, and 2002; federal data on death rates; and factual data regarding quality indicators, such as the ratio of registered nurses to patients and the use of advanced technology. Since the results reflect the doctors' opinions, however, they are, to some degree, subjective. Any institution listed is considered a leading center, and the rankings do not imply that other hospitals cannot or do not deliver excellent care.

1. **Johns Hopkins Hospital**
   Baltimore, MD
   ☎ 800-507-9952/410-955-5000
   www.hopkinsmedicine.org

2. **Cleveland Clinic**
   Cleveland, OH
   ☎ 800-223-2273/216-444-2200
   www.clevelandclinic.org

3. **Mayo Clinic**
   Rochester, MN
   ☎ 507-284-2511
   www.mayoclinic.org

4. **UCLA Medical Center**
   Los Angeles, CA
   ☎ 800-825-2631/310-825-9111
   www.healthcare.ucla.edu

5. **Memorial Sloan-Kettering Cancer Center**
   New York, NY
   ☎ 800-525-2225
   www.mskcc.org

6. **Barnes-Jewish Hospital**
   St. Louis, MO
   ☎ 314-747-3000
   www.barnesjewish.org

7. **Massachusetts General Hospital**
   Boston, MA
   ☎ 617-726-2000
   www.mgh.harvard.edu

8. **New York Presbyterian Hospital**
   New York, NY
   ☎ 212-305-2500
   www.nyp.org

9. **Duke University Medical Center**
   Durham, NC
   ☎ 919-684-8111
   www.mc.duke.edu

10. **UCSF Medical Center**
    San Francisco, CA
    ☎ 888-689-UCSF/415-476-1000
    www.ucsfhealth.org

PROSTATE CANCER TREATMENT AND OSTEOPOROSIS

Physicians and prostate cancer researchers have become increasingly interested in initiating androgen deprivation therapy (also known as hormone therapy; see pages 48–57) in earlier stages of prostate cancer. However, a rise in the number of men receiving hormone therapy is inevitably coupled with an increase in the incidence of side effects, particularly osteoporosis (bone loss). In the article reprinted here from *The Journal of Urology*, Robert W. Ross, M.D., and Eric J. Small, M.D., review the current literature on the identification, evaluation, and treatment of osteoporosis resulting from hormone therapy.

While male hormones, including testosterone, contribute to the development of prostate cancer, they also help maintain bone mineral density. Therefore, blocking male hormones with hormone therapy lowers bone density and increases the risk of osteoporosis and osteoporosis-related fractures. (A common type of medication used for hormone therapy is luteinizing hormone-releasing hormone analogs, here called gonadotropin-releasing hormone agonists.) While the extent of bone loss varies with the type of hormone therapy, bone mineral density decreases by an average of 3% to 5% in the first year of hormone therapy, with smaller decreases in subsequent years. By contrast, over the course of a decade, otherwise healthy men over age 30 experience only a 7% to 12% decrease in bone density. The risk of osteoporosis-related fractures with hormone therapy is less well studied, but research indicates that it may be as high as 28% over seven years. Fractures of the vertebrae appear to be more common than fractures of the hip or upper extremities.

Although the evidence is scant regarding the best ways to prevent and treat osteoporosis that results from prostate cancer treatment, the authors offer some suggestions. First, they recommend an evaluation of bone mineral density when men begin hormone therapy. Then, men should be sure to exercise, take calcium and vitamin D supplements, quit smoking, and severely limit or avoid alcohol consumption—methods that have been effective in preventing osteoporosis in other populations, such as postmenopausal women.

Men taking hormone therapy should then obtain another bone mineral density test one year later to look for evidence of osteoporosis. If the test shows evidence of osteoporosis or low bone mineral density and the man has a long enough life expectancy to be taking hormone therapy for a prolonged time (and therefore has an increased risk of fractures), bisphosphonates may be prescribed. Two bisphosphonate drugs—alendronate (Fosamax) and risedronate (Actonel)—are approved for the treatment of osteoporosis. A third bisphosphonate—zoledronic acid (Zometa)—is approved for treating complications of prostate cancer that has spread to bone, but the drug may also help prevent fractures related to osteoporosis. There is also some evidence that bisphosphonates may slow the progression of prostate cancer that has spread to bones.

0022-5347/02/1675-1952/0
THE JOURNAL OF UROLOGY®

Vol. 167, 1952–1956, May 2002
Printed in U.S.A.

Review Article

OSTEOPOROSIS IN MEN TREATED WITH ANDROGEN DEPRIVATION THERAPY FOR PROSTATE CANCER

ROBERT W. ROSS AND ERIC J. SMALL

From the University of California-San Francisco Comprehensive Cancer Center, University of California-San Francisco, San Francisco, California

ABSTRACT

Purpose: We surveyed the growing literature on osteoporosis secondary to androgen deprivation therapy and provide suggestions regarding its identification and treatment.

Materials and Methods: We reviewed pertinent studies of male osteoporosis, osteoporotic fracture incidence or bone mineral density loss as a possible side effect of prostate cancer treatment and potential therapies for this side effect.

Results: Hypogonadism is a well-known cause of secondary osteoporosis in men. There is evidence of decreased bone mineral density with all types of androgen deprivation therapy, presumably due to its anti-testosterone effect. Bone mineral density loss is 3% to 5% yearly in the first few years of androgen deprivation therapy with an increase in osteoporotic fracture incidence. There are little data on potential treatments, although bisphosphonates and intermittent androgen deprivation therapy may have salutary effects.

Conclusions: Osteoporosis is an important and debilitating side effect of androgen deprivation therapy, although precise estimates of its incidence, degree and cost are not completely elucidated. Until more data are available, it is prudent for all men beginning androgen deprivation therapy to receive calcium and vitamin D, and maintain a moderate exercise regimen. Baseline and at least 1 followup bone density measurement seem appropriate with bisphosphonate treatment a possibility in those in whom osteoporosis develops. More research is needed to explore the effect of bisphosphonates, calcium and vitamin D supplementation, exercise, calcitonin, selective estrogen re-uptake inhibitors, estrogens and intermittent androgen deprivation therapy on the course of androgen deprivation therapy induced osteoporosis. The osteoporotic fracture incidence and bone mineral density should be regularly incorporated into studies involving the hormonal treatment of prostate cancer.

KEY WORDS: prostate, prostatic neoplasms, osteoporosis, androgens, bone and bones

As enthusiasm grows for beginning androgen deprivation therapy earlier for prostate cancer,[1] investigators are exploring the multiple side effects of this therapy. Particularly the side effect of osteoporosis is increasingly recognized as a cause of significant morbidity for these patients and is the basis of this review.

OSTEOPOROSIS IN MEN

While osteoporosis research has derived the bulk of its data from women, recently more attention has focused on men.[2] A definition of male osteoporosis is not well established. In white women osteoporosis was defined by WHO as a bone mineral density measurement of 2.5 standard deviations or more below the young adult mean with osteopenia defined as bone mineral density between 1 and 2.5 standard deviations below this mean.[3] While these reference ranges are also used in studies of male osteoporosis, these ranges have not been validated in men, nor has the use of bone mineral density as a basis for therapy in men been established.[4] When fractures are used as the end point, estimates of the lifetime risk of osteoporosis in men is 13% to 25% versus 50% in women[5] with a seventh of all vertebral compression fractures and a fourth to a fifth of all hip fractures occurring in men.[6]

Bone mineral density can be evaluated by radiological and biochemical testing. The 5 radiological techniques used to measure bone mineral density are dual energy x-ray absorptiometry, quantitative computerized tomography (CT), quantitative radiography, single x-ray absorptiometry and ultrasound. Dual energy x-ray absorptiometry and quantitated CT are most common. Quantitated CT offers the advantage of selectively measuring trabecular bone, which may be a more sensitive method of detecting slight changes in bone mineral density. Moreover, quantitated CT measurements are not influenced by degenerative disease. However, in contrast to dual energy x-ray absorptiometry, quantitated CT can only measure bone mineral density at the spine.[7] Moreover, dual energy x-ray absorptiometry is more precise and subjects the patient to less radiation exposure.[8] These 2 techniques do not differ significantly in their ability to predict future fractures. Similarly the sites of measurement do not seem to differ tremendously in predictive capacity,[9] although some data suggest that bone mineral density at specific sites is slightly superior for predicting fracture at that site. For example, Cummings et al noted that dual energy x-ray absorptiometry values at the hip are a stronger predictor of hip fracture than such values at multiple other sites, including the lumbar spine, Ward's triangle, mid radius and so forth.[10] In a meta-analysis of prospective studies of bone mineral density Marshall et al reported similar results.[11]

Biochemical tests are also done to assess bone formation and resorption. Alkaline phosphatase, osteocalcin and procollagen peptides are used as markers of bone formation. Calcium, hydroxyproline and collagen cross-links, such as pyridinoline and deoxypyridinoline, are used as markers of bone resorption. Deoxypyridinoline is specific for skeletal tissue and urinary levels are useful for measuring changes in bone resorption in response to therapy or throughout a disease course.[7]

In women the most common cause of osteoporosis is idiopathic or essential osteoporosis, which is age related. Men also have gradual, age related bone mineral density loss at about 7% to 12% per decade beginning at age 30 years.[6] In males essential osteoporosis is rare, probably because they have a greater peak bone mass, shorter life expectancy and no menopause equivalent.[12] Eastell et al estimated that more than 50% of men with osteoporosis have a secondary cause.[4] Important secondary causes include hypogonadism, endogenous or exogenous glucocorticoid excess, alcoholism, thyroid and parathyroid disorders, osteomalacia and neoplasm. In fact, Kelepouris et al observed that 64% of the men referred to their bone center after minimally traumatic fractures had at least 1 of these underlying causes.[12] In addition to these secondary conditions, Seeman et al noted that smoking and alcohol consumption were independent risk factors for osteoporosis in men, while obesity was protective with a relative risk of 2.3, 2.4 and 0.3, respectively.[13]

Of all risk factors for osteoporosis in men[5,6,12,14] longstanding testosterone deficiency is perhaps the most important, since it was responsible for at least 30% of cases in 1 review.[6] Jackson and Kleerekoper recommended determining total testosterone in all men who present with minimally traumatic fracture.[6] Stepan et al followed 12 men with a mean age of 28.2 years who underwent bilateral orchiectomy for sexual deviancy.[15] Progressive loss of lumbar bone density was associated with time since orchiectomy, while in healthy controls there was no such loss of bone mineral density. Moreover, this loss was associated with increases in the biochemical indexes of bone resorption, such as urine hydroxyproline. Murphy et al noted a consistently positive relationship of bone mineral density and the free androgen index, that is total testosterone divided by sex hormone binding globulin levels, in an elderly healthy outpatient community.[16] However, this result was not consistently replicated. Slemenda et al reported that bone density in older men was significantly associated with serum estrogen and negatively associated with sex hormone binding globulin.[17] No association was identified with testosterone in nonhypogonadal men.

To our knowledge the mechanism by which testosterone affects bone development and resorption is not completely understood. Androgens mediate osteoblast proliferation and differentiation, and increase bone matrix production and osteocalcin secretion,[14] presumably via the androgen receptor on osteoblasts.[4] Testosterone also has effects on various growth factors, including transforming growth factor-β and insulin growth factor-1, which may be important for osteoblast proliferation.[14] Moreover, the potent estrogen estradiol is produced as a metabolite of testosterone by aromatase. Aromatase is active in bone, raising the issue of whether the protective effects of androgens on bone are mediated by the local production of estrogen intermediates.[14] Men with aromatase deficiency present with delayed bone age, a lack of epiphyseal closure and tall stature,[18] and inhibition of aromatization in older male rats resulted in increased bone resorption and bone loss.[19] It has also been postulated that androgen deprivation results in modulation of the effect of calcitonin, causing resorption via a decrease in the effect of endogenous calcitonin.[15] Thus, the mechanism of the testosterone effect on bone formation is complex and not completely understood. It probably involves direct stimulation of the androgen receptor on osteoblasts, estrogenic intermediaries and down-regulation of growth factors such as transforming growth factor-β.

ANDROGEN DEPRIVATION THERAPY INDUCED OSTEOPOROSIS

For more than a half century physicians have understood the integral role of testosterone as a growth factor for prostate cancer cells.[20,21] Therapies that decrease serum testosterone to castrate levels (androgen deprivation therapies) are used successfully to increase longevity and decrease morbidity due to advanced prostate cancer. Such therapies include orchiectomy, estrogen administration and gonadotropin-releasing hormone (GnRH) agonist administration.[22] Of these treatments estrogen use has fallen out of favor due to its thromboembolic and cardiac toxicity.[23] More recently nonsteroidal antiandrogens, such as flutamide and bicalutamide, which bind to the androgen receptor in prostate cancer cells, have been used to block the adrenal contribution to serum testosterone pools. These therapies have been combined with orchiectomy or GnRH agonists as combined androgen blockade, although the benefits of combined androgen blockade versus simple gonadal deprivation are still being elucidated.[24,25] Intermittent androgen suppression, in which androgen deprivation therapy is given for a set period, followed by an off period until prostate specific antigen increases to a predefined level, is a potentially less morbid and less expensive method of prostate cancer control that is now being evaluated in phase II and III studies.[26] Recent studies suggest that androgen deprivation therapy earlier in the course of prostate cancer may be beneficial.[1,27] Although it appears that such an approach may increase survival, it also increases the duration of the hypogonad state, thereby, increasing the risk of osteoporosis.

GnRH agonists are known to decrease bone mineral density in patients not diagnosed with prostate cancer, presumably via the disruption of sex steroid production. In women this relationship was detected by following young women with endometriosis who were treated with a GnRH analogue, of whom all had significant bone mineral density reductions within 6 months, a result partially explained by the decrease in serum estrogen to post-menopausal levels.[28] In men similar results were noted with GnRH analogues used to treat benign prostatic hypertrophy.[29]

Although the relationship of hypogonadism and male osteoporosis has been appreciated for decades, only recently has research focused on osteoporosis induced by the treatment of prostate cancer. Tables 1 and 2 list these studies. The effects on bone remodeling by prostate cancer treatment is sometimes hard to separate from the effects of metastatic prostate cancer. Prostate cancer metastasis leads to bone disruption and pathological fractures, which are an important cause of morbidity in advanced prostate cancer. However, our focus was on osteoporotic rather than on pathological fractures related to the treatment of prostate cancer.

TABLE 1. *Cohort studies evaluating the effects of androgen deprivation therapy on bone mineral density*

References	Mos. Androgen Deprivation Therapy		
	% 6–9	% 12	% 18–24
Daniell et al[33]		2.4, 3.7	6.5, 10
Eriksson et al[39]		9.6	
Maillefert et al[34]	2.7	3.9	6.6
Berruti et al[48]	1.2		
Diamond et al[36],*	6.5		
Higano et al[47],*	2.7		

Surgical and medical androgen deprivation therapy with percent indicating decrease in femoral neck bone mineral density with time.

* Combined androgen blockade.

TABLE 2. *The effect of androgen deprivation therapy on the osteoporotic fracture incidence*

References	Median Mos. Androgen Deprivation Therapy	% Osteoporotic Fracture
Townsend et al[31]	22.2	5
Modi et al[37]	Greater than 12	50
Ricchiuti et al[35]	44	4
Daniell[30]	60	12

One of the first articles exploring this relationship focused on osteoporosis after orchiectomy. Daniell performed a retrospective chart review of men diagnosed with nonstage A prostate cancer.[30] The initial fracture cumulative incidence rate in the next 7 years in patients treated with orchiectomy versus those who did not undergo androgen deprivation therapy was 28% and 1%, respectively. Moreover, after orchiectomy 48% of the men with at least 9 years of followup had at least 1 osteoporotic fracture. Bone mineral density in 17 men who underwent orchiectomy was compared with that in 23 controls. In castrated men bone mineral density was 17% lower a mean of 64 months later.

In a similar study evaluating medical castration Townsend et al performed a retrospective chart review of 224 patients treated with GnRH agonists.[31] Telephone interviews and medical record searches were used to identify and differentiate pathological and osteoporotic fractures. The group reported a 9% total fracture incidence with a 5% osteoporotic fracture incidence after eliminating fractures within the first 12 months of therapy, fractures associated with trauma and pathological fractures. There was no difference in the mean number of monthly GnRH injections (19.6 and 20.8, respectively) or in prostate cancer stage in the fracture and nonfracture groups.

Wei et al compared 8 men about to begin androgen deprivation therapy with 32 treated for more than 1 year.[32] Of those who had not yet received androgen deprivation therapy 38% had evidence of osteopenia and 25% had evidence of osteoporosis on dual energy x-ray absorptiometry of the lumbar spine and proximal femur. Of the men who had been on androgen deprivation therapy for more than 1 year 50% had evidence of osteopenia and 38% had osteoporosis. These differences did not achieve statistical significance. Patients on androgen deprivation therapy had significantly lower mean bone mineral density in the lumbar spine but not in the proximal femur. In a linear regression model Wei et al observed that lumbar bone mineral density decreased about 0.03 gm./cm.^{2} per year of androgen deprivation therapy. They estimated that osteopenia would develop in a man beginning therapy with average bone mineral density for his weight and race after 48 months of androgen deprivation therapy.

Daniell et al also focused on the rate of bone mineral density loss in men undergoing androgen deprivation therapy in a cohort study following 26 men on androgen deprivation therapy.[33] Bone mineral density was measured at 6-month intervals. In addition, 16 men who had undergone androgen deprivation therapy beginning 3 to 8 years earlier and a control group without prostate cancer were also evaluated. Overall in those who underwent surgical or medical castration average bone mineral density loss was about 4% during years 1 and 2, and 2% per year after year 4. Notably 20% of the men in the medical group were receiving an antiandrogen as well as a GnRH agonist, and a smaller percent were receiving only an antiandrogen. Similarly Maillefert et al evaluated bone mineral density loss in a cohort study of 12 men treated with GnRH agonists who were evaluated after 6, 12 and 18 months of therapy, although at 18 months only 6 remained on treatment.[34] Lumbar and femoral neck bone mineral density was decreased at 6 months by 3% and 2.7%, at 12 months by 4.6% and 3.9%, and at 18 months by 7.1% and 6.6%, respectively. The 18-month bone mineral density losses were statistically significant compared with month zero.

Recently Ricchiuti et al reported data from a retrospective study in which medical records and patient interviews were used to identify 146 consecutive men receiving chronic GnRH agonist therapy for prostate cancer.[35] The median duration of androgen deprivation therapy in these men at data collection was 44 months. In 549 patient-years of androgen deprivation therapy 4 osteoporotic fractures were identified. The relative risk of fracture compared with that in age matched controls without prostate cancer was 2.1.

Modi et al recently described the prevalence of osteoporosis and vertebral fractures in 26 men who had been treated with androgen deprivation therapy for at least 1 year.[37] methods of androgen deprivation therapy varied, including GnRH agonist or orchiectomy, combined androgen blockade and antiandrogen therapy alone. Of these men 38% had osteoporosis and 46% had osteopenia on dual energy x-ray absorptiometry, while 50% had previously unrecognized vertebral fractures. This high fracture rate may reflect an inadvertent selection bias or the inclusion of asymptomatic, clinically unrecognized vertebral fractures.

To our knowledge it is not known whether androgen deprivation therapy with a GnRH agonist and antiandrogen (combined androgen blockade) results in a similar degree of bone mineral density decrease compared with treatment with GnRH agonist or orchiectomy alone. In 12 men treated with combined androgen blockade Diamond reported a 6.6% loss of bone mineral density in the lumbar spine on quantitative CT in 6 months, while on dual energy x-ray absorptiometry femoral neck bone mineral density decreased by 6.5% in the same period.[36] To our knowledge only this study to date has considered combined androgen deprivation therapy exclusively. It is conceivable that the addition of nonsteroidal antiandrogen led to the greater bone mineral density decrease in these patients, although small sample size makes it difficult to reach definitive conclusions.[38]

Briefly, bone mineral density loss is an important concern in androgen deprivation therapy. Since all androgen deprivation therapy strives to decrease serum and tissue testosterone, it is not surprising that there is evidence of decreased bone mineral density regardless of the androgen deprivation strategy. Rates of bone mineral loss vary by study population and type of androgen deprivation therapy but seem to be around 3% to 5% per year in year 1 with a subsequent decrease in annual bone loss thereafter. There are less data on the effect of androgen deprivation therapy on the risk of osteoporotic fractures. Townsend et al reported a 5% rate of osteoporotic fracture after a mean of 22 months from the onset of androgen deprivation therapy,[31] while Ricchiuti et al noted a fracture-free survival rate of 96% at 5 and 10 years.[35] In contrast, Daniell observed a fracture incidence of 28% after 7 years of androgen deprivation therapy.[30] Regardless of the fracture rate in patients with metastatic prostate cancer the risk of osteoporotic fracture is even greater than the risk of pathological fracture.[31] Generally hip and upper extremity fractures impact daily activity more than occult vertebral fractures. Modi et al evaluated the osteoporotic fracture rate associated with androgen deprivation therapy and reported a much higher incidence of vertebral than hip or upper extremity fractures.[37] Thus, prospective studies are needed of the impact of these treatment induced fractures on quality of life.

The interaction of androgen deprivation therapy with other known osteoporosis modulating factors, such as age, smoking, alcohol, obesity and possibly exercise, is not well understood. Ricchiuti et al identified no association of risk factors with the fracture rate, perhaps partially due to the low total number of fractures in their study.[35] Daniell et al noted that after castration average bone mineral loss was 50% greater in obese men and men younger than 75.[33] This finding contradicts the known protective effects of obesity on osteoporosis risk and may reflect larger post-castration decreases in serum estrogen derived from the conversion of testosterone by aromatase in fatty tissue in these castrated patients.

THERAPEUTIC APPROACHES

Several treatment possibilities exist for male osteoporosis in general, including calcitonin,[5] exercise, calcium and vitamin D, and the treatment of underlying disease, such as testosterone for hypogonadism, alcohol cessation and so forth.[4] Recently Orwoll et al assessed the bisphosphonate alendronate for treating male osteoporosis in a randomized, double-blind, placebo controlled trial.[2] This trial excluded men with secondary causes of osteoporosis. In 2 years a significant decrease in bone mineral density loss and a significant decrease in vertebral body fractures was observed in the treatment arm (0.8% versus 7.1%, $p = 0.02$), although there was no decrease in hip or extremity fractures.

Similar approaches have been used for androgen deprivation therapy associated osteoporosis. Eriksson et al compared bone mineral density in 27 men with prostate cancer assigned to orchiectomy or estrogen treatment.[39] A year after orchiectomy bone mineral density decreased at all anatomical sites studied but only achieved statistical significance in the distal radius. In contrast, in patients treated with oral estrogens bone mineral density was unchanged. Data on the tolerability of oral estrogen treatment or on prostate cancer outcomes in the 2 groups was not reported. In a recent abstract Taxel et al randomized 14 men on androgen deprivation therapy for prostate cancer to 1 mg. micronized estradiol or placebo.[40] In men treated with estradiol biochemical markers for bone resorption decreased by 36% after 9 weeks of treatment ($p = 0.002$). These data are interesting in light of our recent preliminary observation that treating prostate cancer with PC-SPES, a putatively estrogenic herbal compound, resulted in anorchid testosterone but not in bone mineral density loss.[41]

Diamond et al treated 12 men with combined androgen blockade for 12 months.[36] During the second 6 months of therapy the patients were also treated with the oral bisphosphonate etidronate and calcium supplementation. After this treatment mean lumbar spine density increased by 7.8%, which was statistically significant compared with the initial 6 months without osteoporosis therapy ($p = 0.001$). Similarly Smith et al randomized 43 men with nonlocalized or recurrent prostate cancer treated with leuprolide to receive intravenous pamidronate or placebo every 12 weeks.[42] Men treated with pamidronate had no change in bone mineral density at the hip and lumbar spine, while at 1 year controls had a mean 1.8% and 3.3% decrease on hip and lumbar spine dual energy x-ray absorptiometry, respectively. These absorptiometry decreases at these sites were significantly greater in the control than in the treatment group ($p < 0.01$). The clinical significance of these results is unclear and these results must be confirmed by others. Nevertheless, these data suggest that bisphosphonates may prevent or reverse some or all bone mineral density loss associated with androgen deprivation therapy. This result is particularly exciting given the preclinical suggestion that bisphosphonates may delay the progression of prostatic skeletal metastases.[43–45] In addition, an early unpublished report of a double-blind, placebo controlled phase III trial suggests that the third generation bisphosphonate zolendronate prevents skeletal related events, defined as pathological fracture, spinal cord compression, the need for radiotherapy or surgery, or a change in therapy because of bone symptoms, in patients with metastatic, hormone resistant prostate cancer.[46] To our knowledge whether this improvement in outcome is due to decreased bone mineral density loss or direct anti-cancer activity is not known.

The effect of intermittent androgen deprivation on bone mineral density was reported by Higano et al.[47] In this series 9 months of combined androgen deprivation therapy was followed by an off period, in which androgen deprivation therapy was withheld until prostate specific antigen increased to a predetermined threshold. Androgen deprivation therapy was then resumed for another 9 months. During the first 9-month period in the 36 enrolled patients mean bone mineral density decreased in the lumbar spine and hip by 4.7% and 2.7%, respectively. Preliminary data on 4 patients suggested that during these off periods bone mineral density stabilized or increased.

CONCLUSIONS AND FUTURE DIRECTIONS

Osteoporosis is an important and debilitating side effect of androgen deprivation therapy, although precise estimates of its incidence, degree and cost are not completely understood. Better understanding of the type of fracture, namely hip versus vertebral, and the impact of fractures on quality of life is required. Possible strategies for prevention and treatment include dual energy x-ray absorptiometry in all men beginning androgen deprivation therapy; exercise for primary and secondary prevention, calcium and vitamin D supplementation in all beginning androgen deprivation therapy, and smoking and alcohol cessation advice for those in whom it is applicable. While to our knowledge these interventions have not been studied in this population, it is prudent to recommend vitamin D and calcium supplementation as well as moderate exercise to all men beginning androgen deprivation therapy.

Until more data are available baseline bone mineral density measurement at the beginning of androgen deprivation therapy and another a year later for following bone mineral density loss is appropriate. Further measurements can be considered at yearly intervals in men with bone mineral density approaching osteoporosis or those with decreased bone mineral density in whom life expectancy warrants it. Men with an osteoporotic fracture or who meet the WHO definition of osteoporosis should discuss about bisphosphonate treatment with their physician. This conversation should acknowledge the lack of data on prostate cancer but the potential for improved bone mineral density and decreased fracture risk. More research is needed to explore the effect of bisphosphonates and intermittent androgen deprivation therapy on the course of androgen deprivation therapy induced osteoporosis. The role of calcium and vitamin D, exercise, calcitonin and selective estrogen receptor modulators require further exploration. Furthermore, osteoporotic fracture incidence and bone mineral density should be regularly incorporated into studies of hormonal treatment for prostate cancer. Randomized controlled trials are needed to define further the scope of this problem as well as cost-effective interventions.

REFERENCES

1. Messing, E. M., Manola, J., Sarosdy, M. et al: Immediate hormonal therapy compared with observation after radical prostatectomy and pelvic lymphadenectomy in men with node-positive prostate cancer. N Engl J Med, **341:** 1781, 1999
2. Orwoll, E., Ettinger, M., Weiss, S. et al: Alendronate for the treatment of osteoporosis in men. N Engl J Med, **343:** 604, 2000
3. Assessment of Fracture Risk and Its Application to Screening for Postmenopausal Osteoporosis. Geneva: WHO, 1994
4. Eastell, R., Boyle, I. T., Compston, J. et al: Management of male osteoporosis: report of the UK Consensus Group. QJM, **91:** 71, 1998
5. Bilezikian, J. P.: Osteoporosis in men. J Clin Endocr Metab, **84:** 3431, 1999

6. Jackson, J. A. and Kleerekoper, M.: Osteoporosis in men: diagnosis, pathophysiology and prevention. Medicine, **69:** 137, 1990
7. Rogers, L. F. and Lenchik, L.: Metabolic, endocrine and related bone diseases. In: Paul and Juhl's Essentials of Radiologic Imaging, 7th ed. Edited by J. Juhl, A. Crummy and K. Kuhlman. Philadelphia: Lippincott-Raven, pp. 199–211, 1998
8. Raisz, L. G., Kream, B. E. and Lorenzo, J. A.: Metabolic bone disease. In: William's Textbook of Endocrinology, 9th ed. Edited by Jean D. Wilson. Philadelphia: W. B. Saunders, pp. 1211–1228, 1998
9. Jergas, M. and Gluer, C. C.: Assessment of fracture risk by bone density measurements. Semin Nucl Med, **27:** 261, 1997
10. Cummings, S. R., Black, D. M., Nevitt, M. C. et al: Bone density at various sites for prediction of hip fractures. Lancet, **341:** 72, 1993
11. Marshall, D., Johnell, O. and, Wedel, H.: Meta-analysis of how well measures of bone mineral density predict occurrence of osteoporotic fractures. BMJ, **312:** 1254, 1996
12. Kelepouris, N., Harper, K. D., Gannon, F. M. et al: Severe osteoporosis in men. Ann Int Med, **123:** 452, 1995
13. Seeman, E., Melton, L. J., O'Fallon, W. M. et al: Risk factors for spinal osteoporosis in men. Am J Med, **75:** 977, 1983
14. Wiren, K. and Orwoll, E.: Androgens and bone: basic aspects. In: Osteoporosis in Men. Edited by E. Orwoll. San Diego: Academic Press, pp. 211–274, 1999
15. Stepan, J., Lachman, M., Zverina, J. et al: Castrated men exhibit bone loss: effect of calcitonin treatment on biochemical indices of bone remodeling. J Clin Endocr Metab, **69:** 523, 1989
16. Murphy, S., Khaw, K., Cassidy, A. et al: Sex hormones and bone mineral density in elderly men. Bone Mineral, **20:** 133, 1993
17. Slemenda, C. W., Longcope, C., Zhou, L. et al: Sex steroids and bone mass in older men. J Clin Invest, **100:** 1755, 1997
18. Morichima, A., Grumbach, M. M., Simpson, E. R. et al: Aromatase deficiency in male and female siblings caused by a novel mutation and the physiological role of estrogens. J Clin Endrocr Metab, **80:** 3689, 1995
19. Vanderschueren, D., Van Herck, E., De Coster, R. et al: Aromatization of androgens is important for the skeletal maintenance of aged male rats. Calcif Tissue Int, **59:** 179, 1996
20. Huggins, C. and Hodges, C. V.: Studies on prostatic cancer I: the effect of castration, estrogen and of androgen injection on serum phosphastases in metastatic carcinoma of the prostate. Cancer Res, **1:** 293, 1941
21. Huggins, C., Stevens, R. E. and Hodges, C. V.: Studies on prostatic cancer II: The effects of castration on advanced carcinoma of the prostate gland. Arch Surg, **43:** 209, 1941
22. Small, E. J.: Hormonal therapy for metastatic prostate cancer. West J Med, **160:** 253, 1994
23. Johansson, J. E., Andersson, S. O., Holmberg, L. et al: Primary orchiectomy versus estrogen therapy in advanced prostatic cancer: a randomized study—results after 7 to 10 years of followup. J Urol, **145:** 519, 1991
24. Crawford, E. D., Eisenberger, M. A., McLeod, D. G. et al: A controlled trial of leuprolide with and without flutamide in prostatic carcinoma. N Engl J Med, **321:** 419, 1989
25. Eisenberger, M. A., Blumenstein, B. A., Crawford, E. D. et al: Bilateral orchiectomy with or without flutamide for metastatic prostate cancer. N Engl J Med, **339:** 1036, 1998
26. Small, E. J. and Reese, D. M.: An update on prostate cancer research. Cur Opin Oncol, **12:** 265, 2000
27. Immediate vs. deferred treatment for advanced prostatic cancer: initial results of the Medical Research Council Trial. Medical Research Council Prostate Cancer Working Party Investigators Group. Br J Urol, **79:** 235, 1997
28. Johansen, J. S., Riis, B. J., Hassager, C. et al: The effect of a gonadotropin-releasing hormone agonist analog (nafarelin) on bone metabolism. J Clin Endocr Metab, **67:** 701, 1988
29. Goldray, D., Weisman, Y., Jaccard, N. et al: Decreased bone density in elderly men treated with the gonadotropin-releasing hormone agonist decapeptyl (D-trp^6-GnRH). J Clin Endocr Metab, **76:** 288, 1993
30. Daniell, H. W.: Osteoporosis after orchiectomy for prostate cancer. J Urol, **157:** 439, 1997
31. Townsend, M. F., Sanders, W. H., Northway, R. O. et al: Bone fractures associated with luteinizing hormone-releasing hormone agonists used in the treatment of prostate carcinoma. Cancer, **79:** 545, 1997
32. Wei, J. T., Gross, M., Jaffe, C. A. et al: Androgen deprivation therapy for prostate cancer results in significant loss of bone density. Urology, **54:** 607, 1999
33. Daniell, H. W., Dunn, S. R., Ferguson, D. W. et al: Progressive osteoporosis during androgen deprivation therapy for prostate cancer. J Urol, **163:** 181, 2000
34. Maillefert, J. F., Sibilia, J., Michel, F. et al: Bone mineral density in men treated with synthetic gonadotropin-releasing hormone agonists for prostatic carcinoma. J Urol, **161:** 1219, 1999
35. Ricchiuti, V. S., Conrad, P. W. and Oefelin, M.: Skeletal fractures associated with androgen-suppression induced osteoporosis—the clinical incidence and risk factors for prostate cancer patients. J Urol, suppl., **165:** 290, abstract 1195, 2001
36. Diamond, T., Campbell, J., Bryant, C. et al: The effect of combined androgen blockade on bone turnover and bone mineral densities in men treated for prostate carcinoma. Cancer, **83:** 1561, 1998
37. Modi, S., Wood, L., Siminoski, K. et al: a comparison of the prevalence of osteoporosis and vertebral fractures in men with prostate cancer on various androgen deprivation therapies: preliminary report. Proc Am Soc Clin Oncol, suppl., **20:** 167b, abstract, 2001
38. Goulding, A. and Gold, E.: Flutamide-mediated androgen blockade evokes osteopenia in the female rat. J Bone Min Res, **8:** 763, 1993
39. Eriksson, S., Eriksson, A., Stege, R. et al: Bone mineral density in patients with prostatic cancer treated with orchiectomy and with estrogens. Calcif Tiss Int, **57:** 97, 1995
40. Taxel, P., Albertson, P., Dowsett, R. et al: Low dose estrogen decreases bone resorption in older men receiving hormonal suppression for prostate cancer. J Urol, suppl., **165:** 291, abstract 1196, 2001
41. Ross, R., Kussmaul, S. and Small, E. J.: The effect of the herbal supplement PC-SPES on bone mineral density in men with prostate cancer. Proc Am Soc Clin Oncol, suppl., **20:** 151b, abstract, 2001
42. Smith, M., McGovern, F. J., Zietman, A. L. et al: Pamidronate to prevent bone loss during androgen-deprivation therapy for prostate cancer. N Engl J Med, **345:** 948, 2001
43. Sun, Y. C., Geldoff, A. A., Newling, D. W. et al: Progression delay of prostate tumor skeletal metastasis effects by bisphosphonates. J Urol, **148:** 1270, 1992
44. Boissier, S., Magnetto, S., Frappart, L. et al: Bisphosphonates inhibit prostate and breast carcinoma cell adhesion to unmineralized and mineralized bone extracellular matrices. Cancer Res, **57:** 3890, 1997
45. Boissier, S., Ferreras, M., Peyruchaud, O. et al: Bisphosphonates inhibit breast and prostate carcinoma cell invasion, an early event in the formation of bone metastases. Cancer Res, **60:** 2949, 2000
46. Lipton, A., Small, E. J., Saad, F. et al: The new bisphosphonate Zomets (zoledronic acid) decreases skeletal complications in both lytic and blastic lesions: a comparison to pamidronate. Cancer Invest, **20:** 45, 2001
47. Higano, C., Stephens, C., Nelson, P. et al: Prospective serial measurements of bone mineral density in prostate cancer patients without bone metastases treated with intermittent androgen suppression. Proc Am Soc Clin Oncol, suppl., **18:** 314a, abstract, 1999
48. Berruti, A., Cerutti, S., Mari, M. et al: Dual energy x-ray absorptiometry in detecting bone loss during androgen deprivation in prostate cancer patients. Proc Am Soc Clin Oncol, suppl., **19:** 333a, 2000

NOTES

NOTES

NOTES

NOTES

NOTES

NOTES

NOTES

NOTES

NOTES

The information contained in this White Paper is not intended as a substitute for the advice of a physician. Readers who suspect they may have specific medical problems should consult a physician about any suggestions made.

Please address inquiries on bulk subscriptions and permission to reproduce selections from this White Paper to Medletter Associates, Inc., 632 Broadway, 11th Floor, New York, NY 10012. The editors are interested in receiving your comments at the above address but regret that they cannot answer letters of any sort personally.

ISBN 0-929661-18-4
ISSN 1542-1716
Tenth Printing
Printed in the United States of America

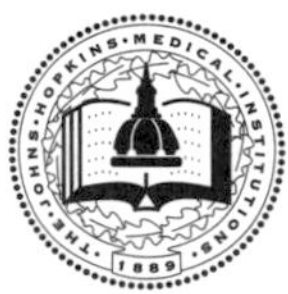

The Johns Hopkins White Papers are published yearly by Medletter Associates, Inc.

Rodney Friedman	Publisher
Devon Schuyler	Executive Editor
Catherine Richter	Senior Editor
Gerald Couzens	Contributing Editor
Paul Candon	Senior Writer
Kimberly Flynn	Writer/Researcher
Liz Curry	Editorial Associate
Abigail Williams	Intern
Leslie Maltese-McGill	Copy Editor
Bonnie Slotnick	Copy Editor
Scott Hunt	Design Production Manager
Robert Duckwall	Medical Illustrator
Tom Damrauer, M.L.S.	Chief of Information Services
Barbara Maxwell O'Neill	Associate Publisher
Helen Mullen	Circulation Director
Tim O'Brien	Circulation Director
Jerry Loo	Product Manager
Darren Leiser	Promotions Coordinator
Joan Mullally	Head of Business Development

VISION

Andrew P. Schachat, M.D.,

Harry A. Quigley, M.D.,

Oliver D. Schein, M.D., M.P.H.

and

Simeon Margolis, M.D., Ph.D.

2003

VISION

Vision disorders such as cataracts, glaucoma, age-related macular degeneration, and diabetic retinopathy can interfere with everyday activities. However, these conditions rarely cause complete blindness; many can be detected early, thanks to modern screening techniques, and treated with drugs or surgical procedures. Advances in the past year include approval of a new device that may improve the surgical treatment of glaucoma and evidence that antioxidant vitamin and zinc supplements may slow the progression to advanced age-related macular degeneration in some people. This White Paper discusses how to protect your vision, what screening tests you should have, and what to do if you are diagnosed with a vision disorder.

■ ■ ■

Highlights:

- What is important in buying a pair of **sunglasses**. (page 7)
- The effect of **hormone replacement therapy** on the eyes. (page 9)
- Steps you can take to **avoid cataract surgery**. (page 11)
- **Choosing the best lighting** if you have low vision. (page 15)
- The use of a **multifocal lens implant** in cataract surgery. (page 17)
- How to know whether **LASIK surgery** is right for you. (page 18)
- Being **nearsighted** appears to raise the risk of glaucoma, according to a new study. (page 24)
- Should **elevated intraocular pressure** be treated if glaucoma is not present? (page 25)
- How to get the most out of your **eye drops**. (page 27)
- A new surgical procedure for open-angle **glaucoma**. (page 30)
- How prevalent is **depression** among people with **macular degeneration**? (page 37)
- Can **antioxidant vitamins and zinc** help preserve your vision? (page 38)
- The latest results with **photodynamic therapy** for macular degeneration. (page 41)
- The relationship between **cholesterol-lowering drugs** and diabetic retinopathy. (page 46)

■ ■ ■

THE AUTHORS

Andrew P. Schachat, M.D., graduated from Princeton University and the Johns Hopkins University School of Medicine. He did his ophthalmology residency at the Wilmer Ophthalmological Institute at Johns Hopkins Hospital and a vitreoretinal and oncology fellowship at the Wills Eye Hospital in Philadelphia. Currently, he is the Karl Hagen Professor of Ophthalmology and director of the Retinal Vascular Center and the Ocular Oncology Service at the Wilmer Institute. In addition, he serves on the editorial boards of *Ophthalmology,* the *Journal of the American Academy of Ophthalmology,* and *The Johns Hopkins Medical Letter, Health After 50.* Dr. Schachat is the editor of the first two volumes of Steven Ryan's *Retina,* a three-volume textbook of retinal disease for ophthalmologists.

In addition, he was a principal investigator on the Macular Photocoagulation Study, the research study that proved the benefit of laser treatment for some patients with age-related macular degeneration, and, more recently, on the trials that showed the safety and efficacy of photodynamic therapy with verteporfin.

■■■

Harry A. Quigley, M.D., is the A. Edward Maumenee Professor of Ophthalmology and the director of both the Glaucoma Service and the Dana Center for Preventive Ophthalmology at the Wilmer Ophthalmological Institute at Johns Hopkins Hospital. He was a founding member of the American Glaucoma Society and served as its secretary for eight years. He was elected chief executive officer of the Association for Research in Vision and Ophthalmology and editor-in-chief of *Investigative Ophthalmology and Visual Science,* the most prestigious journal in vision research.

■■■

Oliver D. Schein, M.D., M.P.H., is the Burton E. Grossman Professor of Ophthalmology at the Wilmer Eye Institute and carries a joint appointment in the Department of Epidemiology at the Johns Hopkins University School of Hygiene and Public Health. Dr. Schein's clinical expertise is in medical and surgical conditions of the anterior segment of the eye involving cataract and complications of cataract surgery, corneal scarring, and corneal surgery. He is an author of the American Academy of Ophthalmology's "Preferred Practice Pattern" on Cataract.

■■■

Simeon Margolis, M.D., Ph.D., received his B.A., M.D., and Ph.D. from the Johns Hopkins University School of Medicine and performed his internship and residency at Johns Hopkins Hospital. He is currently a professor of medicine and biological chemistry at the Johns Hopkins University School of Medicine and medical editor of *The Johns Hopkins Medical Letter, Health After 50.* He has served on various committees for the Department of Health, Education, and Welfare, including the National Diabetes Advisory Board and the Arteriosclerosis Specialized Centers of Research Review Committees. In addition, he has acted as a member of the Endocrinology and Metabolism Panel of the U.S. Food and Drug Administration.

CONTENTS

VISION

If treated early enough, the most common eye disorders—cataracts, glaucoma, age-related macular degeneration, and diabetic retinopathy—can often be slowed or halted with drugs, surgery, or both. In addition, treating vision problems can enhance quality of life by allowing a person to return to such daily activities as driving, grocery shopping, using public transportation, and performing household tasks. Patients can take steps on their own to make it easier to live with any of these disorders, and vision aids are available to enhance diminished visual acuity for those who cannot be treated.

Although the presence of a vision disorder might seem obvious, many people are unaware that they have one. Surveys performed by researchers at Johns Hopkins found that about one third of people with eye disease were unaware of it and that more than one third of people age 65 to 84 had not visited an eye doctor in the last year. Periodic visits to an eye-care specialist are needed to detect conditions (such as glaucoma) early enough to allow effective treatment. Regular check-ups are particularly important for people over age 65, those with risk factors for serious eye disease, individuals in fair or poor general health, and those with diabetes.

ANATOMY OF THE EYE

The eye is a complex structure that sends nerve impulses to the brain when stimulated by light rays reflected from an object. The brain then processes these impulses to create the perception of vision.

The *iris,* the colored circle in the middle of the eye, is the eye's most prominent structure. Also visible from the front are the *pupil,* the opening in the center of the iris that resembles a large black dot, and the *sclera,* part of the outer layer of the eye. The iris is composed of smooth muscles that contract and expand to alter the size of the pupil and control the amount of light that enters the eye. The sclera is the tough, white connective tissue that covers and protects the majority of the eye.

Also at the front of the eye are the *cornea, lens,* and *conjunctiva.* The cornea is a transparent, dome-shaped disk that covers the iris and the pupil. Beneath the cornea is a transparent, elastic structure called the lens. The cornea does about three quarters of the work of focusing light on the retina; the lens does the rest. The conjunctiva is a thin, lubricating mucous membrane that covers the sclera and lines the inside of the eyelids.

Inside the sclera lie two more layers. The middle layer, the *choroid,* contains a dark pigment that minimizes scattering of light inside the eye. It is rich in blood vessels that supply nutrients to the *retina,* the innermost layer of the eye that consists of light-sensitive nerve tissue. The retina functions like film in a camera, receiving an imprint of an image and sending it via the optic nerve to the brain to be "developed."

The *vitreous humor,* a thick, gel-like substance, fills the back of the eyeball behind the lens, while a watery fluid, the *aqueous humor,* is located in front of the lens. These two humors help to maintain intraocular pressure (the internal pressure of the eye), which is needed to prevent the eyeball from collapsing. Intraocular pressure is controlled by specialized cells that produce aqueous humor and by ducts and canals that drain it from the eye.

REFRACTIVE ERRORS

The major role of the lens is to refract and focus light from both distant and near objects. This process is achieved by changes in the shape of the lens (accommodation). For example, to see at a distance, muscle fibers attached to the lens tighten to flatten its shape and focus light coming from a distance onto the retina. For close vision, these muscles relax, and the lens reverts to its naturally rounder shape, which focuses light from close objects onto the retina.

Refractive errors are caused by a deviation in the way light focuses on the retina. The four types of refractive errors are nearsightedness (myopia), farsightedness (hyperopia), astigmatism, and presbyopia. All of these conditions can be corrected with the use of eyeglasses or contact lenses. An increasingly popular alternative to glasses and contacts, especially for nearsightedness, is laser vision correction (see the feature on pages 18–19).

In nearsighted people, the eyeball is too long or the cornea has too much curvature. As a result, light focuses on a point in front of the retina; near objects can be seen clearly but distant ones do not come into proper focus. Nearly 30% of Americans are nearsighted.

If the eyeball is too short or the cornea is too flat, the focal point for light is behind the retina. In this condition, called farsightedness, distant objects can be seen clearly but close ones do not come into proper focus.

Astigmatism occurs when the cornea or lens is slightly irregular in shape. This unequal curvature causes light to focus at different

Common Diseases That Affect the Eye

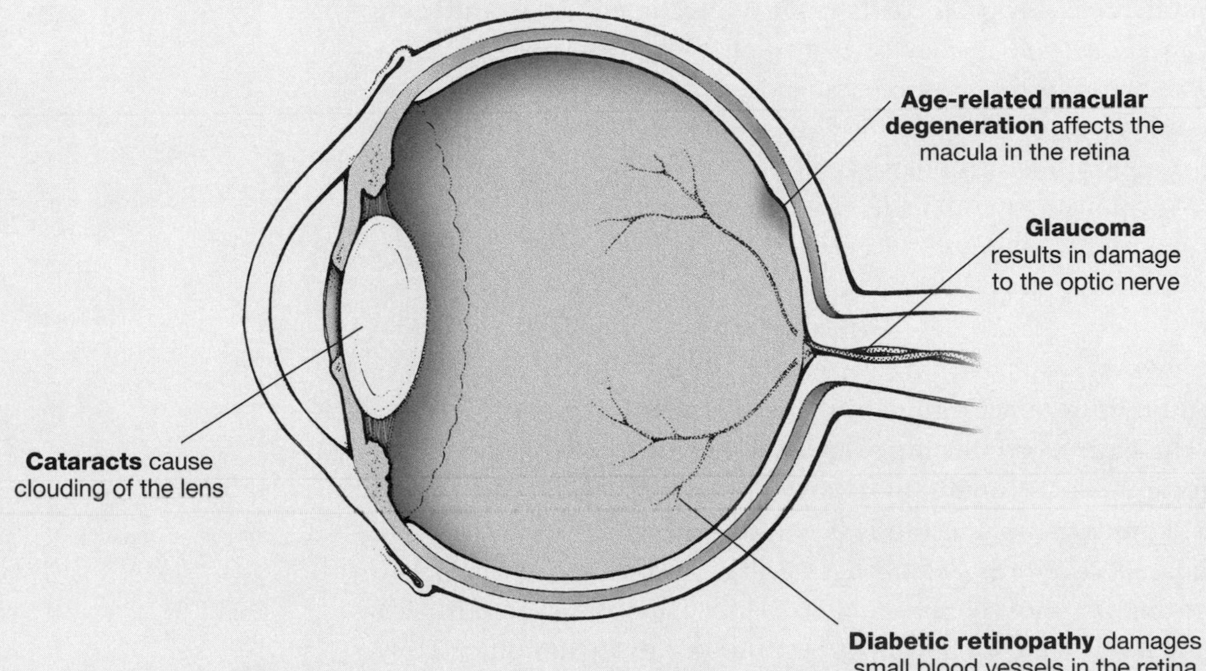

Vision disorders affect different parts of the eye. Cataracts affect the lens in the front of the eye, while age-related macular degeneration (AMD) and diabetic retinopathy injure the retina in the back of the eye. Glaucoma affects the optic nerve, which is also in the back of the eye.

Cataracts. The lens is a clear structure, thickest in the middle, that stretches and contracts to allow the eye to focus the light from objects at various distances. Cataracts are cloudy or opaque areas in the lens. Symptoms include cloudy or filmy vision, impaired night vision, the appearance of halos around lights, and loss of color intensity. Treatment for a severe cataract usually involves surgery to remove the lens and replace it with an artificial one.

Glaucoma. Glaucoma occurs when the fluid within the front of the eye, called the aqueous humor, places pressure on the optic nerve and damages it. Often this damage is caused by elevated pressure within the eye, but sometimes the nerve is damaged by normal pressure. Treatment with medication or surgery reduces the chance of progressive vision loss.

Age-related macular degeneration (AMD). AMD affects the macula, the central, most sensitive part of the retina. The macula is responsible for central vision and for seeing details and colors. The causes of AMD are unknown. As the condition progresses, the eye must rely on peripheral vision because central vision is compromised. There are two types of AMD: dry (non-neovascular) and wet (neovascular). Non-neovascular AMD is much more common, and neovascular AMD is usually much more severe. Patients with the non-neovascular type usually do not lose vision unless they develop advanced non-neovascular AMD with atrophy of retinal cells or develop the neovascular form. In the non-neovascular form, degeneration of the layer of pigment epithelial cells causes the retina to become thinner. In the neovascular form, abnormal blood vessels may begin bleeding. The body heals these blood vessels, but the remaining scar tissue prevents the macula from functioning properly. There is no cure for AMD, though only 1% to 2% of people who have it will lose their vision. The progression of the condition can be arrested in some patients using laser surgery.

Diabetic retinopathy. Over time, people with diabetes often develop damage in the small blood vessels in the retina, a condition called diabetic retinopathy. In the early (nonproliferative) stage of the disease, fluid leaks into the retina from injured blood vessels. This fluid causes swelling of the retina, which may blur vision. In the more advanced (proliferative) stage, new and fragile blood vessels grow into the vitreous humor in the back of the eye. Bleeding from these vessels and the formation of scar tissue can lead to retinal detachment and cause vision loss. Good control of diabetes usually does not reverse the damage, but it does minimize and may prevent progression of the disease. A laser can be used to treat the swelling (macular edema) or bleeding vessels.

points in the eye. The result is blurred or distorted vision.

Presbyopia occurs when the lens gradually loses its ability to accommodate. As we age, the lens gradually becomes thicker and more rigid and is less able to change its shape to bring close objects into focus. Presbyopia is the most common vision disorder, affecting almost all people over age 45. The only treatment is the use of reading glasses. If the person is also nearsighted or has astigmatism, prescription bifocals, trifocals, or contact lenses are required.

Cataracts

A cloudiness or opacification of the lens is called a cataract. Derived from the Latin word meaning waterfall, the term *cataract* arose from the ancient misconception that the symptoms of a cataract are caused by evil liquids that mysteriously flow into the eye.

Cataracts can occur at any age—in fact, babies can be born with them—but are most common later in life. They are present in 50% of people age 65 to 74 and in 70% of those age 75 and older. However, not all cataracts affect vision significantly or require treatment.

Ordinarily, when a person looks at an object, light rays reflected from that object enter the eye through the cornea and the lens, which together focus the light onto the retina to produce a sharp image. When a cataract develops, however, light rays are no longer precisely focused but instead are scattered before reaching the retina.

TYPES OF CATARACTS

The lens is made of protein fibers arranged in a specialized way so that the lens is transparent. It is composed of four distinct structures: At the center is the *nucleus,* which is surrounded by the *cortex,* then the lens *epithelium,* and, finally, the *capsule.* Protein fibers are secreted by the lens epithelium throughout life.

The three common types of cataracts are defined by their location in the lens: nuclear, cortical, and posterior subcapsular (in the rear of the lens capsule). More than one type is often present in the same eye. Posterior subcapsular cataracts are the ones most likely to occur in younger people and may be associated with prolonged use of corticosteroids (such as prednisone), inflammation, or trauma.

The extent of vision damage and how quickly vision is impaired depend not only on the size and density of the cataract, but also its location in the lens. For example, a cataract in the periphery of the cortex has little effect on vision because it does not interfere with the passage of light through the center of the lens, while a dense nuclear cataract causes severe blurring of vision.

CAUSES OF CATARACTS

The cause of most cataracts is unknown, but at least two factors associated with aging contribute to their development. Clumping (aggregation) of lens proteins leads to scattering of light and a decrease in the transparency of the lens. In addition, the breakdown of lens proteins leads to the accumulation of a yellow-brown pigment and clouding of the lens.

Certain chemical changes also take place. These changes include a reduced uptake of oxygen in the lens and a rise in the water content of the lens, which is later followed by dehydration. Amounts of calcium and sodium increase, while potassium, vitamin C, and protein levels decrease during cataract formation. Glutathione, an antioxidant, appears to be deficient in lenses with cataracts. Studies on the use of medications or vitamins to alter the levels of these substances in the lens have not produced promising results, however. Currently, there is no effective drug therapy to prevent cataract formation.

In addition, cigarette smoking, medications such as corticosteroids, eye injuries, sunlight, diabetes, and even obesity and excessive sodium intake can increase the risk of cataracts.

Cigarette Smoking

Cigarette smoking is associated with a higher incidence of cataracts. Studies of male physicians and female nurses found an increased incidence of nuclear and posterior subcapsular cataracts in those who smoked the most. Smoking at least 20 cigarettes a day more than doubled the risk of these cataracts in men; in women, smoking at least 35 cigarettes a day raised the risk by about half. It is not clear why cigarette smoking has an adverse effect on the lens, but it might reduce blood levels of nutrients required for lens maintenance.

Corticosteroids

Long-term use of corticosteroids, especially at high doses, is the most common drug treatment associated with cataracts. In one study of the prolonged use of oral prednisone, cataracts developed in 11% of people taking less than 10 mg a day, in 30% of those taking 10 to 15 mg a day, and in 80% of those taking more than 15 mg a day.

NEW RESEARCH

Former Smokers Remain At Increased Cataract Risk

Smoking cigarettes is known to increase the risk of cataracts. Now a study has found that the likelihood of developing cataracts is lower in people who quit smoking—even decades ago—than in current smokers but remains higher than in people who never smoked.

As part of two large studies, a total of 124,690 doctors and nurses answered health questionnaires every two years beginning as early as 1976. The participants indicated whether they were former, current, or never smokers; current and former smokers indicated how many cigarettes they smoked per day. The participants also listed any cataract surgeries they had undergone.

Compared with current smokers, participants who had quit smoking 25 years earlier had a 20% lower risk of cataract surgery. Those who never smoked had a 36% lower risk than current smokers.

Smoking may increase cataract risk by promoting oxidation in the lens. These results suggest that although quitting smoking lowers the risk of cataracts, smoking may permanently damage the lens. The authors "emphasize the importance of never starting to smoke or quitting early in life."

AMERICAN JOURNAL OF EPIDEMIOLOGY
Volume 155, page 72
January 2002

Short-term use of oral corticosteroids is unlikely to lead to cataracts.

The risk of cataracts was once thought to be unaffected, or even diminished, by inhaled corticosteroids, but recent research suggests otherwise. In one study, patients who had used inhaled corticosteroids had a 50% greater prevalence of nuclear cataracts and a 90% greater prevalence of posterior subcapsular cataracts than those who had not used inhaled corticosteroids. In another study, people using inhaled corticosteroids for more than three years were three times more likely to need cataract surgery than those who did not use these medications. The likelihood of cataract surgery increased with higher doses. These results are of concern for people with asthma, who often rely on inhaled corticosteroids to treat their condition. It is important to remember that the benefits of inhaled corticosteroids for asthma outweigh the long-term risk of cataracts, which are treatable.

Cataracts can also develop from applying topical corticosteroids to the eyelids or using corticosteroid-containing eye drops, although the more common side effect of prolonged topical corticosteroid therapy is elevated pressure in the eye (which may lead to glaucoma). To reduce the chance of these side effects, patients should use topical ocular corticosteroids only under the supervision of an ophthalmologist.

Eye Injuries

Blunt trauma to the eye or damage to the eye from alkaline chemicals can cause opacification of the lens, either immediately or later on. Rapid cataract formation is a common consequence of a penetrating eye injury.

Sunlight and Ionizing Radiation

Population studies have shown that prolonged exposure to the ultraviolet (UV) radiation in sunlight more than doubles the risk of cortical cataracts. In one study, the risk of developing cortical cataracts was two times greater in people with the highest levels of sunlight exposure than in those with low levels. The more sunlight exposure, the higher the risk of cataracts. However, in this same study, nuclear cataracts were not linked to sunlight exposure, possibly because the older lens fibers in the nucleus receive the most sunlight exposure earlier in life, when the body is more able to combat the effects of sunlight. As the eye ages, the nucleus is covered by newer cortical fibers, which receive the most sunlight when the eye is older and less able to protect itself—possibly leading to the formation

Choosing a Pair of Sunglasses

Ultraviolet (UV) rays, the invisible light that causes sunburn, can also damage the eyes. There are three types of UV rays: UVA, UVB, and UVC.

UVC rays are absorbed by the earth's upper atmosphere and do not reach the eyes. UVA rays are mostly absorbed within the lens of eye, and experts are divided on whether they are harmful. Most dangerous are UVB rays, which are absorbed by the cornea and conjunctiva of the eye. Exposure to UVB rays in combination with cold wind and snow can lead to an acute problem called snow blindness—temporary but painful damage to the cornea. In addition, long-term regular exposure to UVB rays increases the risk of cataracts.

Because of the relationship between sunlight and certain diseases of the eye, the American Academy of Ophthalmology recommends wearing sunglasses whenever you are in the sun for an extended period of time. Some medications can make your eyes (as well as your skin) especially sensitive to sunlight. These drugs include: antibiotics such as tetracycline (Achromycin V) and doxycycline (Vibramycin and other brands); the gout drug allopurinol (Aloprim and Zyloprim); psoralen drugs such as trioxsalen (Trisoralen) and methoxsalen (Oxsoralen and Uvadex), which are used for the treatment of vitiligo and T-cell lymphoma; and phenothiazine drugs such as chlorpromazine (Thorazine), which are used to treat mental and emotional disorders. If you are taking any of these medications, wearing sunglasses may help protect your eyes and improve your comfort level.

There are a wide variety of sunglasses on the market, and some offer better protection than others. Here are some things to consider when selecting a pair.

UV Protection

Look for lenses that block 99% to 100% of both UVA and UVB rays. Some lenses say they protect against 400 nanometers, or UV 400, which is the same as 100% protection from UVA and UVB. The American National Standards Institute (ANSI) is the regulatory body that sets standards for sunglasses. To meet ANSI requirements, lenses must block at least 99% of UVA and UVB.

Lens Color

The color of the lens has nothing to do with how much protection it provides, so you can't assume that darker lenses block more UV rays. Choose a tint that is dark enough to keep you from squinting in the sun, but not so dark that it interferes with your vision. Most people find that gray and brown lenses distort colors the least; yellow lenses reduce haze and increase contrast for some people.

Lens Material

Few lenses for nonprescription sunglasses are made of glass. Most are plastic, which is less likely to shatter if hit (for example, with a ball or stone). Polycarbonate plastic lenses are the least likely to break and are the preferred material for athletic activities, but they do scratch easily. Polycarbonate lenses with a scratch-resistant coating are the most durable type.

Lens Style

Most styles provide adequate protection from UV rays, but wraparound lenses help prevent sunlight from reaching your eyes from the sides.

Polarized Lenses

Polarized lenses reduce glare caused by light reflecting from long, flat surfaces, such as water, snow, and pavement. For certain activities, such as driving, skiing, golfing, biking, and boating, polarized lenses may allow you to see more clearly. However, some people find that polarized lenses make it difficult to see liquid crystal displays on dashboards or ATM machines.

Prescription Sunglasses

People who wear glasses to read or see far away may want to consider prescription sunglasses. Almost any pair of frames can be made into sunglasses (with the exception of dramatically curved, wraparound styles). In addition, almost all types of prescription lenses—even progressive lenses for presbyopia—are available tinted and with UV protection. If you don't want to buy or carry around another pair of glasses, tinted clip-on lenses can be worn over your regular glasses.

Photochromic Lenses

Photochromic lenses change from clear when you are indoors to dark-tinted when you are in the sun. While they do allow you to see better in the sun, photochromic lenses usually provide no UV protection unless a special coating is applied to them.

Distortion

Before buying a pair of sunglasses, check to see if they distort your field of vision. While wearing them, look at a rectangular pattern such as floor tiles. As you move your head up and down and from side to side, the lines should continue to appear straight.

Maximizing Protection

You can decrease your sun exposure even further by also wearing a hat with a broad brim. As much as 50% of sunlight comes from overhead, and it can reach your eyes even while wearing sunglasses.

of a cortical cataract. Ionizing radiation (from x-rays, for example) can also cause cataracts.

Diabetes

People with diabetes are at increased risk for cataracts, and these cataracts tend to occur at an earlier age. Some evidence indicates that the accumulation of sorbitol (a sugar formed from glucose) in the lens promotes cataract formation in people with diabetes.

Obesity

Excess weight may also increase the odds of developing cataracts. Proper weight is often determined using body mass index (BMI), a measure of weight in relation to height. To calculate BMI, weight in pounds is multiplied by 704 and divided by the square of height in inches. Overweight is defined as a BMI of 25 to 29.9 and obesity as a BMI of 30 or greater.

In one study of men between the ages of 40 and 84, those with a high BMI had a greater risk of developing cataracts. Specifically, men whose BMI was between 22 and 27.8 had roughly a 50% increase in cataract risk compared with those whose BMI was less than 22. A BMI higher than 27.8 more than doubled cataract risk. Posterior subcapsular cataracts, which reduce visual acuity, were the type of cataract most often associated with a high BMI. Other studies have found similar results in women. Although the reasons for the link between obesity and cataracts is unclear, it is thought that a low calorie intake may reduce cataract formation by decreasing blood glucose levels or improving the antioxidant properties of the blood.

SYMPTOMS OF CATARACTS

The most common symptom of cataracts is a painless blurring of vision. Everything becomes dimmer, as if you were wearing glasses that need cleaning. Most often, both eyes are affected, though one eye is usually more compromised than the other. The impairment usually progresses at a similar rate in the two eyes. Changes can occur in a matter of months or almost imperceptibly over many years. In some cases, double vision occurs. This is caused by the passage of light through a lens that has irregular areas of opacity, which can split the rays of light from a single object and focus them on different parts of the retina. Other possible symptoms of cataracts are the need for increasingly frequent changes in prescriptions for glasses and noting a yellowish tinge to objects.

During the development of a nuclear cataract, some people who previously needed reading glasses for presbyopia are able to read without them, a change referred to as second sight. This minor improvement occurs because the cataract alters the shape of the lens, making it better able to focus on nearby objects. Over time, however, progression of the cataract generally impairs vision further.

Individuals with cortical or posterior subcapsular cataracts often have worse vision in bright light, which causes the pupils to contract and restricts the passage of light to the center of the lens—the part that may be most severely affected by the cataract. For example, such people may have problems with night driving because of the glare of oncoming headlights. (Glare is defined as the light within the field of vision that is brighter than other objects to which the eyes are adapted.)

PREVENTION OF CATARACTS

Since smoking may be responsible for 20% of cataracts, smoking cessation should be thought of as a vital step in cataract prevention. (The many other benefits of quitting smoking include a lower risk of cancer, lung disease, and coronary heart disease.) Other approaches to reducing the risk of cataracts are less certain.

Wearing UV-light-blocking sunglasses and a hat with a wide brim will help reduce exposure of the eyes to UV radiation. This is presumed, but not proven, to reduce the risk of cataracts. For more information on choosing a pair of sunglasses, see the feature on page 7.

Whether consuming particular foods or vitamin supplements or taking medications reduces the risk of cataracts is the subject of considerable debate. Trials of medications, such as aspirin or hormone replacement therapy, have shown no benefit or unclear results. The sidebar at right describes the results of a study that found hormone replacement therapy reduced the risk of nuclear and posterior subcapsular cataracts but not the risk of cortical cataracts.

Some researchers have proposed that antioxidant vitamins might help prevent cataracts. This theory is based on the fact that normal chemical reactions in the eye produce unstable oxygen molecules, called free radicals, which over time can damage various components of the lens. By protecting against these free radicals, antioxidants may prevent their harmful effects. Abundant in fruits and vegetables, antioxidants include beta-carotene, vitamin C, and selenium. A number of studies have found a possible link between high intakes of an-

NEW RESEARCH

Estrogen May Reduce Cataract Risk

Hormone replacement therapy (HRT) after menopause and past exposure to other sources of estrogen (birth control pills and pregnancy) may reduce the risk of certain types of cataracts in women, according to a new study.

As part of a larger population study on eye health, 1,239 women age 65 to 84 were given complete eye examinations. They provided information on their use of HRT and birth control pills and answered questions about their medical history (including pregnancies, hysterectomies, diabetes, high blood pressure, and previous eye surgery).

After adjusting for age and other health factors, women currently using HRT had half the risk of nuclear cataracts as women who had never used HRT. Past use of birth control pills reduced the risk of nuclear cataracts by 30%, and the risk was lowered with each child a woman had. The risk of posterior subcapsular cataracts was reduced with both past and current use of HRT, but HRT use did not protect against cortical cataracts.

Other studies have suggested that HRT may protect against cataracts, but this is the first study to differentiate among cataract types and to suggest an association with estrogen exposure during pregnancy and while taking birth control pills.

ARCHIVES OF OPHTHALMOLOGY
Volume 119, page 1687
November 2001

tioxidants and a reduced incidence of cataracts, but results from the Age-Related Eye Disease Study found no such benefit from antioxidant supplements. This large-scale randomized trial was sponsored by the National Eye Institute of the National Institutes of Health, and the results were published in 2001.

TREATMENT OF CATARACTS

Currently, no nonsurgical treatment cures or slows the development of cataracts, although ongoing studies continue to look for ways to retard the progression of the disease. Some nonsurgical treatments may improve vision in the short term, however. One option is eye drops to dilate the pupil and allow more light to reach the retina. The drawback of this approach is that it increases glare, which may be unacceptable for some people. Nonsurgical management of cataracts is discussed in more detail in the feature on the opposite page.

What To Expect From Cataract Surgery

Surgical removal of a cataract, along with implantation of an intraocular lens, is the most frequently performed surgery in people over age 65. About 1.5 million cataract surgeries are performed each year. It is considered by many doctors to be the most effective surgical procedure in all of medicine.

If the eye is normal except for the cataract, surgery will improve vision in over 95% of cases. Because the new intraocular lens is designed to correct nearsightedness or farsightedness, 85% of patients undergoing cataract surgery attain vision of at least 20/40—good enough to drive a car—one year after the operation. Simply put, 20/40 vision means the ability to see at 20 feet what a normal eye can see at 40 feet. Legal blindness is defined as 20/200 or worse in both eyes. At this level of vision loss, large objects and light are still discernible. With 20/800 vision, getting around without assistance is no longer possible.

Significant postsurgical complications occur in only 1% to 2% of operations (see pages 18–20), but because of the great number of procedures performed, this translates into a large number of patients with such complications.

The success of cataract surgery depends upon a number of factors. One study found that more substantial improvement in visual function after surgery was associated with younger age, poorer preoperative visual function, having a posterior subcapsular cataract, and having neither age-related macular degeneration nor diabetes.

Nonsurgical Management of Cataracts

Not all cataracts require surgery. In fact, surgery is considered mainly for patients whose cataracts significantly interfere with important activities, such as reading or driving. Because surgery to remove cataracts is rarely an emergency and putting off the surgery causes no additional harm, patients whose cataracts do not interfere with day-to-day activities can try the following to improve their vision.

- Reduce glare by wearing sunglasses and a wide-brimmed hat when outdoors.
- Use appropriate indoor lighting. Indoor lighting should be strong, yet not produce glare (see the feature on page 15 for advice on indoor lighting).
- Use a magnifying glass or buy large-print books. Such devices and publications are available through dealers of low-vision products; some of these dealers are listed on page 45.
- Ask your eye care professional about getting a stronger prescription for your eyeglasses or contact lenses.
- Taking a medication that dilates the pupils may be helpful for people with posterior subcapsular cataract. However, many people cannot tolerate the glare that this treatment may cause.

Dissatisfaction with the surgery may be related to unrealistic expectations by patients. For example, some people may incorrectly assume that they will no longer need glasses to read small print or do close handwork.

Proper preparation before surgery will ease recovery after cataract removal. Patients should review what to expect with their ophthalmologist, including how to protect the eye, what medications are needed, what activities are permitted, when to return for follow-up visits, the signs of complications, and how to seek emergency care.

Most patients have minimal discomfort after the operation; a mild painkiller (such as Tylenol) can be taken if needed. Some redness, scratchiness, or slight morning discharge (which can be gently wiped away with a warm washcloth) may be present during the first few days after surgery. In addition, it is common to see a few black spots or shapes (floaters) drifting through the field of vision. A protective patch is generally worn over the eye for 24 hours. Glasses must be worn during the day to avoid eye trauma, and an eye shield is used at night for several days to a few weeks (according to the doctor's instructions) to prevent accidentally rubbing or poking the eye while asleep.

Vision varies widely when the patch is first removed. In most patients, vision remains blurred for several days to weeks, then gradually improves as the eye heals (though some fluctuations are common). In some cases, the sutures left in the eye alter the shape of the cornea and result in temporary blurring or astigmatism. This problem generally goes away on its own, though it may require removal of the sutures, a simple and painless procedure. In general, vision improves faster in those who receive intraocular lens implants rather than waiting for cataract glasses or contact lenses. However, surgery usually changes the corrective prescription for the eye (even in those with lens implants), and new eyeglasses will be needed to correct any remaining near- or farsightedness. New glasses cannot be prescribed, however, until the eye has fully recovered. This usually takes about six weeks, but may take longer in some people.

Whether To Have Cataract Surgery

Immediate removal of a cataract is rarely necessary. Instead, the decision when to have the surgery almost always rests with the patient and is based on the effect of the cataract on the quality of vision, the balance between the operation's benefits and risks, and the presence of other medical conditions that might affect the outcome. In some cases, people with another major vision disorder, such as advanced glaucoma or age-related macular degeneration, may be discouraged from having cataract surgery because it may not improve their vision.

On the other hand, cataract removal might benefit patients with some types of retinal damage. Even though the retinal condition may have impaired central vision, cataract surgery may help the patient regain peripheral vision (the ability to see objects at the edges of the visual field). In other cases, cataract surgery makes it possible to diagnose and treat retinal disease.

Researchers were once concerned that cataract surgery might release lens proteins that could damage the lens in the other eye. But an Italian study found that cataract surgery did not affect the incidence or progression of cataracts in the unoperated eye.

The following are some important questions to consider before deciding on cataract surgery. Answering yes to several of these questions suggests that a cataract is interfering with daily life and that surgery might be beneficial.

- Am I having trouble performing my job duties because I cannot see clearly? Do I have to strain to read computer screens?
- Am I constantly squinting?
- Am I inhibited when participating in activities I enjoy—such as reading, watching television, or going out with friends—because of visual limitations?
- Do I stay in at night because of vision problems?

- Does glare from the sun or car headlights interfere with or prevent me from driving?
- Am I fearful of bumping into something or falling because of my eyesight?
- Do I need help performing daily activities—such as preparing food or doing laundry—because of my vision? Could I be more independent if my vision were improved?
- Am I becoming increasingly nearsighted? Despite frequent prescription changes, do I still have trouble seeing with my glasses?
- Does my eyesight bother me all the time?

Presurgical Tests

A-scan ultrasonography, a test that uses sound to measure the length of the eyeball, is routinely performed prior to cataract surgery. The length of the eye is one component of the equation used to predict the appropriate focusing power of the planned lens replacement (see pages 16–18). If the surgeon cannot see the retina in the back of the eye because the cataract is too opaque, another test called B-scan ultrasonography is used to provide a "view," via reflected sound waves, of structures in the back of the eye. B-scans can also detect such conditions as a detached retina.

In the past, detailed general medical testing and examinations (including blood tests, electrocardiograms, and chest x-rays) were done before cataract surgery. Because the surgery can be performed so safely now, many surgeons request much simpler presurgical evaluations. A 2000 study of more than 18,000 patients at Johns Hopkins found that routine medical testing did not improve outcomes or reduce complications from surgery. Many institutions continue to perform some routine testing, however.

In any case, it is necessary to obtain a general medical history. Then, based on what the history reveals, specific preoperative exams and/or tests might still be recommended. Important details in this medical history include a list of current medications and allergies. For example, use of anticoagulants might preclude certain kinds of surgery, or a patient with a breathing problem may need a chest x-ray. For patients taking aspirin or warfarin (Coumadin), the pros and cons of continuing or discontinuance of these medications around the time of surgery should be discussed with the surgeon. Since cataract surgery is almost always elective, it is generally not performed in the period immediately following a major medical event, such as a stroke or heart attack.

NEW RESEARCH

Cataracts Associated With Increased Mortality in Women

Cataracts are thought to be associated with a higher mortality rate in people with diabetes. A new study suggests that nondiabetic women with cataracts may also have a higher mortality rate.

Researchers assessed the health of 1,502 people age 65 and older from 17 general practice groups in north London. The participants were analyzed in groups based on their age, sex, and whether they had diabetes.

Over the next four years, women without diabetes were significantly more likely to die if they had cataracts than if they did not (40 vs. 25 women per 1,000). This association persisted even after adjusting for age and cardiovascular, respiratory, and other noncancer causes of death. There was no association between cataracts and mortality in nondiabetic men or in people who died of cancer. Among people with diabetes, mortality was significantly elevated during the four years for both men and women with cataracts.

These results suggest that women are exposed to "sex specific" risk factors that increase both their risk of cataracts and death. Further research is needed to identify these factors.

BRITISH JOURNAL OF OPHTHALMOLOGY
Volume 86, page 424
April 2002

Types of Cataract Surgery

Before the 1970s, most surgeons performed cataract operations with the naked eye or with the aid of loupes—specialized glasses that provide a small amount of magnification. Today, microsurgery is the rule.

Before starting any of the cataract removal procedures described below, an operating microscope is placed over the eye undergoing surgery. This microscope magnifies the eye four to six times its normal size. The operation usually takes less than an hour. If both eyes are affected, in almost all cases they are operated on one at a time, with at least several weeks—and more often months—separating the two operations. There are several reasons for the delay. First, it gives the first eye time to recover. Second, should any complications become evident, the surgeon might do the second operation differently. Finally, if the results with the first eye are good enough, the need for a second operation may be eliminated.

About 90% of cataract operations are now performed with a local anesthetic on an outpatient basis. Patients are given a sedative before the surgery to make them feel drowsy on arrival in the operating room. Next, the surgeon administers local anesthesia either by injection or with drops.

Local anesthesia is almost always preferred over general anesthesia, which is associated with nausea, vomiting, and a greater risk of complications. As a result, general anesthesia is used only in unusual circumstances, such as in patients whose extreme anxiety makes surgery difficult or in those rare patients allergic to local anesthetics.

Intracapsular surgery. Intracapsular cataract surgery removes the entire lens—the capsule, the cortex, and the nucleus. The procedure is rarely performed today but is used in some situations—such as when the lens is partially or completely dislocated (owing to a genetic disease, for example). A small incision is made at the side of the cornea. The surgeon inserts a cryoprobe (a rod with an extremely cold tip) through the incision. When the lens is touched by the tip of the probe, it adheres—as a tongue might stick to a cold metal object in the winter—and the surgeon guides the lens out as the probe is withdrawn. The incision is closed with fine sutures.

This procedure can be used in patients who also suffer from glaucoma and are taking a medication, such as pilocarpine (Pilocar and other brands), that narrows the pupil and makes other surgical options more difficult. Overall, intracapsular surgery has a low rate of postoperative complications.

Extracapsular surgery. Extracapsular surgery is now by far the

Lighting for Low Vision

As people age, their lighting requirements change. For example, older people typically need three times as much light as younger people. But lighting needs also vary depending on the health of the eyes. People with glaucoma usually need more light, while those with cataracts typically need lower levels to reduce glare. Using the right amount and type of lighting can help people with low vision make the most of their sight.

Types of Lighting

Four major types of consumer lighting are available. Finding the type of lighting that works best for you may take some trial and error.

Incandescent bulbs. Also called filament bulbs, these are the type most people have in their lamps. Electrical energy produces heat that turns the filament inside the bulb white-hot, which creates light. Incandescent bulbs can be clear, white, frosted, or colored, and they are usually available in 25, 40, 60, 75, 100 watts, or more. (The brightness of the light increases with the wattage). Clear bulbs provide the most light, but many people find they produce too much glare. Frosted and white (or soft white) bulbs are more comfortable to the eyes and produce fewer shadows. Blue bulbs, the most expensive type, produce a light similar to daylight and are preferred by some people.

Fluorescent lighting. This type is used in most commercial buildings and public places, but is also available for home use in some lamps (called PL fluorescent lamps). An electric current excites mercury atoms within the fluorescent bulb. The resulting light is in the ultraviolet range and interacts with a coating on the inside of the bulb to create visible light. Fluorescent bulbs are more expensive than incandescent bulbs, but they last longer, use less electricity, and emit less heat. (Heat can be a problem if the bulb is placed near a person's face or body for close work such as reading or knitting.) Fluorescent bulbs are also advantageous because they distribute light evenly over a large area and produce few shadows. (However, they can cause glare and eye strain, especially if they "flicker.")

Full-spectrum or combination bulbs. These bulbs use both incandescent and fluorescent light to provide the closest substitute for natural light. They are helpful for people with low vision, especially when used in lamps that can be adjusted to shine directly onto a book or activity. However, these bulbs can be difficult to find.

Halogen bulbs. This type of incandescent lighting produces the whitest and brightest light. Some people like halogen lighting because it enhances the contrast between print and background, but others find that it produces too much glare. Halogen bulbs are particularly useful for focusing light on a small area. However, the bulbs emit a lot of heat, are expensive, and use a lot of electricity.

Lighting Your Home

If you have low vision, adjusting the lighting in your home may help you to see more clearly. Here are a few suggestions:

- Have a specific source of light for each task, for example, preparing food, grooming, reading, or doing crafts.
- Position lamps so that the light falls directly onto the task, not into your eyes. Adjustable or clip-on lamps can be helpful for this purpose.
- Use a 60-, 75-, or 100-watt bulb in lamps placed within one foot of your task. A higher-watt bulb may be needed in a floor lamp located farther from the task. Note: Never use a higher wattage bulb than that recommended by the lamp manufacturer.
- Lampshades with white inner linings will reflect the most light onto your task.
- When using task lighting, make sure the rest of the room is well-lit—preferably one third to one fifth as bright—because it can be difficult for your eyes to adjust from light to dark places. For the same reason, try to keep the level of lighting constant throughout your home.
- Bedrooms, staircases, hallways, and bathrooms are common places for falls, so use extra lighting in these areas, especially at night.
- When setting up extra lighting in a room, be sure that there are no trailing wires that can cause someone to trip. In addition, use a power strip rather than a socket adapter, which can be dangerous, if you need to plug in several lamps.

Reducing Glare

Glare is caused by light shining directly into your eyes or reflecting off a surface, such as a piece of paper. The following are ways to minimize glare:

- Position lamps so that the light does not shine into your eyes. For example, place a lamp by your side rather than directly in front of you.
- When reading or working, sit with your back or side to the window instead of facing it so that daylight falls on your work, rather than into your eyes.
- Place drapes or blinds on windows to reduce glare. Sheer or lightweight curtains help reduce glare while still allowing light to enter the room.
- Always use a lampshade. Bare light bulbs are a common source of glare.
- Home furnishings also can be a source of glare. Cover shiny floors with rugs and use fabric to cover glossy furniture.
- Make sure light sources are not directed at mirrors.

most common type of cataract operation because it minimizes trauma to the eye and is associated with fewer postoperative complications than intracapsular surgery. In this form of surgery, the front capsule of the lens is removed, followed by the nucleus and cortical material. The goal is to leave the back capsule of the lens intact. This back capsule forms the ideal support for the intraocular lens. Today, most extracapsular surgery is performed using phacoemulsification.

Phacoemulsification. This type of extracapsular surgery is performed with an ultrasonic device that nearly liquifies the nucleus and cortex so that they can be removed by suction through a tube. Phacoemulsification surgery, which permits a smaller incision than the other techniques, facilitates healing of the surgical wound. Often this surgery requires no stitches for closure of the wound.

Lens Replacement

Once a lens has been removed, the patient is referred to as *aphakic*, which is Greek for "without lens." To see clearly, the refractive power of the lens must be replaced so that light can focus onto the retina. The three most common replacement options are intraocular lens implants, glasses, and contact lenses.

Intraocular lenses. By far the most frequent approach to lens replacement is an intraocular lens implant placed at the time of cataract surgery. The quarter-inch plastic lens implant is placed either just in front of the iris (anterior implant) or just behind it (posterior implant). More than a hundred brands of implants are now manufactured; most of the current implants are posterior ones. These rest against the back wall of the lens capsule and have plastic loops that jut out to hold the implant in position behind the iris. Posterior implants generally can be used only in conjunction with extracapsular surgery or phacoemulsification (although they can be inserted after certain intracapsular procedures). Intraocular lenses have been in wide use since 1977, and most ophthalmologists believe they are very safe, even for children.

Not all patients are able to receive an intraocular lens implant. For example, lens implantation may not be possible in individuals with certain eye diseases, including severe, recurrent uveitis (inflammation of the iris, ciliary body, or choroid); some active cases of proliferative diabetic retinopathy (see pages 46–47); and rubeosis iridis (new blood vessel growth on the iris, which usually occurs in people with diabetes). Most patients with open-angle glaucoma or elevated intraocular pressure are able to receive a lens implant; for those who can, posterior implants are usually preferred.

The most common form of implant is the single-focus lens. Unlike the natural lens of the eye, a single-focus lens cannot alter its shape to bring objects at different distances into ideal focus. Since most single-focus lenses are designed to bring distant objects into good focus, glasses are still required for reading. In general, new glasses cannot be prescribed until about six weeks after the surgery because the measurements needed for the prescription change as the eye heals. Still, if the eye is otherwise normal (for example, no retinal disease), patients with lens implants often have a visual acuity between 20/50 and 20/100 on the day after the operation and as good as 20/20 after several weeks.

Foldable implants have been available since the early 1990s. These implants, which may be made from silicone, acrylic, or a hydrogel, can be inserted into a smaller surgical opening than that required for other types of implants. The smaller opening may cause less trauma to the eye and lead to a quicker recovery.

Other innovations—bifocal and multifocal implants—are being actively investigated (see the sidebar at right). These lenses would work like a pair of bifocal glasses. In addition, recent research suggests that lenses made from a new polyacrylic material may reduce the incidence of opacification of the posterior lens capsule and thus the need for subsequent laser surgery (see page 20).

Implants require no insertion, removal, or care of any kind by the patient. Like any device, however, they have the potential for complications. The most common complication is glare or reduced vision occurring when there is a misalignment between the intraocular lens and the pupil.

Glasses. Although glasses are effective, the ones needed for lens replacement are heavy and awkward. They magnify objects by about 25%, causing objects to appear closer than they actually are—a somewhat disorienting sensation. Because of the thickness and curvature of the lenses, cataract glasses also magnify objects unequally and so have a distorting effect. In addition, they tend to limit peripheral vision. Given these problems, cataract glasses are no longer used after routine cataract surgery.

Contact lenses. Contact lenses provide patients with almost normal vision. Their major drawback is that some people have difficulty handling, removing, and cleaning them. The frequent handling of contact lenses may also increase the long-term risk of eye infections. Because the patient must be able to see when the contacts are not in place, a pair of cataract glasses is also necessary. For all of

NEW RESEARCH

New Lens May Provide Better Vision After Cataract Surgery

The standard treatment for cataracts involves removing the natural lens of the eye and replacing it with a single-focus intraocular lens. However, this lens does not allow the eye to focus easily at different distances, and some people need glasses to see close objects. A new study has found that multifocal intraocular lenses may safely treat the cataract and lessen the need for reading glasses.

The study involved 95 patients (age 14 to 40) without presbyopia who had a cataract in one eye. Fifty-four patients received the multifocal lens, and 41 received the single-focus lens. Nearly all patients achieved good distance vision with glasses, and the need for glasses to see distant objects did not differ between the groups. However, 98% of the multifocal group achieved good close vision, compared with 41% of the single-focus group. Fifty-one percent of the single-focus group needed reading glasses, compared with 9% of the multifocal group. Complications were rare in both groups.

Larger randomized studies with longer follow-up are needed. However, these results suggest that a multifocal lens can treat cataracts and preserve near vision focus in some patients.

OPHTHALMOLOGY
Volume 109, page 680
April 2002

Are You a Good Candidate for LASIK?

Laser in-situ keratomileusis (LASIK), a surgical procedure used to correct refractive errors, has become increasingly popular in recent years. Each year, more than 1.5 million people have the procedure to treat their nearsightedness (myopia), farsightedness (hyperopia), or astigmatism—all of which are caused by errors in the shape of the cornea (the transparent disk that covers the iris and pupil and plays a role in focusing light on the retina).

In LASIK, the surgeon cuts a hinged flap in the outer layer of the cornea, uses a laser to permanently reshape the underlying corneal tissue, and then returns the flap to its original position. Most people who undergo LASIK end up with better vision—and are less reliant on their eyeglasses or contact lenses—than before the surgery. Between 3% and 5% of patients experience complications such as dry eye, glare, halos, or reduced crispness of vision. Less than 1% of people experience more serious complications such as corneal scarring or infection, problems with the flap, or poorer vision than before the surgery.

Despite these encouraging numbers, LASIK is not right for everyone. Careful screening is essential to determine whether the benefits of the procedure outweigh its risks. The American Society of Cataract and Refractive Surgery has issued guidelines on who can, possibly can, and definitely cannot have laser surgery. But bear in mind that even with proper screening, you may experience problems with night vision, or your visual improvement may be temporary. Also, the long-term effects of the procedure are unknown because it has only been used for 11 years.

Ideal Candidates
You are more likely to have a successful LASIK procedure if you:

- Are over 18 years old.
- Have had a stable eyeglass or contact lens prescription for at least two years.
- Have a cornea thick enough for the surgeon to create the hinged flap.
- Have mild to moderate myopia, hyperopia, astigmatism, or a combination of these refractive errors.
- Have no vision-related or other diseases that would limit the effectiveness of the surgery or the ability of your eye to heal properly.
- Fully understand the risks and limitations of LASIK.

Less-Than-Ideal Candidates
Some people may not be perfect candidates for surgery but may still benefit from LASIK. You may be a less-than-ideal candidate if you:

- Have a history of dry eyes. Many people find that this condition becomes worse after surgery.
- Are taking medications (such as corticosteroids or immunosuppressants) or have diseases (such as autoimmune disorders) that can slow or prevent healing.
- Have scarring of the cornea.

Not-Yet-Ideal Candidates
Some people may not be able to have LASIK today but may be better candidates once their medical condition changes or LASIK technology improves. You may fall into this category if you:

- Are pregnant or nursing.
- Are under age 18.
- Have unstable vision.
- Have had ocular herpes within the past year. Eye surgery should not be considered until at least one year after diagnosis.
- Have severe myopia, hyperopia, or astigmatism. Existing technology can only correct certain degrees of refractive error. However, evolving technology may someday be appropriate for more severe errors.

Non-Candidates
LASIK is not an option if you:

- Have cataracts, advanced glaucoma, corneal diseases, corneal thinning disorders, or other eye diseases that affect your vision.
- Have not discussed the benefits and risks of LASIK with your ophthal-

these reasons, contact lenses are not routinely used. Both the contacts and glasses can be prescribed four to eight weeks after surgery.

Possible Complications of Surgery

Though cataract surgery is associated with a low rate of complications, problems may arise, especially in older adults or in those with general health problems. Patients should contact their doctor if any of the following symptoms develop during recovery from surgery: unusual pain or aching; persistent redness; bleeding; excessive tearing or discharge; any sudden vision changes; or seeing many bright

mologist and have not given your informed consent.

• Have unrealistic expectations about what LASIK can do.

Screening Tests
To determine if you are a candidate for LASIK, you need to have a complete eye examination conducted by an eye care professional. During the exam, the eye professional should do the following:

• Dilate your pupils to determine your exact prescription.

• Measure intraocular pressure and examine your retina.

• Measure the curvature of your cornea and pupils.

• Measure the topography (surface) of your eyes.

• Measure the thickness of your cornea.

In addition, the eye professional should collect the following information:

• Your history of wearing glasses. Assessing your eyeglass prescription will help determine whether your vision is stable.

• Your history of wearing contact lenses. Contact lenses can change the shape of the cornea, so you may need to stop wearing them for a period of time before your examination.

• Your history of eye or other diseases.

• Your history of eye problems (for example, lazy eye or double vision) or injury.

• An assessment of your work and lifestyle needs. LASIK can affect depth perception and close or distance vision, so people who rely heavily on these aspects of vision may want to consider a different method of correcting refractive errors.

The results of the eye examination should be reviewed by an ophthalmologist, who should discuss them with you. The ophthalmologist may decide that additional testing is required to determine whether you should undergo LASIK.

Meeting With the Ophthalmologist
Only ophthalmologists are qualified to perform LASIK. If you are considering LASIK, select an experienced refractive surgeon who performs the procedure frequently. For a recommendation, use the "Find an Eye M.D." feature on the Web site of the American Academy of Ophthalmology (www.aao.org).

When you meet with the ophthalmologist, be sure to ask these important questions:

• How long have you been performing LASIK and how many procedures have you performed?

• What is your success rate?

• How many of your patients achieve uncorrected vision in the 20/20 or 20/40 range with one operation?

• How many of your patients need repeat surgeries (enhancements)?

• What are the chances that I will achieve 20/20 vision?

• What is your complication rate?

• What are the possible risks or complications for me?

• What type of after-surgery care is required and who will handle it?

The ophthalmologist may decide that you are not a good candidate for LASIK. If you wish, you can get a second opinion from another ophthalmologist. However, if the second doctor also advises against LASIK, you should take "no" for an answer.

Realistic Expectations
It is important for potential LASIK patients to understand exactly what the procedure can and cannot do. For example, although LASIK does improve vision and lessen the need for glasses or contacts in most patients, it does not give every patient perfect vision. Also, 5% to 15% of patients need repeat surgeries to fully correct vision.

In addition, even when 20/20 vision is achieved, some patients experience a loss in the sharpness or crispness of their vision. Still, the vast majority of properly screened patients are happy with the improvement in their vision from the LASIK procedure.

flashes of light. Full recovery is considered to be the point when the eye is completely healed and vision has stabilized so that a final corrective prescription can be made.

Poor general health is not an impediment to cataract surgery. However, postoperative complications unrelated to the eye, such as an adverse reaction to the anesthetic, are more common in older patients with high blood pressure, diabetes, coronary heart disease (narrowing of the arteries that supply blood to the heart), or other medical problems. Inpatient surgery or an overnight hospital stay after surgery is rarely required. Postoperative death rates for cataract surgery are probably much less than 1 in 10,000.

Eye complications of cataract surgery are more common. For example, some studies have shown a 3% lifetime incidence of retinal detachment after cataract surgery. Retinal detachment is a vision-threatening condition in which the retina becomes separated from the underlying layers of the eye. Disruption of the posterior capsule during or following surgery (such as from laser treatment to clear clouding of the capsule) can increase this risk. Cystoid macular edema (a specific pattern of swelling of the central retina) is one of the most common postoperative complications. This swelling can result in visual impairment that is usually temporary but can occasionally be permanent. If the swelling does not resolve on its own, it may respond to eye drops. Other complications, such as significant bleeding inside the eye or large pieces of the cataract falling into the back of the eye (dropped nucleus), are extremely rare.

In up to 20% of extracapsular surgeries, the posterior capsule of the lens subsequently becomes cloudy and causes vision difficulties similar to those created by the original cataract. Laser treatment (see below) can correct this problem.

In a small minority of patients (about 1 per 1,000), an infection of the vitreous humor—called endophthalmitis—develops following cataract surgery. Patients who notice an increasingly red eye, blurred vision, and pain should see their ophthalmologist promptly. Typically, this condition can be treated with antibiotics and removal of some of the vitreous humor. Chronic low-grade endophthalmitis can also occur long after surgery (and can be difficult to diagnose), but it is very uncommon.

Laser Treatment Following Extracapsular Surgery

A YAG (yttrium, aluminum, and garnet) laser is used if vision is blurred by clouding of the remaining (posterior) portion of the lens capsule following extracapsular surgery. The YAG laser creates a hole in the posterior lens capsule by focusing a burst of energy on it, a procedure called a YAG capsulotomy. Vision clears promptly if the blurring is related to opacification of the posterior capsule.

The risk of retinal detachment rises fourfold with YAG capsulotomy, but is still very rare, affecting 1 in 300 people in the three or four years after surgery. This risk is increased in younger people and extremely nearsighted people. So, just as the initial decision to have cataract surgery is based on balancing possible risks and benefits, similar issues are weighed prior to YAG treatment.

Glaucoma

Glaucoma, the second leading cause of adult blindness in the United States after age-related macular degeneration, usually results from an intraocular pressure (IOP) that is too high for a patient's optic nerve to tolerate. About 3 million Americans have glaucoma and, because the condition does not cause symptoms in its early stages, half of them do not know it. Between 5 and 10 million others are at increased risk for the disorder owing to elevated IOP that is not yet considered glaucoma because it has not caused optic nerve damage.

The two principal forms of glaucoma are closed-angle and open-angle. Closed-angle glaucoma is a relatively uncommon disorder among whites and blacks but is almost as frequent as open-angle glaucoma among people of Chinese descent and some other Asian groups. About 20% of people with closed-angle glaucoma experience acute symptoms such as severe eye pain, nausea, or rapid loss of vision. The other 80% experience no symptoms. Open-angle glaucoma, which accounts for 90% of all glaucoma cases in the United States, is a slow, progressive disease that produces no obvious symptoms until its late stages.

Both types of glaucoma can lead to blindness by damaging the optic nerve. People with glaucoma can have normal IOP but still suffer damage to the optic nerve, since susceptibility to IOP level is quite individual, and risk factors other than IOP play a role. Early detection and treatment can usually control IOP and prevent optic nerve damage.

The occurrence of glaucoma rises with age. In one study, the prevalence of glaucoma was about 1% in the age 40 to 49 group; in those over age 70, it reached 2% to 3% among whites and 10% to 12% among blacks. The likelihood of having open-angle glaucoma is equal in men and women, but closed-angle glaucoma is more common in women.

CAUSES OF GLAUCOMA

Each day, the eye produces about one teaspoon of aqueous humor—a clear fluid that provides nutrients to, and carries waste products away from, the lens and cornea. (In other tissues, these functions are carried out by the blood, but the lens and cornea have no blood supply.) The ciliary body (which surrounds the lens) produces the aqueous humor, which flows from behind the iris through the pupil and

NEW RESEARCH

Age Is a Stronger Glaucoma Risk Factor for Hispanics

Hispanics are more likely than whites (but less likely than blacks) to have glaucoma. In addition, increased age seems to be a more important risk factor for Hispanics than for other ethnic groups, according to a recent study.

Researchers examined the eyes of 4,774 Hispanic people living in two counties in Arizona. Open-angle glaucoma was present in 94 (2%) of them. Gender, blood pressure, and cigarette smoking were not risk factors, but increased age was. Glaucoma incidence rose progressively with age, from 0.5% of participants age 41 to 49 to 13% of those age 80 and older. This increase with age was greater than previous studies had shown for black and white populations.

Only 36 (38%) of the participants with glaucoma knew they had the condition before the study, compared with a 50% undiagnosed rate for black and white populations. As other studies have suggested, relying solely on intraocular pressure to determine the presence of glaucoma would have missed 80% of cases. These cases were found through more detailed eye examinations.

The researchers say more studies are needed to determine the prevalence of glaucoma in other ethnic groups.

JOURNAL OF THE AMERICAN MEDICAL ASSOCIATION
Volume 119, page 1819
December 2001

Glaucoma Drugs 2003

Drug Type	Generic Name	Brand Name	Estimated Cost* (Generic Cost)
Beta-blockers	betaxolol	Betoptic S	0.25%: $6 (0.5%: $5)
	carteolol	Ocupress	1%: $6 ($4)
	levobunolol	Betagan	0.25%: $5 ($3)
	metipranolol	OptiPranolol	0.3%: $4 ($3)
	timolol	Timoptic Ocumeter	0.25%: $4 ($3)
		Timoptic-XE Ocumeter	0.25%: $6 ($3)
Adrenergic agonists	apraclonidine	Iopidine	0.5%: $12
	brimonidine	Alphagan	0.2%: $7
	dipivefrin	Propine	0.1%: $5 ($3)
	epinephrine	Epifrin	0.5%: $3
Miotics	carbachol	Isopto Carbachol	2.25%: $2
	echothiophate	Phospholine Iodide	0.125%: $7
	pilocarpine	Isopto Carpine	2%: $1 ($1)
		Pilocar	2%: $3 ($1)
		Pilopine HS	4% and gel: $38
Carbonic anhydrase inhibitors	acetazolamide	Diamox	250 mg: $56 ($44)
	brinzolamide	Azopt	1%: $5
	dorzolamide	Trusopt Ocumeter	2%: $5
	methazolamide	Neptazane	50 mg: $107 ($79)
Topical prostaglandins	bimatoprost	Lumigan	0.03%: $20
	latanoprost	Xalatan	0.005%: $20
	travoprost	Travatan	0.004%: $18
	unoprostone	Rescula	0.15%: $9

into the anterior (front) chamber of the eye; it then drains from the eye through a spongy network of connective tissue called the trabecular meshwork, where it ultimately enters the bloodstream. An alternate drainage system, the uveoscleral pathway, is located behind the trabecular meshwork. Ordinarily, fluid production and drainage are in balance, and IOP is between 10 and 20 mm Hg (millimeters of mercury, the same units of measurement used for blood pressure).

In those with open-angle glaucoma whose IOP is higher than normal, ophthalmologists suspect that a partial blockage of the trabecular meshwork traps the aqueous humor. Exactly how this happens is unclear. As more aqueous humor is formed than is removed, the blockage causes an increase of IOP. Pressure does not climb high enough in its early stages to cause discomfort or any easily perceived vision changes. When IOP remains elevated or continues to

How They Work	Comments
These eye drops decrease the production of aqueous humor.	Lowered pulse rate, low blood pressure, asthma, fainting, drowsiness, confusion, depression, and dry eyes may occur in some patients. Beta-blockers usually should not be used by people who have severe lung or heart ailments.
These eye drops decrease aqueous humor production and increase its drainage.	Associated with highest rate of allergic reactions. Patients may also experience red eyes, pain, headaches, eye irritation, high blood pressure, or rapid heart rate. The drops may stain contact lenses (except dipivefrin). Used with caution in patients with heart ailments or high blood pressure.
These eye drops or ointment increase drainage of aqueous humor through the trabecular meshwork by constricting the pupil.	Patients may experience dim vision (especially at night) or increased nearsightedness. Echothiophate may cause cataracts, so in general, it is used only when cataracts have been removed.
These oral drugs (acetazolamide and methazolamide) and eye drops (brinzolamide and dorzolamide) decrease the production of aqueous humor.	Up to 50% of patients taking oral carbonic anhydrase inhibitors have side effects, including tingling of hands and feet, stomach upset, depression, kidney stones, and, more rarely, anemia; thus, these drugs are used only when absolutely necessary to avoid surgery and preserve eyesight. Brinzolamide and dorzolamide eye drops do not have such side effects.
These eye drops increase the drainage of aqueous humor from the eye.	A change in eye color is the most noticeable side effect, with about 3% of patients experiencing an increase in brown pigmentation. Other side effects include stinging, burning, redness, and foreign body sensation.

* Average wholesale prices to pharmacists per milliliter for eye drops or for 100 pills. (There are about 30 eye drops per milliliter; the solution strength is given.) If a generic version is available, the cost is listed in parentheses. Costs to consumers are higher. Source: *Red Book, 2002* (Medical Economics Data, publishers).

rise, however, fibers in the optic nerve are compressed and die, leading to a gradual loss of vision over a period of several years. In some people, even a normal level of IOP is sufficient to contribute to optic nerve damage.

Possible genetic clues to open-angle glaucoma have been reported. Mutations causing glaucoma have been identified in the chromosome 1 open-angle glaucoma gene (GLC1A), which directs the production of myocilin. The normal role of myocilin is unknown, but it is a protein that appears to be involved in the function of the eye. Mutations in the gene that directs the production of optineurin have also been associated with glaucoma.

Inhaled corticosteroids—commonly used to treat asthma—and nasal sprays with corticosteroids appear to raise the risk of open-angle glaucoma or elevated IOP, possibly by inhibiting the outflow of aqueous humor. One study found about a 44% increase in risk among patients taking at least 1,500 micrograms of inhaled corticosteroids continuously over at least a three-month period. Asthma patients taking inhaled corticosteroids should not stop their medication but instead should be carefully monitored. Oral corticosteroids may have the same effect. In one study, the risk of high IOP or glaucoma was about 40% greater in users of these drugs than in nonusers. This effect occurred as early as two months after starting therapy and grew in incidence with longer use and higher doses. IOP returned to normal within two weeks of stopping oral corticosteroids. Patients who must use these drugs (for asthma, arthritis, sinusitis, or chronic bronchitis, for example) should have their IOP and vision monitored regularly.

Closed-angle glaucoma is caused by a blockage of aqueous humor at the pupil, leading to a bowing forward of the iris that prevents aqueous humor from reaching the trabecular meshwork. The sudden occlusion of the outflow of aqueous humor induces a rapid buildup of extremely high IOP that can lead to severe, permanent vision damage within a day or two.

SYMPTOMS OF GLAUCOMA

Open-angle glaucoma generally involves both eyes, although the changes in IOP and the extent of damage to the optic nerve often differ between them.

Because of the way the optic nerve is structured, the first nerve fibers damaged are those necessary for peripheral vision. People with advanced open-angle glaucoma can have 20/20 vision when looking straight ahead but may have blind spots (scotomas) for images located to the sides of, above, or below the central visual field. The damaging effects are often undetected by visual field tests (perimetry; see page 26) until as much as 40% of the optic nerve fibers are destroyed. Eventually, the fibers needed for central vision may be lost as well.

Unlike the open-angle form, closed-angle glaucoma sometimes occurs as acute attacks, as IOP rises rapidly to a dangerous level. Signs of an attack include severe pain in the eye, nausea and vomiting, blurred vision, and seeing rainbow-colored halos around lights. The disorder usually affects both eyes, although attacks typically do not occur in both eyes at once; after an initial attack, there is a 40% to 80% chance of a similar attack occurring in the other eye within the next 5 to 10 years if no treatment is provided.

NEW RESEARCH

Nearsightedness Associated With An Increased Risk of Glaucoma

People with myopia (nearsightedness) may be at increased risk for glaucoma, even if they do not have high intraocular pressure (IOP), according to a recent study.

Researchers in Sweden gave eye examinations to 32,918 people (age 57 to 79). After glaucoma was diagnosed in 540 eyes (0.83%), these patients were given more detailed eye exams.

Glaucoma was present in 0.6% of eyes with hyperopia (farsightedness), 0.9% of eyes with normal vision, and 1.5% of eyes with moderate to high myopia. This association was present in both men and women and in all age groups. The effect of myopia varied with IOP: In eyes with an IOP of 15 mm Hg or less, glaucoma occurred four times more often in myopic than in hyperopic eyes. The relationship between myopia and glaucoma declined with increasing IOP; in eyes with an IOP of 31 mm Hg or greater, myopia did not increase the risk of glaucoma. Also, IOP was higher in myopic eyes without glaucoma (16.2 mm Hg) than in hyperopic eyes without glaucoma (15.7 mm Hg).

These findings strengthen the theory that IOP is a risk factor for glaucoma, not a cause, and point to myopia as another important risk factor.

ACTA OPHTHALMOLOGICA SCANDINAVICA
Volume 79, page 560
December 2001

PREVENTION OF GLAUCOMA

A recent study found that some people with elevated IOP may be able to delay or prevent the onset of glaucoma by using IOP-lowering eye drops (see the sidebar at right). However, not everyone who develops glaucoma has an elevated IOP. Therefore, regular glaucoma screening is important.

DIAGNOSIS OF GLAUCOMA

An eye examination for glaucoma involves IOP measurement, viewing of the optic disc, and visual field testing. A common recommendation is for whites to be examined every two years after age 50 and for blacks to be examined every two years after age 40, as optic nerve damage is uncommon before age 50 in whites but can occur as many as 10 years earlier in blacks. Available evidence suggests that cardiovascular disease, diabetes, and high degrees of nearsightedness increase the risk of nerve damage from glaucoma.

IOP is no longer used alone to diagnose glaucoma, because some people with elevated IOP do not develop optic nerve damage and others develop glaucoma despite normal IOP. A high IOP raises the index of suspicion, but other tests are required to make a diagnosis. In one study, individuals with an IOP at or greater than 22 mm Hg or an IOP difference of 5 mm Hg or more between the two eyes had a 17% risk of developing glaucoma in 10 years and a 26% risk in 15 years. By contrast, those with initial IOP measurements below 16 mm Hg had only a 1% and 2% risk of glaucoma within 10 and 15 years, respectively.

Tests for Glaucoma

Ophthalmologists use three types of tests or examinations to screen people at risk for glaucoma, to make the diagnosis, and to follow patients during treatment: tonometry to measure IOP; ophthalmoscopy to inspect the optic nerve; and perimetry to test the visual fields. A high IOP warrants further testing, and the final diagnosis is made by also finding evidence of optic nerve damage typical of glaucoma or by identifying characteristic defects in the visual fields. The distinction between open- and closed-angle glaucoma is made by examining the front part of the eye to check the angle where the iris meets the cornea, using a special technique known as gonioscopy.

Tonometry. Tonometry measures IOP by assessing the amount of force necessary to make a slight indentation in a small area of the

NEW RESEARCH

Eye Drops May Delay Glaucoma In People With Elevated IOP

People with elevated intraocular pressure (IOP) may be able to delay or even prevent the onset of glaucoma by using IOP-lowering eye drops, according to a recent study.

More than 1,600 people (age 40 to 80) who had higher than normal IOP but no evidence of glaucoma were randomized to either observation or treatment with eye drops. Multiple medications were added as necessary to reduce IOP by 20% or more and to achieve an IOP of 24 mm Hg or less. All participants had eye examinations and updated their medical histories every six months.

After five years, IOP had decreased by an average of 23% in the medication group, compared with a 4% decrease in the observation group. Approximately 4% of the medication group and 10% of the observation group developed glaucoma during the follow-up period. There was no evidence that any serious ocular or systemic side effects occurred more often in those treated with eye drops than in the observation group.

This study is the largest so far to show that IOP-lowering eye drops are safe and effective in delaying or preventing glaucoma in people with elevated IOP. The researchers say, however, that not everyone with high IOP is an ideal candidate for medication, and that doctors should consider each patient's individual health status.

ARCHIVES OF OPHTHALMOLOGY
Volume 120, page 701
June 2002

cornea. The most effective way to do this is with applanation tonometry. In this test, anesthetic eye drops are given to numb the eye and slight pressure is applied to the cornea with a small instrument while the doctor looks through a table-mounted microscope (slit lamp). A hand-held device (Tono-Pen) is also relatively accurate. A less-effective test is air puff tonometry, in which IOP is measured with a quick puff of warm air. Anesthetic eye drops are not needed for this procedure because the air-puff tonometer does not touch the eye. Tonometry is painless and poses virtually no risk to the cornea.

Ophthalmoscopy. Examination of the optic nerve is an important part of the initial diagnosis of glaucoma, and periodic photographs of the optic nerve are valuable to follow the progress of the disorder during treatment. To perform ophthalmoscopy, the doctor dilates the patient's pupils with eye drops and then uses an ophthalmoscope—a special instrument with a small light on the end—to magnify and examine the optic nerve. One version, called a slit lamp, is basically a specialized microscope that allows three-dimensional visualization of the optic nerve. The examination is conducted in a darkened room. Signs of a damaged optic nerve are "cupping" in its center and a loss of its normal pink color. A number of imaging systems are now used to supplement ophthalmoscopy, including laser-based image formation and special polarized light reflection measurement.

Perimetry. One reason to perform this test is the suspicion of glaucoma. While the patient looks straight ahead at a bowl-shaped white area, a computer presents lights in fixed locations around the bowl. The patient indicates each time he or she sees the light. Perimetry provides a "map" of the visual fields. The type of vision loss associated with glaucoma is relatively specific, and perimetry can detect the typical visual-field defects that cannot be explained by other disorders. If glaucoma has been diagnosed or is suspected, periodic perimetry examinations are an important part of the follow-up. This test takes about 10 minutes to perform.

Quicker methods that take only two minutes per eye are now being implemented for screening purposes. Among the most promising of these new tests is Frequency Doubling Technology. This test measures damage to the larger retinal ganglion cells, which may be more likely to be damaged by glaucoma.

TREATMENT OF GLAUCOMA

Glaucoma is a chronic disorder that cannot be cured. Open-angle glaucoma can often be treated safely and effectively with medication

Using Glaucoma Eye Drops Correctly

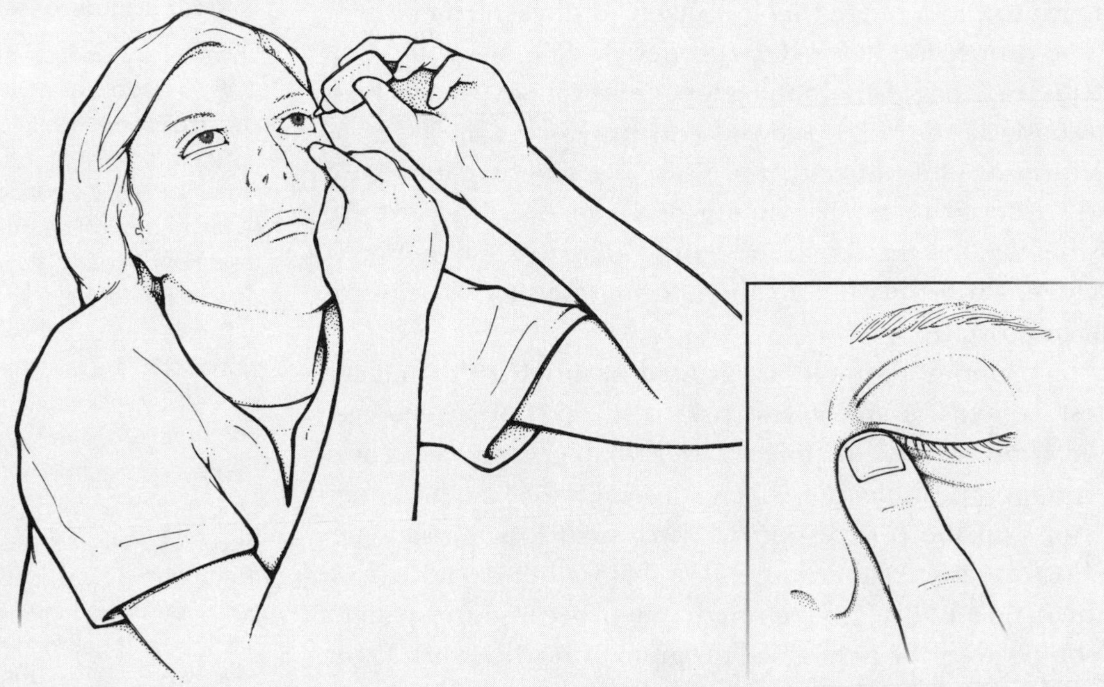

The correct use of eye drops for glaucoma allows the medication to work more effectively and lessens systemic side effects (adverse effects in areas of the body other than the eye). Keep in mind that the following instructions are general suggestions. Your doctor may have different or more specific directions.

First, wash your hands. If you use more than one eye-drop medication, carefully check the label on the bottle to ensure you are using the right one. If the medicine's instructions say to shake before using, shake the bottle. To prevent contamination, be sure the tip of the dropper does not touch anything (for example, your fingers or a countertop) before or after putting the drops in your eye.

Tilt your head back and use the tip of one of your fingers to pull down your lower eyelid to create a pocket. Squeeze a single drop of medicine into the pocket; try not to let the dropper touch your eye or eyelid. Slowly let go of your eyelid and close your eye but don't squeeze it closed too tightly, because this could cause the medicine to run out of your eye. Next, place one of your fingers on the inside corner of your eye (by your nose) for two to three minutes to stop the medicine from entering your nasal ducts. This keeps the medicine in your eye and helps prevent systemic side effects.

If you are required to take more than one eye-drop medication at the same time each day, wait at least five minutes after taking the first medication before using the second one. This delay allows the first medication to be absorbed fully and prevents it from being washed out of the eye by the second medication. If you take a third medication, wait another five minutes after the second medication before taking it.

If you have trouble getting the drops in your eye because of shaking hands, try resting your hand against the side of your face to keep your hand steady. If this doesn't work, buy 1- or 2-lb. wrist weights and place them around your wrists when using the eye drops. These weights are available in sporting goods stores and often can steady a shaking hand enough to allow eye drops to be applied.

or surgery, though lifelong therapy is almost always necessary. Decisions on when to start treatment are based on evidence of optic nerve damage, visual field loss, and risk factors—not just on IOP. Acute closed-angle glaucoma is an ophthalmic emergency. Patients with the symptoms of closed-angle glaucoma (see page 24) should contact their ophthalmologist immediately.

The overall aim in the treatment of any form of glaucoma is to prevent damage to the optic nerve by lowering IOP and consistently maintaining it within a range that is unlikely to cause further nerve damage. The proper target for IOP is generally 25% below the IOP level at the time of diagnosis. In the few patients with extremely high pressure (above 35 mm Hg), the percent decrease in the target is substantially more. Once the target pressure is achieved, patients are monitored to confirm stability of the optic nerve. If progressive damage is detected at the target pressure, a new, lower target pressure is selected. Unfortunately, treatment cannot reverse optic nerve damage or improve vision.

The choice among therapies is dictated by an effort to achieve the greatest benefits at the lowest risk, cost, and inconvenience. Both medical and surgical treatments are available; each has its own complications and possible side effects. In some cases, medical therapy does not stop the progression of visual field loss, possibly because the doctor has selected a target IOP that is not low enough, or because the target IOP is not reached (often because the patient does not comply with the prescribed program of medication). Laser or traditional surgery can be successful even early in the course of treatment. Complications such as the development of cataracts occur in only a small number of patients, and the risk is lower with laser surgery than with traditional surgery.

Although medications are frequently used first, a recent controlled trial found surgery to be a reasonable first option.

Medical Treatment

Periodic follow-up examinations to monitor IOP, visual fields, side effects, and the appearance of the optic nerve are essential during treatment. Follow-up visits may be as frequent as daily or weekly during the initiation or adjustment of treatment for those with severe optic nerve damage or extreme elevations of IOP, or only every three to six months for patients with stable IOP and minimal optic nerve damage.

Research indicates that some people tend not to adhere to their glaucoma treatment regimen. Two main factors contribute to this problem: taking a large number of other prescription medications and having to take the glaucoma medication more than twice a day. Researchers suggest that patients may be confused by the number of prescription drugs they need to take, their ophthalmologist may not have adequately explained the medication's importance, or the patients may have stopped taking the medication on

NEW FINDING

Reducing IOP Delays Progression Of Newly Diagnosed Glaucoma

Lowering intraocular pressure (IOP) in people newly diagnosed with glaucoma has long been thought to prevent vision loss. Now, the results from the first placebo-controlled trial of the treatment of early glaucoma support this theory.

Researchers randomly assigned 255 people (age 50 to 80) with newly diagnosed glaucoma and normal or elevated IOP either to have no treatment (the control group) or to undergo laser trabecular surgery and use betaxolol (Betoptic) eye drops. All participants were examined every three months, and participants in the control group were offered treatment if their glaucoma began to worsen.

After approximately six years, IOP decreased by 5.1 mm Hg (25%) in the treatment group and was unchanged in the control group. Glaucoma progression was more common in the control group (62%) than in the treatment group (45%). Progression occurred after approximately 4 years in the control group and 5½ years in the treatment group. Side effects in the treatment group were rare, although cataracts were more common than in the control group.

The study did not include people with advanced glaucoma and elevated IOP levels, but the researchers theorize that lowering IOP would offer them the same benefit.

ARCHIVES OF OPHTHALMOLOGY
Volume 120, page 1268
October 2002

their own because of its cost or side effects. Patients must understand the need to take their glaucoma medication, how often it should be administered, and what side effects can occur. And they should consult their ophthalmologist before they stop taking a glaucoma medication.

Eye drops. Eye drops are the most common medical treatment for glaucoma because they have fewer systemic effects (effects other than those on the eye) than oral medications. Five types of eye drops are currently used: topical prostaglandins, beta-blockers, carbonic anhydrase inhibitors, adrenergic agonists, and miotics (see the chart on pages 22–23).

Beta-blockers, such as timolol (Timoptic) or levobunolol (Betagan), reduce IOP by diminishing the production of aqueous humor.

The topical prostaglandins bimatoprost (Lumigan), latanoprost (Xalatan), travoprost (Travatan), and unoprostone (Rescula) reduce IOP by increasing outflow of aqueous humor through the uveoscleral pathway. These medications appear to be at least as effective as timolol (Timoptic). The first of these drugs, latanoprost, was approved by the U.S. Food and Drug Administration (FDA) for patients who have experienced significant adverse reactions to other IOP-lowering medications or for those in whom these other medications are ineffective. Owing to their low levels of side effects and their efficacy in lowering IOP, topical prostaglandins are now the most frequently used drugs for glaucoma.

In approval studies, travoprost lowered IOP by 7 to 8 mm Hg in people with an initial IOP of 25 to 27 mm Hg, and bimatoprost lowered IOP to 17 mm Hg or less in two thirds of patients. In a separate study of patients with glaucoma whose IOP was in the normal range, latanoprost lowered IOP by an average of 3.6 mm Hg when patients were given 50 micrograms of the drug once a day for three weeks.

Topical prostaglandins can be used in conjunction with a second medication to produce greater reductions in IOP. One interesting side effect has emerged from research with these drugs: About 3% of patients taking them for six months experience gradual changes in eye color. Other possible side effects include burning, stinging, and increased eyelash growth.

Previously available only as tablets, carbonic anhydrase inhibitors such as dorzolamide (Trusopt) and brinzolamide (Azopt) can be taken as eye drops. Like the tablets, the drops decrease production of aqueous humor. In one study, a 2% solution of dorzolamide reduced IOP by 18%, compared with a 2% reduction experienced

NEW RESEARCH

Medications and Surgery Equally Effective for Early Glaucoma

Medications and surgery appear to be equally beneficial for open-angle glaucoma for at least the first five years after treatment, according to the initial results from an ongoing clinical trial.

Researchers randomly assigned 607 people with newly diagnosed glaucoma either to receive medications (usually beginning with beta-blocker eye drops) or to undergo filtration surgery (trabeculectomy). Further treatment was given as needed to reduce intraocular pressure (IOP).

After up to five years, visual field loss did not differ between the two treatment groups. Visual acuity loss was greater in the surgery group at the beginning of the study, but by the fourth year, it was the same in both groups. The average reduction in IOP was greater with surgery than with medication (48% vs. 35%), but cataract removal was needed more often following surgery than with medical treatment (12% vs. 3%).

The researchers say that their findings to date do not show a need to change current treatment strategies for open-angle glaucoma.

OPHTHALMOLOGY
Volume 108, page 1943
November 2001

New Device To Treat Glaucoma

In July 2001, the U.S. Food and Drug Administration approved a new treatment for people with open-angle glaucoma who are unable to lower their intraocular pressure (IOP) adequately with medication. The treatment involves implanting a small device in the eye. The device, called the AquaFlow Collagen Glaucoma Drainage Device, helps lower IOP by facilitating the drainage of aqueous humor from the eye. The procedure is less invasive than traditional surgery for glaucoma, and early results suggest that it is just as effective.

The Device

The AquaFlow Collagen Glaucoma Drainage Device looks like a tiny cigarette filter. Made of collagen, it is approximately three quarters of an inch long and the width of a pencil lead. The device is implanted into the eye using a type of filtration surgery known as non-penetrating deep sclerectomy. In this procedure, the surgeon cuts a flap in the sclera (the white part of the eye), removes a small area of tissue below the flap, and places the device in the resulting space. Once inserted, the device absorbs some of the aqueous humor and swells. The flap is repositioned to cover the device and then stitched into place. Over the next six to nine months, the device slowly dissolves and is absorbed by the body.

Originally, researchers thought that the AquaFlow device would work like a wick to draw aqueous humor out of the eye. However, they now claim that the device acts as a space-filler to prevent fibrous tissue from covering over the space made by the surgery. Once the device dissolves, they report, a permanent space is created through which aqueous humor can leave the eye, thereby lowering IOP.

Early Results

Clinical trials of the AquaFlow device are now being conducted. In one study carried out at nine sites in the United States, researchers implanted the device into 194 eyes. One year after surgery, 92% of the eyes had an IOP of 21 mm Hg or less, compared with 36% of the eyes before surgery. Also, 66% of the eyes had an IOP of 17 mm Hg or lower, compared with none before the surgery. The device also seemed to reduce the need for glaucoma medications. One year after the surgery, 83% of the eyes required fewer medications than before the surgery. These results are similar to those achieved with traditional filtration surgery, the gold standard surgical treatment for glaucoma. However, no controlled trials have objectively compared the standard surgery with the AquaFlow device.

Complication rates for the AquaFlow procedure are similar to or lower than those for traditional filtration surgery. In the study mentioned above, only 1% of patients experienced complications, but the duration of the study was not long enough to detect long-term problems. Possible complications of the AquaFlow procedure include leaking from the wound, bleeding, retinal detachment,

by placebo patients. Doctors have found that the drops have fewer side effects than the oral form (see pages 31–32).

Adrenergic agonists, such as epinephrine (Epifrin) or dipivefrin (Propine), can increase the outflow of aqueous humor but work primarily by decreasing its production. Brimonidine (Alphagan) and apraclonidine (Iopidine) are adrenergic agonists that reduce IOP by decreasing production of aqueous humor and increasing its drainage through the uveoscleral pathway. Brimonidine appears to lower IOP by 4 to 6 mm Hg and is taken in two or three daily doses.

Miotics, such as pilocarpine (Pilocar) or carbachol (Isopto Carbachol), increase the outflow of aqueous humor by improving its flow through the trabecular meshwork.

In general, eye drops are applied one to four times a day, regularly and on schedule. Drops can cause local side effects, such as burning, stinging, tearing, itching, or redness in the eye. Because some amount of the drug is quickly absorbed into the body, sys-

cataracts, low IOP, infection, inflammation, and swelling or clouding of the cornea. People who have closed-angle glaucoma or are allergic to collagen or products derived from pigs should not undergo the AquaFlow procedure.

One main disadvantage of traditional filtration surgery for glaucoma is that a buildup of fibrous tissue blocks the space created by the surgery, and repeat operations are required. The AquaFlow device claims to prevent this process by occupying the space during the period when the body's natural healing process would try to fill it. Consequently, patients do not need to take medication to halt the healing process, as do some patients after traditional filtration surgery. Traditional surgery can also increase the chance of having an IOP that is too low. But because sclerectomy does not cut all the way through the sclera, this risk is reduced in people who undergo the AquaFlow procedure.

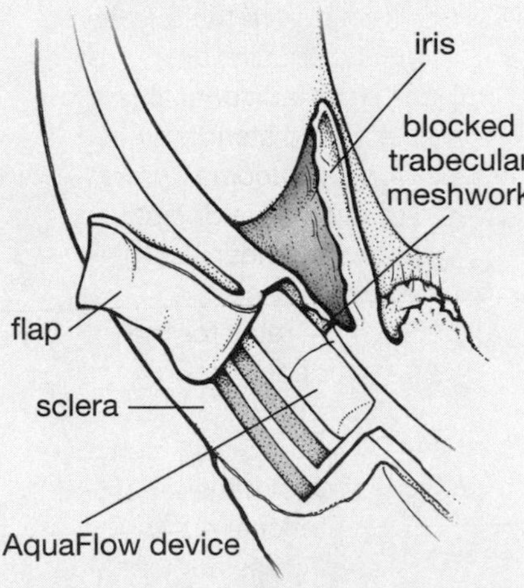

The surgeon cuts a flap in the sclera, removes some tissue, and places the AquaFlow device into the resulting space.

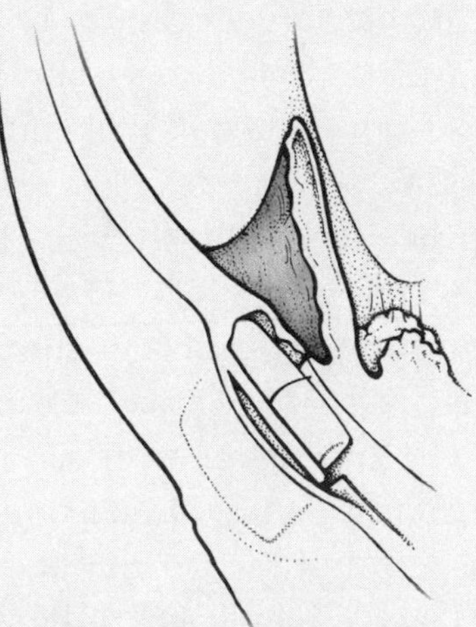

The surgeon closes the flap over the AquaFlow device.

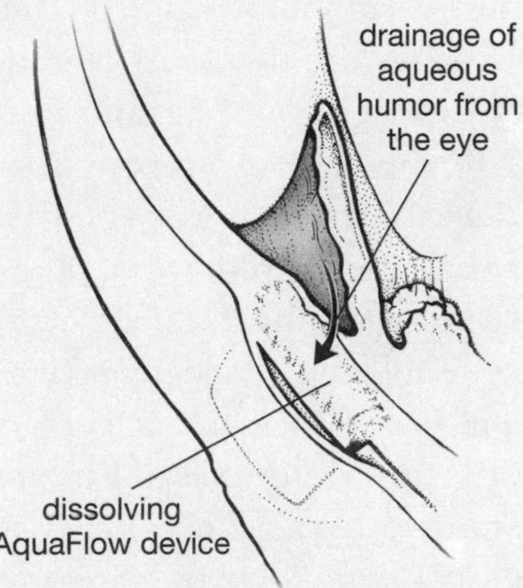

The AquaFlow device slowly dissolves over time, creating a space through which aqueous humor leaves the eye.

temic side effects may occur. For example, beta-blocker drops taken for glaucoma can lower blood pressure at the same time they lower IOP. (Conversely, a beta-blocker tablet taken for high blood pressure may also lower IOP.) Obviously, doctors must tailor therapy to the individual needs of each patient, taking into account the presence of such conditions as high blood pressure.

For more information on using eye drops correctly, see the feature on page 27.

Oral medications. Acetazolamide (Diamox) and methazolamide (Neptazane), both carbonic anhydrase inhibitors, are the only glaucoma medications that are taken orally. Because of their side effects, they are generally used only when optic nerve damage continues or seems likely to continue despite topical treatment at the greatest tolerable dose. The drugs initially lower IOP by 20% to 30%, on average, but significant systemic side effects (such as numbness or tingling in the extremities, malaise, and loss of appetite) and occasional serious complications (such as depression, kidney stones, diarrhea, and damage to blood cells) can limit their utility.

Surgery

About 10% of patients with open-angle glaucoma undergo surgery. They choose surgery either by preference or because they experience serious side effects from medications, do not comply with or respond adequately to drug treatment, are unable to take their medications properly, or have medical conditions or allergies that do not permit maximal drug therapy. While surgery cannot restore lost vision, the two most common surgical procedures—laser trabecular surgery and filtration surgery—can reduce IOP by improving the drainage of aqueous humor.

Laser trabecular surgery. In this procedure, 80 to 100 tiny laser burns are made in the area of the trabecular meshwork. The procedure increases the drainage of aqueous humor, possibly by stimulating the metabolic activity of trabecular cells. The procedure takes about 15 minutes and is performed on an outpatient basis using eye drops for anesthesia. Eye pressure must be tested one hour after surgery because IOP may rise as a result of the treatment. Postoperative complications are minimal and include eye inflammation, blurred vision, and minimal discomfort, which usually last for only about 24 hours.

It takes up to six weeks to determine whether the procedure has been effective. If the procedure reduced IOP, medications can sometimes be continued at lower doses. As with many treatments, however, the effect of surgery diminishes with time in some people. About 40% of patients treated with lasers need an additional medical treatment or some other form of surgery within five years.

Filtration surgery. Filtration surgery (trabeculectomy) uses conventional surgical instruments to open a passage through the trabecular meshwork, so that aqueous humor can drain into surrounding tissues. The operation takes about 20 minutes, is performed on an outpatient basis under local anesthesia, and is relatively safe and long-lasting. In general, a protective eye patch must be worn for one day, and patients are advised to avoid driving, bending over, and any type of strenuous activity for at least a week. If necessary, the drainage flap can be loosened or tightened after the surgery with a new laser procedure, called suture lysis, or with special adjustable sutures.

Researchers are studying whether antimetabolites (substances that block biological processes) such as mitomycin (Mutamycin) or fluorouracil (Efudex) will improve results from filtration surgery. These drugs, applied during or in the days after surgery, interfere with normal wound healing so that the openings created by the procedure do not close. Currently, these antimetabolites are used in less favorable cases, such as in patients who have had unsuccessful prior surgery or younger patients who tend to have strong wound-healing abilities and therefore have a smaller chance of effective filtration surgery.

About half of patients can discontinue glaucoma medications completely after filtration surgery; 35% to 40% still need some medications; and 10% to 15% will need some additional type of surgery, such as cyclodestructive or shunt surgery (see below). Filtration surgery poses some risk of infection and bleeding in the eye and requires a longer recovery period than laser surgery. About one third of patients experience worsening of cataracts within five years. It is not clear whether the surgery itself causes the cataracts or whether they would have occurred anyway, but they can be surgically removed when necessary.

About 1% of patients who undergo filtration surgery get a bacterial infection; symptoms include pain, redness, a sticky discharge, and blurred vision. Although the infection is usually controlled with antibiotics, it can become very serious. Late-onset infections may be an increasing problem, particularly as antimetabolites are used more often. Therefore, patients should be sure to discuss follow-up plans with their doctor and know what symptoms to watch for.

Shunts. If filtration surgery is unsuccessful, one alternative is the creation of a new passage to drain excess aqueous humor using a shunt of plastic tubing. The effectiveness of shunts (or tube-shunts) is being studied widely. In one study, a shunt called the Baerveldt implant lowered IOP in 72% of patients with previously uncontrolled glaucoma.

Cyclodestructive surgery. This form of surgery destroys the ciliary body (which produces aqueous humor) using a laser. Patients may experience some pain and inflammation after surgery; recovery time depends on the type and extent of surgery. This procedure does not require an incision, so normal activity can be resumed earlier than after some filtration operations. Visual recovery, however, may be slower than for the other types of surgery. Cyclodestructive surgery is generally used only when other measures have failed, because it has a less predictable outcome and poses a greater risk to the eye (for example, inflammation, cataracts, or an IOP that is too low for a prolonged time).

NEW RESEARCH

Filtration Surgery for Glaucoma Increases Risk of Cataracts

Surgical treatment for glaucoma increases the risk of cataracts, and a new study has now quantified the risk.

Between 1988 and 1992, 591 patients with glaucoma that could not be controlled with medication were randomized to undergo either laser trabecular surgery or filtration surgery (trabeculectomy). Additional surgical procedures were performed as needed.

During a follow-up period of 7 to 11 years, cataracts developed in half of the eyes. Eyes treated with filtration surgery (either first or after laser surgery) were 80% more likely to develop cataracts than eyes treated with laser surgery alone. The risk of cataracts was only increased by 50% in eyes that underwent filtration surgery without complications, but the risk was more than doubled when complications occurred. Cataracts were nearly three times more likely in eyes that required a second filtration surgery. Diabetes and increased age also increased the risk of cataracts.

The researchers stress that many of the patients who underwent treatment did not experience cataracts, that cataracts occurred in patients assigned to both treatment groups, and that having laser surgery before filtration surgery did not increase the eventual risk of cataracts.

ARCHIVES OF OPHTHALMOLOGY
Volume 119, page 1771
December 2001

Treatment of Closed-Angle Glaucoma

During an acute attack of closed-angle glaucoma, IOP may be high enough to damage the optic nerve or obstruct one of the blood vessels feeding the retina. Unless the pressure is relieved promptly, blindness can occur within a day or two. The goals of treatment are to protect the optic nerve by rapidly stopping the attack, to protect the other eye, and to carry out definitive treatment—making a hole in the iris (iridotomy) or, much more rarely, a surgical filtering operation to allow a path for the flow of aqueous humor. These procedures are effective for acute cases, and repeat treatment is rarely necessary. A preventive iridotomy in the other eye is always recommended because of the high likelihood that it will be involved in a future acute attack. In some patients, a chronic form of closed-angle glaucoma may require eye drops or filtration surgery.

Age-related Macular Degeneration

In the United States, age-related macular degeneration (AMD)—also referred to as senile macular degeneration—is the leading cause of severe and irreversible loss of central vision in people over age 50, affecting 1.7 million Americans. Although there are various definitions of severe vision loss, a commonly accepted one is a decline in visual acuity to 20/200 (which corresponds to seeing only the big "E" on an eye chart) or less.

As the name suggests, the prevalence of severe vision loss from AMD increases with age, and most patients with visual impairment from AMD are age 60 or older. Some features of AMD can be detected in up to one fourth of people over age 65 and in one third of those over age 80. Slightly more than 2% of individuals age 65 or older are blind in one or both eyes because of AMD. Fortunately, however, most cases of AMD do not result in serious vision loss.

ANATOMY OF THE RETINA

The retina is the light-sensitive layer of nerve tissue that lines the inner eye. It is made up of millions of tiny nerve receptor cells called cones and rods. Light rays reflected from an object are focused by the cornea and lens onto the retina; the cones and rods send impulses through the optic nerve to the brain in response to light.

The most sensitive portion of the retina is a small area at its cen-

How To Enlarge Text on the Internet

A variety of options are available to make computers more accessible to people with low vision, including talking software and large print keyboards. But one of the simplest steps you can take is to enlarge the text in your Web browser. The three major Web browsers (Netscape, Explorer, and AOL) all have settings that allow for text enlargement. The steps involved in enlarging text depend on which version of the software you use, and whether you use a PC or a Mac.

On Mac computers, there's an easy way to enlarge text on your Explorer browser: hold down the Apple key and then press "+" to enlarge text or "–" to reduce it. Once your new settings are in place, they should remain fixed until you reset them.

When printing from a PC or Mac, keep in mind that the larger font size will appear on the page. You may wish to use the Print Preview option to be certain that everything fits. Print Preview is located under File in the menu bar.

The instructions below are for enlarging text on a PC.

For newer versions of Netscape (4.0 and higher):

1. Select **Edit** from the menu bar.
2. Choose **Preferences**.
3. From the left-hand list, click **Appearance** and then click **Fonts**.
4. Using pull-down menus, adjust the size and font according to your preference.
5. Click **OK** to save your changes.

For older versions of Netscape (3.0 and lower):

1. Select **Options** from the menu bar.
2. Click **General Preferences**.
3. Choose **Fonts**.
4. Click **Choose Font** to change the size and font of your text.

The latest version of Explorer (5.0):

1. Choose **Tools** from the menu bar.
2. Select **Internet Options**.
3. Click the **General** tab and then click **Accessibility**.
4. Check the box **Ignore font sizes specified in Web pages**, then click OK.
5. Adjust text size further by choosing **View** from the menu bar.
6. Go down to **Text Size**.
7. Select **Large** or **Larger**.

For Explorer version 4.0:

1. Choose **View** from the menu bar.
2. Go down and click **Internet Options**.
3. Select the **General** tab in the dialog box and click the **Fonts** button.
4. Using the **Font Size** pull-down menu, select a larger text size.
5. Be sure to click **OK** on both dialog boxes to save your changes.

For Explorer version 3.0:

1. Select **View** from the menu bar.
2. Choose **Fonts**.
3. Set your font size from the choices listed ("Largest," for example).

For America Online 4.0:

1. Double click **My AOL** from the menu bar.
2. Choose **Preferences** from the pull-down menu.
3. Scroll down to the **Font** icon and use the pull-down menus to select a new font or change its size.
4. You may manipulate other appearance options by clicking the **General** icon.

ter, called the macula, which is about one fiftieth of an inch across and is responsible for central and fine-detail vision. In the middle of the macula is a small indentation, the fovea. It contains the highest concentration of cones (the most sensitive receptors of light) and is the area of most acute vision. When you look directly at an object, the light rays focus onto the fovea. Central and detailed vision depend on an intact macula. If function of the macula is lost, the eye must rely on peripheral vision, which is less sensitive. As a result, activities such as reading normal-sized print are impossible without low-vision aids.

CAUSES OF AGE-RELATED MACULAR DEGENERATION

The two forms of AMD are non-neovascular (also known as nonexudative, atrophic, or dry) and neovascular (exudative or wet). The causes of both types are unknown. In addition to age, risk factors include farsightedness, cigarette smoking, a light-colored iris, and a family history of the disorder. High blood pressure appears to be a risk factor for neovascular AMD.

About 90% of people with AMD have the non-neovascular form, characterized by a breakdown or thinning of macular tissues. Most often, non-neovascular AMD is characterized by atrophy of retinal tissues and the formation of drusen, which are small accumulations of debris underneath the retina. Although this form of the disease cannot be prevented or reversed, the changes occur slowly and may stabilize for periods of time; often vision is not impaired.

Neovascular AMD, the more serious form of the disorder, is the primary cause of AMD-related vision loss. It may develop at any time in people with non-neovascular AMD. Vision loss from neovascular AMD results from either the growth of new blood vessels (neovascularization) in the choroid layer of the eye (the layer between the retina and the sclera) or the subsequent detachment of the layer of pigment epithelial cells just beneath the retina. The new blood vessels tend to leak and exude fluid (including lipids, or fats) under the retina, hence its old name "exudative AMD." Patients with more or larger drusen and more pigment change in the macular area have a greater chance of developing the neovascular form. Those with neovascular AMD in one eye have a 20% to 60% chance that the other eye will become similarly affected within the next five years.

Neovascular AMD can be further classified by either the location of the new blood vessels or the pattern of fluid leakage on fluorescein angiography (a diagnostic technique).

The location is described in terms of the proximity of the neovascularization to the fovea. New vessels most distant from the fovea are termed extrafoveal; those at the fovea itself are called subfoveal; and vessels in between are named juxtafoveal. An overgrowth of connective tissue, which accompanies the neovascularization, produces the scarring that is responsible for loss of vision. If the condition is left untreated, severe vision loss occurs in three years in about 60% of eyes with extrafoveal neovascularization and in two years in 70% of eyes with either juxtafoveal or subfoveal neovascularization.

The pattern of fluid leakage is described as classic or occult. Classic new vessels tend to leak more than occult new vessels in the early frames of the angiogram, and the extent tends to be better delineated.

A defect in a gene called ABCR may play a role in AMD. A study recently found that 16% of people with AMD had a mutation in this gene, compared with only 0.5% of people in the general population without the disease. ABCR directs the production of a protein found in the rods of the retina; the gene is mutated in a rare hereditary cause of macular abnormalities, called Stargardt disease, that occur in children and young adults. This first evidence of a genetic cause of AMD might lead to new methods for earlier diagnosis or new strategies for prevention and treatment.

SYMPTOMS OF AGE-RELATED MACULAR DEGENERATION

In most cases, AMD produces no symptoms. When symptoms occur, they usually appear as an otherwise unexplained distortion of objects and mild loss of visual acuity that develops gradually (non-neovascular); less often, symptoms can be severe and occur in a matter of days or weeks (neovascular). A grayness, haziness, or blank spot may appear in the area of central vision; words may be blurred on a page; straight lines may appear to have a kink in them; and objects may seem smaller than they are. Alternatively, color vision may become dimmer, since the receptors involved in color discrimination (cones) are most dense in the fovea.

Vision distortion can be detected by self-monitoring with an Amsler grid, a diagram of a box subdivided into smaller boxes by a series of cross-connecting perpendicular lines. Patients hold the grid at reading distance, fix one eye on its center, and cover the other eye. Indications of early stages of AMD include minor blurring or wavy or distorted lines. More advanced cases are indicated by gray areas or blind spots around the center of the visual field. The Amsler grid alone, however, is not a reliable indicator of AMD. Because many patients may not notice gradual changes in vision, they are advised to monitor their vision in several ways, such as during reading, while watching television, and by noting the appearance of various objects.

NEW RESEARCH

Macular Degeneration May Increase Risk of Depression

People with advanced age-related macular degeneration (AMD) may be at higher risk for depression than people without vision problems, according to a recent study.

Researchers examined the eyes of 151 people age 60 and older with AMD who lived independently. The participants also answered questions about their general health, chronic medical conditions, the impact of AMD on their lives, and symptoms of depression.

Forty nine (33%) of the participants met the criteria for a depressive disorder, approximately twice the rate found in independent older people in the general population. There was a strong correlation between depression and disability, but even people who were not depressed were more likely to be disabled if their vision was poor.

The researchers say the rates of depression and disability in people with AMD are similar to those of people who have cancer or have had a stroke. The authors recommend that primary care physicians and ophthalmologists consider interviewing their patients for depressive symptoms, that people with AMD who are depressed undergo treatment, and that low-vision rehabilitation be available to help reduce disability.

OPHTHALMOLOGY
Volume 108, page 1893
October 2001

Dietary Supplements for Macular Degeneration

In October 2001, researchers from the Age-Related Eye Disease Study (AREDS) reported in the *Archives of Ophthalmology* that taking a combination of antioxidant vitamins and zinc reduced the rate of progression of age-related macular degeneration (AMD) in some people. Because of the media attention surrounding this study, you may have questions about whether you should take vitamins and minerals to protect your vision. So just what did the researchers find, and who might benefit from nutritional supplements?

The Study

The AREDS researchers studied 3,640 people, age 55 to 80, who had no AMD, early AMD in one or both eyes, intermediate AMD in one or both eyes, or advanced AMD in one eye. For an average of six years, the participants took one of the following four treatments daily: 1) placebo pills; 2) antioxidants (500 mg of vitamin C, 400 IU of vitamin E, and 15 mg of beta-carotene); 3) zinc (80 mg of zinc oxide plus 2 mg of copper as cupric oxide to prevent the loss of copper that can occur with the use of zinc); or 4) antioxidants plus zinc.

Neither antioxidants nor zinc, alone or in combination, reduced the risk of developing AMD in people without the disease or slowed its progression in those with early AMD. However, in people with intermediate AMD or advanced AMD in one eye who took both antioxidants and zinc, the risk of progression to more advanced AMD was reduced by about 25%; in addition, these individuals lowered their risk of vision loss from AMD by 19%.

Who Does Supplementation Help?

Currently, experts recommend the AREDS supplements (antioxidants plus zinc) only for people with intermediate AMD in one or both eyes or advanced AMD in one eye. An evaluation by an eye care professional is needed to determine if you are in one of these categories. The supplements will not prevent someone without AMD from developing the disease or prevent someone with early AMD from developing intermediate AMD; so, these individuals should not take the supplements to protect their vision. Also, the AREDS researchers only reported the effects of the supplements in eyes with non-neovascular AMD. In an unplanned analysis, they did find some slowed progression in eyes with neovascular AMD, but these results were uncertain and warrant further research. Furthermore, the AREDS supplements do not prevent the development of cataracts.

Precautions

Because the AREDS supplements contain larger dosages of vitamins and minerals than those present in a normal diet or a typical multivitamin tablet, you should check with your primary care physician before starting to take the supplements. This caution applies especially to people receiving treatment for diabetes, heart disease, or cancer. In addition, the AREDS supplements may interfere with over-the-counter or prescription medications or interact with other dietary supplements or herbal preparations.

Another important precaution is

PREVENTION OF AGE-RELATED MACULAR DEGENERATION

Some studies indicate that certain factors within an individual's control might play a role in the development of AMD. These include dietary supplements, diet, and exposure to sunlight.

The Age-Related Eye Disease Study found that a dietary supplement with high levels of antioxidants and zinc significantly reduced the risk of developing advanced AMD. (For more about this study, see the feature above). Other studies have suggested that eating fruits and vegetables high in carotenoids, especially those high in beta-carotene (carrots, spinach, and cantaloupes, for example), might help prevent AMD.

Avoiding excessive exposure to sunlight has been found to be protective in some studies. In the Beaver Dam Eye Study, people who spent at least five hours a day engaged in leisure activities outdoors in

that smokers and people who recently stopped smoking should avoid taking beta-carotene (one of the vitamins in the AREDS supplements) because research has shown that it increases the risk of lung cancer in smokers. Such individuals should talk with their doctor or eye care professional to individualize their treatment. Typically, only the zinc and copper from the AREDS supplements are advised until the person has been a nonsmoker for about two years.

While the study did find that the supplements were generally well tolerated, prostate and urinary tract problems that required a hospital stay were slightly more common in people who took zinc than in those who did not (7.5% vs. 5%).

Also, the results of another study suggest that certain antioxidants may interfere with the beneficial effects of statin drugs, which are used to reduce high levels of low density lipoprotein (LDL or "bad") cholesterol. The study, from the November 29, 2001 issue of *The New England Journal of Medicine,* found that patients with coronary artery disease who took the statin drug simvastatin (Zocor) along with niacin had reduced narrowing of their coronary arteries, while those who took antioxidants (vitamins E and C, beta-carotene, and selenium) in addition to these medications had a small increase in arterial narrowing. At this time, however, there is not enough evidence to tell people who take statins to avoid antioxidant supplements.

The Supplements

The eye care company Bausch and Lomb, which supplied the supplements to the AREDS researchers, now offers the antioxidant plus zinc preparation to consumers under the brand name Ocuvite PreserVision. This supplement contains the same levels and combination of supplements that were found effective in the AREDS study. The recommended intake is two tablets twice daily. A 30-day supply costs around $16.

A second company, Vitamin Science, is currently marketing a similar supplement called VisiVite Original Formula. While this preparation contains the same combination of supplements used in the AREDS study, the levels of the individual nutrients are not exactly the same. Therefore, it is unclear whether this preparation will give the same results as Ocuvite PreserVision. A 30-day supply costs about $18.

Vitamin Science also sells VisiVite Smoker's Formula, which contains lutein instead of beta-carotene. (Some evidence indicates that lutein, a carotenoid similar to beta-carotene, may play an important role in vision, but a product containing lutein was not available 10 years ago when AREDS was planned.) Again, because the preparation is not exactly the same as the one used in the AREDS research, no one can be sure exactly how well it works. The price is the same as for VisiVite Original Formula.

About 67% of people in AREDS chose to take a daily multivitamin in addition to their assigned supplement, and they did so without experiencing any problems. If you are already taking a daily multivitamin, there is no need to stop if you begin to take the AREDS supplements.

the summer in their teens and 30s had twice the rate of AMD as those who spent fewer than two hours outside each day. People who wore hats and sunglasses tended to have a lower rate of AMD.

Based on such findings, it appears to be worthwhile to take steps to protect the eyes from UV rays (see the feature on page 7) and to eat plenty of fruits and vegetables rich in carotenoids. Taking vitamin and mineral supplements to prevent advanced AMD may also be helpful in some people.

The more large drusen one has, the greater the risk of developing a leaky blood vessel. Researchers have found that laser treatment can cause many of the drusen to regress, but it is not yet known whether this reduces the risk of developing neovascular AMD. A large study is now examining this question.

A study of 1,222 people published in 2000 suggested that people with high blood pressure may be at increased risk for neovascular AMD. This might explain why a 2001 analysis of more than 20,000 men in the Physicians' Health Study found that aspirin reduced the risk of AMD, but only among men who had high blood pressure.

DIAGNOSIS OF AGE-RELATED MACULAR DEGENERATION

Non-neovascular AMD is diagnosed when the doctor observes drusen or other pigment changes in the macula during an ophthalmoscopic examination. Angiography generally is not required for this form of AMD. A diagnosis of neovascular AMD is suspected when a person notes the onset of new symptoms and an eye examination shows an exudate (fluid deposit) or hemorrhage in the macular area. The diagnosis is confirmed by fluorescein angiography. This test must be performed and interpreted promptly because neovascular AMD can progress within days.

An angiogram is an examination of blood vessels. In fluorescein angiography, a special dye called fluorescein is injected into a vein in the arm. Photographs of the retina are taken as the dye circulates through the blood vessels of the eye. The light from the camera flash is passed through a blue filter; the resulting blue light stimulates the fluorescein to emit a yellow-green light from the vessels in the retina and choroid and from any fluid that has leaked from damaged vessels. This procedure is associated with some risks (death in about 1 in 225,000 patients and serious medical complications in 1 in 2,000 patients), as well as a small chance of nausea or vomiting. But the test is essential to prove the diagnosis of neovascular AMD and to identify the sites of neovascularization.

A newer test, indocyanine green angiography, which uses a similar procedure but a different dye, may be employed if the fluorescein angiogram does not adequately delineate the abnormal vessels. This green dye can sometimes provide a clear image despite such barriers as hemorrhages or changes in pigmentation.

In some cases, it may be necessary first to remove cataracts that obstruct the view of the back of the eye to aid in the diagnosis and treatment of AMD and other retinal disorders, such as diabetic retinopathy. Removal of cataracts alone can improve vision in some patients, even when retinal treatment is not possible.

TREATMENT OF AGE-RELATED MACULAR DEGENERATION

Neovascular AMD can be treated about 20% of the time, though many low-vision aids can help patients go about their daily activities despite vision loss in both eyes. Non-neovascular AMD is usually not treated; instead, patients are followed for the possible development of neovascular AMD. In addition, based on results from the Age-Related Eye Disease Study, people with intermediate non-neovascular AMD in one or both eyes or advanced non-neovascular AMD in one eye should consider taking supplemental antioxidants and zinc to slow the progression of the disease (see the feature on pages 38–39).

Photocoagulation

The standard treatment of neovascular AMD when the new blood vessels are outside the center of the retina is coagulation of the new blood vessels with a laser, a procedure referred to as photocoagulation. Because of its difficulty, the procedure must be carried out by an ophthalmologist with special training and experience. However, such treatment has not proven useful in patients with poorly demarcated new vessels.

Photocoagulation does decrease the risk of vision loss when well-demarcated new vessels can be identified in extrafoveal, juxtafoveal, or subfoveal sites, according to the Macular Photocoagulation Study. In study patients with extrafoveal AMD, severe vision loss occurred after 18 months in 60% of untreated eyes but in only 25% of treated eyes. Although benefits persisted for five years after treatment, they diminished over time. The recurrence rate after successful photocoagulation was 10% at one to two months, 24% after six months, and 54% after three years. The risk of severe vision loss was also diminished after photocoagulation of juxtafoveal and subfoveal vessels.

The high recurrence rate of AMD after photocoagulation necessitates careful follow-up and periodic fluorescein angiography. Immediate reexamination is required if new symptoms of vision loss or distortion are noted. A close watch must be maintained on the other eye as well. Some people use an Amsler grid for self-monitoring, but this method is not very reliable for either picking up on or ruling out AMD.

Photodynamic Therapy

The FDA approved photodynamic therapy for treating neovascular AMD in 2000. Photodynamic therapy appears to stop the leakage of abnormal blood vessels with minimal damage to the retina (one of the dangers with photocoagulation). This approach halts further vision loss and may improve visual acuity in some patients. Because it does not repair retinal tissue that is already damaged, photodynamic

NEW RESEARCH

Photodynamic Therapy for AMD May Provide Long-Term Benefit

Photodynamic therapy, used to stop the leakage of abnormal blood vessels in people with neovascular age-related macular degeneration (AMD), appears to halt vision loss up to three years after treatment. Two-year results from this clinical trial led by researchers at Johns Hopkins were published previously.

In the original study, 402 participants with neovascularization received photodynamic therapy, and 207 participants had a sham procedure (the control group). After two years, 53% of the treatment group had no further vision loss, compared with 38% of those in the control group.

From the end of the second year to the end of the third year, participants from the treatment group who had predominantly classic neovascularization experienced little change in visual acuity and few or no additional side effects from the procedure. During this time, these individuals needed an average of 1.3 repeat treatments.

The researchers conclude that photodynamic therapy offers a safe, long-lasting benefit, especially for people with predominantly classic neovascularization (the more aggressive type of AMD). Repeat treatments, as needed, also appear safe and effective.

ARCHIVES OF OPHTHALMOLOGY
Volume 120, page 1307
October 2002

Making the Most of Your Appointment with an Eye Care Professional

A small amount of preparation can help you get the most out of your appointment with an eye care professional. Below is a list of things to do before and questions to ask during an eye care appointment. Much of the advice could apply to a meeting with almost any health care professional.

Before the Appointment

Information to write down:

• Any vision symptoms, for example, vision loss or double vision; halos, flashes of light, or floaters; trouble seeing in dim light or at night; recurrent eye infections; misaligned or crossed eyes; bulging in either eye; watery or inflamed eyes; excessive crusting on or near the eyelids; or swollen or red-rimmed eyelids.

• Eye surgeries or injuries. Include the date, where you were treated, the doctor who treated you, and the name of the procedure or the nature and extent of the injury.

• Other health conditions. These could include chronic health problems, such as allergies, diabetes, or heart disease, as well as any operations you have had that did not involve your eyes.

• Any family history of eye problems or eye disease.

• Information about any prescription or over-the-counter medications, herbal supplements, or vitamins you are taking. Be sure to include doses.

What and who to bring:

• The glasses and/or contacts you are currently using.

• Any questions you want to ask. Choose the three most important ones in case time runs short.

• Your spouse, a family member, or a friend to help listen to the information provided by the eye care professional and to ask questions.

• A pen and pad to take notes during the exam. Write down important information, especially if you typically have trouble remembering later on what the eye care professional said during the appointment.

During the Appointment

General questions:

• If the eye care professional uses terms you do not understand, be sure to ask him or her to explain them in a less technical way.

• Ask for the names of any tests, why they are necessary, and what to expect during them.

Questions about your diagnosis:

• What is the scientific name of your diagnosis and what does it mean in layperson's terms?

therapy usually cannot restore lost vision.

Photodynamic therapy is a two-step procedure that can be performed in a doctor's office. It involves injection of a light-sensitive drug called verteporfin (Visudyne) into the patient's arm. The drug selectively binds to proteins in the tissue affected by abnormal blood vessel growth.

A low-powered laser is then beamed into the eye to activate the drug and produce a toxic, reactive form of oxygen that destroys the abnormal tissue, but leaves normal tissue intact. The growth of abnormal vessels is stopped and vision loss is stabilized.

In two randomized trials led by researchers at Johns Hopkins, 402 patients with abnormal vessel growth received photodynamic therapy as needed (determined by fluorescein angiography done every three months), and 207 patients received placebo therapy (laser therapy without verteporfin).

After one year, further vision loss was halted in 61% of patients who received photodynamic therapy compared to 46% of those who did not. These results were maintained two years after treatment, according to a report published in 2001. Adverse side effects, including pain, swelling, hemorrhage, and inflammation at the injection

• How did the condition develop?
• Will the condition progress and what are the chances you will lose your vision?
• What treatments are available, and what are the benefits and drawbacks of each?
• Ask your eye care professional to develop a treatment plan for you. This plan may include what treatment option to try first and what to do if the first option is not successful.

Questions regarding medications or supplements:

• Ask your doctor for the generic and brand name of any medication prescribed. Also inquire about the dose and the number of times each day (and the time of day) you are to take it. The same applies to dietary supplements your eye care professional may recommend.
• Ask if there are any special instructions for taking the medication.
• If your insurance does not cover the drug, ask if there is a less expensive option or if a generic drug can be prescribed.
• Ask about which symptoms will likely improve with treatment and when you might see the improvement.
• Inquire about what side effects are common and which ones are serious enough to warrant contacting a doctor.
• Ask what to do if you forget to take a dose.
• Ask how long you will need to take the medication.

Questions to ask if surgery is recommended:

• Ask the doctor how your vision may improve after surgery, as well as the risks of the procedure.
• Is the procedure necessary, and are there any risks in delaying it?
• Who will perform the surgery, and where will the surgery take place (for example, in the hospital or in the doctor's office)?
• Can the surgery be performed under local anesthesia, or is general anesthesia necessary?
• How long is the recuperation period? What types of activities will you be able and unable to do?

Questions to ask if your vision problem cannot be corrected:

• Ask your doctor whether low vision aids can help you see better.
• Inquire about any local agencies, such as Lighthouse International (see page 55), that provide vision rehabilitation programs and other resources for people with low vision. Low vision specialists can give you advice about which low vision aids would be best for you.
• Ask if there are any local support groups for people with your condition.

site, occurred in 13% of patients treated with verteporfin compared with 3% of those treated with placebo therapy. Photosensitivity reactions were seen in around 1% of patients. The three-year data are discussed in the sidebar on page 41.

In the studies, the benefit of photodynamic therapy was greater in patients with predominantly classic disease (the more aggressive type). In such patients, about 60% of eyes treated with photodynamic therapy stabilized, vs. 30% of eyes treated with placebo therapy. In patients with occult disease, about 46% of eyes treated with photodynamic therapy stabilized, vs. 33% of eyes treated with placebo therapy.

Photodynamic therapy is currently FDA approved only for patients with predominately classic disease, but it also appears to be helpful for patients with occult disease. A study of nearly 300 people published in the *American Journal of Ophthalmology* in 2001 found that verteporfin therapy was just as effective in people with occult disease alone as it was in those with evidence of classic disease.

Other Treatments Under Study

A variety of treatments are being evaluated for patients whose pattern of new blood vessels is not amenable to laser photocoagulation or photodynamic therapy. These include medical therapy with different antiangiogenic drugs (drugs that may cause the abnormal vessels to shrink), steroid injections and implants, and low-dose radiation. However, a recent study suggests that radiation may not be effective in people with new blood vessel growth at the fovea (see the sidebar at right).

Other potential new therapies may offer hope to people with neovascular AMD. For example, the abnormal vessels can be removed surgically from beneath the retina, and researchers are investigating this method with the hope that the scar that forms after surgery may be smaller than the scar from natural healing. A smaller scar could preserve more vision. This procedure, called subfoveal surgery, is currently being evaluated in a nationwide trial led by researchers at Johns Hopkins.

Several years ago, Johns Hopkins researchers began investigating macular translocation, a surgical technique to move the retina. For patients with subfoveal neovascularization (under the fovea), the retina is detached, moved, and reattached so that the subfoveal vessels may become extrafoveal, where they then can be treated without harming central vision. Early results showed improvement in up to one third of patients. However, interest in macular translocation has dwindled since the advent of photodynamic therapy.

Low-Vision Aids

Despite timely detection and treatment (if indicated), AMD leads to low vision in some patients. A number of low-vision optical aids can optimize remaining vision.

The perceived benefits of these aids—such as a pair of high-power reading glasses (available at a local drugstore)—depend on the expectations of patients. Patients with unrealistic expectations are likely to be disappointed, while many with more realistic hopes will recognize significant benefits. Also essential is proper training in the use of these devices. Many devices to aid vision are available through low-vision clinics and low-vision rehabilitation services.

In addition to these aids, the Low Vision Enhancement System (LVES) has been developed by collaborators at Johns Hopkins, the National Aeronautics and Space Administration (NASA), and the Veterans Administration. The LVES is a battery-powered, head-mounted (to free the user's hands) video device with a camera and a handset that allows the user to control the magnification, contrast, and bright-

NEW RESEARCH

Radiation Does Not Prevent Vision Loss From AMD

Radiation is not effective in preventing vision loss in patients with a specific type of age-related macular degeneration (AMD), according to a recent study.

Researchers randomly assigned 203 patients with AMD (age 60 or older) to either observation or radiation therapy. All patients had subfoveal neovascularization (new vessel growth at the fovea, the part of the eye responsible for the most acute vision).

Near visual acuity was better in the radiation group at six months, but this benefit was no longer present one and two years after treatment. Radiation, at the dose used in this study, did not appear to damage the retina, but the treated patients had a mild decrease in tear formation. With longer follow-up, retinal damage or cataract progression might become apparent.

When the researchers considered the results of all the vision tests given to the participants, there was a slight benefit in favor of the treatment group. However, this benefit was not strong enough to recommend radiation as an effective treatment for subfoveal neovascularization.

ARCHIVES OF OPHTHALMOLOGY
Volume 120, page 1029
August 2002

Where To Find Low Vision Products

Numerous products are available to help people with low vision function better in a variety of situations. Some of the more complex low-vision aids (for example, telescopes) require an evaluation or prescription from an ophthalmologist, optometrist, or low-vision specialist. These specialists can recommend equipment that is appropriate for you and provide training in its use. Some of the more basic products (such as talking clocks and large-print playing cards) can be purchased without a consultation with a vision specialist and require no special training.

Listed below are seven companies that supply low-vision aids and related items to consumers. To view their products, call them for a catalog or go to their Web sites. Some provide on-line shopping while others do not. If you have any questions about whether a certain low-vision product is right for you, contact a vision specialist first to determine what best fits your needs.

The American Printing House for the Blind
1839 Frankfort Ave.
P.O. Box 6085
Louisville, KY 40206-0085
☎ 800-223-1839
www.aph.org
This company sells a variety of low-vision devices, as well as large-print and daily living items, through its APH Adult Life Products catalog. Products are also sold on-line, but the customer must set up a Web account with the company first.

Bernell
4016 North Home St.
Mishawaka, IN 46545
☎ 800-348-2225
www.bernell.com
This company sells magnifiers, telescopes, and other vision-related products, which can be purchased on-line.

Beyond Sight
5650 South Windermere St.
Littleton, CO 80120
☎ 303-795-6455
www.beyondsight.com
Beyond Sight sells a wide selection of products for people with visual impairment, including computers, talking clocks, magnifiers, kitchen items, audio books, and other devices. Items can be purchased on-line.

Gold Violin
3342 Melrose Ave. NW
Roanoke, VA 24017
☎ 877-648-8465 (toll-free number)
www.goldviolin.com
In conjunction with Lighthouse International, Gold Violin sells various low-vision products like talking watches and calculators, magnifiers, and screen readers. On-line shopping is available.

Goodkin Border & Associates
1862 Veterans Memorial Hwy.
Austell, GA 30168
☎ 800-759-6275
www.gbacorp.com
This company offers low-vision magnifiers, computer products, and other electronic devices, which it sells through its consumer catalog. On-line shopping is not available.

Independent Living Aids
200 Robbins Ln.
Jericho, NY 11753
☎ 800-537-2118
www.independentliving.com
Independent Living Aids sells a wide range of products, including cooking aids, computer equipment, electronics, household and personal care items, magnifiers, and miscellaneous items for people with low vision. Customers can shop on-line.

National Association for the Visually Handicapped
- 22 West 21st St., 6th Fl.
  New York, NY 10010
  ☎ 212-889-3141
- 3201 Balboa St.
  San Francisco, CA 94121
  ☎ 415-221-3201

www.navh.org
The National Association for the Visually Handicapped supplies a variety of low-vision devices ranging from magnifiers, writing aids, and lamps to large-print watches, calculators, and playing cards. On-line shopping is available.

ness of an image seen on a monitor.

Also available is the V-max from Enhanced Vision Systems; it uses a color camera instead of the monochrome display of the LVES. The control box for the V-max is also smaller and simpler to use than that of the LVES. While helpful, these devices are expensive and can be unwieldy. Other systems now in development will be smaller, be lighter, and display higher-quality images. Recently, the manufacturers of the LVES developed a smaller, lighter device called the Aurora imaging system.

Diabetic Retinopathy

About 16 million Americans have diabetes, a condition characterized by abnormally high levels of glucose (sugar) in the blood. Although no cure exists for diabetes, consistent control of blood glucose levels can greatly reduce the risk of complications. Blood glucose control is accomplished by careful adherence to a program of diet, exercise, and, if necessary, medication. High blood glucose levels can damage small blood vessels in the retina, a condition called diabetic retinopathy. This is more common in people with poorly controlled diabetes. Between 600,000 and 700,000 Americans have diabetic retinopathy severe enough to cause vision loss.

CAUSES OF DIABETIC RETINOPATHY

There are two forms of diabetes: type 1 and type 2. In type 1 diabetes, a careful eye exam reveals mild retinal abnormalities an average of seven years after the onset of diabetes, but damage that threatens vision usually does not develop until much later. Retinopathy may be seen relatively earlier after patients are diagnosed with the more common type 2 diabetes. Because its onset is subtle, retinal changes may have already taken place by the time diabetes is first recognized. In fact, a third of the people with type 2 diabetes do not know they have the disorder. Although people with type 2 diabetes are less likely to have severe retinopathy and vision loss than people with type 1 diabetes, at least 70% of those with type 2 diabetes develop some retinopathy within 10 years of the onset of the disease.

In the early, or nonproliferative, stages of diabetic retinopathy, the retinal blood vessels develop weak spots that bulge outward (microaneurysms) and may leak fluids (exudates) and blood (hemorrhages) into the surrounding retinal tissue. These initial abnormalities usually cause no visual symptoms, and, in many people, the disease progresses no further.

Macular edema—a swelling around the macula caused by leakage and accumulation of fluid—occurs with increased frequency in people with diabetes. The swelling around the macula alters the position of the retina and causes blurred vision. Loss of vision is greater when the center of the macula is affected.

The most dangerous form of diabetic retinopathy is proliferative retinopathy, characterized by neovascularization—the growth of

NEW RESEARCH

Statin Drug May Slow Progress Of Diabetic Retinopathy

Taking a statin drug for high cholesterol may slow the progression of diabetic retinopathy in people with diabetes, according to a recent study from India.

Fifty people with type 1 or type 2 diabetes, good glucose control, high cholesterol, and diabetic retinopathy were randomly assigned to receive either 20 mg a day of simvastatin (Zocor) or a placebo. The participants' visual acuity was assessed before the study and every 30 days thereafter. At days 1, 90, and 180, the participants gave blood samples and had complete eye examinations.

After six months, cholesterol was 33% lower in the simvastatin group and unchanged in the placebo group. Visual acuity worsened in seven patients in the placebo group and none in the simvastatin group, and diabetic retinopathy worsened in seven patients in the placebo group and improved in one patient in the simvastatin group.

High cholesterol appears to increase the formation of the hard exudates in the retina that worsen visual acuity. High levels of low density lipoprotein (LDL) cholesterol have been shown to be toxic to retinal cells in animals and may be in humans, as well. Larger studies with longer follow-up are needed to confirm the benefit of statins for people with diabetic retinopathy.

DIABETES RESEARCH AND CLINICAL PRACTICE
Volume 56, page 1
April 2002

small, new blood vessels into the vitreous humor. Acute loss of vision can occur owing to bleeding into the vitreous humor from the rupture of these fragile blood vessels or from the development of fibrous bands of scar tissue that can pull the retina away from the back of the eye (retinal detachment).

Researchers may have found at least one of the culprits responsible for diabetic proliferative retinopathy. One study detected in eye fluid a substance called vascular endothelial growth factor (VEGF), secreted by the endothelial cells (cells lining blood vessels) in the eye in response to damage caused by diabetes. VEGF, which promotes the abnormal growth of blood vessels characteristic of proliferative retinopathy, was detected in 51% of the patients with retinopathy but in only 7% of those with eye diseases that are not associated with the growth of new blood vessels, such as cataracts. Better understanding of the exact role of VEGF in proliferative retinopathy could lead to improved screening tests and treatments. A clinical trial testing oral VEGF inhibitors is under way.

And a recent study suggests that elevated levels of blood lipids—cholesterol and triglycerides—may increase the risk of visual impairment in people with diabetic retinopathy. In the study, which included more than 2,700 people, those with either high total or low density lipoprotein (LDL, or "bad") cholesterol levels were two times more likely to have hard exudates (waxy yellow deposits in the eye) than those with normal levels.

SYMPTOMS OF DIABETIC RETINOPATHY

The early stages of diabetic retinopathy generally cause no symptoms, so periodic eye exams are necessary to screen diabetic patients. Even proliferative retinopathy is initially asymptomatic. Symptoms only develop when there is bleeding—the patient sees spots or showers of small spots called floaters, which can be so severe as to block vision entirely. Abrupt bleeding into the vitreous humor can also cause sudden vision loss in one eye. If blood vessel changes cause macular edema or closure of the small vessels supplying the macula (macular nonperfusion), patients may notice blurring of vision. In addition, formation of scar tissue on the macula due to proliferative retinopathy can blur vision. Symptoms of retinal detachment include a wavy or watery quality to overall vision, the appearance of a dark shadow in part of the peripheral field of vision, and sudden blindness in one eye.

NEW RESEARCH

Blood Pressure Reduction May Halt Progression of Diabetic Retinopathy

Several studies have already shown that reducing high blood pressure in people with type 2 diabetes can reduce their risk of complications such as diabetic retinopathy. Now research suggests that type 2 diabetes patients with normal blood pressure can also benefit from lowering their blood pressure.

This study included 480 people with type 2 diabetes who had diastolic blood pressures between 80 and 89 mm Hg. The participants received blood pressure-lowering medication (nisoldipine [Sular] or enalapril [Vasotec]) or a placebo.

The mean blood pressure during the study was 128/75 mm Hg in the medication group and 137/81 mm Hg in the placebo group. After five years, diabetic retinopathy had progressed in 34% of patients in the medication group, compared with 46% of the placebo group. Proliferative retinopathy developed in 4% of those on the placebo but in none of the subjects in the medication group. The medication group also had a slower onset or progression of kidney disease and had fewer strokes. Nisoldipine and enalapril had similar beneficial effects on diabetic complications.

The researchers conclude that aggressive blood pressure control should be encouraged for all people with type 2 diabetes, not just those with high blood pressure.

KIDNEY INTERNATIONAL
Volume 61, page 1086
March 2002

Reducing the Risk of Diabetic Retinopathy

Diabetic retinopathy, a potential long-term complication of diabetes, is an eye disorder caused by damage to blood vessels in the retina, the light-sensitive tissue at the back of the eye. Mild forms of the disorder are common: Almost all people with type 1 diabetes and more than 70% of people with type 2 diabetes will experience some degree of retinopathy.

Without treatment, diabetic retinopathy can progress from mild ("nonproliferative") forms to more serious ("proliferative") disease, which can lead to blindness. People with diabetes can take several steps to help reduce their risk of developing retinopathy or having it progress.

Have Regular Eye Exams

Regular visits to an ophthalmologist are essential to detect early retinal damage so it can be monitored and, if necessary, treated with laser therapy or vitrectomy. An annual eye exam is recommended for people who have had type 1 diabetes for more than five years. Everyone with type 2 diabetes should have an eye exam as soon as diabetes is diagnosed, and annually thereafter. The exam should include drops to dilate the pupil. If retinopathy is suspected or known, it should be monitored by an ophthalmologist who specializes in diseases of the retina.

Control Blood Glucose

The most important way to prevent diabetic retinopathy is to keep blood glucose levels as close to normal as possible. This is because high blood glucose levels can damage blood vessels in the retina.

Two large studies have shown the benefits of tight glucose control. In the Diabetes Control and Complications Trial (DCCT), people with type 1 diabetes who gave themselves multiple insulin injections (or continuous insulin infusions) each day reduced their risk of developing diabetic retinopathy by 76% and their risk of having existing retinopathy progress by 54%, compared with people who followed a less rigorous treatment program. In addition, the United Kingdom Prospective Diabetes Study (UKPDS) found that people with type 2 diabetes who controlled their blood glucose levels with medication were 30% less likely to have retinopathy that required laser treatment than people who relied on diet and exercise alone.

The best way to achieve tight glucose control is to measure your blood glucose levels frequently with a glucose monitor and to follow the advice of a doctor who manages diabetes aggressively. It is also important to have a hemoglobin A1c (HbA1c) test every three to six months to evaluate your blood glucose control. Experts recommend that people with diabetes maintain an HbA1c level below 7%. The DCCT found that every 10% reduction in elevated HbA1c levels was associated with a 39% reduction in the risk of diabetic retinopathy.

Tight glucose control is difficult to achieve, and it can be dangerous for some people because of an increased risk of hypoglycemia (low blood glucose levels). Talk to your doctor about the level of glucose control that is best for you.

Control Blood Pressure

High blood pressure can also damage blood vessels in the retina. Research shows that keeping blood pressure as close to normal as possible can help prevent the onset and progression of retinal damage.

In one study of people with type 1 diabetes and mild retinopathy, the retinopathy was more likely to have worsened in the patients who had a high diastolic blood pressure (the bottom number in a blood pressure reading) three years earlier. Every 10 mm Hg increase in diastolic blood pressure raised the risk of more severe retinopathy by 24%.

PREVENTION OF DIABETIC RETINOPATHY

Results from the landmark Diabetes Control and Complications Trial (DCCT) indicate that careful control of blood glucose levels can delay or prevent diabetic retinopathy in people with type 1 diabetes. Although the study did not include people with type 2 diabetes, most diabetes specialists believed the results would hold true for them as well. And indeed, a small study in Japan and the larger, long-term United Kingdom Prospective Diabetes Study (UKPDS) both showed that excellent glucose control also decreased retinopathy in type 2 diabetes. Controlling blood pressure also reduces the risk. For more in-

Elevated systolic blood pressure (the top number in a blood pressure reading) may also increase the likelihood of diabetic retinopathy. In another study, every reduction of 10 mm Hg in systolic blood pressure decreased the incidence of retinopathy and other diabetic complications by 12%.

Blood pressure reduction may even help diabetic patients who do not have high blood pressure. One study looked at people with type 2 diabetes who had a blood pressure below 140/90 mm Hg. When their blood pressure was lowered to approximately 128/75 mm Hg with medication, they had less progression of diabetic retinopathy over a five-year period than people whose blood pressure averaged 137/81 mm Hg (see the sidebar on page 47).

Experts recommend that people with diabetes keep their blood pressure at or below 130/80 mm Hg to prevent long-term complications. To achieve this goal, patients must control their weight, follow a low-fat diet rich in fruits and vegetables and low in sodium, engage in regular physical activity, and in many cases take one or more blood pressure-lowering medications.

Control Cholesterol Levels

Studies have reached conflicting conclusions as to whether high blood cholesterol is associated with the development or progression of diabetic retinopathy, although there is universal agreement that it will increase the risk of heart disease. One study of 485 patients found that elevated cholesterol levels were not associated with more severe cases of diabetic retinopathy. However, another study of 50 patients found that those who were given simvastatin (Zocor), a cholesterol-lowering drug, were less likely to have their diabetic retinopathy worsen than patients given a placebo (see the sidebar on page 46).

High blood cholesterol also seems to increase the risk of vision loss in people with diabetic retinopathy. People with diabetes who have high cholesterol have a higher risk of hard exudates (waxy yellow deposits that form in the eye). These hard exudates can accumulate in the macula and cause a decrease in central and fine-detail vision. The Early Treatment Diabetic Retinopathy Study, a trial of about 3,700 people with diabetic retinopathy, found that patients with high total blood cholesterol levels (240 mg/dL or more) were twice as likely as patients with normal total blood cholesterol levels (less than 200 mg/dL) to have hard exudates.

Lowering blood cholesterol levels is already a priority for people with diabetes because of their increased risk of heart attack and stroke, and preserving vision may be an added benefit of taking steps to lower cholesterol. These steps include maintaining a healthy body weight, eating a diet low in saturated fat, engaging in regular exercise, and, if necessary, taking medication.

Stop Smoking

Some—but not all—studies find that smoking cigarettes is a risk factor for diabetic retinopathy. Even if there is no direct link, the blood pressure-raising effect of smoking can increase the risk of retinopathy. If you need help quitting, talk to your doctor. He or she can recommend a smoking cessation program or prescribe a nicotine replacement therapy.

Recognize the Warning Signs

Diabetic retinopathy usually has no symptoms. However, any of the following visual changes could indicate retinal damage, and you should contact your eye doctor immediately if you experience any of them:

- sudden loss of vision in one eye;
- blurred vision;
- problems reading;
- double vision;
- pain in one or both eyes;
- pressure in your eyes;
- the appearance of spots or floaters;
- problems seeing things with your peripheral vision.

formation on reducing the risk of diabetic retinopathy, see the feature above.

DIAGNOSIS OF DIABETIC RETINOPATHY

Early laser treatment can usually spare vision by stopping the growth of new blood vessels on the retina. Because even advanced retinopathy can be asymptomatic, it is crucial for all people with type 1 diabetes to begin seeing an ophthalmologist (not an optometrist) for regular eye exams no later than five years after the diagnosis of the disorder. Significant retinopathy may be present at the time of diagnosis of type 2 diabetes, so an eye examination is advised at that time. All patients with diabetes should then have a follow-up examination at least once a year. More frequent follow-ups are recommended if more than minimal retinopathy is detected. For some, an eye examination by a primary care physician may be used to augment the regular screenings by an ophthalmologist. It is important, however, that such examinations do not substitute for periodic visits to an ophthalmologist.

After eye drops are used to dilate the pupils (which takes 15 to 30 minutes), the retina is directly viewed with an ophthalmoscope. The ophthalmologist will look for signs of edema, exudates, new blood vessel growth, hemorrhages, or other abnormalities. Because the drops cause the eyes to be extremely sensitive to light, patients should bring a pair of sunglasses with them; if driving, they may prefer to ask someone else to drive them home afterward. Fluorescein angiography (see page 40) is also used to examine the retina for blood vessel changes.

TREATMENT OF DIABETIC RETINOPATHY

Results from the DCCT and the UKPDS indicate that good blood glucose control lessens the risk that retinopathy will progress to a more severe stage. Treating other conditions, such as high blood pressure and abnormal cholesterol levels, may also slow progression. In most cases, no treatment is required for nonproliferative retinopathy, but retinal changes are carefully monitored for the development of macular edema or proliferative disease. There are two treatments for proliferative retinopathy: laser photocoagulation for macular edema or proliferative changes, and vitrectomy for advanced abnormalities.

Laser photocoagulation. Photocoagulation, using lasers to promote closure of new blood vessels, can halt or retard vision loss in most patients if it is performed before too much damage has occurred. In patients with macular edema, focal laser photocoagulation can target individual blood vessels. Panretinal photocoagulation, which creates a grid-like pattern across a larger area of the retina, is used to treat proliferative retinopathy. Laser treatment leads to regression of new blood vessels and reduces by half the chance of eventual blindness in those with proliferative retinopathy. Laser treatment improves vision in only about 10% of patients with macular edema. But even when vision does not improve, photocoagulation can cut in half the chance of further deterioration. Although complications are rare, vision loss can result from the treatment.

Vitrectomy. If the extent or location of the damage makes photocoagulation ineffective, or if the vitreous humor is too clouded with blood, vision may be improved or stabilized by vitrectomy, a surgical procedure that removes the vitreous humor and replaces it with a saline solution. Photocoagulation can also be carried out during vitrectomy with a special laser that is inserted into the eye. Roughly 70% of those who have vitrectomies notice improvement or stabilization of their vision, and some recover enough vision to resume reading and driving.

Experimental treatments. Several treatments are being tested for diabetic retinopathy, including a steroid-releasing device that is implanted in the eye and a class of oral medications called protein kinase C inhibitors, but so far none of these have been proven to be effective. ■

GLOSSARY

A-scan ultrasonography—A test that uses sound waves to measure the length of the eyeball.

adrenergic agonist eye drops—A treatment for glaucoma. The eye drops reduce intraocular pressure by decreasing the production of aqueous humor and increasing its drainage through the uveoscleral pathway.

age-related macular degeneration—A loss of central vision caused by changes in the macula. Commonly abbreviated as AMD and sometimes referred to as senile macular degeneration.

anti-angiogenic drugs—An experimental therapy for age-related macular degeneration that shrinks blood vessels in the eye.

aqueous humor—A watery fluid that is located in front of the lens and provides nutrients to the lens and cornea.

B-scan ultrasonography—A test that uses sound waves to view structures in the back of the eye.

beta-blocker eye drops—A treatment for glaucoma. The eye drops reduce intraocular pressure by decreasing the production of aqueous humor.

bifocals—A pair of glasses with lenses that correct both distant and near vision.

capsule, lens—The outermost structure of the lens.

carbonic anhydrase inhibitors—Medications used to treat glaucoma that decrease the production of aqueous humor. Available in both oral and eye drop forms.

cataract—A cloudiness or opacification of the lens that can lead to visual impairment.

choroid—A layer of the eye inside the sclera. It contains a dark pigment that minimizes scattering of light inside the eye.

ciliary body—A part of the eye that surrounds the lens and produces aqueous humor.

closed-angle glaucoma—A type of glaucoma caused by a blockage near the iris that prevents aqueous humor from reaching the trabecular meshwork. It results in a rapid buildup of extremely high intraocular pressure that can lead to severe, permanent vision damage within a day or two.

color blindness—An inability to perceive or distinguish between certain colors.

cones—Nerve cells in the retina that are activated only in bright light and by one of three colors: red, blue, or green.

conjunctiva—A thin, lubricating mucous membrane that covers the sclera and lines the inside of the eyelid.

cornea—The transparent, dome-shaped disk covering the iris and pupil.

cortex, lens—The second innermost structure of the lens. It surrounds the nucleus, and its outer edge is lined with epithelium.

cortical cataract—A cataract affecting the cortex of the lens.

cyclodestructive surgery—A treatment for glaucoma that destroys the ciliary body with laser treatment or other methods.

cystoid macular edema—A specific pattern of swelling of the central retina.

diabetes—A disease characterized by abnormally high glucose (sugar) levels in the blood.

diabetic retinopathy—Damage to small blood vessels in the retina resulting from chronic high blood glucose levels; more common in people with poorly controlled diabetes.

drusen—Small accumulations of debris underneath the retina.

endophthalmitis—An infection of the vitreous humor that develops in a small number of patients after cataract surgery or other kinds of eye surgery.

epithelium, lens—Cells that line the outer surface of the lens cortex.

extracapsular surgery—Cataract surgery that removes the capsule, cortex, and nucleus of the lens while sparing the posterior capsule.

exudate—Fluid deposit.

filtration surgery—A treatment for glaucoma that uses conventional surgical instruments to open a passage through the clogged trabecular meshwork, so that excess aqueous humor can drain into surrounding tissues.

floaters—Black spots or shapes that drift through the field of vision.

fluorescein angiography—A diagnostic procedure for age-related macular degeneration and other retinal diseases. A special dye, called fluorescein, is injected into a vein in the arm. Photographs of the retina are taken as the dye circulates through the blood vessels of the eye.

glare—The light within the field of vision that is brighter than other objects to which the eyes are adapted.

glaucoma—An eye disease that results in damage to the optic nerve. It is not always caused by elevated intraocular pressure.

gonioscopy—A technique used to distinguish between open- and closed-angle glaucoma. It involves an examination of the front part of the eye to check the angle where the iris meets the cornea.

hemorrhage—Leakage of blood from blood vessels.

hyperopia—Farsightedness.

hypoglycemia—Low blood glucose (sugar) levels.

insulin—A hormone that controls blood glucose levels.

intracapsular surgery—Cataract surgery that removes the entire lens (capsule, cortex, and nucleus). The procedure is rarely performed today. Unlike extracapsular surgery, the posterior capsule is not spared.

intraocular lens implant—A plastic lens that replaces the lens removed during cataract surgery.

intraocular pressure (IOP)—The pressure exerted by the fluids inside the eyeball.

iridectomy—Removal of part of the iris.

iridotomy—Creation of a hole in the iris with a laser or other method.

iris—The colored circle in the middle of the eye that controls the amount of light that enters the eye.

laser trabecular surgery—A treatment for glaucoma that involves making 80 to 100 tiny laser burns in the area of the trabecular meshwork. The procedure increases the drainage of aqueous humor.

legal blindness—Vision that is 20/200 or worse in both eyes. (20/200 vision is the ability to see at 20 feet what a normal eye can see at 200 feet.)

lens—A transparent, biconvex structure that is responsible (in conjunction with the cornea) for the eye's ability to focus light.

Low Vision Enhancement System—An aid for low vision that includes a battery-powered, head-mounted video device, a camera, and a handset, which allow the user to control the magnification, contrast, and brightness of an image seen on a monitor.

macula—A small area at the center of the retina that is responsible for central and fine-detail vision.

macular edema—A swelling of the macula caused by leakage and accumulation of fluid. It occurs with increased frequency in people with diabetes.

macular nonperfusion—Closure of the small blood vessels supplying the macula.

microaneurysms—Weak spots that bulge outward from blood vessels, including those of the retina.

miotics—Eye drops used to treat glaucoma. They increase the outflow of aqueous humor by improving its flow through the trabecular meshwork.

mydriatic eye drops—Drops that dilate the pupil and allow more light to reach the retina. Used as a short-term treatment for cataracts.

myopia—Nearsightedness.

neovascular age-related macular degeneration—A form of age-related macular degeneration in which new blood vessels grow in the choroid layer of the eye.

neovascularization—The growth of new blood vessels.

non-neovascular age-related macular degeneration—A form of age-related macular degeneration characterized by a breakdown or thinning of macular tissues. It is characterized by the formation of drusen and atrophy of retinal tissues and often does not impair vision.

normal-tension glaucoma—Damage to the optic nerve by glaucoma despite normal intraocular pressure.

nuclear cataract—A cataract affecting the nucleus of the lens.

nucleus, lens—The center structure of the lens. It is surrounded by the cortex.

opacification—The process of becoming impenetrable by light.

open-angle glaucoma—The most common form of glaucoma. It usually produces no obvious symptoms until its late stages.

ophthalmoscopy—Examination and visualization of the interior structures of the eye, especially the retina, using a specialized instrument.

perimetry—A test used to determine a person's visual field. While the person looks straight ahead at a bowl-shaped white area, a computer presents lights in fixed locations around the bowl. The patient indicates each time he or she sees the light.

peripheral vision—The ability to see objects at the edges of the visual field.

phacoemulsification—A type of extracapsular surgery that is performed with an ultrasonic device, which nearly liquefies the nucleus and cortex so that they can be removed by suction through a tube.

photocoagulation—The older, standard treatment for neovascular age-related macular degeneration when the new blood vessels are outside the center of the retina. The procedure involves closing the new blood vessels with a laser.

photodynamic therapy—A newer treatment for age-related macular degeneration that involves the intravenous administration of a special drug to sensitize blood vessels in the eye to light. A low-power laser, directed at the abnormal vessels, activates the drug and closes the vessels in a way that causes less damage to the retina than standard laser treatment.

GLOSSARY—continued

posterior subcapsular cataract—A cataract in the rear of the lens capsule.

presbyopia—An inability to focus on near objects.

pupil—The opening in the center of the iris that resembles a large black dot.

retina—The innermost layer of the eye that consists of light-sensitive nerve tissue.

retinal detachment—A vision-threatening condition in which the retina becomes separated from the underlying layers of the eye.

rods—Nerve cells in the retina that are sensitive to dim light.

rubeosis iridis—New blood vessel growth on the iris. It usually occurs in people with diabetes.

sclera—The white outer layer that covers and protects most of the eye.

scotoma—A blind spot in the visual field.

shunt (or tube-shunt)—Used in the treatment of glaucoma when filtration surgery is unsuccessful. A shunt creates a new passage to drain excess aqueous humor.

subfoveal surgery—A procedure that surgically removes the abnormal blood vessels beneath the retina in people with age-related macular degeneration.

tonometry—A method of measuring intraocular pressure by determining the amount of force needed to make a slight indentation in a small area of the cornea.

topical prostaglandin eye drops—A treatment for glaucoma. The eye drops reduce intraocular pressure by increasing the outflow of aqueous humor through the uveoscleral pathway.

trabecular meshwork—A spongy network of connective tissue through which aqueous humor drains from the eye. Blockage of the meshwork causes a buildup of intraocular pressure.

uveitis—Inflammation of the uvea, the part of the eye that contains the iris, ciliary body, and choroid.

uveoscleral pathway—An alternative drainage system for aqueous humor. It is located behind the trabecular meshwork.

vitrectomy—A surgical procedure that removes the vitreous humor and replaces it with a saline solution.

vitreous humor—A thick, gel-like substance that fills the back of the eyeball behind the lens.

YAG laser—A type of laser that contains yttrium, aluminum, and garnet. It is used to clear blurred vision that may occur after extracapsular surgery.

HEALTH INFORMATION ORGANIZATIONS AND SUPPORT GROUPS

American Academy of Ophthalmology
P.O. Box 7424
San Francisco, CA 94120-7424
☎ 415-561-8500
www.aao.org
Largest association of ophthalmologists in the United States. For information on a variety of eye-related diseases and their prevention and treatment, describe your ailment(s) and send a self-addressed, stamped business envelope.

American Council of the Blind
1155 15th St. NW, Suite 1004
Washington, DC 20005
☎ 800-424-8666
202-467-5081
www.acb.org
National information clearinghouse that also offers group insurance plans and other services.

American Optometric Association
243 North Lindbergh Blvd.
St. Louis, MO 63141
☎ 314-991-4100
www.aoanet.org
A professional group of doctors of optometry that provides more than 50 pamphlets and fact sheets on eye-care topics, especially vision problems corrected by eyeglasses and contact lenses. Specify your topic(s) of interest and send a self-addressed, stamped business envelope.

Association for Macular Diseases, Inc.
210 East 64th St.
New York, NY 10021
☎ 212-605-3719
www.macula.org/association/about.html
Not-for-profit corporation devoted solely to macular disease. Membership includes a support group and a newsletter devoted to medical advances, new developments in low-vision aids, and advice on coping strategies.

The Foundation Fighting Blindness
11435 Cronhill Dr.
Owings Mills, MD 21117-2220
☎ 800-683-5555
800-683-5551 (TDD)
www.blindness.org
Supports research and provides education about retinal degeneration. Publishes a newsletter entitled *Fighting Blindness News*.

Glaucoma Research Foundation
200 Pine St., Suite 200
San Francisco, CA 94104
☎ 800-826-6693
415-986-3162
www.glaucoma.org
National nonprofit organization committed to protecting the sight of people with glaucoma through research and education. Call the toll-free number for free publications.

Lighthouse International
111 E. 59th St.
New York, NY 10022
☎ 800-829-0500
212-821-9200
www.lighthouse.org
National nonprofit vision rehabilitation organization that conducts research and offers educational opportunities and direct services for people with vision loss.

National Association for the Visually Handicapped
22 W. 21st St., 6th Fl.
New York, NY 10010
☎ 212-889-3141
www.navh.org
Volunteer health agency dedicated to serving the partially sighted. Publishes a newsletter, medical updates, and other publications. Services include sale and/or referral of currently available vision aids and an extensive library of large-print books.

National Eye Institute Information Office
2020 Vision Pl.
Bethesda, MD 20892-3655
☎ 800-869-2020 (for publications)
301-496-5248
www.nei.nih.gov
Part of the National Institutes of Health. Provides information packets on a variety of eye ailments and answers inquiries over the phone. Supports more than 75% of the vision research conducted in the United States.

Prevent Blindness America
500 E. Remington Rd.
Schaumburg, IL 60173
☎ 800-331-2020
www.prevent-blindness.org
Provides public and professional education through community programs, patient services, and research.

Vision Foundation
23A Elm St.
Watertown, MA 02472
☎ 617-926-4232
Provides peer support, information, resources, and specialized rehabilitation instruction for people in the process of losing their sight.

Vision World Wide, Inc.
5707 Brockton Dr., Suite 302
Indianapolis, IN 46220-5481
☎ 800-431-1739
317-254-1332
www.visionww.org
Provides publications in large print, audiocassette, or on computer disk. Call the toll-free number for information and referral services.

LEADING HOSPITALS FOR OPHTHALMOLOGY

U.S. News & World Report and the National Opinion Research Center, a social-science research group at the University of Chicago, recently conducted their 13th annual nationwide survey of 1,484 physicians in 17 medical specialties. The doctors nominated up to five hospitals they consider the best from among 6,045 U.S. hospitals. This is the current list of the best ophthalmology hospitals, as determined by the doctors' recommendations from 2000, 2001, and 2002. Since the results reflect the doctors' opinions, they are, of course, subjective. Any institution listed is considered a leading center; nevertheless, the rankings do not imply that other hospitals cannot or do not deliver excellent care.

1. **Johns Hopkins Hospital (Wilmer Eye Institute)**
   Baltimore, MD
   ☎ 410-955-5080
   www.wilmer.jhu.edu

2. **University of Miami (Bascom Palmer Eye Institute)**
   Miami, FL
   ☎ 305-243-2020
   www.bpei.med.miami.edu

3. **Wills Eye Hospital**
   Philadelphia, PA
   ☎ 215-928-3000
   www.willseye.org

4. **Massachusetts Eye and Ear Infirmary**
   Boston, MA
   ☎ 617-573-5520
   www.meei.harvard.edu

5. **UCLA Medical Center (Jules Stein Eye Institute)**
   Los Angeles, CA
   ☎ 310-825-5000
   www.medsch.ucla.edu/som/jsei

6. **University of Iowa Hospitals and Clinics**
   Iowa City, IA
   ☎ 800-777-8442/319-384-8442
   www.uihealthcare.com/uihospitalsandclinics

7. **USC Medical Center (Doheny Eye Institute)**
   Los Angeles, CA
   ☎ 323-442-6335
   www.usc.edu/hsc/doheny

8. **Duke University Medical Center**
   Durham, NC
   ☎ 919-684-8111
   www.mc.duke.edu

9. **Mayo Clinic**
   Rochester, MN
   ☎ 507-284-2511
   www.mayoclinic.org

10. **Barnes-Jewish Hospital**
    St. Louis, MO
    ☎ 314-747-3000
    www.barnesjewish.org

AGE-RELATED MACULAR DEGENERATION AND VITAMIN E

Recently, much attention has been paid to the idea of using vitamin and mineral supplements to protect vision. In 2001, the Age-Related Eye Disease Study (AREDS) found that a combination of antioxidants (beta-carotene and vitamins C and E) plus the mineral zinc reduced the rate of progression of age-related macular degeneration (AMD) in some people with AMD (see the feature on pages 38–39). Participants taking antioxidants alone or zinc alone did not fare as well as those taking both antioxidants and zinc; however, AREDS did not address which individual components of the antioxidant regimen were responsible for the protective effect.

Case studies and cross-sectional studies that have looked at the effect of antioxidant supplementation and AMD have reached inconclusive or contradictory findings. The following study, reprinted from the *British Medical Journal*, is the first randomized, controlled trial to examine the relationship between vitamin E supplementation and AMD. The results suggest that vitamin E may not be the key ingredient in the antioxidant-vitamin mixture.

As part of a larger study on vitamin E, cataracts, and AMD, researchers randomly assigned more than 1,000 healthy people between the ages of 55 and 80 to take either 500 IU of vitamin E or a placebo daily for four years. The participants had eye examinations before the study began and then annually. Lens and retinal photographs were taken at each examination; the initial and final photographs for each participant were compared at the end of the study.

At the end of four years, 9% of the vitamin E group and 8% of the placebo group had developed early AMD. In those who already had AMD before the study began, the disease had progressed in 19% of the vitamin E group and 18% of the placebo group. Also, similar numbers of participants in both groups had decreased visual acuity (a loss of more than two lines on the eye chart). Participants taking vitamin E had no more adverse effects than those in the placebo group.

The researchers are unsure whether vitamin E has no protective effect against AMD or whether it needs to be taken for longer periods or in combination with other antioxidants to have an effect. Another possibility is that vitamin E may only help people who are at high risk for AMD or are susceptible to retinal damage or oxidation (such as smokers).

"Our findings may mean that vitamin E does not have an important role in protecting against macular degeneration," the authors write. "This last conclusion would be consistent with the variable and often contradictory results obtained from previous cross-sectional studies."

Papers

Vitamin E supplementation and macular degeneration: randomised controlled trial

Hugh R Taylor, Gabriella Tikellis, Luba D Robman, Catherine A McCarty, John J McNeil

Abstract

Objective To determine whether vitamin E supplementation influences the incidence or rate of progression of age related maculopathy (AMD).
Design Prospective randomised placebo controlled clinical trial.
Setting An urban study centre in a residential area supervised by university research staff.
Participants 1193 healthy volunteers aged between 55 and 80 years; 73% completed the trial on full protocol.
Interventions Vitamin E 500 IU or placebo daily for four years.
Main outcome measures Primary outcome: development of early age related macular degeneration in retinal photographs. Other measures included alternative definitions of age related macular degeneration, progression, changes in component features, visual acuity, and visual function
Results The incidence of early age related macular degeneration (early AMD 3) was 8.6% in those receiving vitamin E versus 8.1% in those on placebo (relative risk 1.05, 95% confidence interval 0.69 to 1.61). For late disease the incidence was 0.8% versus 0.6% (1.36, 0.67 to 2.77). Further analysis showed no consistent differences in secondary outcomes.
Conclusion Daily supplement with vitamin E supplement does not prevent the development or progression of early or later stages of age related macular degeneration.

Introduction

Age related macular degeneration (AMD) is now the leading cause of blindness and loss of vision in developed countries.[1 2] This is due to the increased life expectancy and "greying" of the population and the successful control and treatment of other causes of blindness, such as ophthalmia neonatorum, cataract, or diabetic retinopathy. Population based studies have shown that the age specific prevalence of AMD rapidly increases in people aged over 60 years.[3-5] Two thirds of people in their 90s will have AMD, and one quarter will have the most severe form (late), which is associated with serious loss of vision.[2]

The cause or causes of AMD are unknown, and treatment is only partially effective and appropriate in only a few.[6] There is no effective method of prevention. A genetic basis for AMD has been suggested,[7] and the genes for some similar macular disorders that occur in younger people have been described.[8 9] Associations with several measures of cardiovascular disease and its associated risk factors are inconsistent.[10 11] Cigarette smoking is a significant risk factor for both the incidence and progression of AMD.[4] Exposure to sunlight may contribute to its development,[12] but this association is inconsistent.[5 13]

Many of the early changes of AMD occur at the level of the retinal pigment epithelium and failure to repair oxidative damage may be an early step in its development. Case-control and cross sectional studies have examined the association between intake or plasma concentrations of antioxidant vitamins and AMD.[14 15] The findings have been inconclusive and sometimes contradictory. It is unclear whether this reflects the lack of a biological linkage or methodological difficulties in study design, dietary ascertainment, or biochemical measurements of vitamin E.

A recent study investigated the effects of the combined antioxidant vitamins A, C, and E and zinc on the development of cataract and AMD. The results showed some partial protective effect of antioxidant supplements on the progression of moderately advanced AMD, but only when both eyes were affected.[16] We undertook a prospective randomised controlled trial to examine whether a high dose supplement of vitamin E influenced the development of AMD.

Methods

Study design

One of the major arms of the vitamin E, cataract, and age related maculopathy trial (VECAT) looked at vitamin supplementation and incidence and progression of AMD. Volunteers were recruited mainly through community advertising and by post between January 1995 and April 1996.[17] From the 1906 people who were screened by telephone, 1289 (69%) were examined and 1204 (93%) of these were enrolled and randomised. We excluded 11 participants after randomisation as they were outside the required age range at enrolment. All remaining eligible participants were those aged between 55 and 80 years in whom the lens and retina of at least one eye could be photographed. We excluded those with bilateral cataract surgery, advanced bilateral cataract, other seri-

Centre for Eye Research Australia, University of Melbourne, Locked Bag 8, East Melbourne, Victoria, Australia, 8002
Hugh R Taylor *professor*
Gabriella Tikellis *research fellow*
Luba D Robman *senior research fellow*
Catherine A McCarty *associate professor*
Department of Epidemiology and Preventive Medicine, Monash University, Room 306, Building ALF, Alfred Hospital, Caulfield, Victoria, Australia, 3145
John J McNeil *professor*
Correspondence to: H R Taylor h.taylor@unimelb.edu.au

bmj.com 2002;325:11

ous disease, or sensitivity to vitamin E or who were taking steroids or anticoagulant treatment.

We obtained written informed consent. The project was approved by the standing committee on ethics in research on humans at Monash University (project 50/91).

Annual follow up examinations were planned within one month of the anniversary of enrolment. Follow up ended in January 2000. A standardised eye examination was performed that has been described in detail elsewhere.[18] It included the measurement of best corrected visual acuity, visual function (VF-14), slit lamp examination, and funduscopy and photography through dilated pupils.

Randomisation

Participants randomly received either 500 IU natural vitamin E (335 mg d-α tocopherol) in a soybean oil suspension encapsulated in gelatin or a matched placebo capsule containing only the soybean oil. Study numbers were allocated sequentially by the study coordinator as participants were enrolled in the study. Participants were then randomly allocated to treatment group. This random allocation was performed by using a "permuted blocks" allocation scheme. The allocation list was stored at a remote site.

Bulk medications were dispensed into labelled jars by a person not involved in the study. Vitamin E and placebo were dispensed on different days to avoid confusion. Identical containers were used. The jars were packed in numerical order and then dispensed by study personnel.

Vitamin E and placebo capsules were of identical appearance and taste. Neither study staff nor examiners or participants were aware of the treatment allocation, although all knew that participants would be randomly assigned to receive either vitamin E or placebo.

The number of bottles and capsules returned by participants during the course of the study were documented as one measure of compliance. Participants were encouraged to report any adverse effects immediately and were asked specifically about adverse events and compliance during quarterly telephone calls or letters and at the annual examination. Adverse effects were investigated and periodically reported to the data monitoring and safety committee for review.

Outcomes

The primary outcome of the study was the development of early AMD (fig 1). Secondary outcomes were the progression of early AMD, the development of late AMD (fig 2), changes in visual acuity (the number of letters read on the LogMAR chart), and changes in visual function (VF-14 score).

Grading of age related macular degeneration

The clinical assessment of AMD was performed with 90 and 78 dioptre lenses and was graded according to the international classification.[19] One frame simultaneous stereophotographs of the macula were taken with a Nidek 3-DX fundus camera (Nidek, Japan) with Kodachrome 64 ASA colour film. These photographs were graded independently for AMD by trained graders according to the international classification.[19 20] Sets of circles were used to estimate drusen size and the area affected with drusen or abnormalities in retinal pigmentary. At the end of the study we reassessed the initial and final photographs for any change with a "side by side" comparison in a masked and randomised fashion.

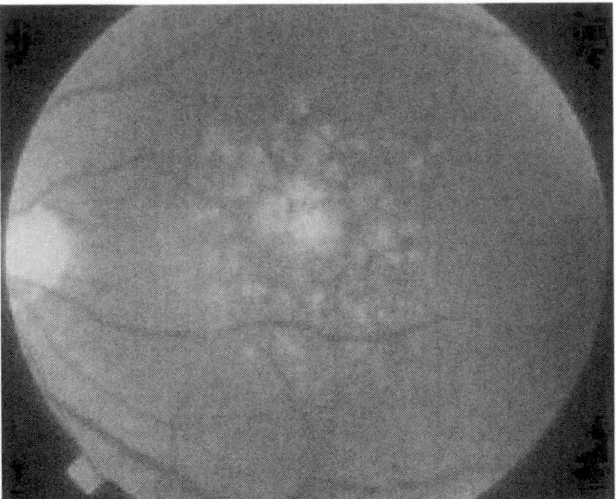

Fig 1 Early age related macular degeneration (AMD), characterised by numerous drusen of various sizes and types that extend across macular. Larger soft drusen types are of particular concern because of risk of developing into late AMD

The grading of retinal photographs was performed over five years. Two people graded the baseline slides (grading was in the proportion 70:30). Slides for the remaining four years of follow up were graded by GT. To prevent systematic bias or drift we carried out retraining followed by observer trials every three months, when 10% of randomly selected slides were regraded. All cases of late AMD were also included in this masked regrading. We assessed agreement between observers by unweighted kappa statistics: κ ranged from 0.77 (95% confidence interval 0.30 to 1.00) for hyperpigmentation to 0.86 (0.40 to 1.00) for soft distinct drusen and 1.00 for soft indistinct drusen, hypopigmentation, and late AMD. Cases in which the retinal changes were questionable or uncertain were referred to a retinal specialist for adjudication.

Because the international classification and grading system for age related maculopathy and age related

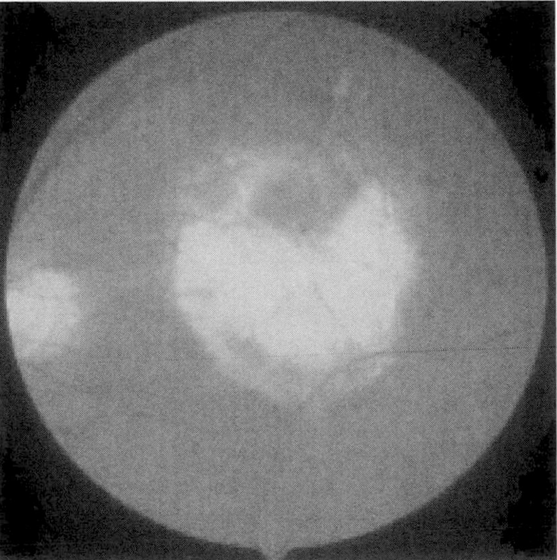

Fig 2 Late age related macular degeneration (AMD): exudative end stage. Extensive fibrovascular scar that covers macula results in severe loss of vision

macular degeneration is somewhat ambiguous about the inclusion of soft intermediate drusen and pigmentary changes[4 5 19] we modelled several different definitions of early AMD (table 1). Early AMD-3 was the primary outcome.

We considered that AMD progressed through six stages: (a) no drusen or only hard drusen; (b) intermediate drusen or hyperpigmentation without hypopigmentation; (c) soft drusen or pigmentary change; (d) soft drusen and pigmentary change; (e) geographic atrophy; and (f) neovascular AMD. We defined progression as movement from a lower stage to a higher stage. Participants were categorised by their worse eye.

We defined the incidence of early AMD as the appearance of early AMD in at least one eye of participants who did not have AMD in either eye at baseline.

Late AMD included neovascular AMD with serious or haemorrhagic detachment of the retinal pigment epithelium or sensory retina, characteristic haemorrhages, or subretinal fibrous scars.[19] We defined atrophic late AMD as a central areolar zone of retinal pigment epithelial atrophy with visible choroidal vessels, at least 175 μm in diameter, in the absence of signs of neovascular AMD in the same eye.[19]

Sample size

The VECAT study was initially designed to evaluate cataract, and the original estimation of sample size was based on a four year progression rate of 15% for nuclear cataract.[21] One thousand people allocated in a 1:1 ratio to vitamin E or placebo would detect a 15% reduction (type I error of 0.01, power 0.95), with allowance for a 10% annual loss due to death or withdrawals.

Given a sample size of 1000 people we calculated the power to detect changes in the incidence and progression of early AMD from published data.[3 22] Power calculations were based on baseline data with type 1 error of 0.05 and a power of 0.80. The final statistical power of this study to detect a 50% reduction in the incidence of early AMD (early AMD 3) was 82%. The power to detect a 50% reduction in the progression of early AMD was 98%. However, the power to detect a change in the incidence or progression of individual features of AMD such as soft drusen and pigment changes was lower (≤70%).

We used the nQuery Advisor software program, release 2.0 (Statistical Solutions, Crosse's Green, Cork, Ireland) for all power calculations.

Data analysis

Data were entered directly on to either a computer or self coding forms. Open ended responses were coded later. Double data entry was used. Data were cross checked for inconsistencies. The allocation code was not broken until all the data cleaning had been completed and the dataset "locked." Analyses were based on intention to treat. However, we performed subanalyses including only those who continued on protocol—that is, those who took the study capsules to the end of the study. We used SPSS 8.0 (SPSS, Chicago, IL) in the data analyses.

The safety committee assessed adverse events each year. The study was to be stopped if serious adverse effects occurred that were attributed to vitamin E. There was no interim analysis of the outcomes for the duration of the study.

Table 1 Definitions used to model early age related macular degeneration

Feature	Grading of photographs	Clinical grading
Early AMD 1	Soft intermediate or soft distinct or soft indistinct or pigment changes (hyperpigmentation or hypopigmentation)	Not applicable
Early AMD 2	Soft intermediate or soft distinct or soft indistinct and pigment changes (hyperpigmentation or hypopigmentation)	Not applicable
Early AMD 3*	Soft distinct or soft indistinct or pigment changes (hyperpigmentation or hypopigmentation)	Large/soft drusen or non-geographical RPE atrophy
Early AMD 4	Soft distinct or soft indistinct and pigment changes (hyperpigmentation or hypopigmentation)	Large/soft drusen and non-geographical RPE atrophy

RPE=retinal pigment epithelium. *Primary outcome.

Table 2 Comparison of baseline characteristics between two groups of participants. Figures are numbers (percentage) of participants unless otherwise stated

Characteristic	Treatment group: Vitamin E	Placebo
Mean age (years)	65.72	65.73
Women	321/595 (54)	349/598 (58)
Current smokers	14/589 (2.3)	10/597 (1.7)
Ever smoked	285/594 (48)	292/595 (49)
Best corrected visual acuity (≥40 letters on LogMAR)	593/595 (99)	597/598 (99)
Blue iris colour	255/593 (43)	252/596 (42)
Cortical opacity (≥2)	97/595 (16)	69/597 (12)
Nuclear opacity (≥2)	26/594 (4)	25/596 (4)
Any posterior subcapsular opacity	18/595 (3)	18/597 (3)
Mean VF-14 score	92.5807	92.7431
Early AMD	104/595 (17.5)	110/598 (18)
Late AMD	3/595 (0.5)	5/598 (0.5)
Family history:		
Cataract	167/595 (28)	175/598 (29)
AMD	11/595 (2)	11/598 (2)
Glaucoma	52/595 (9)	58/598 (10)
Blindness	41/595 (7)	34/598 (6)
Mean visible light exposure	21.04	20.14
Mean ultraviolet light exposure	0.55	0.52
Previous intake of vitamin E supplementation	156/553 (28)	133/542 (25)
Median dietary intake of vitamin E (mg/day)	3.62	3.72
Body mass index ≥27	248/595 (42)	220/598 (37)
Hypertension	226/595 (38)	196/598 (33)
Hyperlipidaemia	151/595 (25)	141/598 (24)
Ischaemic heart disease	67/595 (11)	54/598 (9)
Diabetes	29/595 (4.9)	21/598 (3.5)

Results

Characteristics of participants

We enrolled 1193 participants (fig 3). The groups were highly comparable with no differences in baseline characteristics except for a small excess in the number with cortical lens opacities in the vitamin E group (χ^2=5.6, P=0.02, table 2).

The rate of compliance with the study protocol for treatment and examinations was high and similar for both groups (tables 3 and 4). In the vitamin E group eight people were excluded from final data analysis: six developed diabetic retinopathy, one had myopic degeneration, and one had missing data. Six people were excluded from the placebo group: two developed adult vitelliform macular degeneration and four had missing data.

Mean serum vitamin E concentrations at baseline were 39.4 (SD 20.9) μmol/l in the vitamin E group and 35.3 (6.6) μmol/l in the placebo group. At two and four years respectively, the concentrations were 63.8

Table 3 Reasons for withdrawal or discontinued intervention

	Withdrawn		Discontinued intervention	
	Vitamin E	Placebo	Vitamin E	Placebo
Died	11	7	0	0
Adverse reaction	4	7	12	10
After cataract extraction	1	1	2	2
Relocated	4	5	1	0
Health related	24	21	13	7
Personal	23	24	8	12
Wanted to take own vitamin E	4	1	12	9
Contraindication to vitamin E	4	3	12	11
Changed studies	0	0	0	1
Unknown	3	3	14	18
Total	78	72	74	70

Table 4 Annual status of study participants

	Vitamin E			Placebo		
Time point	On protocol	Off protocol*	Withdrawn	On protocol	Off protocol*	Withdrawn
Baseline	595	0	0	598	0	0
1 year	533	34	28	525	33	40
2 years	497	44	54	496	48	54
3 years	468	58	69	483	51	64
4 years	443	74	78	456	70	72

*Off protocol indicates ceased study medication but underwent annual examination.

(21.6) μmol/l and 58.3 (25.6) μmol/l in the vitamin E group and 32.0 (SD 8.8) μmol/l and 31.4 (SD 8.9) μmol/l for the placebo group (at two years Student's t=6.82, P>0.001; at four years t=4.98, P>0.001).

We assessed compliance by counting left over capsules, and 78% of participants had a compliance rate of 80% or higher based on intention to treat analyses. There was no difference in compliance between the two groups (χ^2=3.61, df=1, P=0.46). We measured plasma concentrations in a subgroup of participants to assess compliance with treatment allocation.

Adverse events

We classified adverse events according to the body system affected. No serious adverse events were reported, though 678 people reported at least one adverse event.

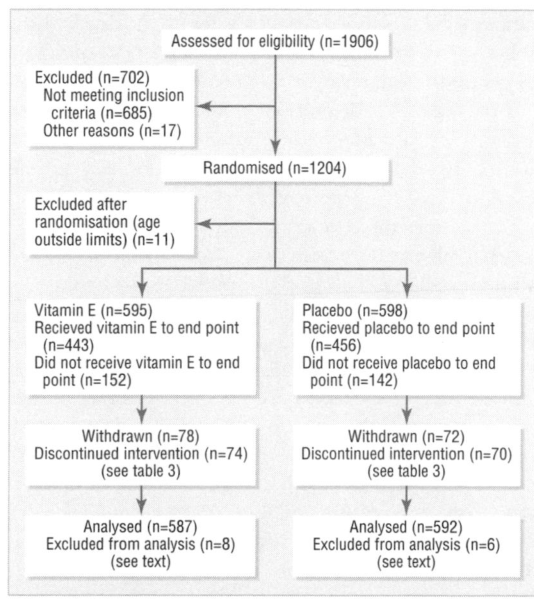

Fig 3 Randomisation of participants for vitamin E, cataract, and age related maculopathy (VECAT) study

There was no significant difference between overall number and type of adverse event between the two groups (χ^2=1.82, df=7, P=0.97). A total of 174 adverse events were potentially related to the use of study capsules, 91 (15%) in the vitamin E group and 83 (14%) in the placebo grpup (χ^2=0.48, df=1, P=0.49). Ophthalmic adverse events were reported by 105 (18%) in the vitamin E group and 90 (15%) in the placebo group (χ^2=1.44, df=1, P=0.23).

Early AMD

Incidence—There was no difference in the four year incidence of early AMD in the two treatment groups over the four years (table 5). This was true for each definition tested and for both grading of photographs and clinical grading. Similarly, there was no difference between the incidence of the separate features of early AMD and treatment, except for hypopigmentation. Hypopigmentation was significantly less common in those on vitamin E, although the clinical significance of this is unclear. In addition, there were no differences between the groups in the prevalence of early AMD, its component features, or late AMD at baseline or at four years by either grading of photographs or clinical grading (tables 6 and 7).

Progression—According to grading of photographs 95 of 491 (19%) in the vitamin E group showed progression compared with 90 of 506 (18%) in the placebo group (relative risk=1.09, 0.84 to 1.42). By clinical grading, we observed progression in 40 of 508 (7.9%) in the vitamin E group and 31 of 514 (6.0%) in the those placebo group (1.31, 0.83 to 2.07). We saw no difference in the rate of progression of drusen types by treatment group (hard drusen being replaced by soft drusen, intermediate soft drusen being replaced by soft distinct or indistinct drusen, or the increase in area of either soft distinct or soft indistinct drusen; data not shown).

A masked "side by side" comparison of photographs from baseline and at four years showed no significant difference between the two groups (table 8). There was slightly more progression in the vitamin E group, which was only marginally significant (1.26, 1.01 to 1.57).

Additional analysis

Analysis of best corrected visual acuity and visual function data showed no differences between the groups (data not shown). Similar numbers of people lost more than nine letters (two lines) of visual acuity (59 in vitamin E group, 57 in placebo group).

Further analyses included all cases of AMD, geographic atrophy alone, and neovascular AMD alone. Subgroup analyses included current smokers, those with a family history of AMD, and those with a high ocular exposure to visible light or to ultraviolet-B radiation. In none of these analyses was there a difference between the two treatment groups. Similarly, no difference was found when we repeated the analyses and controlled for the baseline presence of cortical lens opacities.

Finally, a multiple logistic regression analysis that included potential confounders of incidence or progression showed no association between the study intervention and the incidence or progression of early AMD.

Table 5 Four year incidence* of features related to early AMD, AMD, and late AMD. Figures are numbers (percentage) of participants with feature and risk ratios (95% confidence interval)

	Grading of photographs			Clinical grading		
	Vitamin E	Placebo	Risk ratio (95% CI)	Vitamin E	Placebo	Risk ratio (95% CI)
Soft intermediate drusen	78/403 (19)	73/397 (18)	1.05 (0.80 to 1.39)	NA	NA	NA
Soft distinct drusen	29/482 (6)	28/487 (6)	1.05 (0.60 to 1.82)	NA	NA	NA
Soft indistinct drusen	7/451 (2)	7/466 (2)	1.03 (0.77 to 1.38)	NA	NA	NA
Hypopigmentation	6/470 (1)	16/481 (3)	0.38 (1.16 to 0.93)	NA	NA	NA
Hyperpigmentation	21/459 (5)	32/470 (7)	0.68 (0.41 to 1.14)	NA	NA	NA
Early AMD 1	79/339 (23)	70/330 (21)	1.10 (0.82 to 1.47)	NA	NA	NA
Early AMD 2	10/480 (2)	14/489 (3)	0.73 (0.33 to 1.62)	NA	NA	NA
Early AMD 3†	35/409 (9)	34/418 (8)	1.05 (0.69 to 1.61)	28/387 (7)	25/386 (7)	1.12 (0.66 to 1.90)
Early AMD 4	6/488 (1)	9/498 (2)	0.68 (0.25 to 1.88)	9/495 (1)	5/495 (1)	0.56 (0.20 to 1.64)
Late AMD	4/494 (1)	3/504 (1)	1.36 (0.67 to 2.77)	3/507 (1)	3/510 (1)	1.00 (NA)

NA=Not applicable to clinical grading.
*Incidence=absence of particular lesion at baseline and presence of this lesion in at least one eye at four years.
†Primary outcome.

Table 6 Prevalence of early and late AMD assessed by photograph grading at baseline and at four years. Figures are numbers (percentage) of participants

	Baseline				Four years			
	Vitamin E	Placebo	χ^2 (df=1)	P value	Vitamin E	Placebo	χ^2 (df=1)	P value
Early AMD 1	192/587 (33)	205/593 (35)	0.46	0.50	167/504 (33)	155/512 (30)	0.96	0.33
Early AMD 2	20/587 (3)	24/593 (4)	0.38	0.56	14/504 (3)	22/512 (4)	1.72	0.19
Early AMD 3	104/587 (18)	111/593 (19)	0.20	0.66	87/504 (17)	88/512 (17)	0.01	0.98
Early AMD 4	11/587 (2)	11/593 (2)	0.06	0.98	7/504 (1)	10/512 (2)	0.49	0.48
Late AMD	3/587 (0)	4/593 (1)	NA	1.00*	5/504 (1)	4/512 (1)	NA	0.75*

NA=not applicable.
*Fisher's exact test.

Table 7 Prevalence of early and late AMD as assessed by clinical grading at baseline and at four years. Figures are numbers (percentage) of participants

	Baseline				Four years			
	Vitamin E	Placebo	χ^2 (df=1)	P value	Vitamin E	Placebo	χ^2 (df=1)	P value
Early AMD 3	151/595 (25)	149/598 (25)	0.03	0.85	104/508 (21)	95/514 (19)	0.65	0.42
Early AMD 4	19/595 (3)	18/598 (3)	0.03	0.86	14/508 (3)	14/514 (3)	0.01	0.98
Late AMD	3/508 (1)	4/593 (1)	NA	1.00*	4/508 (1)	4/514 (1)	NA	1.00*

NA=not applicable.
*Fisher's exact test.

Discussion

In this four year study of the effect of vitamin E supplementation of the development and progression of early age related macular degeneration (early AMD-3) we found no protective or deleterious effect of the daily dietary supplementation of 500 IU vitamin E on incidence or progression. Further analysis of the incidence of individual features of early AMD also showed no protective effect of supplementation except for a decrease in retinal hypopigmentation. However, the clinical significance of this finding is unclear and it may be due to chance alone. The secondary analyses of visual acuity and visual function also failed to show an intervention effect.

To our knowledge this is the first prospective randomised controlled trial to evaluate vitamin E supplementation and age related macular degeneration.

Table 8 Progression as determined by "side by side" comparison of baseline and four year photographs. Figures are numbers (percentage) of participants

	Vitamin E	Placebo
Better	20/493 (4)	28/505 (6)
Same	337/493 (68)	366/505 (73)
Worse	136/493 (28)	111/505 (22)

The strengths of this study include the sample size, the high rates of compliance and follow up, the prospective and randomised design, and photographic documentation. Weaknesses in the study were the relatively short follow up (four years) and the relatively low proportion of cigarette smokers.

We saw no deleterious effects associated with vitamin E supplementation, and the adverse effects that were reported occurred with a similar frequency in each group. This is consistent with data from another recent report about vitamin E supplementation.[23]

The physicians health study showed that physicians who used either vitamin E or multivitamins had a 13% and 10% reduction in the risk of AMD respectively, although this finding was not significant.[24] Since we completed our study results from the age related eye disease study (AREDS) have become available.[16] That study examined the effect of a combination of antioxidants (vitamin C 500 mg/day; vitamin E 400 IU/day; β carotene 15 mg/day) with and without zinc (80 mg as zinc oxide and copper and 2 mg as cupric oxide). They found a reduction in the progression of photographic signs of AMD but only in those with moderately advanced disease in both eyes. They found no effect on earlier or later stages of AMD or in those with

What is already known on this topic

Age related macular degeneration is the leading cause of loss of vision and blindness in elderly people; for people aged ≥90 years, two out of every three will be affected and one in four will become blind

Currently, there are no methods of prevention or treatment in most cases, though a third of cases are due to cigarette smoking

Antioxidant vitamins have been suggested as a possible prevention

What this study adds

Daily supplementation with 500 mg vitamin E for four years did not alter the incidence or progression of AMD

unilateral disease. They did not examine the effect of vitamin E supplementation on its own.

Implications

The lack of a protective effect of vitamin E supplementation is somewhat disappointing. Possibly our follow up period was too short and vitamin E may need to be taken for a long time, if not for the whole of life, or in combination with other antioxidants. There may be a long time lag between the time of damage and the appearance of clinical signs. In addition, antioxidants may be effective only in certain subgroups of people who are at particular risk or who have a high exposure to retinal damage or oxidation, such as those with a genetic susceptibility, cigarette smokers, or those with a high ocular light exposure.[25] Alternatively, our findings may mean that vitamin E does not have an important role in protecting against macular degeneration. This last conclusion would be consistent with the variable and often contradictory results obtained from previous cross sectional studies.

Contributors: HRT, GT, LDR, JJM, and CAM wrote the paper. JJM, HRT, Martha Sinclair, and the late Chris Silagy designed the study. JJM, HRT, CAM, LDR, Sinead K Garrett, MS, Flavia Cicuttini, Kath Ogden, and Adrian Thomas were members of the study's steering committee. The Data Safety and Monitoring Committee was chaired by the late Professor Chris Silagy. JJM, HRT, CAM were overall supervisors for the VECAT study. CAM was the trial epidemiologist. SKG was study coordinator. Hugo Stephenson designed and managed the software used for data collection. GT, LDR, and SKG conducted the study. Alex Harper was the external retinal consultant. LDR was the study ophthalmologist, was responsible for all fundus photography and clinical eye examinations, and was internal adjudicator for fundus grading. GT was responsible for all macular grading, development of grading protocol, participant interviews and medical examinations, and assessment of compliance to study protocol. Lynne Rodereda and Trudy Mai contributed to the data collection. LDR, GT, Kath Ogden, and Nicole Doherty contributed to the finalisation of the dataset. GT, LDR, and CAM (statistical supervisor) were responsible for data analysis. HRT is guarantor.

Funding: The VECAT study was funded in part by grants from the National Health and Medical Research Council, the Jack Brockhoff Foundation, the Eirene Lucas Foundation, the Stoicesco Foundation, the Carleton Family Charitable Trust, Je Hope Knell Trust Fund, Smith and Nephew, Australia, and Henkel Australia.

Competing interests: None declared.

1 Evans J, Wormald R. Is the incidence of registrable age-related macular degeneration increasing? *Br J Ophthalmol* 1996;80:9-14.
2 VanNewkirk M, Weih LM, McCarty CA, Taylor HR. Cause-specific prevalence of bilateral visual impairment in Victoria, Australia: the visual impairment project. *Ophthalmol* 2001;108:960-7.
3 Klein R, Klein BEK, Jensen SC, Meuer SM. The five-year incidence and progression of age-related maculopathy: the Beaver Dam eye study. *Ophthalmology* 1997;104:7-2.
4 Smith W, Assink J, Klein R, Mitchell P, Klaver CC, Klein BE, et al. Risk factors for age-related macular degeneration: pooled findings from three continents. *Ophthalmology* 2001;108:697-704.
5 McCarty CA, Mukesh BN, Fu CL, Mitchell P, Wang SS, Taylor HR. Risk factors for age-related maculopathy: the visual impairment project. *Arch Ophthalmol* 2001;119:1455-62
6 Bressler NM. Age related macular degeneration. New hope for a common problem comes from photodynamic therapy. *BMJ* 2000;321:1425-7.
7 Heiba IM, Elston RC, Klein BE, Klein R. Sibling correlations and segregation analysis of age-related maculopathy: the Beaver Dam study. *Genet Epidemiol* 1994;11:51-67.
8 Allikmets R, Shroyer NF, Singh N, Seddon JM, Lewis RA, Bernstein PS, et al. Mutation of the Stargardt disease gene (ABCR) in age-related macular degeneration. *Science* 1997;227:1805-7.
9 Stone EM, Lotery AJ, Munier FL, Heon E, Piguet B, Guymer RH, et al. A single EFEMP1 mutation associated with both Malattia Leventinese and Doyne honeycomb retinal dystrophy. *Nat Genet* 1999;22:199-202.
10 Hyman LG, Lilienfeld AM, Ferris FL 3rd, Fine SL. Senile macular degeneration: a case-control study. *Am J Epidemiol* 1983;118:213-27.
11 Vingerling JR, Dielemans I, Bots ML. Age-related macular degeneration is associated with atherosclerosis: the Rotterdam study. *Am J Epidemiol* 1995;142:404-9.
12 Taylor HR, West S, Munoz B, Rosenthal FS, Bressler SB, Bressler NM. The long-term effects of visible light on the eye. *Arch Ophthalmol* 1992;110:99-104.
13 Mitchell P, Smith W, Wang JJ. Iris color, skin sun sensitivity, and age-related maculopathy. The Blue Mountains eye study. *Ophthalmology* 1998;105:1359-63.
14 Delcourt C, Cristol JP, Tessier F, Leger CL, Descomps B, Papoz L. Age-related macular degeneration and antioxidant status in the POLA study. *Arch Ophthalmol* 1999;117:1384-90.
15 West S, Vitale S, Hallfrisch J, Munoz B, Muller D, Bressler S, Bressler NM. Are antioxidants or supplements protective for age-related macular degeneration? *Arch Ophthalmol* 1994;112:222-7.
16 Age-Related Eye Disease Study Research Group. A randomized, placebo-controlled, clinical trial of high-dose supplementation with vitamins C and E and beta carotene for age-related cataract and vision loss. *Arch Ophthalmol* 2001;119:1439-52.
17 Garrett SKM, Thomas AP, Cicuttini F, Silagy C, Taylor HR, McNeil JJ. Community-based recruitment strategies for a longitudinal interventional study: the VECAT experience. *J Clin Epidemiol* 2000;53:541-8.
18 Robman LD, Tikellis G, Garrett SKM, Harper CA, McNeil JJ, Taylor HR, et al. Baseline ophthalmic findings in the vitamin E, cataract and age-related maculopathy (VECAT) study. *Aust N Z J Ophthalmol* 1999;27:410-6.
19 Bird AC, Bressler NM, Bressler SB, Chisholm IH, Coscas G, Davis MD, et al. The International ARM Epidemiological Study Group. An international classification and grading system for age-related maculopathy and age-related macular degeneration. *Surv Ophthalmol* 1995;39:367-74.
20 Tikellis G, Robman LD, Harper A, McNeil JJ, Taylor HR, McCarty C. Methods for detecting age-related maculopathy: a comparison between photographic and clinical assessment. *Clin Experiment Ophthalmol* 2000;28:367-72.
21 West S, Munoz B, Schein OD, Vitale S, Maguire M, Taylor HR, et al. Cigarette smoking and risk for progression of nuclear opacities. *Arch Ophthalmol* 1995;113:1377-80.
22 Bressler NM, Muñoz B, Maguire MG, Vitale SE, Schein OD, Taylor HR, et al. Five-year incidence and disappearance of drusen and retinal pigment epithelial abnormalities: Waterman study. *Arch Ophthalmol* 1995;113:301-8.
23 Yusuf S, Dagenais G, Pogue J, Bosch J, Sleight P. Heart Outcomes Prevention Evaluation Study Investigators. Vitamin E supplementation and cardiovascular events in high-risk patients. *N Engl J Med* 2000;342:154-60.
24 Christen WG, Ajani UA, Glynn RJ, Manson JE, Schaumberg DA, Chew EC, et al. Prospective cohort study of antioxidant vitamin supplement use and the risk of age-related maculopathy. *Am J Epidemiol* 1999;149:476-84.
25 Meagher EA, Barry OP, Lawson JA, Rokach J, Fitzgerald GA. Effects of vitamin E on lipid peroxidation in healthy persons. *JAMA* 2001;285:1178-82.

(Accepted 9 January 2002)

NOTES

NOTES

The information contained in this White Paper is not intended as a substitute for the advice of a physician. Readers who suspect they may have specific medical problems should consult a physician about any suggestions made.

Please address inquiries on bulk subscriptions and permission to reproduce selections from this White Paper to Medletter Associates, Inc., 632 Broadway, 11th Floor, New York, NY 10012. The editors are interested in receiving your comments at the above address but regret that they cannot answer letters of any sort personally.

ISBN 0-929661-26-5
ISSN 1542-1910
Tenth Printing
Printed in the United States of America

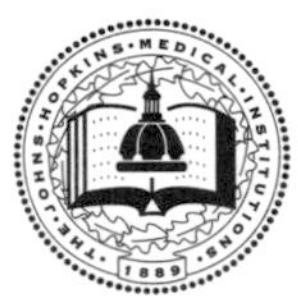

The Johns Hopkins White Papers are published yearly by Medletter Associates, Inc.

Index Abbreviations
HYP=Hypertension and Stroke
LUN=Lung Disorders
MEM=Memory
NUT=Nutrition and Weight Control
PRO=Prostate Disorders
VIS=Vision